616.8

MFT Library Services
North Manchester
N01976

Clinical Neurology

Graeme J. Hankey
MBBS, MD, FRCP (Lond), FRCP (Edin), FRACP
Consultant Neurologist and Head of Stroke Unit
Department of Neurology, Royal Perth Hospital
and Clinical Professor
Department of Medicine, University of Western Australia
Perth, Australia

Joanna M. Wardlaw
MBChB, MD, FRCP, FRCR
Professor and Honorary Consultant Neuroradiologist
Department of Clinical Neurosciences, University of Edinburgh
Western General Hospital
Edinburgh, UK

WITHDRAWN FROM STOCK

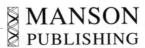

MANSON
PUBLISHING

First softcover edition 2008

Copyright © 2002, 2008 Manson Publishing Ltd

ISBN 978-1-84076-097-2

All rights reserved. No part of this publication may be reproduced, stored in a retrieval system or transmitted in any form or by any means without the written permission of the copyright holder or in accordance with the provisions of the Copyright Act 1956 (as amended), or under the terms of any licence permitting limited copying issued by the Copyright Licensing Agency, 33–34 Alfred Place, London WC1E 7D, UK.

Any person who does any unauthorized act in relation to this publication may be liable to criminal prosecution and civil claims for damages.

A CIP catalogue record for this book is available from the British Library.

For full details of all Manson Publishing Ltd titles please write to:
Manson Publishing Ltd
73 Corringham Road
London NW11 7DL, UK

Tel: +44 (0)20 8905 5150
Fax: +44 (0)20 8201 9233

Website: www.mansonpublishing.co.uk

Commissioning editor: Jill Northcott
Project manager: Paul Bennett
Text editor: Ruth C Maxwell
Layout: Top Draw (Tableaux)
Electronic artwork: MTG
Cover design: Patrick Daly
Color reproduction: Tenon & Polert Colour Scanning Ltd, Hong Kong
Printed by: Replika Press Pvt Ltd, Kundli, India

Contents

Foreword

Education and learning in clinical neurology involve a process of integration. The student or trainee in the clinical neurosciences must learn detailed information concerning the clinical presentation, pathology, radiology, electro-diagnosis, and, finally, treatment of neurologic diseases. There are many excellent texts where these components are separately reviewed. *Clinical Neurology* is a work where each area has been integrated into a practical approach to the patient. There is a high level of integration that brings together clinical presentation, appropriate diagnostic studies and treatment. The text is concise and, where appropriate, a bulleted topic format is used. This makes information easy to retrieve. High-quality illustrations present anatomic drawings, radiographs and pathologic specimens. This approach logically leads the reader through different clinical scenarios from presentation to diagnosis and treatment.

The reader will be introduced to the principles of neurologic diagnosis at the beginning of the book. This detailed but concise initiation will be particularly useful to the senior student or trainee in neurology. This is followed by an introduction to all of the major types of study used to aid in the diagnosis of patients with neurologic disease. The book is organized to be practically useful. Drs Hankey and Wardlaw present material which is organized according to the presenting complaint of the patient or according to a logical pathophysiologic and anatomic classification scheme. For each disorder there is a clear definition, discussion of etiology, clinical features, and investigations.

The authors have extensive experience as clinical educators. This leads to a clarity of presentation that is ideal for the advanced student or trainee in neurology. Program or course directors responsible for clinical education in neurology will find this text extremely useful. It can be used directly as the major source work for a course in advanced clinical neuroscience.

This is an important addition to the textbooks that are available in clinical neurology. The overall quality of production ensures that this will be a durable educational text in neurology.

Anthony J Windebank, MD
Dean, Mayo Medical School
Neuroscience Research – Guggenheim 1501
Mayo Clinic and Mayo Foundation
Rochester
Minnesota
USA

Preface

Neurology is an exciting and evolving clinical science. Since we began our training in neurology (GJH) and neuroradiology (JMW) in the 1980s, the understanding and practice of clinical neurology and neuroradiology have been transformed. Traditionally, the essence of neurology was the rigorous application of meticulous clinical skills to localize the presence (or absence) and precise location of neurological lesions. Clinical findings were correlated with pathological findings at autopsy, but understanding of disease mechanisms was poor and therapeutic options were limited. Indeed, most neurological disorders like stroke, epilepsy, Alzheimer's disease, multiple sclerosis, and motor neuron disease were considered untreatable. Neurology was thus regarded by many outside the specialty as rather erudite and nihilistic.

However, in the past 15 years, advances in neuroimaging, basic neuroscience, molecular genetics, and the consequent development and evaluation of therapies have brought new meaning and life to the clinical features elicited at the bedside. Furthermore, new diseases with potentially devastating consequences have emerged, and traditional rigid boundaries between neurology and psychiatry have blurred with increased recognition of the interaction between mind and body. Thus, clinical neurology has emerged as one of the most exciting frontiers in medicine. The array of new and emerging diagnostic and therapeutic options include:

- Superb, safe, and noninvasive diagnostic imaging of the vasculature and the structure, metabolism and function of the brain and spinal cord by magnetic resonance. This has added a new dimension to clinico-pathologic correlation, optimized diagnosis, exposed new insights into pathophysiology, and facilitated new treatments.
- Advances in catheter technology and interventional neuroradiology. The better availability of these less invasive techniques is changing the focus of neurosurgery, neurology and neuroimaging.
- The introduction of DNA analysis as a diagnostic and prognostic tool. The enormous advances in molecular biology have revolutionized our understanding of the pathogenesis of many inherited and degenerative neurologic conditions and facilitated accurate diagnosis, predictive testing, and genetic counselling.
- Effective treatments have been recognized in large, randomized controlled clinical trials for many neurologic disorders, such as acute migraine, stroke, limb spasticity and other movement disorders, partial epilepsy, multiple sclerosis, Parkinson's disease, Alzheimer's disease, Guillain–Barré syndrome and other immune-mediate peripheral neuropathies, myopathies, and myasthenia gravis. However, many treatments are still not very effective and there is enormous opportunity for improvement.

The fact that many previously untreatable diseases are now known to be not only treatable but preventable, has raised new optimism for the probability that treatments will emerge for other currently incurable neurologic disorders. To take full advantage of the breadth of techniques, knowledge and skills now available requires increased collaboration between neurologists, neuroradiologists and other clinical neuro disciplines.

These developments have been one of the prompts to writing this book. Where appropriate and possible, we have incorporated them, but only if their clinical effectiveness is supported by high quality evidence. For therapies, the level of evidence required is a systematic review of all (published and unpublished) randomized trials, as published and regularly updated in the *Cochrane Library* and *Clinical Evidence*. Where such evidence is not available, we have indicated so, and offered empirical recommendations based on the best available evidence and our own experience.

Another prompt has been our impression of a void in middle-sized clinical neurology texts which have some flesh added to the raw, skeletal content of many handbooks, yet which are not as bulky as comprehensive texts which we find difficult to carry, read and use. We have therefore taken this rapidly changing field and focused on the essentials. The book is written and illustrated for students of clinical neurology, particularly neurologists-in-training and practicing neurologists, who wish to have ready access to a comprehensive, up-to-date, and evidence-based guide to the understanding, diagnosis and management of common and important neurologic disorders.

We have included more than 800 illustrations in the text. Many are images taken from our own patients, whom we would like to thank for allowing us to photograph them or the outcome of their investigations. Furthermore, we would also like to thank Professor John Best, Dr Andrew Chancellor, Professor Byron Kakulas, Dr Robin Sellar, Mr Matthew Wade, and the Department of Medical Illustrations, Royal Perth Hospital, for all providing illustrations, as indicated throughout the book, and Dr Peter Silbert for helpful comments on sections of the text. Finally, we would like to thank our families and colleagues for supporting us in this endeavour. We hope you enjoy the book and welcome any comments and criticisms.

Graeme J Hankey
Joanna M Wardlaw

Abbreviations

α-TTP   α-tocopherol-transfer protein
AAG   allergic angiitis and granulomatosis of Churg–Strauss
ACA   anticardiolipin antibody
ACE   angiotensin-converting enzyme
ACh   acetylcholine
AChR   acetylcholine receptor
ACTH   adrenocorticotropic hormone
AD   Alzheimer's disease
ADCA   autosomal dominant cerebellar ataxia
ADD   attention deficit disorder
ADEM   acute disseminated encephalomyelitis
ADH   antidiuretic hormone
ADL   activities of daily living
ADP   adenosine diphosphate
AF   atrial fibrillation
AF-MSA   autonomic failure with multiple system atrophy
AF-PD   autonomic failure with Parkinson's disease
AGE   advanced glycation end product
AHC   anterior horn cells
AIDP   acute inflammatory demyelinating polyradiculoneuropathy
AIDS   acquired immunodeficiency syndrome
AION   anterior ischemic optic neuropathy
ALD   adrenoleukodystrophy
ALS   amyotrophic lateral sclerosis
AMAN   acute motor-sensory axonal neuropathy
AMN   adrenomyeloneuropathy
AMSAN   acute motor-sensory axonal neuropathy
ANCA   antineutrophil cytoplasmic antibody
ANNA   anti-neuronal nuclear antibody
AP   antero-posterior
APA   antiphospholipid antibodies
APCA-1   anti-Yo antibody
APLAb   antiphospholipid antibody syndrome
ApoE   apolipoprotein E
APP   amyloid precursor protein
APTT   activated partial thromboplastin time
AR   Argyll Robertson
ARR   absolute risk reduction
ASA   arylsulfatase A
ATP   adenosine triphosphate
AVM   arteriovenous malformation
anti-AChRAb   anti-acetylcholine receptor antibody

ßA4   beta amyloid
BAEP   brainstem auditory evoked potential
BAL   British anti-lewisite
BBB   blood–brain barrier
BCG   bacille Calmette–Guerin
bd   twice daily
BMD   Becker's muscular dystrophy
BP   blood pressure
BSE   bovine spongiform encephalopathy
BTX-A/F   botulinum toxin A/F

CADASIL   cerebral autosomal dominant arteriopathy with subcortical infarction and leukoencephalopathy
CAM   computer assisted myelography
CANOMAD   chronic ataxic neuropathy, ophthalmoplegia, M protein, agglutination, anti-disialosyl antibodies
CAVATAS   Carotid And Vertebral Artery Transluminal Angioplasty Study
CBF   cerebral blood flow
CCA   common carotid artery
cDNA   complementary deoxyribonucleic acid
CEA   carcino-embryonic antigen
CGRP   calcitonin gene-related peptide

CHOP   cyclophosphamide, doxorubicin, vincristine and prednisone-based therapy
CIDP   chronic inflammatory demyelinating polyneuropathy
CJD   Creutzfeldt–Jakob disease
CK   creatine kinase
CLAM   cholesterol-lowering agentmyopathy
CMAP   compound muscle action potential
CMT   Charcot–Marie–Tooth disease
CMV   cytomegalovirus
CNS   central nervous system
CO_2 carbon dioxide
CoA   coenzyme A
COMT   catechol-O-methyltransferase
COX   cyclo-oxygenase
CPAP   continuous positive airway pressure
CPEO   chronic progressive external ophthalmoplegia
CPH   chronic paroxysmal hemicrania
CPT   carnitine palmitoyl transferase
CREST   calcinosis, Raynaud's phenomenon, esophageal dysmotility, sclerodactyly and telangiectasis
CSDH   chronic subdural hematoma
CSF   cerebrospinal fluid
CT   computerized tomography
CTS   carpal tunnel syndrome
CVST   cerbral venous sinus thrombosis
CXR   chest x-ray

DBS   deep brain stimulation
DDAVP   desmopressin
DGC   dentate granule cell
DLBD   diffuse Lewy body disease
DMD   Duchenne's muscular dystrophy
DML
DNA   deoxyribonucleic acid
Dpt   dilute prothrombin time
DRG   dorsal root ganglia
DRPLA   dentato-rubro-pallido-luysian atrophy
dRVVT   dilute Russell's viper venom time
DSA   digital subtraction angiography
DSM IIIr   *Diagnostic and statistical manual of mental disorders – revised*
DVT   deep vein thrombosis
DWI   diffusion-weighted imaging
DZ   dizygotic

EBV   Epstein–Barr virus
ECA   external carotid artery
EKG (ECG)   electrocardiograph
ECOG   electrocorticography
ECST
ECT   electroconvulsive therapy
EEG   electroencephalogram/electroencephalograph
EGFR   epidermal growth factor receptor
EITB   enzyme-linked immunoelectrotransfer blot
ELISA   enzyme-linked immunosorbent assay
EM   electronmicroscopy
EMG   electromyography/electroencephalogram
EPH   episodic paroxysmal hemicrania
EPP   end-plate potential
EPT   enhanced physiological tremor
ERG   electroretinogram
ESR   erythrocyte sedimentation rate
ET   essential tremor

FAME   familial adult myoclonic epilepsy
FAST   functional assessment staging test
FBP   full blood picture
FDG   fluorodeoxyglucose

FFI   fatal familial insomnia
FHM   familial hemiplegic migraine
FPP   familial (primary) periodic paralysis
FSH   follicle stimulating hormone
FSHD   facio-scapulo-humeral muscular dystrophy
FTA   fluorescent treponemal antibody test
FTA-ABS   fluorescent treponemal antibody absorption

GABA   gamma amino butyric acid
GAP   guanosine triphosphatase-activating protein
GBS   Guillain–Barré syndrome
GCA   giant cell arteritis
GCI   glial cytoplasmic inclusions
GI   gastrointestinal
GLT   glutamate transporter gene
GP   general practitioner
GPI   glycoprotein I
GPl   lateral globus pallidus
GPm   medial/internal globus pallidus
GSS   Gerstmann Straussler Scheinker syndrome
GTCS   generalized tonic-clonic seizures
GTE   glycerol trierucate
GTO   glycerol trioleate oil
GTP   guanine triphosphate

5-HT   5-hydroxytryptamine
5-HT3   5-hydroxytryptophan-3
HAART   highly active antiretroviral therapy
HACEK   *Haemophilus* spp., *Actinobacillus actinmycetemcomitans, Cardiobacterium hominis, Fikenella corrodens, Kingella* spp.
HCG   human chorionic gonadotrophin
HCl   hydrochloric acid
HD   Huntington's disease
HDL   high-density lipoprotein
H&E   hematoxylin and eosin
HE   hepatic encephalopathy
HexA   hexosaminidase A
HexB   hexosaminidase B
hGH   human growth hormone
HHT   hereditary hemorrhagic telangiectasia
Hib   *Haemophilus influenzae* type b
HIV   human immunodeficiency virus
HIV-CMC   human immunodeficiency virus-associated cognitive/motor complex
HLA   human leukocyte antigen
HMPAO   hexamethylpropylenamine oxime
HMSN   hereditary motor and sensory neuropathy
HNA   hereditary neuralgic amyotrophy
HNPP   hereditary neuropathy with liability to pressure palsies
HR   heart rate
HSAN   hereditary sensory and autonomic neuropathy
HSE   herpes simplex virus encephalitis
HSP   hereditary spastic paraparesis
HS-tk   herpes simplex thymidine kinase
HSV   herpes simplex virus
HTI   hemorrhagic transformation of the infarct
HTLV   human T lymphocyte virus

IA-DSA   intra-arterial digital subtraction angiography
IBM   inclusion body myositis
iC   interstitial nucleus of Cajal
ICA   internal carotid artery
ICH   intracerebral hemorrhage
ICP   intracranial pressure
ICU   intensive care unit
IF   intrinsic factor
IFN   interferon
Ig   immunoglobulin
IIH   idiopathic intracranial hypertension
i.m.   intramuscular
INR   internal normalized ratio
IOH   idiopathic orthostatic hypotension
IQ   intelligence quotient
i.v.   intravenous
IV DSA   intravenous digital subtraction angiography
IVIG   intravenous immunoglobulin

JCV   JC virus

JME   juvenile myoclonic epilepsy

KCT   kaolin clotting time
K–F   Kayser–Fleischer
KSS   Kearns–Sayre syndrome

LA   lupus anticoagulant
LACI   lacunar infarct
LCM   lymphocytic choriomeningitis
LDL   low-density lipoprotein
LEMS   Lambert–Eaton myasthenic syndrome
LG   lymphomatoid granulomatosis
LGMD   limb-girdle muscular dystrophies
LH   luteinizing hormone
LHON   Leber's hereditary optic neuropathy
LP   lumbar puncture

MAG   myelin associated glycoprotein
MAO   monoamine oxidase
MAOI   monoamine oxidase inhibitor
MAP   microtubule-associated protein
MBP   myelin basic protein
MCA   middle cerebral artery
MCTD   mixed connective tissue disease
MELAS   mitochondrial encephalomyopathy, lactic acidosis, and stroke-like episodes syndrome
MEPP   miniature end-plate potential
MERRF   myoclonic epilepsy with ragged-red fibers
Mct   methionine
MFS   Miller Fisher syndrome
MG   myasthenia gravis
MGUS   monoclonal gammopathy of uncertain significance
MI   myocardial infarction
MJD   Machado Joseph disease
MLD   metachromatic leukodystrophy
MLF   medial longitudinal fasciculus
MMSE   Mini-Mental State exam
MNCV   motor nerve conduction velocities
MND   motor neuron disease
MPTP   N-methyl-4-phenyl-1,2,3,6,-tetrahydropyridine
MR   magnetic resonance
MRA   magnetic resonance angiography
MRC   Medical Research Council
MRI   magnetic resonance imaging
mRNA   messenger ribonucleic acid
MS   multiple sclerosis
MSA   multiple system atrophy
MSU   mid-stream urine
MT   metallothionein
mtDNA   mitochondrial deoxyribonucleic acid
MTS   mesial temporal sclerosis
MUP   motor unit potentials
MZ   monozygotic

NAIP   neuronal apoptosis inhibitory protein
NASCET   North American symptomatic carotid endarterectomy trial
NCV   nerve conduction velocities
NF   neurofibromatosis
NGF   nerve growth factor
NMDA   N-methyl-D-aspartate
NMS   neuroleptic malignant syndrome
NNT   number needed to treat
NO   nitric oxide
NP   Niemann–Pick
NP-C   Niemann–Pick disease type C
NPH   normal pressure hydrocephalus
NRT   nucleus reticularis thalami
NSE   neuron-specific enolase
NTD   neural tube defect
nvCJD   new variant Creutzfeldt–Jakob disease

OCP   oral contraceptive pill
OFSM   oculo-facial-skeletal myorhythmia
OMM   oculomasticatory myorhythmia
OPCA   olivopontocerebellar atrophy
OR   odds ratio

P100   positive wave at 100 ms
PA   pernicious anemia

PACI   partial anterior circulation infarct
PaCO$_2$ partial pressure of carbon dioxide
PAF   pure autonomic failure
PAN   polyarteritis nodosa
PAS   periodic acid-Schiff
PCA   posterior communicating artery
PCA-1   type 1 anti-Purkinje cell antibody
PCR   polymerase chain reaction
PCV   procarbazine, lomustine, and vincristine
PD   proton density
PD   Parkinson's disease
PDE   phosphodiesterase
PDW   proton density weighted
PDWI   proton density weighted image
PE   pulmonary embolism
PED   paroxysmal exertion-induced dyskinesia
PEG   percutaneous endoscopic gastrostomy
PET   positron emission tomography
PGI$_2$ prostacyclin
PGL   phenolic glycolipid
PHD   paroxysmal hypnogenic dyskinesia
PI   protease inhibitor
PICH   primary intracerebral hemorrhage
PKD   paroxysmal kinesogenic dyskinesia
PL   phospholipid
PLED   periodic lateralized epileptiform discharge
PME   progressive myoclonic epilepsies
PML   progressive multifocal leukoencephalopathy
PMR   polymyalgia rheumatica
PNKD   paroxysmal non-kinesogenic dyskinesia
PNS   peripheral nervous system
p.o.   by mouth (per os)
POCI   posterior circulation infarct
POEMS   polyneuropathy, organomegaly, endocrinopathy,
    monoclonal paraproteinemia, and skin hyperpigmentation
PPRF   paramedian pontine reticular formation
PrP   prion protein
PROMM   proximal myotonic myopathy
PS-1/2   presenilin-1/2
PSA   prostatic specific antigen
PSD   periodic synchronous discharge
PSP   progressive supranuclear palsy
PSS   progressive systemic sclerosis
PTHRP   parathyroid hormone-related protein
PVC   procarbazine, lomustine, and vincristine
PVS   permanent vegetative state
PWI   perfusion-weighted image

Q-SART   quantitative sudomotor axon reflex test

RA   rheumatoid arthritis
RBC   red blood cells
RCT   randomized controlled trial
REM   rapid-eye movement
RFLP   restriction fragment length polymorphism
RIA   radioimmunoassay
riMLF   rostral interstitial nucleus of the medial longitudinal
    fasciculus
RNA   ribonucleic acid
ROM   rifampicin, ofloxacin and minocycline
RPR   rapid plasma reagin
rRNA   ribosomal ribonucleic acid
RRR   relative risk reduction
RT   reverse transcriptase
rt-PA or r-tPA   recombinant tissue plasminogen activator

SAE   subcortical arteriosclerotic encephalopathy
SAF   scrapie-associated fibrils
SAH   subarachnoid hemorrhage
SBMA   androgen receptor
SC   sickle cell
SCA   spinocerebellar atrophy subtype
SCLC   small cell lung cancer
SDH   succinate dehydrogenase
SDS   Shy–Drager syndrome
SE   status epilepticus
SFEMG   single fiber electromyography
SIADH   syndrome of inappropriate antidiuretic hormone

SLE   systemic lupus erythematosus
SMA   spinal muscular atrophy
SMN   survival motor neuron protein
SMN^T survival motor neuron gene
SNAP   sensory nerve action potential
SNc   substantia nigra pars compacta
SND   striatonigral degeneration
SNr   substantia nigra reticulata
SOD   Cu/Zn superoxide dismutase
SPECT   single photon emission computed tomography
SS   Sjögren's syndrome
SSCP   single strand conformation polymorphism
SSEP   somatosensory evoked potentials
SSPE   subacute sclerosing panencephalitis
SSRI   selective serotonin reuptake inhibitor
SSS   sick sinus syndrome
STIR   short time inversion recovery
STN   subthalamic nucleus
SUDEP   sudden unexplained death in epilepsy
SUNCT   short-lasting unilateral neuralgiform headache with
    conjunctival injection and tearing

T1W   T1 weighted
T2W   T2 weighted
TA   Takayasu's arteritis
TACI   total anterior circulation infarct
TACS   total anterior circulation syndrome
TB   tuberculosis
TCD   transcranial doppler ultrasound
TD   Tourette disorder
tds   three times daily
TENS   transcutaneous electrical nerve stimulation.
TETA   triethylene tetramine dihydrochloride
TF   tissue factor
TFPI   tissue factor pathway inhibitor
TG   therapeutic gain
TIA   transient ischemic attacks
TNF   tumor necrosis factor
TOE   transesophageal echocardiography
tPA   tissue plasminogen activator
TPHA   *Treponema pallidum* hemagglutination test
TPI   *Treponema pallidum* immobilization test
TPP   thyrotoxic periodic paralysis
tRNA   transfer ribonucleic acid
TS   Tourette syndrome
TSH   thyroid stimulating hormone
TSC   tuberous sclerosis complex
TST   thermoregulatory sweat test
TT   thrombin time
TTE   transthoracic echocardiography
TTP   thrombotic thrombocytopenic purpura

UCH   ubiquitin carboxy-terminal hydrolase
UL   upper limb
UMN   upper motor neuron

VC   vital capacity
VDRL   Venereal Disease Research Laboratory slide flocculation
    test
VEP   visual evoked potential
VGCC   voltage-gated calcium channels
VHL   von Hippel–Lindau disease
Vim   ventrointermediate nucleus
VL   ventrolateral thalamus
VLCFA   very long chain saturated fatty acids
VMA   vanillylmandelic acid
VSD   ventricular septal defect
vWF   von Willebrand factor
VZV   varicella-zoster virus

WADA   intracarotid amytal test
WBC   white blood cells
WD   Wilson's disease
WFNS   World Federation of Neurological Surgeons
WG   Wegener's granulomatosis
WH   Werdnig–Hoffman
WHO   World Health Organization

Neurologic Diagnosis

THE NEUROLOGIC HISTORY

The purpose of the assessment of a patient with a suspected neurologic disorder is to answer the following questions:

- Is there a neurologic lesion?/Is this a neurologic disorder? *Syndromic diagnosis.*
- What is the level of the neurologic lesion in the neuraxis? *Anatomic diagnosis.*
- Where is (are) the neurologic lesion(s)? *Anatomic diagnosis.*
- What is the nature/cause of the neurologic lesion(s)? *Pathologic diagnosis.*
- What are the patient's impairments, disabilities and handicaps? *Functional diagnosis.*
- What is the likely outcome? *Prognosis.*
- What can be done about it? *Treatment.*

The history must be taken; a relevant, succinct history is rarely given by the patient. The narrative history should be emphasized, not a long list of complaints and detailed systemic enquiry. Brief notes should be recorded as the history unfolds, recording what the patient actually said rather than your interpretation, to ensure greater reliability. While taking the history, the clinician must indirectly assess the patient's mental status, and consider the circumstances under which the symptoms occurred (e.g. seizure). Concurrently, observe the patient for signs of underlying disease that may be relevant to the presenting complaint (**1–3**). If an adequate history is not available from the patient, or needs verification, other useful sources include family members, friends, employers, observers of any events, and previous medical records.

The clinical history is the most important and productive part of the neurologic assessment. Although the physical examination is often used to localize the lesion accurately and elicit physical signs suggestive of the cause, the history provides most of the information about the presence or absence and nature/cause of the lesion. Therefore, if time is at a premium it is preferable to be selective with the examination rather than with the history, using the history to select or target the appropriate examination.

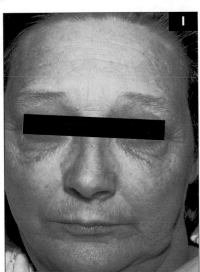

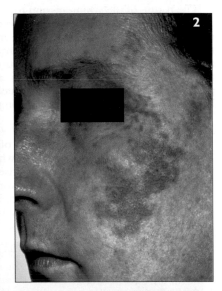

1 This patient, who complained of altered sensation in the feet and hands, is also noticeably pale. The cause of her sensory neuropathy and pallor was pernicious anemia.

2 Capillary hemangioma (port wine stain) on the left side of the face in the distribution of the ophthalmic and maxillary divisions of the left trigeminal nerve in a patient with Sturge–Weber syndrome who presented following his first epileptic seizure.

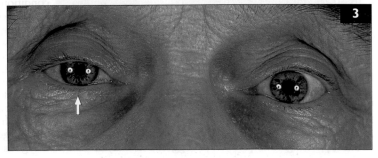

3 Right Horner's syndrome (ptosis of the right eyelid and miosis of the right pupil, arrow) due to right lateral medullary infarction.

look at the eyes (**8–11**). Is there evidence of:
- Abnormal facial appearance.
- Ptosis or facial asymmetry.
- Reduced blink frequency, facial expression and voice volume of Parkinsonism.
- Abnormal posture.
- Wasting or fasciculation.
- Tremor or other involuntary movements.

Also determine whether the patient is right or left handed (i.e. which is likely to be the dominant hemisphere for language).

MENTAL STATE (HIGHER MENTAL FUNCTION)
The patient's alertness, speech, and intelligence can be assessed during history-taking; taking the clinical history and evaluating the competence of the patient to give an accurate history involves an assessment of higher mental functioning. So, a formal assessment of higher mental function is not necessary in every patient. However, if suspicions are aroused or the presenting complaint demands it, a standardized test of higher mental function should be undertaken. One of the many available is the Mini Mental State examination (*Table 1*).

The Mini Mental State examination is only a screening test however, and fails to assess other higher mental functions, particularly non-verbal functions. Other aspects to consider include:

Consciousness (see p.44)

Orientation in time, place and person

Attention
- Concentration: digit span (normal: 6±1 forwards [i.e. abnormal <5 digits forward], 4±1 backwards [i.e. abnormal <3 digits backwards]).
- Persistence: serial recitation (months of year backwards, serial 7s); word list generation (words beginning with a letter; normal >12/minute).
- Resistance to interference: alternating sequences: +o+o+o.

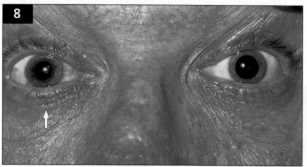

8 The patient's right eye is affected by ischemic oculopathy (arrow). Note the congested sclera, cloudy cornea, new vessel formation (neovascularization) around the limbus of the iris (rubeosis iridis) and mid-dilated pupil, which indicate chronic anterior segment ocular ischemia due to carotid occlusive disease. (Reproduced with permission from Hankey GJ and Warlow CP [1994] *Transient Ischaemic Attacks of the Brain and Eye*. WB Saunders.)

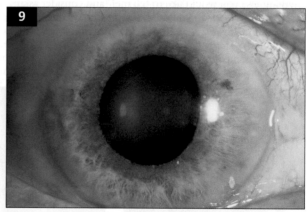

9 Close-up view of the right eye in **8** showing rubeosis iridis more clearly.

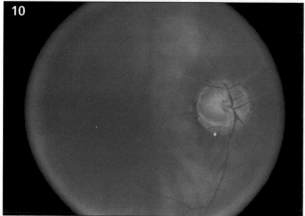

10 Fundus of the severely ischemic right eye of the patient in **8** showing attenuated vessels and pallor of the retina due to retinal edema caused by severe ischemia.

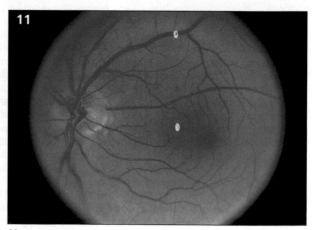

11 Fundus of the normal left eye of the patient in **8**.

Table 1 Mini-mental state examination

	Maximum score		Maximum score
Orientation		*Language*	
What is the Time? Day? Month? Year? Season?	5 points	Name two objects (e.g. a pencil and a watch).	2 points
What is the name of this Ward? Hospital? Town? State? Country?	5 points	Repeat a short phrase (e.g. 'No ifs, ands or buts').	1 point
		Execute a three-stage command, scoring 1 point for each stage (e.g. 'With the index finger of your left hand touch the tip of your nose and then your left ear.').	3 points
Registration			
Name three objects (e.g. car, dog, book) and then ask patient to repeat these. The number of objects repeated correctly is the score. Endeavor, by further attempts and prompting, to have all three repeated, so as to test recall later.	3 points	Read and obey the following 'Close your eyes'.	1 point
		Write a sentence of your own choice (the sentence must make sense and contain a subject and verb).	1 point
Attention and calculation		Copy a diagram showing two intersecting pentagons.	1 point
Subtract 7 from 100, and then 7 from the result. Repeat this five times, scoring 1 point for each correct subtraction. If the patient cannot/will not do this: spell 'world' backwards.	5 points	Total score	30 points
Recall		Scoring 23 or less denotes cognitive impairment (76% detection rate, 4% false positive). (Adapted from Dick *et al.*, *J. Neurol. Neurosurg. Psychiatry*, 1984; **47**: 496.)	
Name the three objects repeated in the registration test. Score 1 point for each correct answer.	3 points		

Memory
- Retrograde: information (e.g. 'who is the Prime Minister/President, how many weeks in a year, dates of World War 1 and II, define an island').
- Anterograde: verbal: register and recall three objects after 3 minutes; non-verbal: Rey Osterrieth complex figure test.

Other functions of intellect
- Calculation: serial 7s, or more simple calculations.
- Abstraction: similarities (e.g. orange and banana, dog and horse), proverbs (e.g. 'hunger is the best gravy').
- Praxis:
- Constructional: draw a clock, cube, flower; block design.
- Ideomotor: buccofacial, limbs, body: 'show how you would blow out a match, use a comb to comb your hair, use a toothbrush to brush your teeth'.
- Visual–spatial perception: line bisection, star cancellation.
- Right–left orientation.

Communication
- Verbal:
- Spontaneous speech: 'describe what you can see in this picture'.
- Oral comprehension: one, two and three stage commands.
- Repetition: 'If I were here then she could be there'.
- Naming: objects, body parts, lists of animals, words beginning with a letter (e.g. 'A').
- Reading: 'point to the word 'X' on the card'.
- Writing: write 'ocean', 'groceries', 'some water is not good to drink'.
- Articulation: labial sounds ('pa'), lingual sounds ('ta'), palatal sounds ('ka').
- Non-verbal: prosody: use of intonation, gesture, appropriate turn-taking.
- Handedness: language is a function of the dominant hemisphere (the left hemisphere in 96% of right-handers and more than 50% of left-handers).

- Dysphasia is a disturbance of language function, causing difficulty understanding or expressing spoken or written language.
- Dysarthria is a disturbance of articulation of speech.

Affect: mood and motivation, response to questions, attitude to others

Perception
- Illusions: misinterpretation of sensory stimuli (e.g. confusional state).
- Delusions: incorrect beliefs that are held with conviction.
- Hallucinations: sensory perceptions unrelated to sensory stimuli.

SKULL
Size and shape.

SPINE
- Deformity.
- Tuft of hair in lumbosacral region (underlying spina bifida).
- Tenderness: spinal, paraspinal.
- Range of motion.

CRANIAL NERVES
Nerve I (olfactory nerve)
- Olfactory sensation is seldom impaired in isolation.
- As testing is time consuming, it need not be done unless there is a history of head trauma or possible dementia.

Nerve II (optic nerve)
Visual acuity
- Only relevant if the patient has a history of ocular problems or visual symptoms.
- Record visual acuity in right and left eyes at 6 m (20 ft) from a Snellen's chart, with the patient wearing spectacles if necessary.

Color vision

Color vision can be assessed at the bedside, ideally by testing each eye with pseudoisochromatic plates. A more simple convention is to take the bright-red top from a bottle of the mydriatic solutions, place it over a small flashlight, and present it to each eye. To a patient with optic nerve disease, the color red will appear pale or brownish. The degree of color desaturation can be roughly quantified by asking the patient to express the value of the color as a percentage of the value of the color perceived by the normal eye.

Visual fields

Test first; patients may be dazzled for minutes after pupil tests and ophthalmoscopy.

Screen by confrontation, in which the patient is asked to look at the examiner's eyes. Check the upper temporal quadrants by simultaneously wiggling your right and left index fingers in the upper temporal visual fields of the patient and yourself, ensuring that your moving fingers are an equal distance between you and the patient so that you both have the same visual field. Ask the patient to point (if they can) to which fingers are moving: the right, left, or both. If any doubt, repeat the test, wiggling one finger at a time and then both fingers. Repeat in the lower temporal quadrants. This technique detects conventional hemianopic and quadrantanopic field defect as well as visual inattention.

If there is a visual field defect, the nasal and temporal fields should be tested individually and the margins of any defect discerned with the use of a 5 mm (0.2 in) white and red pin head.

Central vision and the size of the blind spot should also be tested by confrontation and using a pin head. Confrontation testing is however only a screening technique. Quantitative perimetry (colloquially known as 'formal' fields) is more accurate and precise.

Pupillary responses

Note the size and shape of each pupil, and the direct and consensual response of each pupil to stimulation by light and accommodation.

Argyll **R**obertson pupils are '**A**ccomodation **R**etaining' (pneumonic to remember that the accomodation reflex is preserved in Argyll Robertson pupils, i.e. they both have the initials 'AR'); i.e. accommodation reflex present but light reflex absent.

Horner's syndrome consists of miosis, ptosis and anhidrosis.

Ask the patient if the light appears equally bright when shone in both eyes. If there is a difference, look for a relative afferent pupillary defect. With the patient's gaze fixed in the distance, shine the light in one eye and note both pupils constrict. Move the light to the other eye. During the light beam's transit across the nose, both pupils dilate slightly. In normal eyes, both pupils constrict again when the beam of light falls onto the other eye. If the patient has a relative afferent pupillary defect, the pupil (and also the contralateral pupil) continues to dilate when the light beam falls on it. This usually indicates retinal or optic nerve dysfunction, but may be observed with lesions as posterior as the optic tract. The extreme example of an afferent pupillary defect is the amaurotic pupil of the completely blind eye. The term Marcus Gunn pupil is often used but what we now call a relative afferent pupillary defect is not what Marcus Gunn described.

While the iris is illuminated, look for inflammation, arcus senilis and a Kayser–Fleischer ring; the latter may require closer examination with the ophthalmoscope or slit lamp, but can even be seen by looking at the limbus through an auroscope from which the attached ear piece has been removed.

Fundoscopy

Perform fundoscopy in all patients. Ask the patient to fix on an external object with one eye while the other eye is being examined. The examiner's head must remain vertical so as not to obscure the line of vision of the patient's fixating eye. Note any abnormalities on the surface of the eye and the lens (e.g. cataract). Then focus on the:

- Optic disc: note its color – pale in optic atrophy, pink and congested in papilledema (**12**). N.B. Temporal pallor of the optic disk is a normal finding in many discs, but it indicates optic atrophy when it is associated with decreased visual acuity, a field defect, and an abnormality of color vision.
- Optic cup: diminished in papilledema (**12**), enlarged in glaucoma.
- Venous pulsation in the optic cup: absent if intracranial pressure exceeds retinal venous pressure.
- Disc margins: blurred in papilledema (**12**). If the disc cannot be seen, look even harder and change focus because a swollen, red disc of papilledema may not be obvious among the background red retina. In addition, its surface will not be in focus when focusing on the retina, because it is heaped up, as if looking from above at a large mountain coming out of the sea.
- Retinal vessels: narrow and tortuous with arteriovenous nipping in hypertension; microaneurysms with diabetes; cholesterol, platelet or calcific emboli in arterioles (**13–16**), distension or collapse of veins.
- Retinal surface: exudates, hemorrhages (**17**), retinitis pigmentosa, choroiditis.

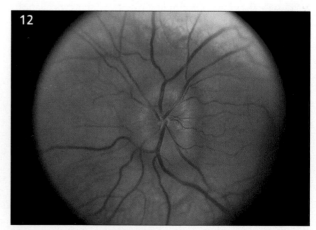

12 Ocular fundus showing papilledema in a patient with headache due to idiopathic intracranial hypertension. Note the congested swollen optic disc, loss of the physiological cup, blurred disc margins and congested retinal veins. (Courtesy of Mr M Wade, Department of Medical Illustrations, Royal Perth Hospital, Australia.)

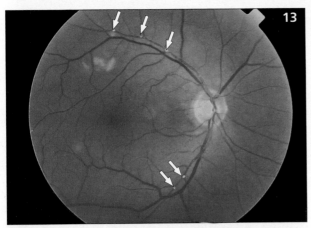

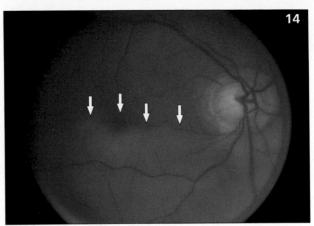

13 Fundus examination showing cholesterol emboli (arrows) as bright, orange-yellow, refractile, crystalline, glinting lipid emboli, so-called Hollenhorst cholesterol plaques. They are usually unilateral, multiple and found at the bifurcation of retinal arterioles. They frequently arise from ulcerated atherosclerotic plaque in the ipsilateral carotid system. (Reproduced with permission from Hankey GJ and Warlow CP [1994] *Transient Ischaemic Attacks of the Brain and Eye*. WB Saunders.)

14 Ocular fundus of a patient with inferior temporal branch retinal artery occlusion showing pallor of the inferior half of the retina (arrows) due to cloudy swelling of the retinal ganglion cells caused by retinal infarction. (Courtesy of Mr M Wade, Department of Medical Illustrations, Royal Perth Hospital, Australia.)

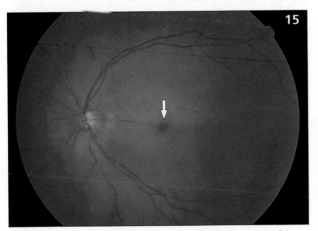

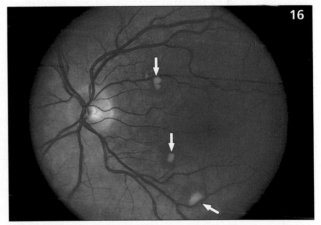

15 Ocular fundus showing narrow arterioles and veins, pallor of the retina, and a cherry-red spot over the fovea (arrow) due to accentuation of the normal fovea, which is devoid of ganglion cells, by the opalescent halo, in a patient with central retinal artery occlusion. (Courtesy of Mr M Wade, Department of Medical Illustrations, Royal Perth Hospital, Australia.)

17 Ocular fundus showing a retinal hemorrhage (arrow) due to thrombocytopenia in a patient who presented with a symptomatic intracerebral hemorrhage.

16 Ocular fundus showing multiple small retinal infarcts due to fat emboli (arrows). (Courtesy of Mr M Wade, Department of Medical Illustrations, Royal Perth Hospital, Australia.)

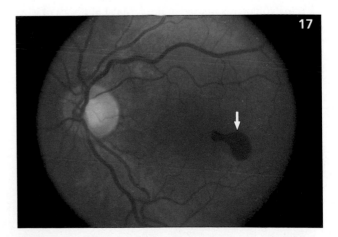

Nerves III, IV, and VI (oculomotor, trochlear, and abducens nerves)

Ask the patient to look straight ahead at a target (e.g. the tip of a hat pin or pen; the use of a finger may miss subtle diplopia) and examine the eyes in the primary position of gaze, noting the position of each eye (whether the eyes are conjugate or not), whether there are any involuntary movements of the eyes (e.g. nystagmus [vertical, rotational, horizontal], opsoclonus, ocular bobbing, fixational instability: square wave jerks), the size of the palpebral fissures (whether there is ptosis or lid retraction on one or both sides) and whether there is any fatiguability with prolonged gaze.

Ask if the patient sees one or two targets. If they have double vision, assess this with a simple 'cover-uncover' test that is accurate if one extraocular muscle is weak but can be misleading if two or more muscles are weak:

- Find the position of the target that causes maximum separation of the images.
- Holding the target steady in your right hand, cover one of the patient's eyes with your left thumb (pronating your wrist and resting the dorsum of your distal left fingers [flexed at the metacarpophalangeal joints] against the patient's lower central forehead), and ask which (if any) object disappears – the outer (more peripheral) object is seen by the defective eye and the inner (more central) object is seen by the 'good' eye.
- Swing your left thumb to cover the patient's other eye and the other object should disappear. If the same object disappears, the patient has not understood the test or the diplopia is monocular (i.e. intraocular pathology such as vitreous hemorrhage; or functional).

Ask the patient to follow a slowly moving target (no faster than 30° per second, otherwise smooth pursuit will be normally interrupted by saccadic intrusions) to examine ocular pursuit in each of the nine cardinal positions of gaze (straight ahead, left, right, up, down, up and to the right, up and to the left, down and to the right and left) and during convergence and accommodation. Ocular pursuit should be smooth, maintaining the target fixed on the macular, but may be interrupted by saccadic intrusions (jerky, cogwheel or saccadic pursuit) in various disease states such as extrapyramidal or cerebellar dysfunction. If double vision occurs in any position of gaze carry out the 'cover–uncover' test described above. Nystagmus unrelated to vestibular disease seldom produces symptoms and should be closely looked for (see pp.107, 110, 138).

Look voluntarily in each of the cardinal positions of gaze to test voluntary/saccadic eye movements that are generated from frontal eyefields in Brodmann's area 8 of the contralateral frontal cortex (**18, 19**). A frontal lobe lesion may result in a conjugate horizontal gaze palsy to the opposite side and so the eyes will be deviated to the side of the lesion due to unopposed action of the contralateral frontal lobe.

Nerve V (trigeminal nerve)
Corneal response
- Need not be tested routinely because it can be unpleasant to the patient, carry a risk of corneal damage, and be unreliable.
- Perform only if you really want to assess the integrity of the trigeminal nerve (e.g. other cranial nerve damage or suspected acoustic neuroma or syringobulbia).
- Use cotton wool.

Facial sensation
Not necessary to test rigorously unless the patient complains of facial sensory disturbance; patients usually know when they have a disturbance of spinothalamic or trigeminothalamic sensation because, for example, when they have a shave or shower they may note the temperature of the water feels different. Patients have much greater difficulty in discerning a loss of other sensory modalities.

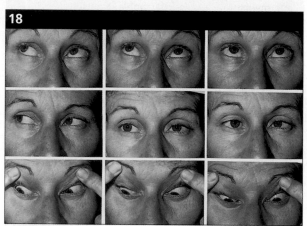

18 Eye movements in each of the nine cardinal positions of gaze showing a left esotropia and left gaze palsy (in each eye, but dysconjugate) due to an ischemic stroke involving the abducens nuclear complex in the left low pons. The patient had non-insulin dependent diabetes mellitus. (Courtesy of Mr M Wade, Department of Medical Illustrations, Royal Perth Hospital, Australia.)

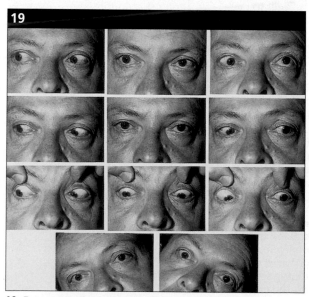

19 Eye movements in each of the nine cardinal positions of gaze showing bilateral ptosis, skew deviation due to hypotropia of the right eye, and a supranuclear upward gaze palsy due to an ischemic stroke in the left midbrain (causing a nuclear oculomotor palsy) and left thalamus caused by an embolus to the top of the basilar artery, occluding the P1 segment of the left posterior cerebral artery. (Courtesy of Mr M Wade, Department of Medical Illustrations, Royal Perth Hospital, Australia.)

Masticatory muscles
- The bulk of the temporalis and masseter should be examined by inspection and palpation; ask the patient to clench their jaw and feel the muscle bulk.
- To test pterygoid muscle power, ask the patient to open the mouth fully. A unilateral trigeminal motor neuropathy will manifest with deviation of the lower jaw (chin) to the paretic side. Bilateral weakness, which may be suspected if the patient needs to support the jaw with their hand during conversation, may be seen in myasthenia gravis and myopathies such as dystrophia myotonica.
- Less severe weakness may be detected by trying to close the opened jaw with the heel of your palm.

Jaw jerk
Unreliable and unhelpful as a screening test but it has a role in determining the level of bilateral corticospinal tract lesions; if brisk it suggests bilateral lesions above the mid-pons (a trigeminal nerve reflex: stretching and contraction of the masticatory muscles).

Nerve VII (facial nerve)
Facial muscle power will have been assessed informally during history-taking: facial asymmetry, dysarthria. Ask the patient to:
- Raise their eyebrows (or look up to the ceiling): the frontalis muscle is spared in contralateral upper motor neuron (supranuclear) lesions due to bilateral hemispheric representation.
- Smile and show their teeth: weak in lower and upper motor neuron lesions of VII, and note any asymmetry.
- Grimace by making a maximal effort to draw the lower lip and angle of the mouth downward and outward, at the same time tensing the skin over the anterior surface of the neck, to test the platysma. The examiner generally needs to demonstrate the test and instruct the patient to mimic him or her.

Altered, and even unpleasant taste, may be a symptom of facial palsy.

Nerve VIII (auditory and vestibular nerve)
Rub your thumb and middle finger together repetitively in both hands, about 2–3 cm (0.8–1.2 in) away from both of the patient's ears. Ask the patient if they hear the sound and if there is any asymmetry. Alternatively, rub your thumb and middle finger together repetitively next to one ear (to produce a masking sound) and whisper quietly in, or hold a ticking clock adjacent to, the other ear (the testing ear) at varying distances.

If there is any difficulty hearing, conduct the Rinne and Weber tuning fork tests and inspect the external auditory meatus and tympanic membrane. The Rinne test involves striking the 256 Hz tuning fork and holding the vibrating tuning fork about 2–3 cm (0.8–1.2 in) from the ear. Ask the patient if they can hear it. Then place the base of a vibrating tuning fork behind the ear, over the mastoid process and ask the patient if they can hear it and whether the sound is louder 'in the front' (outside the ear) or 'at the back' (over the mastoid process). It is normally louder in the front (positive Rinne test), but if not (negative Rinne test), this suggests conductive hearing loss, due to blocked ears or a middle ear defect, for example. For the Weber test, the vibrating tuning fork is placed over the vertex of the head in the midline and the patient is asked where they hear the buzzing sound. Normally, it is heard in the middle of the head. If it lateralizes to one side this suggests either conductive hearing loss on that side (diminished masking of external sounds) or sensorineural hearing loss on the other side (poor bone conduction to that side). The Rinne and Weber tests are not always reliable. Vestibular nerve function is tested by eye movement and balance tests.

Nerves IX and X (glossopharyngeal and vagus nerves)
Inspect the palate and ask the patient to say 'Ah'. If the palate moves to one side this indicates a lesion of the vagus nerve (motor to the palate) on the contralateral side; the contracting palatal muscles pull the palate up and ipsilaterally. If the palate does not move this may be due to bilateral supranuclear, nuclear or infranuclear vagus nerve lesions, depressed consciousness, or even a disturbance of neuromuscular junction or muscle function.

It is not necessary to test the gag reflex because it is unpleasant to the patient and is rarely abnormal in the presence of normal palatal movement (i.e. it is very unusual to have a palatal sensory deficit due to a IXth nerve palsy without a palatal motor deficit due to a Xth nerve palsy).

Nerve XI (accessory nerve)
- Ask the patient if they have neck pain; cervical spondylosis is common and neck pain may not only be uncomfortable but cause spurious weakness.
- Place the palm of your right hand over the patient's left mandible and ask the patient to turn their head to the left against your resistance to test the power of the right sternocleidomastoid. Repeat on the other side.
- Place your hand on the patient's forehead and ask them to push forward. This should usually be performed with the patient lying supine because it may evoke neck pain. Painless weakness is suggestive of motor neuron disease, myasthenia gravis, or a myopathy such as dystrophia myotonica and polymyositis.
- Ask the patient to elevate (shrug) the shoulders, observing and palpating any asymmetry of contraction of the upper trapezius muscles, and test muscle strength by attempting to depress the shoulders by pushing down on both shoulders against the patient's resistance. The lower portion of the trapezius can be tested by having the patient brace the shoulders backward and down. Unilateral paralysis of the trapezius is evidenced by inability to elevate and retract the shoulder and by difficulty in elevating the arm above the horizontal. The trapezial ridge is depressed, exposing the levator scapulae; the scapula appears rotated, the upper end laterally and down, the lower end up and in.

Nerve XII (hypoglossal nerve)
Ask the patient to:
- Open the mouth: inspect the tongue while it is at rest in the floor of the mouth, noting any wasting or fasciculation.
- Protrude the tongue: observe any deviation (toward the side of a nuclear/infranuclear lesion, away from the side of a supranuclear lesion).
- Move the tongue quickly from side to side: this is slow with pyramidal or extrapyramidal disease.

Tongue power can be tested by asking the patient to push the tongue into the cheek on each side but there is no reliable test for tongue power.

Anal reflex

The tip of the finger, covered with a glove, is inserted into the anal ring, and contraction of the anal ring is felt as the skin around the anus and the perineum is scratched or pricked with a pin; or the contraction simply may be observed without being palpated. This is a test specifically of the external or voluntary anal sphincter. In the presence of a flaccid paralysis of the external anal sphincter, the normal tonus of the internal sphincter is felt to give way on insertion of the finger. As the finger is withdrawn, the anus remains open or patulous. This does not indicate a loss of internal anal sphincter function.

Coordination

- Heel–knee–shin test: the patient lifts one leg, places it on the opposite knee and runs it down the shin.
- Rapid tapping movement of the feet against the examiner's hand.
- Toe–finger test

N.B. Tests of coordination require reasonable muscle power.

Sensation

As for the upper limbs.

Stance and gait

- Ask the patient to walk 10 m (33 ft), turn around, and walk back.

Note the speed of initiation of gait, the posture, stride length, heel strike, and extent and symmetry of arm swing. As the patient turns, pay particular attention to the number of steps taken to turn and any evidence of slight overbalancing that may occur with extrapyramidal or cerebellar lesions. Dystonic movements and tremor are also often enhanced by walking. Pyramidal tract lesions cause the foot to drag and the toes to scuff (spastic foot drop) because of involuntary plantar flexion and inversion of the foot to varying degrees. The knee flexes less than normal (or not at all) and with unilateral lesions in particular, the pelvis rocks to the normal side to help raise the dragged foot from the floor and overcome weakness of the hip abductors (a Trendelenburg-type gait).

Flaccid foot drop is manifest by the feet having to be lifted high to avoid catching the toes on the floor. If the foot is also stamped on the floor, joint position sense is likely to be impaired. Foot drop may be bilateral (e.g. distal [sensori-]motor, sciatic or peroneal neuropathies) or unilateral. A high-stepping gait and stamping is a classical sign of tabes dorsalis.

Ask the patient to:

- Walk heel-to-toe to test tandem gait; patients with a lesion of the cerebellar vermis may only manifest truncal ataxia and have no evidence of limb ataxia on finger–nose and heel-knee-shin testing.
- Walk on the toes (to detect weakness of the gastrocnemii due to a sciatic nerve or S1 nerve root lesion, for example, that may be difficult to elicit otherwise).
- Walk on the heels (to detect weakness of tibialis anterior due to a peroneal nerve or L4/L5 root, or pyramidal tract lesion for example).

- Squat down and arise from a squat (to detect proximal hip girdle muscle weakness).
- Stand still with feet together, first with eyes open and then shut, and notice any change in stability that may reflect impaired joint position sense (Romberg's sign). If uncertain about the result, challenge the patient by standing behind them and, when the patient is stable with eyes open, tell the patient you are going to pull back on the shoulders and ask them to try to remain upright (if they cannot, they will fall back into your arms). If they manage to remain upright, repeat this with the patient's eyes closed.

N.B. If the patient can walk, and if the history suggests a disturbance of gait or lower limb function, it is often preferable to begin the lower limb examination by asking the patient to stand and walk.

Functional consequences

It is important to observe the functional consequences of any neurologic impairment on the patient's activities of daily living, such as dressing, feeding, grooming, and walking.

CONCLUDING THE CONSULTATION

Frequently patients have certain ideas about what their symptoms are due to (and they may well be right) or they may be fearful that they have a certain diagnosis (such as one that afflicted a friend or family member, such as a brain tumor). By asking the patient 'What do you think the problem is?' can sometimes be helpful in management (e.g. if the patient says they think it is due to stress and you agree with them), and sometimes it allows the clinician to be able to reassure the

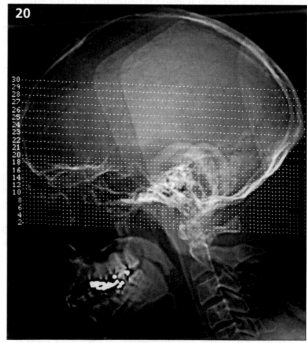

20 'Scout' view for a CT brain scan. This consists of a lateral view of the skull (usually) with lines representing the axial image positions superimposed. Note the number at the left-hand end of each line corresponds with the axial image of that number.

patient that they have not got what they a fearing. Alternatively, the patient may be asked: 'Do you have any concerns about what the problem/diagnosis might be?', or 'Has anyone suggested what the problem/diagnosis might be?'.

One of the most frequent complaints patients and families make about doctors is that the doctor did not explain (or they could not understand) what had happened and what was likely to happen. So conclude the consultation by asking the patient: 'Do you have any questions or would you like to discuss anything else?'.

IMAGING THE BRAIN

COMPUTERIZED TOMOGRAPHY (CT) SCANNING
Advantages

CT (20–24) is a great technique, particularly for acutely ill patients, due to its rapidity, ease of access to the patient, and relatively wide availability. It is useful in acute neurology in patients with headache, focal neurologic deficit, loss of consciousness, and suspected subarachnoid hemorrhage, hydrocephalus, brain tumor, stroke, brain abscess, prior to lumbar puncture and for demonstrating cerebrospinal fluid (CSF) leaks, and for paranasal sinus and mastoid diseases. It is vital following head and spine trauma, facial fractures, skull base bone lesions and for post-operative neurosurgical complications. In the spine it is most useful in trauma, for lumbar discs, and combined with myelography for thoracic and cervical lesions.

21–23 Axial views from a normal CT brain scan taken on soft tissue window settings, at the level of the fourth ventricle (**21**), the third ventricle (**22**) and the bodies of the lateral ventricles (**23**).

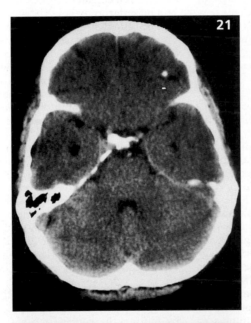

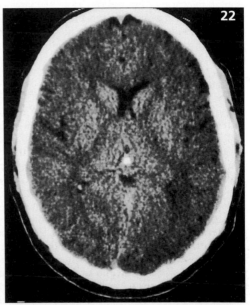

24 Axial view of the skull base from a normal CT brain scan imaged on bone window settings to display bone detail optimally (but at the expense of soft tissue detail).

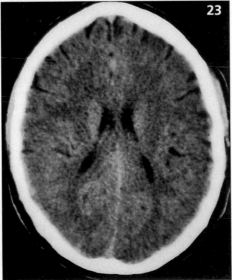

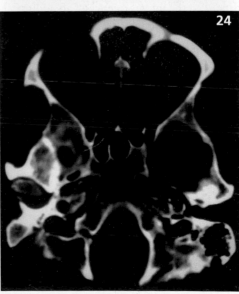

Disadvantages

CT uses ionizing radiation (an average brain CT scan exposes the patient to the equivalent of a year of background radiation!). It is not so good for demonstrating white matter diseases (such as multiple sclerosis [MS]), encephalitides, small lesions in the temporal lobes and posterior fossa (because of streak artefact from the adjacent bones) and spinal cord lesions.

Technique

A standard CT brain scan consists of 10 to 15 axial slices from the foramen magnum to the vertex at about 1.0 cm intervals (0.5 cm slice intervals through the posterior fossa). Modern scanners will produce many more thinner slices very quickly, but there is the danger of increasing radiation without necessarily increasing diagnostic yield.

The basic scan can be modified to include thinner slices at narrower intervals to show greater detail (e.g. in the pituitary fossa or orbits), or at different scan angles (e.g. coronal), or after an injection of intravenous iodinated x-ray contrast (e.g. iopamidol), or using different scan parameters to demonstrate bone optimally. A standard scan takes less then 2 minutes to perform with modern technology (not including the time taken to get the patient into and out of the scanner).

Precautions

Patients who are, or might be pregnant should not undergo CT unless absolutely essential. If CT is essential, the abdomen and pelvis should be shielded with lead aprons.

Patients with previous allergic reaction to iodinated contrast should not be given contrast again (although it is worth checking out the patient's story in some detail as often so-called 'allergic reactions' are in fact something else). Patients with atopic history are more likely to have a de novo contrast reaction than those without an atopic history.

Scan techniques these days are complicated with lots of different possible ways of conducting the investigation. In order to get the answer to the patient's problem with imaging, it is essential to give the radiologist ALL the relevant information or you may end up having to repeat the scan because it was not done in the correct way (to demonstrate whatever disease condition) the first time, thus exposing the patient to the inconvenience of an additional scan plus an extra year's worth of background radiation! The same applies to all radiologic investigations. There is no such thing as a simple and hazard-free radiologic test. So use them wisely!

Appearance of various tissues on CT

The appearance of a tissue on CT depends on how much radiation it absorbed as the x-ray beam passed through it, which in turn is dependent on the atomic number of its main components. The higher the atomic number, the greater the absorption. Densely calcified structures like bone absorb most radiation so look white; fresh blood is less white; gray matter is gray but whiter than white matter; white matter is gray but a bit darker; CSF (basically water) looks black; fat looks even blacker; and air (which absorbs virtually no radiation) looks very black.

HOW TO REVIEW A CT SCAN

Most scans, be they CT or MR, are displayed in more or less the same way on the hard copy. The hard copy is printed onto radiographic film and transilluminated to view. There are usually about 12 images on each film. Usually the scan starts at the posterior fossa and works up to the vertex. A 'scout' view (like a lateral skull x-ray) showing where in the patient the image slices have been taken, is usually displayed at the start or the end of the sequence of images (**20**).

Usually the right side of the patient is on the left side of the film, but check! – some scanners display the other way round. A large 'R' or 'L' should indicate which is which.

Each image shows the patients name, and often a date of birth, and the date of the scan – all useful information: 50 year old females have a different range of disease from 20 year old males.

To read the images, follow a system much as you would do to examine the patient, that way you will not miss things. Start at the bottom of the head and work up: look at the orbits, skull base including neural foramina, and petrous bones. Then look at the intracranial structures: the IVth ventricle should lie slightly closer to the front of the posterior fossa than the back (**21**). It should also be in the shape of a 'frown'. If it is nearer the back or starts to 'smile', there may be a mass distorting it.

The brain stem and midbrain and surrounding CSF spaces should be symmetrical. The pituitary fossa, IIIrd ventricle, basal ganglia, lateral ventricles, cerebral white matter and cortex should all be symmetrical with similar appearance of the frontal, parietal, temporal and occipital lobes. It is worth 'eyeballing' these lobes and the basal ganglia in turn, this helps to highlight subtle abnormalities (and make obvious ones more visible for the learner). If you do all this each time, you will not miss anything.

Finally, if you cannot see anything wrong, double check the orbits, pituitary fossa, posterior fossa and basal ganglia (review areas where people tend to miss things), and possibly suggest that the patient be given contrast.

The review of spine images is on similar principles but the scout view is very useful as it helps you keep your bearings. There is nothing worse than getting the disc level wrong. Count carefully and use the slice number to line up with the numbering on the scout view. Really helpful scanners display a mini scout view in the corner of each scan image.

MAGNETIC RESONANCE (MR) IMAGING (MRI)

The principles behind how you produce a picture of the brain by putting the patient into a strong magnetic field are completely beyond the scope of this book and will not be discussed further. It is more important for the neurology student to know about the advantages and disadvantages of MR and a few basics about what tissues look bright or dark. The principles of reading an MR scan (**25–28**) are the same as for a CT scan, except that there are usually far more images to go through (so rather more daunting) including a midline sagittal set (which are useful for impressing your tutors by looking for herniation of the cerebellar tonsils). Thus apply the principles outlined above and you will not go far wrong.

Advantages

The principal advantages of MR are its great ability to demonstrate soft tissue detail especially in the brain and spinal cord, muscles, ligaments and cartilages.

In neurology it is very useful for demonstrating suspected white matter diseases (such as MS, encephalitis, metabolic disease), cervical and thoracic cord disease, metastatic involvement of the spine, lumbar discs (though CT is good for that too), precise delineation of tumors, posterior and pituitary fossa diseases.

It can be used to show blood vessels (arteries and veins) inside the head and in the neck (MR angiography [MRA]), perfusion and diffusion of fluids in the brain and metabolites in the brain (using advanced techniques such as MR spectroscopy).

Images can be obtained in any plane, at millimeter intervals, with paramagnetic contrast for demonstration of areas of blood–brain barrier breakdown, and using all sorts of fancy sequences to highlight different features.

Disadvantages

Having a cardiac pacemaker or intracranial aneurysm clip or metallic intraocular foreign body are all absolute contra-indications to MR (the pacemaker will stop working, the aneurysm clip may move and tear the artery and the ocular foreign body may move causing an intraocular hemorrhage).

Relative contraindications include other metallic prostheses or foreign bodies, or tattooed-in eyeliner (contains metallic particles which can cause burns). All patients are carefully screened for these factors and x-rayed if necessary to exclude intraocular foreign bodies. Welders particularly are prime suspects for intraocular foreign bodies. Deodorants and talcs and eye makeup must be removed as they may contain metallic bits.

Claustrophobic patients may have difficulty going into the very enclosed space of the scanner (though modern scanners are becoming more open access).

25 T1W midline sagittal view of the brain. Note the brain appears as a rather bland gray texture and CSF is black. Subcutaneous fat is white.

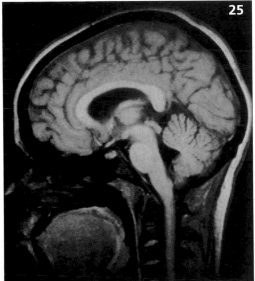

26 T2W axial view of the brain. Note the CSF appears white, the gray matter appears whitish and white matter dark. The gray matter is easily differentiated from the white.

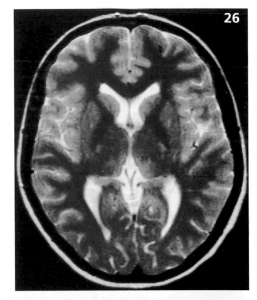

27 Proton density (PD) weighted axial view of the brain. Note the CSF is grayish and difficult to distinguish from brain, gray matter is whiter than white matter.

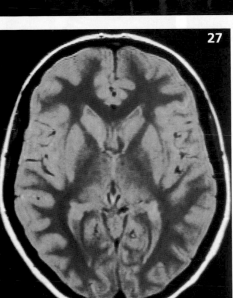

28 Magnified T1W coronal image of the pituitary gland (long arrow), optic chiasm (arrow head), pituitary stalk (short arrow), and internal carotid arteries (asterisks).

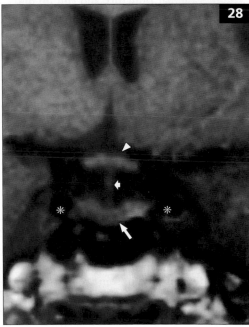

COMPLICATIONS

- Herniation of the medial temporal lobe through the tentorial opening (transtentorial herniation) or of the medulla through the foramen magnum (coning), leading to medullary compression and death (**45**). This is the most serious complication but can be avoided by never doing a LP if there is clinical evidence of raised intracranial pressure (see p.477), or focal cerebral or posterior fossa signs. If there is raised intracranial pressure with shift of the intracranial contents, or obstruction to CSF flow, then removing CSF by LP, or continuing leakage of CSF after the LP, may create a lower pressure in the vertebral canal than in the intracranial compartments, leading to mass movements and herniation of the brain. On the other hand, if there is diffusely raised intracranial pressure with free flow of CSF through all parts of the intracranial and spinal CSF compartments, which can only be discerned with CT or MRI scan, then LP should be safe.
- Spinal nerve root damage, usually caused by inserting the needle lateral to the midline.
- Low-pressure headache (30% [1–70%] of LPs) due to continuing CSF leakage through the hole in the dura. It is present only after sitting or standing for minutes to hours and is relieved by lying down. If the headache comes on suddenly or is accompanied by drowsiness, then perform a CT scan to see if an intracranial subdural or subarachnoid hemorrhage is present. Treatment otherwise involves the patient lying flat in bed with the foot of the bed elevated and drinking plenty of fluids. If the headache persists then it can be stopped in some patients by an autologous blood 'patch' in the epidural space over the site of the presumed dural hole or, as a last resort, by open surgery to seal the dural leak. Strategies to minimize the incidence of post-LP syndrome are to use a needle of small diameter and atraumatic shape, and to reinsert the stylet before removing the needle. Otherwise a strand of arachnoid that may have entered the needle with the outflowing CSF may be threaded back through the dural defect and facilitate prolonged CSF leakage along the arachnoid.
- Infection of the CSF, or an epidural abscess, if sterile precautions are not taken or if the needle is inserted through inflamed or infected skin.
- Transient back stiffness. If persistent, consider a spinal hemorrhage.
- Spinal hemorrhage (epidural, subdural, or subarachnoid). This may manifest as severe back and/or nerve root pain, nerve root compression or spinal cord compression, but is very rare unless the patient has a bleeding diathesis (e.g. platelet or coagulation defect).
- Intracranial subdural and subarachnoid hemorrhages are very rare.

INDICATIONS

- Diagnosis: suspected subarachnoid hemorrhage, meningitis, encephalitis, MS, dementia and idiopathic intracranial hypertension.
- Investigation: previously to introduce contrast media such as metrizamide for myelography and CT scanning, radioisotopes for ventriculo-cisternography, and air for pneumoencephalography; MRI has superseded these.
- Treatment: to introduce local spinal anesthetics and occasionally antibiotic or antitumor agents into the subarachnoid space, and to remove regularly CSF to lower the CSF pressure in idiopathic intracranial hypertension.

CONTRAINDICATIONS

- Intracranial space-occupying lesion (e.g. abscess, hematoma, tumor), particularly in the posterior fossa.
- Obstructive hydrocephalus.
- Generalized brain edema with obliteration of the CSF cisterns around the upper brainstem.
- If a CT scan is not available, then LP is contraindicated in patients with clinical features suggestive of the above three conditions (e.g. papilledema and/or focal neurologic signs and/or coma). If bacterial meningitis is suspected, it is essential to treat the patient immediately and empirically with broad spectrum antibiotics (after collecting blood cultures) rather than risk brain herniation by performing a lumbar puncture in order to obtain CSF and isolate the organism (see p.273).
- Infection of the skin in the lumbar region.
- Bleeding diathesis.

NORMAL VALUES

- Pressure. Less than 250 mm of CSF/water, and usually less than 200 mm, if the patient is relaxed and there is free flow of CSF (the CSF fluctuates in the manometer with respiration and coughing). Falsely low CSF pressure may be due to removing too much CSF before measuring the CSF pressure, a CSF leak around the needle, transtentorial herniation and brainstem coning.
- Red blood cells: normally the CSF is clear with no red blood cells (RBC). If the CSF is bloody it should be centrifuged immediately and the supernatant examined by spectrophotometry (or, if not available, the naked eye). Yellow (xanthochromic) pigmentation is due to the breakdown of products of hemoglobin (e.g. oxyhemoglobin and bilirubin), and is seen in patients with subarachnoid hemorrhage (at least 12 hours before), jaundice or a very high CSF protein. Pinkish pigmentation is due to hemoglobin from disintegrated RBCs.

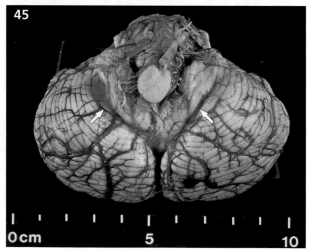

45 A potential complication of lumbar puncture if the patient has an intracranial mass lesion. Photograph of the under-surface of the cerebellum showing swelling and grooving of the inferior mesial parts of both cerebellar hemispheres (mainly the ventral paraflocculi or tonsillae) (arrows) which have herniated, with the medulla, through the foramen magnum, and compressed the medulla. (Courtesy of Professor BA Kakulas, Royal Perth Hospital, Australia.)

- White blood cells: <5 lymphocytes per mm^3 and no polymorphs. If the CSF is contaminated by blood from a traumatic tap, one alternative is to repeat the CSF after a few hours (through a different lumbar interspace) or to calculate the number of white blood cells (WBC) that have been introduced into the CSF from the traumatic bleed by using the following formula: (WBC in peripheral blood/RBC in peripheral blood) × RBC CSF.

  As there are about 1000 times more RBC in the peripheral blood than WBC, this formula is usually about 0.001 × RBC CSF. An estimate of the true CSF WBC count can then be made by subtracting the number of WBC introduced from the number observed but, as this tends to be an over-estimate, it is best to consider a definite excess CSF WBC count as the ratio of observed CSF WBC to calculated number of WBC introduced exceeding 10.
- Glucose: normally more than 50% of the simultaneous blood glucose.
- Protein: 0.15–0.45 g/l (15–45 mg/dl), depending on the laboratory. A very high CSF protein concentration causes the CSF to clot (Froin's syndrome).
- Immunoglobulin G (IgG) is a component of the CSF protein, normally making up less than 15% of the total protein.
- IgG/albumin ratio in the CSF is normally less than about 0.25.
- IgG index ([CSF IgG/serum IgG]/[CSF albumin/serum albumin]) is a better measure of CSF IgG because it takes into account the serum level of IgG and albumin; if the IgG level in the blood is abnormal, it is otherwise difficult to interpret the level of IgG in the CSF.
- Oligoclonal bands: perhaps a more sensitive measure of locally synthesized immunoglobulin in the CSF. Polyacrylamide gel electrophoresis separates two or more gamma globulins (IgG) in the CSF on the basis of their charge and size, which appear as two or more bands. Need to check that no similar bands are present in the serum.

Causes of an increase in CSF IgG and oligoclonal bands
- Increased IgG in the blood and breakdown of the blood-brain barrier.
- Contamination of the CSF by red cells.
- Multiple sclerosis.
- Meningitis.
- Encephalitis.
- Acute post-infectious encephalomyelitis.
- Subacute sclerosing panencephalitis.
- Cerebral infarction.
- Brain tumors.
- Neurosyphilis.
- Sarcoidosis.
- Cerebral systemic lupus erythematosus.
- Acute inflammatory demyelinating polyradiculoneuropathy (Guillain–Barré syndrome).

CSF taken from the cervical spinal canal and the ventricles contains fewer cells and has a lower protein concentration (up to 0.15 g/l [15 mg/dl]) than lumbar canal CSF, but the glucose concentrations are similar in the different compartments.

ELECTROENCEPHALOGRAPHY (EEG)

DEFINITION
The EEG is a recording, by means of electrodes attached to the scalp, of the electric field generated by the spontaneous neuronal activity of the underlying brain. The recording reflects the electric currents that flow in the extracellular space and these in turn reflect the summated effects of innumerable excitatory and inhibitory synaptic potentials that occur in cortical neurons. The spontaneous activity of cortical neurons is influenced by subcortical structures, especially the thalamus and rostral brainstem reticular formation.

TECHNIQUE
Electrodes (usually 21), which are solder or silver–silver chloride discs 0.5 cm (0.2 in) in diameter, are placed equidistantly over the surface of the scalp according to an international convention (10–20 System) (**46**). They are attached to the scalp by means of adhesive material such as collodion or bentonite (bentoquatam, quaternium-18 bentonite), using EKG paste under the electrode to make contact with the scalp. They are wired up to separate amplifying units, or 'channels'. Potential electric differences between pairs of electrodes or combinations of electrodes can be recorded, amplified, and displayed on an oscilloscope or digital screen or a paper trace moving at a standard speed of 3 cm/s. The resulting EEG or voltage-versus-time graph appears as a number of parallel wavy lines, each representing one channel.

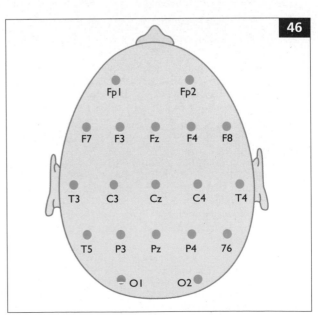

46 The international 10–20 electrode system.

Patients are usually examined in the awake state, lying or sitting down in a quiet room with their eyes closed. The resting electrocerebral activity is recorded for about 30 minutes, during which time a number of 'activating' procedures are usually carried out:

- Sleep: the patient is allowed to fall asleep, because sleep may enhance potentially epileptogenic or epileptiform activity.
- Hyperventilation: the patient is asked to breathe deeply 20 times a minute for 3 minutes, evoking hypocapnia, alkalosis and cerebral vasoconstriction. The rhythm slows and a paroxysm of spike wave activity or another abnormality may be induced.
- Photic stimulation: a powerful flashing light (stroboscope) is placed about 40 cm (16 in) from the patient's eyes and flashed at varying frequencies of 1–20 per second with the patient's eyes open and closed. The EEG over the occipital region may show waves corresponding to each flash of light (evoked response or photic driving) or to abnormal discharges (e.g. a photoparoxysmal response).

Other techniques that can be used to identify epileptic foci include:

- Sleep recordings, which may reveal abnormalities not evident when the subject is awake or in light sleep.
- Prolonged (6–8 hours) telemetric recordings.
- Video EEG.

RECORDINGS
Normal EEG recordings
Awake
Amplitude: 50–200 μV.
Waveforms/rhythms:

- Alpha waves: 8–13 per second (Hz), 50 μV sinusoidal waves, recorded over the occipital region when the eyes are closed and are attenuated or suppressed completely by eye opening or mental activity. The occipital alpha rhythm depends on synchronous discharge of cells in the visual cortex.
- Beta waves: 14–22 Hz, low amplitude (10–20 μV) is recorded maximally and symmetrically from the frontal regions.
- Theta waves: 4–7 Hz, is prominent in children, gradually diminishing during adolescence. A small amount of theta activity may be normal over the temporal regions, somewhat more so in older people (over 60 years of age).
- Delta waves: 1–3 Hz, 50–350 μV is a normal finding only in early childhood; it is not present in the normal waking adult.
- Mu rhythm: of alpha frequency but has a characteristic appearance like the Greek letter μ or the top of a picket fence, and is distributed asymmetrically in the central regions of the head.
- Lambda waves: generated in the occipital region by saccadic eye movements when the eyes are open.

Sleep
The alpha rhythm slows symmetrically and characteristic waveforms (vertex sharp waves and sleep spindles) appear. If sleep is induced by benzodiazepine or barbiturate drugs, an increase in fast frequencies occurs normally.

Abnormal EEG recordings
- Absent brain waves – generalized 'electrocerebral silence': the electric activity of the cortical mantle measured at the scalp is absent or less than 2 μV. This may be due to artefacts (which can be identified as the gains are increased), hypothermia or acute intoxication with anesthetic levels of drugs, such as barbiturates, and severe diffuse cerebral ischemia and hypoxia.
- Absent brain waves – localized: indicates a large area of brain softening, tumor or extra- or subdural hematoma. This is rare because most lesions are not large enough to abolish brain waves or prevent recording of abnormal waves arising from the borders of the lesion.
- Slow waves (delta or theta) – generalized: encountered in coma and any diffuse brain disorder such as a metabolic/toxic disturbance.
- Slow waves – localized: recorded over the site of any focal brain lesion such as a hemorrhage, infarct, herpes simplex encephalitis, tumor.
- Spikes or sharp waves: transient high-voltage waveforms that have a pointed peak at conventional paper speeds and a duration of 20–70 ms. Spikes or sharp waves that occur interictally are referred to as epileptiform discharges.
- Spike discharges or sharp waves – localized: indicate a potentially epileptogenic focus.
- Combined spike and slow wave (spike wave) discharges – generalized: 'typical' if well formed at 3 Hz; 'atypical' if of higher or lower frequency than 3 Hz and if their pattern includes multiple spikes (polyspike wave complexes) (**47**). Such patterns are commonly associated with epilepsy.
- Periodic discharges: may occur regularly in certain pancortical diseases such as Creutzfeldt–Jakob disease (CJD), subacute sclerosing panencephalitis (SSPE) and metabolic encephalopathies.

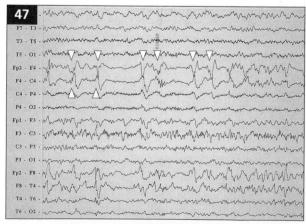

47 16 channel electroencephalograph of a patient who was confused but able to answer simple questions, showing epileptiform features in a patient with non-convulsive status epilepticus (arrowheads).

ROLE

- Accurate diagnosis of epilepsy (see p.71).
- Determine the nature of some pancortical disturbances: SSPE, CJD.
- Confirm the clinical localization of some brain lesions (imaging techniques do this better).
- Monitor progress (e.g. HSE).

An EEG should only be requested if there is a clear question to be answered and the question is answerable by means of EEG. A succinct and relevant clinical history is crucial to accurate interpretation of the recording.

INTERPRETATION

Considerable training, skill and caution is required to interpret accurately the EEG. There is considerable variation in the normal EEG and all too often minor deviations can be erroneously diagnosed as abnormal or, even worse, as indicative of epilepsy or other brain disorders.

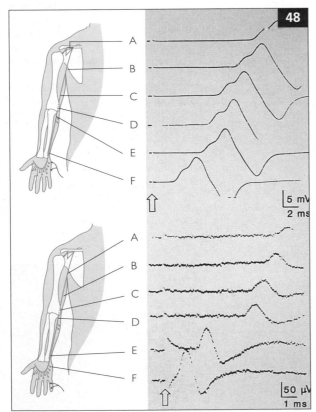

48 Upper diagram illustrates the CMAP recorded from the hypothenar eminence after electrically stimulating the ulnar nerve at various points in the upper limb: the supraclavicular fossa (A), axilla (B), above and below the elbow (C, D, E) and wrist (F).

Lower diagram illustrates the SNAP recorded from various points in the upper limb after electrically stimulating the ulnar nerve in the little finger (orthodromic conduction). Note the different time and voltage scale compared with motor nerve conduction studies above.

NERVE CONDUCTION STUDIES

These involve percutaneous stimulation of peripheral nerve fibers and recording of the compound muscle and sensory nerve action potentials.

MOTOR NERVE CONDUCTION STUDIES

An accessible motor or mixed sensori-motor nerve (e.g. the median nerve at the wrist) is stimulated electrically through surface electrodes applied to the skin and the resulting compound muscle action potential (CMAP) is recorded by surface electrodes on the skin over the motor end point of the muscle (e.g. abductor pollicis brevis) (**48**). The CMAP is filtered, amplified and displayed graphically on a digital screen. The amplitude of the CMAP is measured in millivolts and reflects the number of depolarized muscle fibers. A reduced CMAP amplitude may indicate:

- Fewer motor fibers in the motor nerve (axonal neuropathy).
- Fewer muscle fibers in a motor unit (denervated muscle).
- Temporal dispersion of conduction velocities (demyelinating neuropathy).

The delay (latency) between the time that the stimulus was delivered to the time of onset of the CMAP is measured in milliseconds (e.g. the distal motor latency for median nerve stimulation at the wrist may be 3.6 ms in a patient). If the same nerve is stimulated again, but at a more proximal point (e.g. the cubital fossa), the distance measured between the two stimulus sites (e.g. 200 mm) can be divided by the difference in latency for the two responses (7.6 ms–3.6 ms = 4 ms) to produce a conduction velocity in m/s (e.g. 50 m/s).

In newborn infants the motor conduction velocity is about one-half that of adults and increases with age to reach 'adult values' at about 3–5 years. The conduction velocity is a measure of the conduction in the fastest conducting fibers in the nerve; the large diameter, well myelinated nerves. Small myelinated and unmyelinated nerve fibers are not assessed. Nerve conduction velocity is also influenced by temperature, decreasing by about 1.9 m/s per °C below normal temperature. Because proximal nerve fibers have a larger diameter and are a little warmer than distally, conduction velocities are a little faster in proximal nerve segments. Limb temperature must be known and controlled before nerve conduction studies can be carried out and interpreted reliably.

Normal distal motor latency to onset of CMAP	*ms*
Median nerve (wrist to abductor pollicis brevis, 6–8 cm)	<4.2
Ulnar nerve (wrist to abductor digiti minimi, 6–8 cm)	<3.5

Normal motor conduction velocities	*m/s*
Median nerve in forearm	>49
Ulnar nerve in forearm	>51
Common peroneal nerve (extensor digitorum brevis)	>41
Tibial nerve	>40

SENSORY NERVE CONDUCTION STUDIES

Antidromic conduction in accessible sensory or mixed sensori-motor nerves can be assessed by electrically stimulating the sensory nerve proximally (e.g. the median or ulnar nerve at the wrist) and recording the resulting sensory nerve action potential (SNAP) distally (e.g. from ring electrodes around the index or little fingers respectively) (**48**). Alternatively, orthodromic sensory conduction can be assessed by electrically stimulating the distal sensory fibers (e.g. of the median nerve in the index finger) through surface (ring) electrodes applied to the skin and recording the SNAP by surface electrodes on the skin over the nerve more proximally (e.g. the median nerve at the wrist).

The SNAP reflects the number of nerve fibers that have responded to the stimulus and conducted to the recording point. Lesions of the sensory nerves distal to the dorsal root ganglia lead to a reduction or loss of the amplitude of the SNAP. Sensory nerve action potentials are of very small amplitude (10–20 μV) compared with CMAPs (2–20 mV), and consequently sensory nerve conduction velocities are more technically demanding and less reliable than motor nerve conduction studies. Sensory nerve conduction velocity can be calculated by recording the SNAP at two separate points over a nerve.

Normal sensory action potentials

	Latency to peak (ms)	Amplitude (μV)
Median nerve	<3.5	>15
(wrist to index finger, 12–14 cm)		
Ulnar nerve	<3.1	>10
(wrist to little finger, 10–12 cm)		
Sural nerve	<4.0	>6
(point B, 14 cm)		

These values depend on the age of the patient. The temperature of the limb and the distance between the electric stimulus and the recording site need to be controlled.

PATHOLOGIES
Four pathologic processes may affect peripheral nerves.

Wallerian degeneration
This follows mechanical injury (e.g. transection or crush) or ischemia (e.g. vasculitis) of nerve fibers (**49**).

Neuropathology
- Within 4–5 days, both the axon and myelin distal to the site of injury degenerate.
- The degenerating myelin forms linear arrays of ovoids and globules along the degenerating axon.
- The axon of the proximal segment regenerates forming sprouts which grow distally, and some re-innervate the surviving distal neurilemmal tubes of the Schwann cell basement membrane, inside which the Schwann cells have divided and arranged themselves in line. The regenerating axons are then myelinated by the Schwann cells but the nerve fibers are smaller in diameter and have shorter internodal lengths than originally.

Neurophysiology
- Following nerve transection, the fibers continue to conduct impulses at normal or near normal conduction velocities until about 1–4 days later when the fibers become totally inexcitable and conduction ceases altogether.
- Conduction may be restored following nerve fiber regeneration but conduction velocities are rarely as fast as previously.

Axonal degeneration
Follows most metabolic, toxic and nutritional diseases of peripheral nerves, which result in a disturbance of the metabolism of the cell body, or perikaryon, that impedes fast axonal transport and other functions so that the most distal parts of the axon (which may be up to 1 m (3.3 ft) from the cell body) are affected first and die back from the periphery ('dying-back neuropathy').

Neuropathology
Axonal degeneration of the distal portion of the nerve fiber, similar to the Wallerian degeneration.

Neurophysiology
The intact proximal segments conduct normally but conduction fails over the distal degenerating part of the axon in the same way that it does in Wallerian degeneration.

Segmental demyelination
Follows primary damage of the myelin sheath by a disturbance of Schwann cell metabolism (e.g. some hereditary neuropathies), a direct immune-mediated attack on the myelin or the Schwann cell (e.g. Guillain–Barré syndrome), or toxic damage to the myelin sheath (e.g. diphtheria toxin).

Neuropathology
- Demyelination usually begins paranodally and tends to affect peripheral nerves proximally (e.g. the roots) and very distally at the nerve terminal more than (or, as much as) intervening regions.
- The axon remains intact unless demyelination is severe, causing secondary axonal degeneration.
- Remyelination occurs when Schwann cells divide and form new internodes of irregular length with thin myelin sheaths.
- Repeated episodes of demyelination and remyelination results in the formation of concentric layers of Schwann cell cytoplasm around the axon ('onion-bulb' formations).

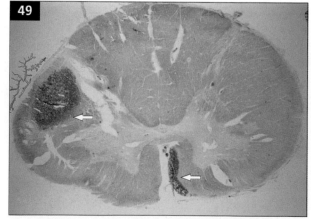

49 Autopsy specimen of the thoracic spinal cord in cross section showing evidence of Wallerian degeneration of the contralateral and ipsilateral corticospinal tracts (arrows) secondary to a more proximal corticospinal tract lesion (i.e. internal capsule lacunar infarct).

Neurophysiology
- Demyelination may result in slowing of conduction, conduction block, inconsistent and incomplete transmission of rapid trains of impulses, and increased susceptibility to changes in temperature.
- In normal myelinated fibers, impulses conduct rapidly from one node of Ranvier to the next by saltatory conduction.
- In demyelinated nerve fibers conduction between nodes is delayed or, as with unmyelinated nerve fibers, conduction becomes continuous across the demyelinated segments. The delay in conduction results in slowing of conduction velocity, temporal dispersion, and therefore a slightly lower amplitude of the action potential.
- Conduction block is present when a proportion of nerve fibers fail to transmit any electric impulses across a demyelinated segment. When the stimulating electrodes are moved proximally along the nerve segment, the CMAP attenuates by more than 50% in area and amplitude between a distal and proximal site of stimulation, indicating failure of conduction in at least some nerve fibers. Conduction block may be caused by focal nerve compression and inflammatory neuropathies.

Neuronopathy or primary nerve cell degeneration
- Primary destruction of nerve cell bodies in the anterior horn cells (e.g. spinal muscular atrophy, poliomyelitis, amyotrophic lateral sclerosis) or dorsal root ganglia (e.g. hereditary, Friedreich's ataxia, paraneoplastic).
- The peripheral sensory axons degenerate distally and the ascending sensory tracts in the posterior columns and other spinal tracts degenerate proximally. As the cell bodies are destroyed, there is no recovery.

LATE WAVES
F-waves
F-waves are late, small motor responses that are evoked by a supramaximal stimulus of a motor nerve. The stimulus to the nerve (e.g. the median nerve at the wrist) not only activates motor fibers that travel orthodromically to produce the initial direct muscle action potential but also activates motor fibers that travel antidromically to the anterior horn cells. Here, some anterior horn cells may be activated to produce a later orthodromic response. So, after a latency longer than that for the direct motor response, a second small muscle action potential is recorded (F-wave). The latency of the F-wave is a measure of the time of conduction in motor fibers from the site of stimulation to the motor neuron and then back again to the recording site, and can be a measure of conduction in the proximal segments of nerves and spinal roots. The consistency of the response to serial stimuli (e.g. 10 electric shocks) is also recorded as a measure of conduction but the validity of this measure remains controversial.

H-reflex
H-reflex is a monosynaptic reflex evoked by low intensity, submaximal electric stimulation of a motor nerve (e.g. posterior tibial nerve), insufficient to produce a direct motor response, which selectively activates the largest fibers in the nerve, the afferent Ia fibers originating from the muscle spindles. This produces impulses that ascend the Ia sensory fibers to the spinal cord, where they synapse with the anterior horn cells, and are then transmitted down the motor fibers to the muscle, producing a muscle contraction (H-wave) after a latency that is much longer than that of the direct motor response (M-wave).

Thus, the H-reflex is the electric representation of the tendon reflex circuit and provides a means of quantitating reflex changes; it is decreased or absent in most peripheral neuropathies and increased in upper motor neuron disorders. It is rarely assessed nowadays in routine neurophysiologic practice.

REPETITIVE STIMULATION STUDIES
Normally, if repeated supramaximal electric stimuli are delivered to a nerve (e.g. the ulnar nerve at the wrist) at rates of up to 25 per second (which most patients would not be able to tolerate), each motor response (CMAP) will have the same form and amplitude. If the stimulus continues at this rate for more than 60 seconds or so, fatigue will occur and a decrement in successive CMAPs appears.

In myasthenia gravis, the initial CMAP produced by electric stimulation is normal (or reduced) but supramaximal stimulation at 2 Hz results in a decrement in amplitude of the first four responses (**50**). In the Lambert–Eaton myasthenic syndrome, post-exercise facilitation is seen a marked increase from initial very low amplitude potentials toward normal amplitude motor unit potentials after 10 seconds of exercising the relevant muscle. This is also a feature of botulism.

CENTRAL MOTOR CONDUCTION
Central motor conduction down the corticospinal tract can be measured by electromagnetic stimulation of the motor cortex and recording the CMAPs and latencies in distal limb muscles.

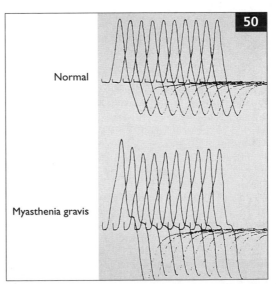

50 Repetitive nerve stimulation studies. Compound muscle action potentials evoked by repetitive electrical stimulation of the ulnar nerve at the wrist at 4 Hz in a normal person (top) and a patient with myasthenia gravis (bottom). Myasthenia gravis is characterized by a decrement in amplitude of the first four responses.

ELECTROMYOGRAPHY (EMG)

The recording through a needle or surface electrode of electric activity from muscles. The signals are amplified and displayed visually on a screen and broadcast audibly through a loudspeaker.

NORMAL MUSCLE ACTIVITY
Insertional activity
When the needle is moved gently within the muscle, a brief burst of electric activity occurs (**51**).

At rest
No electric activity from muscle fibers at rest (**52**).

Muscle activation
- With slight voluntary activation of muscle the smallest motor neuron in the motor neuron pool will begin to fire slowly, producing a stereotyped recurrent individual motor unit action potential discharge on the screen and over the loudspeaker.
- With increasing voluntary effort, more and larger motor units are activated. Initially these are identifiable as individual potentials on the screen and over the loud-speaker but as more and more units are recruited they begin to overlap and produce a 'recruitment pattern'.
- With maximum effort, a full recruitment pattern is seen.

ABNORMAL MUSCLE ACTIVITY
Insertional activity:
- Increased in denervation and many forms of muscle disease.
- Decreased in advanced denervation or myopathy where muscle fibers have been largely replaced by fat and connective tissue.

At rest (spontaneous)
Fibrillation potentials are characterized by an initial positive (downward) deflection followed by a largely negative deflection of 100–300 μV in amplitude and 1–2 ms in duration (**52, 53**). They represent the spontaneous contraction of a single muscle fiber that has lost its nerve supply. If a motor neuron or nerve fiber is destroyed by disease or when its axon is interrupted, the distal part of the axon degenerates over several days. Within 10–14 days from the time of denervation, all of the muscle fibers connected to the branches of the dead axon (the motor unit) begin to generate random spontaneous biphasic or triphasic action potentials (fibrillation potentials) and positive sharp waves (see below).

Fibrillation potentials may also be recorded in some primary muscle diseases with muscle fiber splitting, inflammation or vacuolation (e.g. Duchenne muscular dystrophy, polymyositis, inclusion-body myositis), because the terminal innervation of some muscle fibers is damaged by the disease process. Fibrillation potentials continue until the muscle fiber is re-innervated by progressive proximal–distal regeneration of the interrupted nerve fiber, by the outgrowth of new axons from nearly healthy nerve fibers (collateral sprouting), or until the atrophied muscle fibers degenerate and are replaced over many years by connective tissue. Fibrillation potentials may take the form of positive sharp waves (**51, 53**), which are spontaneous,

initially positive diphasic potentials of longer duration and slightly greater amplitude than the biphasic or triphasic spikes of fibrillation potentials.

Fasciculation potentials are single motor unit action potentials produced by spontaneous discharges in degenerating nerve fibers (**52**). Such contractions of a motor unit or part of a motor unit may be large enough to cause a brief visible twitching or dimpling under the skin. Commonly they are several millivolts in amplitude, last from 5 to >15 ms and usually fire irregularly. They are evidence of motor nerve fiber irritability and not necessarily nerve fiber destruction or motor unit denervation. They may occur in normal people in the calves and hands, and may be induced by low temperature and low serum calcium levels. However, their occurrence in isolation in a relaxed muscle is characteristic of motor nerve fiber degeneration, and this can be confirmed by the presence of associated fibrillation

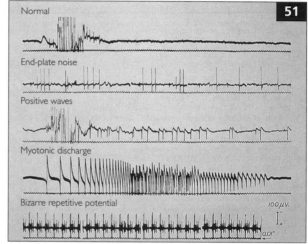

51 Insertional activity. Diagram illustrating the electric activity that may be evoked by insertion of a needle electrode into muscle.

The top tracing shows the normal brief discharge of electric activity (insertion potentials) that last little longer than the movement of the needle. Insertional activity may be prolonged in denervated muscle, myotonic disorders, and as a normal variant; and may be reduced in periodic paralysis during paralysis and if muscle is replaced by connective tissue or fat (e.g. chronic, end-stage myopathy).

'End-plate noise' and associated muscle fiber action potentials is electric activity evoked when the needle is in contact with motor end plates and irritates small intramuscular nerves. 'Positive waves' are evoked in denervated muscle.

'Myotonic discharges' are the action potentials of muscle fibers firing in a prolonged fashion after external excitation. The potentials take two forms (positive waves and brief spikes) depending on the relationship of the recording electrode to the muscle fiber, and wax and wane in amplitude and frequency (40–100 per second) due to an abnormality in the muscle fiber membrane, caused by cholesterol-lowering agents (CLAM), myotonic dystrophy, myotonia congenita, paramyotonia, hyperkalemic periodic paralysis, polymyositis and acid maltase deficiency.

'Bizarre repetitive potentials', now referred to as 'complex repetitive discharges' are action potentials of groups of muscle fibers discharging in near synchrony at high rates (3–40 per second). They occur in a wide range of chronic neuropathies (e.g. poliomyelitis, motor neuron disease, spinal muscular atrophy, radiculoneuropathies) and chronic myopathies (chronic polymyositis, Duchenne dystrophy, limb-girdle dystrophy).

potentials and certain changes in the motor unit potentials (see below).

Myokymia: persistent spontaneous rippling and quivering of muscles at rest, due to groups of repetitive firing potentials, each group firing at its own rate. Often associated with radiation nerve damage.

Myotonia: high frequency repetitive discharges which generally have a positive sharp waveform and wax and wane in frequency and amplitude, producing a 'dive-bomber' sound over the loudspeaker (**51**). Elicited during voluntary muscle contraction and mechanically by movement of the needle electrode. After muscle contraction, a prolonged afterdischarge occurs for up to several minutes, consisting of long trains of fibrillation-like potentials, corresponding to the clinical feature of failure of voluntary relaxation of muscle following forceful contraction.

Complex repetitive discharges: spontaneous repetitive potentials with a bizarre configuration that start and stop abruptly. A sign of chronicity (>6 months) in chronic neurogenic processes and some neuromyopathies.

Continuous muscle fiber activity (neuromyotonia): high frequency (up to 300 Hz) repetitive discharges of varying wave forms. Successive discharges show decrements in amplitude. These discharges probably originate in the distal peripheral nerve, where activity of afferent nerve fibers excites distal motor terminals.

Voluntary muscle activation

Upper motor neuron lesion: poor drive from the upper motor neuron results in few motor units being activated and hence poor recruitment of motor unit potentials. This pattern of recruitment may also be seen in patients who do not (e.g. hysteria), or cannot (e.g. due to joint pain), make an adequate voluntary effort.

Lower motor neuron lesion: after denervation of certain muscle fibers and motor units within a muscle, the surviving nerve fibers that innervate other motor units within the muscle begin to sprout new nerve twigs from nodal points and terminals of undamaged axons, and re-innervate some or all of the denervated fibers. This process results in the addition of more muscle fibers to the surviving motor units, which appear on the EMG and large amplitude, long duration, complex (polyphasic) potentials, which are characteristic of partial denervation and subsequent

52 Spontaneous electric activity in voluntarily relaxed muscle.

Normal: no electric activity. *Fibrillations:* action potentials of single muscle fibers that are twitching spontaneously and usually regularly at rates of 0.5–15 per second in the absence of innervation. They take two forms (positive waves and brief triphasic or biphasic spikes).

Fasciculation: action potential of a group of muscle fibers innervated by an anterior horn cell that discharges in a random, irregular fashion. They may arise from any portion of the lower motor neuron, from the cell body to the nerve terminal.

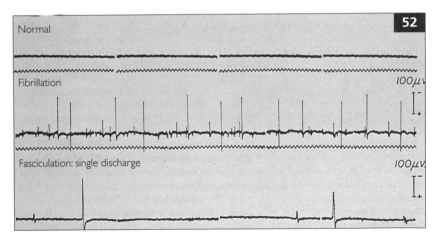

53 Needle electromyographic recording of a resting muscle showing abnormal spontaneous fibrillation potentials (upward spikes) and positive sharp waves (downward spikes).

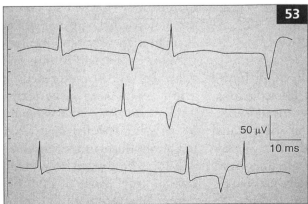

SOMATOSENSORY EVOKED POTENTIALS (SSEPs)

Consecutive electric stimuli are applied, at frequencies of 1.8 Hz, 2.1 Hz or a little faster (but not a multiple of 60, to avoid 60 Hz artefact), to sensory or mixed peripheral nerves (e.g. the posterior tibial, median and ulnar nerves) while recording the evoked potentials from electrodes (for the upper limb) over Erb's point above the clavicle, the dorsal root entry zone, the spinal cord at C2, and the scalp overlying the contralateral parietal cortex, and (for the lower limb) over the lumbar and cervical spine and the contralateral sensory cortex. Characteristic waveforms, designated by the symbol P (positive) or N (negative) and a number indicating the interval of time from stimulus to recording (e.g. N9), are produced in each of these locations, and averaged by computer (**59, 60**).

The integrity of the large sensory nerve fibers and their central pathways though the posterior columns, medial lemniscus, and thalamus to the parietal cortex are tested. Delay between the stimulus site and Erb's point or lumbar spine indicates peripheral nerve disease; delay from Erb's point (or lumbar spine) to C2 implies an abnormality in the appropriate nerve roots or in the posterior columns; delay of subsequent waves recorded from the parietal cortex infer lesions in the medial lemniscus or thalamoparietal connections.

SSEPs are used in cases of suspected MS and cervical spondylitic myelopathy and in monitoring the integrity of the spinal cord during spinal cord operations such as scoliosis surgery. They are abnormal in up to 70% of patients with clinically definite MS (**61**), but are not as sensitive as VEPs and MRI brain and spinal cord in detecting central demyelination.

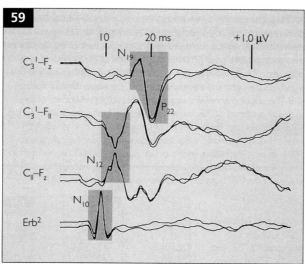

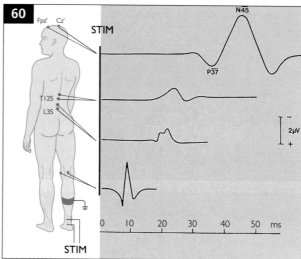

59, 60 Normal short-latency somatosensory evoked potentials. **59** Stimulation of the median nerve at the wrist initially evokes a sharp, predominantly negative potential over Erb's point at about 10 ms (bottom channel) as the sensory and retrograde motor compound action potentials pass beneath it in the brachial plexus at midclavicle, behind the sternomastoid. The next response is a surface negative bifid peak (N_{12}) over the second cervical vertebra (C_2) with instrumental phase reversal (channels 2 and 3). Finally a potential is recorded over the contralateral parietal lobe somatosensory cortex (C_3: 2 cm [0.8 in] behind C_3), with a negative peak at about 19 ms (N_{19}) and a positive wave at about 22 ms (P_{22}). **60** Stimulation of the posterior tibial nerve at the ankle and recording somatosensory evoked potentials at the popliteal fossa, spine and scalp.

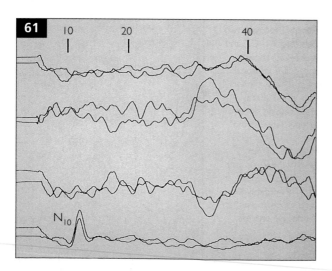

61 Abnormal short-latency somatosensory evoked potentials. Stimulation of the median nerve at the wrist in a patient with multiple sclerosis and loss of proprioception in the hands evokes potentials initially over Erb's point at about 10 ms (bottom channel), but then the potentials over the second cervical vertebral (N_{12}) and cortex (N_{19}) are not clearly seen.

FURTHER READING

NEUROLOGIC EXAMINATION

Acierno MD (2001) Ophthalmoscopy for the neurologist. *The Neurologist* 7: 234–251.

Blessing WW (2000) Alternating two finger tapping as part of the neurological motor examination. *Aust. NZ. J. Med.*, **30**: 506–507.

Mayo Clinic and Mayo Foundation (1981) *Clinical Examinations in Neurology* 5th edn. W.B. Saunders, Philadelphia.

Pandit RJ, Gales K, Griffiths PG (2001) Effectiveness of testing visual fields by confrontation. *Lancet,* **358**: 1339–1340.

Weaver DF (2000) A clinical examination technique for mild upper motor neuron paresis of the arm. *Neurology*, **54**: 531–532.

IMAGING THE BRAIN

Rudkin TM, Arnold DL (1999) Proton magnetic spectroscopy for the diagnosis and management of cerebral disorders. *Arch. Neurol.*, **56**: 919–926.

Costa DC, Pilowsky LS, Ell PJ (1999) Nuclear medicine in neurology and psychiatry. *Lancet,* **354**: 1107–1111.

IMAGING THE CEREBRAL CIRCULATION

Bendszus M, Koltzenburg M, Burger R, *et al.*, (1999) Silent embolism in diagnostic cerebral angiography and neurointerventional procedures: a prospective study. *Lancet,* **354**: 1594–1597.

Keir SL, Wardlaw JM (2000) Systematic review of diffusion and perfusion imaging in acute ischemic stroke. *Stroke*, **31**: 2723–2731.

Markus HS (1999) Transcranial Doppler ultrasound. *J. Neurol. Neurosurg. Psychiatry*, **67**: 135–137.

LUMBAR PUNCTURE AND CSF EXAMINATION

Serpell MG, Rawal N (2000) Headaches after diagnostic dural punctures. *BMJ*, **321**: 973–974.

Steigbigel NH (2001) Computed tomography of the head before a lumbar puncture in suspected meningitis – is it helpful? *N. Engl. J. Med.*, **345**: 1768–1770.

Thomas SR, Jamieson DRS, Muir KW (2000) Randomised controlled trial of atraumatic versus standard needles for diagnostic lumbar puncture. *BMJ*, **321**: 986–990.

ELECTROENCEPHALOGRAPHY

Blume WT (2001) Current trends in electroencephalography. *Curr. Opin. Neurol.* **14**: 193–197.

Fish D (2001) Anticipation of epileptic seizures from standard electro-encephalographic recordings. *Lancet* **357**: 160–161.

- Resting position of the eyes and spontaneous eye movements (*continued*):
- Dysconjugate eyes: nuclear or infranuclear oculomotor or abducens nerve lesion, or internuclear ophthalmoplegia (medial longitudinal fasciculus).
- Regular conjugate horizontal eye movements ('ping-pong gaze'): brainstem lesion.
- Eyes jerk backwards into orbits (retractory nystagmus): midbrain lesion.
- Intermittent downward jerking of the eyes (ocular bobbing): low pons lesion.
- Spontaneous nystagmus: rare in comatose patients because the fast phase is a corrective saccade generated by the frontal cortex and requires intact and interactive vestibular pathways, cerebral cortex and oculomotor system.
- Oculocephalic reflex: rotating the patient's head from side to side in a comatose patient with an intact brainstem evokes conjugate eye movements in the opposite direction to the head movement, so that the eyes move in the orbit but remain 'focused', looking straight ahead ('doll's eye movements'). If the oculovestibular reflex is interrupted, due to brainstem dysfunction, the eyes move dysconjugately, or do not move in the orbits, remaining in the mid-position of the head, 'looking' in the direction of the head movement.
- Oculovestibular responses: after examining the intact tympanic membranes, 50–200 ml of ice cold water is instilled into one of the external auditory meati. If the oculovestibular reflex is intact, the eyes deviate tonically toward the irrigated ear. In a conscious patient (or psychogenic coma) with intact corticopontine fibers, the frontal cortex tries to drive the eyes back to mid-position thus generating the fast phase of nystagmus away from the side of stimulation. Tonic and conjugate deviation of the eyes toward the irrigated ear, without corrective ocular saccades (the fast phase), indicates an intact brainstem and a supratentorial cause for the coma. If the response is dysconjugate, or absent, brainstem dysfunction is the likely cause of the coma. Both external auditory meati should be irrigated independently; simultaneous irrigation will evoke vertical conjugate eye movement and corrective saccades (nystagmus).
- Corneal response: may be absent in light coma due to drug intoxication but otherwise is usually retained until deep coma and then its absence is a poor prognostic factor.
- Respiration:
- Post-hyperventilation apnea: bilateral hemispheric disturbance.
- Long-cycle Cheyne–Stokes respiration: diencephalic dysfunction.
- Central neurogenic hyperventilation: low midbrain and upper pons lesions.
- Short-cycle Cheyne–Stokes respiration: medullary dysfunction.
- Yawning, vomiting, hiccough: brainstem dysfunction.

Ophthalmoscopy: look for papilledema, sub-hyaloid hemorrhages, retinal emboli, diabetic or hypertensive retinopathy. The absence of papilledema or venous pulsation does not exclude raised intracranial pressure.

Motor function
- Glasgow coma scale.
- Lateralizing features are important (facial grimace; limbs).
- Seizures: focal or generalized.
- Multifocal myoclonus: diffuse cortical irritation due to anoxia or metabolic disturbance.
- Muscle tone, deep tendon reflexes, and plantar responses: abnormal with corticospinal tract lesions and also sometimes with hepatic and hypoglycemic encephalopathy.

DIFFERENTIAL DIAGNOSIS
Coma or not?
Confusion
Confusion is often caused by acute metabolic or toxic disturbances, particularly in the elderly (e.g. hypoxia, hypercapnia, fluid and electrolyte disturbance, hypoglycemia, drug intoxication, and drug withdrawal), or sleep deprivation, pain and as a transient phenomenon after seizures. It needs to be differentiated from dysphasia, amnesia, acute psychosis, the retardation of severe depression and dementia.

Delirium
Delirium is commonly caused by metabolic and toxic disorders but can be mimicked by degenerative brain disease, acute psychosis and hypermania.

Stupor
Stupor needs to be differentiated from catatonic schizophrenia or severe retarded depression. The EEG is always abnormal in stupor due to organic disease.

Persistent vegetative state (see p.52)

Locked-in syndrome (see p.55)

Brain death (see p.51)

Etiology of the coma
Coma with focal neurologic signs or evidence of head injury
- Supratentorial or infratentorial mass lesion (vascular, inflammatory, neoplastic).
- Hypoglycemic encephalopathy.
- Hepatic coma.

Coma with meningism but no focal/lateralizing neurologic signs
- Subarachnoid hemorrhage.
- Meningo-encephalitis.

Coma without focal/lateralizing neurologic signs or meningismus
Metabolic/toxic encephalopathy:
- Hypoxic encephalopathy.
- Hyponatremia. Altered consciousness and seizures, without focal neurologic signs.
- Hypoglycemic encephalopathy:
- Altered consciousness.
- Focal neurologic signs, such as hemiparesis, may be present.
- Excess sympathetic adrenergic activity (pallor, sweating, dilated pupils, tremor, tachycardia).
- Underlying diabetes, alcoholism, hypopituitarism, hypothyroidism or pancreatic islet cell tumor.

- Hyperglycemia, hyperosmolality and acidosis:
- Diabetic ketoacidosis: dehydration, hyperosmolality, acidosis, and deep sighing respirations (Kussmaul breathing).
- Hyperosmolar coma, with dehydration but no ketoacidosis: older patients taking oral hypoglycemic drugs or small doses of insulin
- Non-ketotic lactic acidosis in diabetic patients taking hypoglycemic agents such as metformin. The blood sugar may or may not be elevated.
- Hyperglycemia may not be the cause of the coma; it may be a consequence of other causes of coma such as stroke, head injury and meningitis.
- Renal failure (uremia).
- Liver failure (hepatic encephalopathy, see p.452):
- Confusion or delirium.
- Asterixis: an inability to maintain the arms outstretched with the hands and fingers held dorsiflexed because of periodic inhibition of contraction of the wrist and finger extensors causing recurrent lapses in posture of the hands at the wrists, giving rise to the appearance of a 'liver flap'.
- Hypocalcemia:
- Tetany and seizures: underlying renal failure and hypoparathyroidism.
- Hypercalcemia:
  Dehydration, weakness, nausea, anorexia, and vomiting: Underlying primary hyperparathyroidism or malignancy, or prolonged immobilization.
- Hypothermia and hypothyroidism:
- History of prolonged immersion in water or exposure to the cold.
- Hypothyroidism: coma can be precipitated by cold, infection or withdrawal of thyroid medication. Clinical features include obesity, coarse myxedema facies, low body temperature and delayed relaxation of the ankle jerks.
- Thiamine deficiency (Wernicke's encephalopathy [see p.460]):
  Malnourished chronic alcoholics, recent increased glucose intake.
- Confusion, ophthalmoplegia (bilateral abducens nerve palsies), nystagmus and ataxia, but some present in coma. Peripheral neuropathy may present.

Drug overdose:
- History and circumstances of discovery.
- A discrepancy between marked depression of brainstem responses and relatively light coma is present in some patients.
- Pin-point pupils suggest opiate poisoning.

Subarachnoid hemorrhage (see p.249): neck stiffness is usually, but not always, present.

Meningo-encephalitis (see p.273): fever, neck stiffness may be absent in a deeply comatose patient.

Generalized epilepsy (nonconvulsive status or post ictal state):
- History of epilepsy.
- Evidence of tongue biting and incontinence.

Non-neurologic (malingering or hysteria):
- Normal rate and depth of respiration, pupillary reactions, muscle tone, deep tendon and abdominal reflexes, and plantar responses.
- Attempts to open the patient's eyes may be resisted.

- Slow, roving eye movements are not evident.
- Irrigation of the ears with ice-cold water is noxious and usually evokes nausea, sometimes with vomiting, and nystagmus with the fast phase beating away from the side of the irrigated ear (which is a cortical response to the tonic deviation of the eyes toward the irrigated ear, that is mediated by the brainstem reflex).

INVESTIGATIONS
Coma with focal neurologic signs or evidence of head injury
- CT or MRI brain scan: supratentorial or infratentorial mass lesion.
- Blood glucose.
- Liver function tests.

N.B. Lumbar puncture (LP) is contraindicated in the presence of space-occupying lesions that increase the pressure in one brain compartment, particularly the infratentorial compartment, because it may lower pressure in the spinal canal and increase the pressure differential across different brain compartments and precipitate herniation of brain, particularly through the foramen magnum ('coning') (see p.31).

Coma with meningism but no focal/lateralizing neurologic signs
- CT brain scan: subarachnoid blood, or focal collections of blood or pus.
- LP, depending on results of CT scan, to examine CSF for blood, inflammatory cells, and micro-organisms.

Coma without focal or lateralizing neurologic signs or meningismus:
- Full blood count and ESR.
- Urea and electrolytes.
- Plasma and urine osmolality.
- Blood glucose.
- Red blood cell transketolase.
- Thiamine.
- Liver function tests.
- Calcium and phosphate.
- Thyroid function tests.
- Arterial blood gases.
- Drug and toxin screen in blood and urine.
- EEG: triphasic waves of hepatic and uremic encephalopathy, non-convulsive status epilepticus or a post ictal recording.
- CT or MRI brain may be necessary but the chance of finding a focal abnormality is low.
- LP may occasionally be indicated to exclude an inflammatory or infectious cause.

MANAGEMENT
Establish brain death with certainty using recognized criteria
- Diagnosis (Wijdicks, 2001).
- Exclusion of potential confounding factors: metabolic, endocrine and toxic causes. Wait at least four half-lives of elimination of the relevant drug in the absence of factors known to delay excretion. This is usually 3 or 4 days. Evidence of delayed excretion may necessitate confirmatory cerebral vessel radiocontrast or radionuclide angiography.
- Observation (6–48 hours depending on the age of the patient).
- Examination:
- Proof of extensive brain damage.
- Exclusion of reversible causes of coma.
- Clinical examination of brainstem reflexes: pupillary, corneal, oculocephalic, oculovestibular, gag, cough.
- Assessment of somatic responses.
- Demonstration of apnea despite arterial $PaCO_2$ >8 kPa (60 mmHg) with pH <7.30.
- Repeat examination (more than 2 hours after first examination).
- Certification by two practitioners.

Prepare and discuss with the family or family spokesperson
- The underlying condition.
- What constitutes brain death.
- Why and how it has occurred.
- Differences between brain death and permanent vegetative state.

Provide emotional and practical support
Continual contact between the family and:
- A responsible decision maker.
- The intensive care/ward staff providing hour-by-hour care.

When counselling
- Sit close enough to be easily seen and heard in an area where you will not be disturbed.
- Avoid physical barriers such as tables or desks.
- Achieve and sustain eye contact.
- Extend a comforting touch to the relative's shoulder or hand, if appropriate.

Allow time for acceptance of the situation
- Do not rush or pressurize a decision.
- Do not become impatient with requests to cover the same ground many times.
- Do not withhold information.
- Do not peripheralize the family in the decision processes.
- Do not over-promote the issue of organ donation.

Involve the family centrally in final decision making and participation in the 'switch off' process if requested

After brain death is determined, life support is removed
- Do not withdraw contact after the 'switch off'.

PERMANENT VEGETATIVE STATE (PVS)

DEFINITION:
- A condition of 'wakefulness without awareness'.
- The absence of any adaptive response to the external environment and any evidence of a functioning mind which is either receiving or projecting information, in a patient who has long periods of wakefulness.

The vegetative state
- A clinical condition of unawareness of self and environment in which the patient breathes spontaneously, has a stable circulation, and shows cycles of eye closure and eye opening which may simulate sleep and waking.
- May be a transient stage in the recovery from coma or it may persist until death.

The continuing or persistent vegetative state
- The vegetative state has continued for more than 4 weeks and it has become increasingly unlikely that the condition is part of a recovery phase from coma.

The permanent vegetative state
- A diagnosis based on a high degree of clinical certainty that the continuing vegetative state is irreversible; usually a continuing vegetative state for more than 12 months after head injury and more than 6 months following other causes of brain damage.
- Avoiding this state is one of the most important aspects of attempting to assess prognosis early in coma.

EPIDEMIOLOGY
Prevalence: 10 000 to 25 000 adults and 400–1000 children in the USA.

PATHOPHYSIOLOGY
- Severe damage to part or all of the cerebral hemispheres, with an intact brainstem.
- Can occur with damage to the more rostral part of the brainstem.

PATHOLOGY
Three main patterns:
- Diffuse axonal injury, typically as a sequel to severe closed head trauma, giving rise to degeneration of the white matter throughout the cerebral hemispheres.
- Extensive laminar necrosis of the cerebral cortex, following global cerebral hypoxia or ischemia (69).
- Thalamic necrosis, occasionally.

ETIOLOGY
- Head injury.
- Hypoxic-ischemic encephalopathy: cardiac arrest, carbon monoxide poisoning.
- Stroke: ischemic or hemorrhagic.
- Hypoglycemia.
- Intracranial infection.
- Brain tumor.
- End stage of degenerative brain disorders: Alzheimer's disease.

CLINICAL FEATURES
- Inattentive and unaware of the surroundings but breathes spontaneously, without mechanical support, and has a stable circulation.
- At times the eyes are closed and the patient appears asleep, at other times the eyes are open and they seem to be awake.
- May be aroused by painful or prominent stimuli, opening the eyes if they are closed, increasing the respiratory rate, or occasionally grimacing or moving the limbs.
- When the eyes are open the eyelids may blink in response to any threat to the eye.
- A range of spontaneous movements may occur such as roving eye movements, chewing, teeth-grinding, groaning, grunting and even swallowing is possible. More distressingly, patients may smile, shed tears, moan or scream, without any discernible reason. Sometimes, the head and eyes turn fleetingly to follow a moving object or sound.
- Body posture may be decorticate or decerebrate.
- Brainstem reflexes (pupillary, oculocephalic [doll's eye], corneal and gag) are usually preserved.
- Primitive reflexes such as pouting and sucking reflexes, grasp reflex, and withdrawal reflexes to pain may be present.
- Painful stimuli may provoke an extensor or a flexor response.
- Plantar responses are commonly extensor.

N.B. Any unambiguous sign of conscious perception or deliberate action (e.g. any evidence of communication, including a consistent response to command, or any purposeful movement) is incompatible with the diagnosis of vegetative state. Careful prolonged observation is required before concluding that a patient's wakefulness is unaccompanied by awareness.

DIAGNOSIS
Two medical practitioners experienced in assessing disturbances of consciousness and awareness should separately assess the patient (this includes discussion with other medical and nursing staff, relatives and carers about the reactions and responses of the patient, and to ensure that the patient is not sentient) and document their findings and conclusions in the medical record. If there is any uncertainty about the diagnosis of the permanent vegetative state, then a re-assessment should be undertaken at a later date.

DIAGNOSTIC CRITERIA
Preconditions
- A cause for the syndrome has been established.
- Persisting effects of sedative, anesthetic and neuromuscular blocking drugs have been excluded by the passage or time or by appropriate analysis of body fluids.
- Reversible metabolic causes have been corrected or excluded as the cause.

Clinical criteria
All three of:
- No evidence of awareness of self or environment at any time. No volitional response to visual, auditory, tactile or noxious stimuli, and no evidence of language comprehension or expression.
- Cycles of eye closure and eye opening which may simulate sleep and waking shall be present.
- Hypothalamic and brainstem function is sufficiently preserved to ensure the maintenance of respiration and circulation.

Other clinical features include:
- Spontaneous blinking.
- Inconsistent, non-purposeful reflex movements in response to external stimuli:
  - Apparent smiling.
  - Facial 'grimacing' to painful stimuli.
  - Watering of the eyes.
  - Startle myoclonus.
  - Occasional movements of the head and eyes towards a peripheral sound or movement.
  - Purposeless movement of the limbs and trunk.
- Retained pupillary and corneal responses (usually).
- Absence of visual fixation and ability to track moving objects with the eyes or show a 'menace' response.
- Roving eye movements may be present.
- Conjugate or dysconjugate tonic eye movement, without corrective saccades (nystagmus) in response to ice water caloric testing.
- Variable deep tendon reflexes (reduced, normal or brisk) and plantar responses.
- Clonus and other signs of spasticity may be present.
- Incontinence of bladder and bowel.

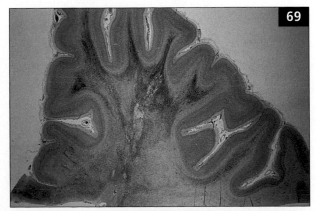

69 Microscopic section of a part of a cerebral hemisphere showing laminar necrosis and demyelination in the white matter due to carbon monoxide poisoning. (Courtesy of Professor BA Kakulas, Royal Perth Hospital, Western Australia.)

DIFFERENTIAL DIAGNOSIS

- Locked-in syndrome (see p.55): a brainstem lesion disrupts the voluntary control of movement but arousal and the content of awareness are not abolished. Patients are able to communicate by movement of the eyes or eyelids.
- Coma (see p.44): most patients who are in 'coma' for weeks, months or years are in a continuing vegetative state.
- Brain death (see p.51): implies the irreversible loss of all brainstem functions. It is, in a sense, the converse of PVS, in which brainstem function survives while the function of the cerebral hemispheres is lost or gravely impaired. Brain death is followed, within hours or days, despite intensive care, by cardiac arrest.
- Akinetic mutism: a state of profound apathy with evidence of preserved awareness and attentive visual pursuit, giving an unfulfilled 'promise of speech'. The responsible lesions often involve the medial frontal lobes.
- Psychogenic unresponsiveness.

The differentiation of these conditions from the vegetative state is based on clinical findings (*Table 3*).

INVESTIGATIONS

- CT or MRI head scan: may show non-specific focal or diffuse abnormalities, brain atrophy, and hydrocephalus.
- Single photon emission computed tomography (SPECT) and positron emission tomography (PET): show a reduction in cerebral metabolism.
- Neurophysiology studies: EEG, somatosensory evoked potentials (SSEPs), and electrodermal techniques; very variable results. Often these studies provide evidence of some cortical activity, reminding us that an accurate clinical diagnosis of vegetative state does not imply cortical silence. They are of little value in predicting outcome, other than early EEG evidence of burst suppression and SSEP evidence of an absent N20 potential.

No findings are diagnostic of the permanent vegetative state.

PROGNOSIS

- Determined by the age of the patient, underlying cause and the duration of the vegetative state.
- The outlook is better in children, and after traumatic (as opposed to non-traumatic) brain injury. If the cause is not head injury, there is very little hope of recovery of sentience after 3 months and none after 6 months.
- If the cause is head injury, a longer time should elapse (e.g. 6 months) before being confident that the chances of recovery are extremely low (and almost non-existent after 12 months).

Table 3 Differentiation of vegetative state from other conditions

Condition	Locked-in syndrome	Vegetative state	Coma	Brain death
Self-awareness	Present	Absent	Absent	Absent
Cyclical eye opening	Present	Present	Absent	Absent
Glasgow coma scale				
Eye opening	4	4	1–2	1
Motor response	1	1–4	1–4	1–2
Verbal response	1	1	1–2	1
Motor function	Eye movement preserved in the vertical plane and able to blink volitionally	No purposeful movement	No purposeful movement	None or only reflex spinal movement
Pain sensation	Yes	No	No	No
Respiratory function	Normal	Normal	Depressed or varied	Absent
EEG activity	Normal or minimally abnormal	Polymorphic delta or theta —sometimes slow alpha	Polymorphic delta or theta	Electrocerebral silence or theta
Brain metabolism	Minimal/moderate reduction	≥50% reduction	≥50% reduction	Absent or great reduction
Prognosis	Depends on cause Recovery unlikely	Depends on cause and duration	Recovery, vegetative state, or death within 2–4 weeks	No recovery

MANAGEMENT

Establish the diagnosis of a permanent vegetative state by (1) identifying the clinical state of the patient, (2) the cause for the syndrome, and (3) the lapse of time. Because many patients entering a vegetative state emerge from it within a few weeks or months, supportive early management is usually appropriate. The diagnosis of a permanent vegetative state implies that recovery cannot be achieved and further therapy is futile. It merely prolongs an insentient life for the patient and a hopeless vigil for relatives and carers.

Medical care

- Appropriate nursing or home care.
- Maintain oxygenation, circulation and nutrition.
- Correct complicating factors such as infection and hypoglycemia.
- Sensitive discussion with, and education of, relatives and carers about the cause, clinical state, 'hopeless' prognosis, and implications, including the possibility of withdrawing artificial means of administering food and fluid.
- Decisions to withdraw nutrition, hydration and other life-sustaining medication such as insulin for diabetes, should currently be referred to the court before any action is taken.
- Decisions not to intervene with cardio-pulmonary resuscitation or prescribe antibiotics are clinical decisions, but they should take account of, and respect, the views of the relatives, carers and patient, if known, whether formally recorded in a written document (or advance directive) or not.
- The role of sensory stimulation remains uncertain, despite the writings of Hippocrates: 'the patient in a state of coma should be spoken to in a loud voice, splashed with cold water and exposed to bright light'.

LOCKED-IN SYNDROME

DEFINITION

A de-efferented state whereby patients are aware of themselves and their environment but are unable to respond due to loss of motor and speech function.

PATHOGENESIS

- A supranuclear (upper motor neuon) lesion of the descending corticospinal tracts, usually in the ventral portion of the brainstem (commonly the pons), below the level of the IIIrd cranial nerve nuclei, causes paralysis of the muscles innervated by the lower cranial nerves and peripheral nerves.
- A widespread nuclear or infranuclear (lower motor neuon) disease of motor nerves.

ETIOLOGY

Ventral brainstem lesion

- Infarction or hemorrhage (commonly hypertensive patients) (**70, 71**).
- Tumor.
- Demyelination (multiple sclerosis).
- Central pontine myelinolysis, following profound hyponatremia (see p.457).
- Head injury.

Polyneuropathy

- Critical illness polyneuropathy.
- Acute onset post-infectious polyradiculoneuropathy (Guillain–Barré syndrome).

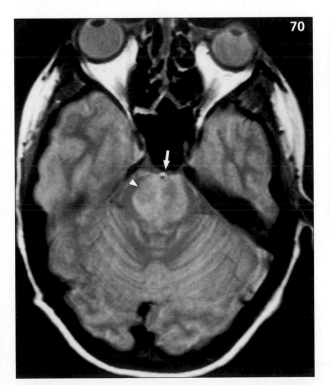

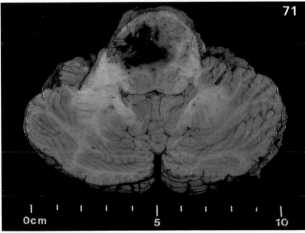

71 Autopsy specimen of a cross section of the midpons and cerebellum in the axial plane of a patient who was 'locked-in' showing hemorrhagic infarction in the ventral pons bilaterally.

70 Proton density weighted axial MR scan showing high signal in the basilar artery (due to thrombus, arrow) and increased signal in the pons due to pontine infarction (arrowhead) in a patient who presented 'locked-in'.

CLINICAL FEATURES
- Unable to speak.
- Unable to move the limbs.
- Awareness and consciousness are preserved because the brainstem tegmentum, including the reticular formation and oculomotor nerves and pathways are spared.
- Able to open the eyes and move them, (particularly in the vertical plane) and blink, in order to try and communicate.

INVESTIGATIONS:
- CT or MRI brain scan: ventral pontine or midbrain lesion.
- Other investigations, as appropriate, to ascertain the cause (e.g. serum sodium, EEG, EMG).

DIAGNOSIS
Diagnosis is clinical, based on the presence of total paralysis of the limbs and muscles innervated by the lower cranial nerves, but with the ability of the patient to open and close the eyes voluntarily and in response to commands, and to respond to verbal and sensory stimuli by blinking.

TREATMENT
General (see Coma, p.44)
Patients can see, hear and feel everything (including pain and itch) so are sensitive to what staff are saying. They are also very frustrated that they cannot move.
- Prevention of complications of immobility: pneumonia, deep vein thrombosis, contractures, urinary tract infection.
- Rehabilitation: physiotherapy, swallowing and speech therapy, occupational therapy, psychologic support and therapy.

Specific
Correct the underlying cause (e.g. hyponatremia; see Central pontine myelinolysis, p.457).

PROGNOSIS
Prognosis is poor. Some patients recover, usually with residual limb spasticity.

NARCOLEPSY

DEFINITION
A syndrome of excessive sleepiness and abnormally regulated rapid-eye-movement (REM) sleep.

EPIDEMIOLOGY
- Prevalence: 1 in 500 000 (Israel), 1 in 5000 (USA, Europe), 1 in 600 (Japan).
- Age: 5–50 years, usually 15–35 years.
- Gender: M=F.

PATHOLOGY
Unknown.

ETIOLOGY AND PATHOPHYSIOLOGY
- Inherited susceptibility: probably dominant with variable penetrance.
- Linked strongly to certain Class II HLA antigens: HLA-DR2 and HLA-DQw1 antigens in 98–100% of patients. Classic narcolepsy (narcolepsy associated with cataplexy) has almost a 100% association with the DRw15 subtype of the HLA-DR2 antigen, the DQw6 subtype of the HLA-DQw1 antigen, and the HLA-Dw2 subtype of the HLA-D antigen.
- The 'narcolepsy-susceptibility' gene has not been located exactly but is likely to be just outside the HLA-DQ and HLA-DR subregions on the short arm of chromosome 6.
- The occurrence of normal periods of REM sleep at the onset of sleep or within 10 minutes thereafter is the most characteristic and striking physiologic abnormality, and probably indicates impaired sleep–wake regulation rather than an excessive need for REM sleep.
- The mechanism may be abnormalities of monoaminergic and cholinergic functioning in the brain (e.g. impaired release of norepinephric neurotransmitters).
- Abnormalities in the orexin (hypocretin) neurotransmitter system are directly involved in the pathogenesis of narcolepsy in two animal models. Decreased levels of orexin A in the CSF are found in narcoleptic patients, and an association of a rare polymorphism in the *prepro-orexin* gene with narcolepsy in a cohort of 178 patients has been reported recently.
- Hypnagogic hallucinations, sleep paralysis and cataplexy appear to be associated manifestations of REM sleep that intrude into wakefulness.

CLINICAL FEATURES
Excessive sleepiness (rather than increased sleep)
- Brief (a few to 30 minutes), irresistible episodes of daytime sleep, sometimes associated with dreaming, and preceded by increasing drowsiness.
- Most apparent in boring, sedentary situations.
- Partially alleviated by mental stimulation and motor activity.
- Cannot be fully relieved by any amount of sleep.
- Patients usually feel refreshed after a sleep attack.
- Chronic excessive daytime sleepiness between attacks of sleep.
- The degree of sleepiness usually remains stable after the first few months.
- Increased sleepiness after several years suggests the presence of an additional disorder, such as sleep apnea.

Cataplexy
- Attacks, lasting from a few seconds to several minutes, of sudden reduction or loss of muscle tone, usually precipitated by excitement, emotion (such as surprise, anger, laughter) and athletic activities. Severe attacks cause complete paralysis except for the respiratory muscles. More common partial episodes cause patients to drop objects, sit down, stop walking, and even lose sphincter control (e.g. fecal incontinence).
- Consciousness is almost always maintained.
- Most attacks last less than 1 minute.
- Prolonged episodes may be associated with hallucinations.
- Rarely, cataplexy that is almost continuous ('status cataplecticus') may occur.
- Sleep paralysis (60% of patients).
- Brief episodes of inability to move during the onset of sleep or on awakening.
- Patient may feel as if he or she is struggling to move.
- Lasts up to 10 minutes.

Hypnagogic hallucinations (60% of patients)
- Hallucinatory experiences, usually visual but can be auditory or tactile, that accompany the onset of sleep or awakening.
- May have a dream-like quality but awareness of surroundings is preserved.
- May accompany sleep paralysis or occur independently.

Other symptoms
- Automatic behavior (up to 80% of cases): episodes of semi-purposeful activity, such as writing off the edge of the page, putting clothes in the refrigerator, usually during monotonous or repetitive behavior, and for which the patient is amnesic.
- Brief lapses in speech and concentration.
- Disrupted nocturnal sleep.
- Memory disturbances, due to impaired attention and fluctuating levels of alertness.
- Blurred or double vision (10–14%).
- Depression (?due to altered central monoamine function).

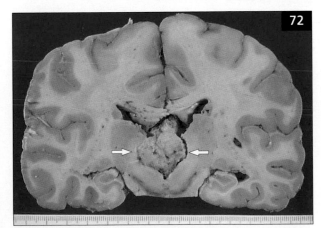

72 Macroscopic appearance of the brain, coronal section through the thalami and upper midbrain showing a pineal germinoma occupying the third ventricle (arrows) and compressing the rostral midbrain in a patient who presented with recurrent episodes of daytime sleepiness and was initially considered to have narcolepsy.

DIFFERENTIAL DIAGNOSIS
Epilepsy
Although a single episode may be clinically indistinguishable from a complex partial or absence seizure, the 'sleep-like' appearance of the patient and the association of the episodes with drowsiness and passive situations helps to distinguish automatic behavior from the repetitive stereotyped behavior that accompanies epileptic seizures.

Schizophrenia
Patients with narcolepsy and prominent hallucinations may be misdiagnosed as schizophrenic.

Daytime sleepiness
- Sleep apnea: obstructive sleep apnea is characterized by recurrent episodes of partial or complete upper airway obstruction during sleep (causing habitual snoring and witnessed apneas) which are terminated by arousal. The recurrent arousals have a destructive effect on sleep and so the common symptoms are excessive daytime sleepiness, and impairment of mood, memory and concentration. Consequently, the patients' work, family and social lives are disrupted and the risk of accidents is increased. Obstructive sleep apnea affects about 4% of middle-aged men and half as many women. Predisposing factors include male gender, increasing age, obesity, alcohol and sedative abuse, family history, specific upper airway abnormalities (nasal obstruction, tonsillar/adenoidal hypertrophy, micrognathia, retrognathia, Marfan's syndrome), endocrine diseases (hypothyroidism, acromegaly) and neuromuscular diseases (decreased ventilatory drive, decreased upper airway muscle tone). Treatment strategies include modification of predisposing factors; reduction of weight, smoking, alcohol and sedatives; modification of sleeping posture; nasal continuous positive airway pressure (CPAP); dental splints; and surgery (nasal [if obstructed], palatal, mandibular/maxillary).
- Insufficient sleep.
- Medication effects.
- Diencephalic lesions: tumors in the region of the third ventricle (**72**).

Excessive sleepiness without REM-sleep abnormalities or cataplexy
- Narcolepsy which progresses with time to include abnormalities of REM sleep and cataplexy.
- Atypical depression.
- Irregular sleep schedules.
- Idiopathic hypersomnia (a diagnosis of exclusion, having excluded depression, insufficient sleep, and abnormalities of REM sleep).

REM sleep at onset of sleep
- Endogenous depression.
- Sleep deprivation: sleep apnea, disturbances of the sleep-wake schedule.
- Drug and alcohol withdrawal.
- Some structural brain lesions.

INVESTIGATIONS

- Multiple sleep latency test (**73**): monitors the time to the onset of sleep and the type of sleep that occurs during attempts to sleep at 2 hourly intervals throughout the day. More than 80% of patients with narcolepsy have a mean sleep latency of less than 5 minutes and at least two REM periods at the onset of sleep during the procedure.
- MRI brain scan is sometimes indicated to exclude the most unlikely possibility of a diencephalic structural lesion.

DIAGNOSIS

- Excessive sleepiness and frequent REM periods at the onset of sleep.
- Confirmation with a formal multiple sleep latency test is essential in view of the long term implications of the diagnosis.

TREATMENT

Narcolepsy

- Avoid occupations and situations where nodding off to sleep is a danger to the patient or to others, such as driving.
- Take regular 15–20 minute naps.

Stimulants:
- Enhance the synaptic availability of noradrenaline.
- Methylphenidate 10–60 mg/day, or
- Dextroamphetamine 5–50 mg/day.
- Higher doses offer little additional benefit and increase the risk of adverse effects.
- Pemoline or protriptyline may be tried if methylphenidate and dextroamphetamine are not successful or not tolerated.
- Modafinil (an alpha1-adrenergic agent) 100 mg bd, mazindol (an imidazole derivative), and selegiline (a monoamine oxidase-type B inhibitor) improve daytime alertness and may have fewer adverse effects than amphetamine.
- Narcoleptics are not immune to the problems associated with the chronic use of stimulants.

Cataplexy and sleep paralysis

- Tricyclic antidepressants (e.g. imipramine, clomipramine, protriptyline) in low doses (10–50 mg): act by inhibiting reuptake of noradrenaline and serotonin rather than cholinergic blockade.
- Specific serotonin reuptake inhibitors (e.g. fluoxetine): may be as effective with fewer anticholinergic adverse effects.
- Noradrenaline reuptake inhibitors (e.g. viloxazine).
- Gamma-hydroxybutyrate (sodium oxybate): increases slow-wave sleep and REM sleep; effective in some.
- Abrupt discontinuation of tricyclic agents can lead to a rebound increase in cataplexy.
- Gradual withdrawal of tricyclic antidepressants followed by a drug holiday sometimes helps restore efficacy.

Disturbed nocturnal sleep

- Short acting hypnotic (e.g. temazepam) one or twice a week; regular nightly use is rarely beneficial.

CLINICAL COURSE AND PROGNOSIS

- Sleepiness usually precedes cataplexy by several months but 6–10% of patients experience cataplexy initially, and 10–15% do not develop cataplexy until 10 years or more after the onset of sleepiness.
- The degree of sleepiness usually remains stable after the first few months and rarely lessens. Increased sleepiness after several years suggests the presence of an additional disorder, such as sleep apnea.
- Cataplexy, hypnagogic hallucinations, and sleep paralysis improve or disappear with age in about one-third of patients.

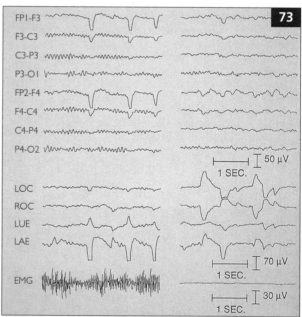

73 Electroencephalography (EEG) of a middle-aged male with episodes of loss of consciousness (sleep attacks) and automatic behavior (mini-sleeps). Multiple sleep latency test gave evidence of narcolepsy with short sleep latency (2 minutes) and sleep-onset REM periods (REM latency 1 minute). Typical features during REM sleep include rapid eye movements, absent muscle artefact, and drowsy EEG pattern.

LOC: left outer canthus; ROC: right outer canthus; LUE: left under eye; LAE: left above eye. Ocular electrodes were referential to A1A2.

(Reproduced with permission from the editor (Elaine Wyllie, MD) and publisher (Williams & Wilkins) of Wylie E (ed) (1997) *The Treatment of Epilepsy: Principles and Practice*, 2nd edn. Williams & Wilkins, Baltimore.)

SYNCOPE

DEFINITION
A transient loss of postural tone and consciousness resulting from an acute reduction in blood flow to the brain.

EPIDEMIOLOGY
- Incidence: The most common non-epileptic cause of loss of consciousness.
- Age and gender: any age and either sex.

PATHOPHYSIOLOGY
Basic neurophysiology
The conscious state depends on the integrity of the brainstem reticular activating system interacting (through its ascending pathways) with both cerebral hemispheres. Therefore, to disturb consciousness, the function of the brainstem or both cerebral hemispheres needs to be disturbed (see Coma, p.44).

Basic vascular physiology:
- Blood flow to the brain depends on the mean arterial blood pressure and the intracranial pressure.
- Blood pressure is the product of the cardiac output (heart rate × stroke volume) and total peripheral resistance.
- Blood flow in the brain is maintained by autoregulation in response to minor changes in systemic blood pressure. However, sudden, dramatic reductions in blood pressure below a mean arterial BP of about 8 kPa (60 mmHg) result in a parallel fall in brain perfusion, resulting in a gradual loss of consciousness.

Altered heart rate
Bradyarrhythmia
Primary:
- Complete heart block (Stokes–Adams attack).
- Atrial fibrillation.
- Sinus arrest.

Secondary:
- Carotid sinus hypersensitivity (head turning, neck massage).
- Swallow syncope: swallowing can activate a vagal reflex. It may indicate an underlying structural abnormality of the esophagus, glossopharyngeal neuralgia, digoxin toxicity, or ischemic heart disease.
- Stretch syncope.
- Ice-cream syncope: cold food held in the mouth can activate a vagal reflex.
- Prostatic syncope: rectal examination may activate a vagal reflex.
- Vaso-vagal attack: often precipitated by emotion.
- Baroreceptor dysfunction (age, hypertension, prolonged bed rest, autonomic neuropathy).

Tachyarrhythmia
Supraventricular tachycardia:
- Wolff–Parkinson–White syndrome.
- Prolonged QT syndrome.
- Complex partial seizures (very rare).

Ventricular tachycardia.

Reduced stroke volume
Acute reduction
Low blood volume:
- Acute fluid loss: burns, vomiting, diarrhea, dehydration.
- Hemorrhage.
- Addison's disease.
- Diuretics.
- Very low salt diet.

Obstruction to venous return to the heart:
- Cough/micturition/defecation.
- Cardiac tamponade.

Impaired outflow from the heart: acute myocardial infarction.

Obstruction to outflow from the heart:
- Pulmonary embolus.
- Aortic dissection.

Chronic reduction
Impaired outflow from the heart:
- Cardiomyopathy: dilated.
- Congenital heart disease.

Obstruction to outflow from the heart:
- Atrial myxoma or ball valve thrombus (impaired ventricular filling).
- Hypertrophic obstructive cardiomyopathy.
- Aortic stenosis (syncope on exertion).

Reduced peripheral resistance
Central autonomic neuropathy
- Multiple systems atrophy (see p.435).
- Parkinson's disease.
- Primary autonomic failure.
- Spinal cord injury.

Peripheral neuropathy
- Diabetic neuropathy.
- Guillain–Barré syndrome.
- Tabes dorsalis.
- Amyloid neuropathy.
- Acute porphyria.
- Autonomic ganglionitis and neuritis.

Other
- Vaso-vagal (the most common cause of syncope).
- Drugs: vasodilators (e.g. glyceryl trinitrate, prazosin, hydralazine, calcium channel blockers) and other anti-hypertensives (e.g. diuretics, ganglion blockers), levodopa, bromocriptine, antidepressants, phenothiazines, sedatives.
- Large meal (dilatation of splanchnic vessels).
- Heat (dilatation of cutaneous vessel).
- Anemia.
- Hyponatremia.
- Old age and prolonged recumbency.

Drop attacks

- Spontaneous episodic raised intracranial pressure may impair brain perfusion (e.g. colloid cyst of the third ventricle [74, 75], posterior fossa tumor). Usually associated headache and visual obscurations
- Cryptogenic drop attacks: abrupt episodes of falling to the ground without any warning, precipitating factor, or loss of awareness. Usually in middle-aged women and benign.

Metabolic disorders

- Hypoglycemia: usually diabetes but may be caused by insulinoma, Addison's disease, and post-gastrectomy. Tends to occur after fasting. Associated symptoms may include sweating and a sensation of hunger.
- Pheochromocytoma: episodic release of catecholamine may lead to transient palpitations, headache, sweating, and hypotension. Many patients have postural hypotension due to chronic excess secretion of catecholamines, but rarely causes syncope.
- Hyperventilation-induced alkalosis.

Sleep disorders

- Narcolepsy: excessive daytime sleepiness (see p.57).
- Cataplexy: sudden onset of focal or generalized loss of muscle tone, often precipitated by emotion such as laughter, and resulting in either episodic limb weakness or sudden collapse from an upright position (see p.57).
- Obstructive sleep apnea.

Psychiatric

Pseudoseizures.

INVESTIGATIONS

The history, physical examination and EKG are the core of the diagnostic workup. In most patients, there is an obvious precipitant and no investigations are required, or at most an EKG and hemoglobin. For example, syncope in the elderly often results from polypharmacy and abnormal physiologic responses to daily events. The need for further investigations are determined by the certainty of the clinical diagnosis and nature of the clinical findings.

Cardiologic

Indicated in patients with known or suspected heart disease (e.g. history of congestive heart failure or ventricular arrhythmia), exertional syncope, and recurrent syncope.

Non-invasive

- EKG: to exclude complete heart block, an aberrant conduction pathway, and an acute cardiac event (76, 77).
- 24-hour ambulatory or patient activated EKG recording (Holter monitoring): can be useful if the attacks are frequent enough to be captured and the patient is known to have, or is suspected of having, heart disease. However, it may fail to detect arrhythmias if they do not occur during the monitoring period, and increasing the period of monitoring only slightly improves sensitivity. If an arrhythmia is detected (e.g. frequent ventricular ectopic beats) but it is associated with no symptoms, it does not prove that the arrhythmia is the cause of the syncope. Nevertheless, the arrhythmia may point to an underlying structural heart disease.
- Echocardiography: if valvular heart disease, outflow obstruction or cardiomyopathy is suspected.
- Carotid sinus stimulation under EKG control: aims to detect carotid sinus hypersensitivity but is of limited use. Should be performed with the patient lying supine. A period of more than 3 seconds of asystole on EKG monitoring is positive, although this response is non-specific, being present in up to 20% of the asymptomatic population.
- Upright tilt table testing: a method of diagnosing vaso-vagal syncope in patients with frequent recurrent undiagnosed syncopal events but no heart disease and patients with recurrent syncope and heart disease but no evidence of arrhythmias. The technique involves constant EKG recording and blood pressure monitoring while the patient is brought from a supine to an upright position

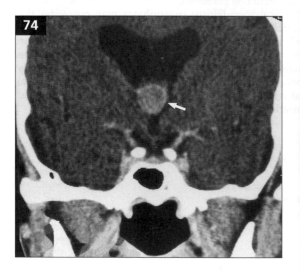

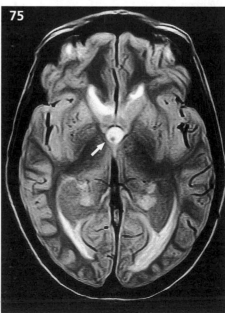

74 Contrast-enhanced CT brain scan, coronal plane, showing a colloid cyst of the third ventricle as a round hyperintense mass lesion (arrow), causing obstructive hydrocephalus.

75 T2W MRI brain scan, axial plane, showing a colloid cyst of the third ventricle (arrow).

(e.g. 70° head-up tilt) in a series of stages, and maintained in that position, in the absence of drugs for up to 40 minutes. The test is positive if there is syncope or presyncope in association with hypotension and/or bradycardia. The sensitivity of this test is up to 70% but the specificity is uncertain. If there is no abnormal response, an isoprenaline (isoproterenol) infusion can be given to improve sensitivity further (at the expense of specificity). It is commenced at 1 μg per minute and the rate progressively increased every 5 minutes by a further microgram per minute at successive tilts. The isoprenaline (isoproterenol) infusion initially increases the heart rate and then the rhythm may change from sinus to another rhythm (e.g. junctional rhythm), resulting in a fall in blood pressure and symptoms of syncope. The symptoms resolve with resumption of the supine posture. The test is again positive if there is syncope or presyncope in association with hypotension and/or bradycardia.

Invasive
- Electrophysiologic studies: directly assess intracardiac conduction and the presence of inducible supraventricular and ventricular arrhythmias by intracardiac stimulation. Although invasive, the morbidity is low (1–2%) and mortality very low. May be indicated if recurrent and disabling syncopal episodes, clinical suspicion of an arrhythmia, abnormal resting EKG, arrhythmias on Holter monitoring, and structural heart disease.

Blood
Basic laboratory tests are not usually helpful and should be minimized:
- Hemoglobin level may reveal anemia.
- Serum urea and electrolytes and glucose may reveal the most common metabolic causes.
- Prolonged fast to exclude hypoglycemia.
- Short tetracosactrin (cosyntropin) test, if abnormal urea and electrolytes, to exclude Addison's disease.

Urine
24-hour urine collection for vanillylmandelic acid to exclude pheochromocytoma.

Neurologic
Neurologic investigation is rarely helpful unless additional neurologic symptoms or signs are present.
- CT or MRI brain scan: if drop attacks or suspected Arnold–Chiari malformation, hydrocephalus, colloid cyst of the third ventricle, or subdural hematoma.
- EEG (combined with simultaneous EKG monitoring): if suspected seizure disorder. A positive EEG may support the diagnosis of epilepsy but a negative study does not exclude it.
- Nerve conduction studies and EMG: if neuropathy suspected.
- Autonomic function tests.

Biopsy
Rectal: if amyloidosis suspected (rare).

Psychiatric
Occasionally a psychiatric assessment may be useful in patients with otherwise unexplained frequent syncopal events and no injury, as patients with anxiety disorders, panic reaction and somatization disorders may report syncope as a symptom.

DIAGNOSIS
The key to the diagnosis of syncope is a sound clinical history from the patient and an eyewitness.

TREATMENT
Aims to identify and correct the specific underlying cause:
- In most patients, whose syncope was due to the simultaneous occurrence of several predisposing factors (e.g. dehydrated, tired, hot and stuffy room), an explanation and reassurance is all that is required.
- Attend to any heart disease: e.g. pacemaker insertion may help patients with complete heart block and carotid sinus hypersensitivity.
- Correct any metabolic and hormonal deficiencies.

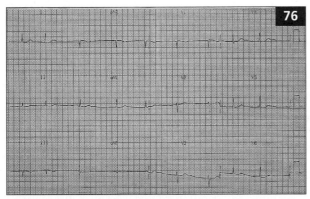

76 Electrocardiograph (EKG) showing slow atrial fibrillation with a ventricular rate of about 45 per minute.

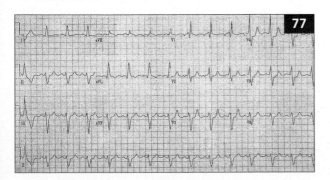

77 Electrocardiograph (EKG) showing bifascicular block (a combination of right bundle branch block and left anterior hemiblock) due to coronary artery disease in a 70 year old male who presented with three episodes of collapse due to cardiac syncope related to paroxysmal bradycardia. Electrophysiologic studies failed to induce clinically significant tachycardia and the patient responded well to permanent pacemaker insertion. Bifascicular block can develop into complete conduction block due to trifascicular block or complete AV block.

Postural hypotension

- Stop any drugs that may cause postural hypotension (if possible), particularly in the elderly. These include diuretics (particularly in hot weather), α-adrenoreceptor blockers (e.g. prazosin), psychotropic drugs with α-adrenoreceptor blocking activity (tricyclic antidepressants, antipsychotics, including prochlorperazine [Stemetil]); α-methyldopa, nitrovasodilators (e.g. glyceryl trinitrate, including long-acting formulations), and antiparkinsonian drugs (L-dopa, bromocriptine).
- Avoid large meals, especially when accompanied by alcohol.
- Change posture, from supine to standing, slowly (avoid sudden changes).
- Waist-high supportive garments (e.g. elasticated stockings) or antigravity suits may be helpful for venous pooling but can be uncomfortable.
- Elevate the head of the bed at night.
- High salt diet.
- Prophylactic medication such as the mineralocorticoid fludrocortisone in low dose; sympathomimetics such as ephedrine; caffeine; non-steroidal anti-inflammatory drugs such as indomethacin, if there is no contraindication; ergot alkaloids, theophylline, β-adrenoreceptor antagonists with intrinsic sympathomimetic activity; disopyramide and octreotide (somatostatin analogue). Insertion of a pacemaker may be indicated for cardiogenic syncope if medical therapy fails.

- Advise patients with recurrent syncope to avoid precipitating factors (e.g. large meals) and circumstances that may lead to injury if they do lose consciousness and to stand slowly. Driving should be restricted until free of recurrent syncopal episodes for up to 1 year if the cause of the loss of consciousness has not been elucidated and treated appropriately.

PROGNOSIS

Depends upon the underlying cause; benign in many cases, a warning sign of sudden death in a minority of others. Sudden death occurs within the next year in about 20% of patients with syncope due to ischemic or structural heart disease. The spontaneous remission rate is high and the rate of sudden death is low in patients with unexplained syncope after intensive investigation.

FURTHER READING

COMA

Bateman DE (2001) Neurological assessment of coma. *J. Neurol. Neurosurg. Psychiatry*, **71 (suppl 1)**: i13–i17.

Bates D (1993) The management of medical coma. *J. Neurol. Neurosurg. Psychiatry*, **56**: 589–598.

Bates D (2001) The prognosis of medical coma. *J. Neurol. Neurosurg. Psychiatry*, **71 (suppl 1)**: i20–i23.

Cartlidge N (2001) States related to or confused with coma. *J. Neurol. Neurosurg. Psychiatry*, **71 (suppl 1)**: i8–i19.

Fisher CM (1995) Brain herniation: a revision of classical concepts. *Can. J. Neurol. Sci.*, **22**: 83–91.

Johnson MH (2001) Assessing confused patients. *J. Neurol. Neurosurg. Psychiatry*, **71 (suppl 1)**: i7–i12.

Meagher DJ (2001) Delirium: optimising management. *BMJ*, **322**: 144–149.

Mercer WN, Childs NL (1999) Coma, vegetative state, and the minimally conscious state: Diagnosis and management. *The Neurologist*, **5**: 186–193.

Overell J, Bone I, Fuller GN (2001) An aid to predicting prognosis in patients with non-traumatic coma at one day. *J. Neurol. Neurosurg. Psychiatry*, **71 (suppl 1)**: i24–i25.

Ropper AH (1986) Lateral displacement of the brain and level of consciousness in patients with an acute hemispheral mass. *N. Engl. J. Med.*, **314**: 953–958.

Wijdicks EFM, Miller GM (1997) MR imaging of progressive downward herniation of the diencephalon. *Neurology*, **48**: 1456–1459.

BRAIN DEATH

Bernat JL (1992) Brain death. *Arch. Neurol.*, **49**: 569–570.

De Tourtchaninoff M, Hantson P, Mahieu P, *et al.*, (1999) Brain death diagnosis in misleading conditions. *Q. J. Med.*, **92**: 407–414.

Hachinski V (1992) Brain death or loss of human brain life? *Arch. Neurol.*, **49**: 572.

Inwald D, Jakobovits I, Petros A (2000) Brain stem death: managing care when accepted medical guidelines and religious beliefs are in conflict. *BMJ*, **320**: 1266–1268.

Lövblad K-O, Basssetti C (2000) Diffusion-weighted magnetic resonance imaging in brain death. *Stroke*, **31**: 539–542.

Pugh J, Clarke L, Gray J *et al* (2000) Presence of relatives during testing for brain stem death: Questionnaire study. *BMJ*, **321**: 1505–1506.

Wijdicks EFM (2001) The diagnosis of brain death. *N. Engl. J. Med.*, **344**: 1215–1221.

Younger SJ (1992) Defining death. *Arch. Neurol.*, **49**: 570–572.

PERMANENT VEGETATIVE STATE

Andrews K (1999) The vegetative state – clinical diagnosis. *Postgrad. Med. J.*, **75**: 321–324.

Kennard C, Illingworth R (1995) Persistent vegetative state. *J. Neurol. Neurosurg. Psychiatry*, **59**: 347–348.

McLean SAM (2001) Permanent vegetative state and the law. *J. Neurol. Neurosurg. Psychiatry*, **71 (suppl 1)**: i26–i27.

Review by a working group convened by the Royal College of Physicians and endorsed by the conference of Medical Royal Colleges and their Faculties of the United Kingdom (1996) The Permanent Vegetative State. *J. R. Coll. Physicians Lond.*, **30**: 119–121.

Zeman A (1997) Persistent vegetative state. *Lancet*, **350**: 795–799.

NARCOLEPSY

Aldrich MS (1990) Narcolepsy. *N. Engl. J. Med.*, **323**: 389–393.

Aldrich MS (1998) Diagnostic aspects of narcolepsy. *Neurology*, **50** (Suppl 1): S2–S7.

Broughton RJ, Fleming JAE, George CFP, *et al.* (1997) Randomized, double-blind, placebo-controlled crossover trial of modafinil in the treatment of excessive daytime sleepiness in narcolepsy. *Neurology*, **49**: 444–451.

Douglas NJ (2001) The sleepy patient. *J. Neurol. Neurosurg. Psychiatry*, **71 (suppl 1)**: i3–i6.

Fry JM (1998) Treatment modalities for narcolepsy. *Neurology*, **50** (Suppl 1): S43–S48.

Gencik M, Dahmen N, Wieczorek S, *et al* (2001) A *prepro-orexin* gene polymorphism is associated with narcolepsy. *Neurology*, **56**: 115–117.

Guilleminault C, Brooks SN (2001) Excessive daytime sleepiness. A challenge for the practising neurologist. *Brain*, **124**: 1482–1491.

Krahn LE, Black JL, Silber MH (2001) Narcolepsy: new understanding of irresistible sleep. *Mayo Clin. Proc.*, **76**: 185–194.

SYNCOPE

Arthur W, Kaye GC (2000) The pathophysiology of common causes of syncope. *Postgrad. Med. J.*, **76**: 750–753.

Kapoor WN (2000) Syncope. *N. Engl. J. Med.*, **343**: 1856–1862.

Linzer M, Yang EH, Estes M III, Wang P, Vorperian VR, Kapoor WN, for the Clinical Efficacy Assessment Project of the American College of Physicians (1997) Diagnosing syncope. Part 1: Value of history, physical examination, and electrocardiography. *Ann. Intern. Med.*, **126**: 989–996.

Linzer M, Yang EH, Estes M III, Wang P, Vorperian VR, Kapoor WN, for the Clinical Efficacy Assessment Project of the American College of Physicians (1997) Diagnosing syncope. Part 2: Unexplained syncope. *Ann. Intern. Med.*, **127**: 76–86.

Mathias CJ, Kimber JR (1998) Treatment of postural hypotension. *J. Neurol. Neursurg. Psychiatry*, **65**: 285–289.

Parry SW, Kenny RA (1999) Tile table testing in the diagnosis of unexplained syncope. *Q. J. Med.*, **92**: 623–629.

Epilepsy

EPILEPSY

DEFINITION
Epileptic seizure

A paroxysmal, stereotyped disturbance of consciousness, behavior, emotion, motor function, perception or sensation (which may occur singly or in any combination), that results from cortical neuronal discharge.

Epilepsy

A condition in which epileptic seizures recur, usually spontaneously.

EPIDEMIOLOGY
- Incidence: 20–70 per 100 000 per year.
- Prevalence: 0.5–1.0% of the population (active epilepsy).
- Cumulative/lifetime (or total) prevalence:
  Single seizure (including seizure with acute illness, but not febrile seizure): 3%.
- Active epilepsy and/or on treatment: 4–5 per 1000.
- N.B. These figures exclude febrile convulsions, which occur in about 5% of children.

Table 6 International classification of seizures

	Prevalence in adults
Partial seizures (beginning focally)	55%
• Simple partial seizures (without impaired consciousness)	5%
– With motor symptoms	
– With somatosensory or special sensory symptoms (e.g. olfactory, auditory, visual hallucinations)	
– With autonomic symptoms	
– With psychological symptoms	
• Complex partial seizures (with impaired consciousness)	15%
– Simple partial onset followed by impaired consciousness	
– Impaired consciousness at onset	
• Partial seizures evolving into secondary generalized seizures	35%
Generalized seizures (convulsive or non-convulsive)	35%
• Absence seizures	
– Typical	1%
– Atypical	
• Myoclonic seizures	1%
• Clonic seizures	
• Tonic seizures	
• Tonic-clonic seizures	30%
• Atonic seizures	
• Status epilepticus	
Unclassifiable/undifferentiated epileptic seizures	10%

- Age: any age. Peak incidence in early childhood and a second peak in the elderly (over-60 age group).
- Gender: slight excess among males.

CLASSIFICATION
Epileptic seizures are now classified as generalized and partial, based on clinical and electroencephalograph (EEG) distinctions. This classification replaces such imprecise terms as 'grand mal' and 'petit mal'.

N.B. Epilepsy may manifest itself in the form of more than one seizure type in the same patient. In addition,

Table 7 International classification of epilepsies and epileptic syndromes

Localization-related (local, focal, or partial) epilepsies and syndromes
- Idiopathic epilepsy with age-related onset:
- Benign childhood epilepsy with centro-temporal spikes
- Childhood epilepsy with occipital paroxysms
- Symptomatic epilepsy

Generalized epilepsies and syndromes
- Idiopathic epilepsy with age-related onset (listed in order of age of onset):
- Benign neonatal familial convulsions
- Benign neonatal non-familial convulsions
- Benign myoclonic epilepsy in infancy
- Childhood absence epilepsy (formerly known as pyknolepsy)
- Juvenile absence epilepsy
- Juvenile myoclonic epilepsy (formerly known as impulsive petit mal)
- Epilepsy with generalized tonic-clonic seizures (GTCS) on awakening
- Other idiopathic epilepsies
- Idiopathic or symptomatic epilepsy (listed in order of age of onset):
- West's syndrome (infantile spasms)
- Lennox–Gastaut syndrome (childhood epileptic encephalopathy)
- Epilepsy with myoclonic-astatic seizures
- Epilepsy with myoclonic absence seizures
- Symptomatic epilepsy
- Non-specific syndromes:
- Early myoclonic encephalopathy
- Early infantile epileptic encephalopathy with suppression burst.
- Specific syndromes:
- Epileptic seizures complicating other disease states (such as cerebral malformations, inborn errors of metabolism, and disorders presenting as progressive myoclonic epilepsy)

Continued on page 66

seizures of one type may be easy to control in some patients but difficult to treat in others.

Epileptic syndromes are determined by: seizure type(s), age of onset, EEG findings (interictal and ictal) and associated findings (e.g. family history, neurologic signs). They provide information about the likelihood of identifying an underlying cause, the prognosis, and the appropriate investigations and management, including medications, lifestyle modification and genetic counselling.

ETIOLOGY
Epilepsy (like stroke) is a symptom of an underlying disorder(s) of the brain. The likely causes vary depending on the type of epilepsy and the age of the patient (i.e. more likely to be idiopathic in young people, whereas in the elderly about half are idiopathic, a third due to vascular diseases, and the majority of the remainder due to tumors and other structural lesions).

Idiopathic
In about two-thirds of epilepsies no specific cause is found (idiopathic epilepsies). Idiopathic generalized absence epilepsies:
* Age-dependent onset between childhood and adolescence.
* Distinct phenotypic expression.
* Frequent familial clustering.
* Abnormal EEG in about 10% (but up to 30%) of otherwise healthy family members.

Genetic factors
Inheritance of epilepsy is predominantly polygenic and multifactorial.

Generalized epilepsy
Siblings or children of people with generalized epilepsy have up to a 10% risk of developing epilepsy.
* Primary generalized epilepsies:
– 30–50% of cases may have a genetic basis.
– 5–10% of children whose parents or siblings have a primary generalized epilepsy develop epilepsy.
– Usually inherited as an autosomal dominant trait, probably polygenic.

– Benign familial neonatal convulsions – chromosomes 8q and 20q.
– Benign familial infantile convulsions – chromosome 19.
* Juvenile myoclonic epilepsy – possibly HLA region of chromosome 6p (controversial: see p.86).
* The 'spike wave trait': an autosomal dominantly inherited tendency to develop paroxysms of spike wave complexes, usually at 3 Hz, but infrequently associated with clinical seizures.
* Some progressive myoclonic epilepsies are inherited as a recessive trait (see p.87).

Partial epilepsy
Siblings of people with focal epilepsy have a <5% risk of epilepsy.

Simple (single gene) inheritance
* Uncommon single gene disorders: tuberous sclerosis, familial cavernous angiomas (chromosome 7q), familial periventricular heterotopia (chromosome Xq28).
* Autosomal dominant nocturnal frontal lobe epilepsy:
– One family was found to have a missense mutation in a gene on chromosome 20 which is closely related to the neuronal nicotinic acetylcholine receptor alpha 4 subunit, which is important for modulating glutamate.
– Incomplete penetrance.
– Onset usually in childhood.
– Aura often present on awakening; tonic spasms or hyperkinetic motor symptoms.
* Autosomal dominant partial epilepsy with variable foci.
* Familial temporal lobe epilepsy: dominantly inherited.
* Autosomal dominant rolandic epilepsy with speech dyspraxia.

Complex (polygenic or multifactorial) inheritance:
* Idiopathic partial epilepsies: benign partial epilepsy of childhood with centro-temporal spikes (benign rolandic epilepsy).
* Cryptogenic/symptomatic partial epilepsies: temporal lobe epilepsy.
* Situation-related seizures: siblings of people with febrile seizures have an 8% risk of epilepsy.

Perinatal factors
The contribution of perinatal damage to the development of partial epilepsy is difficult to assess but is probably less important than previously thought. Perinatal causes include birth trauma, intracranial hemorrhage, hypoxia and hypoglycemia.

Structural cerebral cortex lesions
Interfere with function of the cortex or lead to cortical gliosis.

Congenital
* Hamartomas.
* Arteriovenous malformations (cavernous angiomas) (**78**).
* Tuberous sclerosis (**79**).
* Storage diseases: cerebral lipidosis.
* Neuronal migration disorders causing cortical malformations.
* Generalized (agyria, pachygyria/lissencephaly and band heterotopias).
* Unilateral hemispheric (hemimegalencephaly).
* Focal (cortical dysplasia, polymicrogyria, schizencephaly, focal heterotopias).

Trauma
- Birth injury (trauma or hypoxia).
- Head injury (cortical contusion more than laceration).

Vascular
- Ischemic or hemorrhagic stroke.
- Cerebral edema: hypertensive encephalopathy.

Infection
- Meningitis.
- Abscess.
- Encephalitis.

Tumor
Primary and secondary.

Degenerative
Alzheimer's disease.

Metabolic/toxic factors
Epileptic seizures may be caused, or exacerbated by, many disturbances to cellular metabolism, such as hyperthermia, hypoxia, hypocapnia, hyponatremia, uremia, hypocalcemia, hypoglycemia, liver failure, porphyria, pyridoxine deficiency, drugs (e.g. solvents, cytotoxic drugs [e.g. nitrogen mustard drugs and ifosfamide]), drug and alcohol withdrawal, fatigue, pregnancy and toxins (e.g. insecticides and heavy metals).

PATHOPHYSIOLOGY
Focal epilepsy
- Gliosis or a local deficiency of inhibitory neuro transmitters (gamma aminobutyric acid [GABA], glycine and taurine) lead to a failure of normal modulation of dendrites of neurons from surrounding cells.
- Shortening of dendrites bring excitatory inputs closer to the cell body.

- Depolarization waves (paroxysmal depolarization shift) affect dendrites of epileptic neurons.
- Electric current flows from neutral cell bodies in layers 5 and 6 of the cerebral cortex to depolarized dendrites in the superficial layer of the cortex, which is recorded by EEG scalp electrodes as a negative spike discharge.
- The epileptic discharge also activates inhibitory feedback circuits which repolarize the cell bodies while the dendrites are recovering from depolarization, resulting sometimes in a surface-negative slow wave following the spike discharge; current flows from the hyperpolarized cell body to the neutral dendrites, causing a surface-negative slow wave in the EEG.
- Spike wave complexes may remain localized, spread over the cortex via association fibers, or spread to the opposite cerebral hemisphere through the corpus callosum causing a 'mirror focus' or a generalized epileptic seizure.

Generalized epilepsy
- Thalamo-reticular and thalamo-cortical projections combine with inhibitory intra-thalamic projections to generate a rhythmic discharge.
- Absence seizures result from synchronous burst-firing generated in the thalamocortical circuit, which is made up of three principal neuronal populations: neocortical pyramidal cells, thalamic relay neurons, and the exclusively GABAergic neurons which form nucleus reticularis thalami (NRT). The frequency of burst-firing between reciprocally interconnected thalamic relay neurons and neocortical pyramidal neurons is synchronized by NRT neurons. GABAergic neurotransmission is important in the generation of synchronous burst-firing in the thalamo-cortical circuit. PET scanning in patients with generalized epilepsies shows thalamic activation.

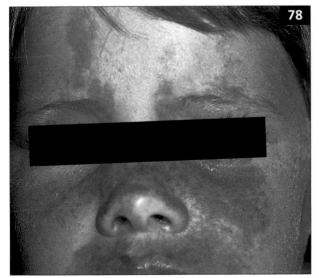

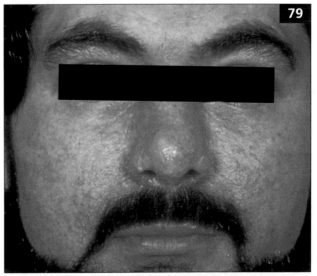

78 Facial photograph of a young male with Sturge–Weber disease and epilepsy due to a left fronto-parietal venous hemangioma of the meninges over the left fronto-parietal lobes and atrophy of the underlying subcortex. Note the deep red port wine nevus (hemangiomatous malformation) not only within but also outside the distribution of the left trigeminal nerve.

79 Photograph of the face of a patient with epilepsy due to tuberous sclerosis. Note the diffuse small adenoma sebaceum (pink, wart-like angiofibromas) over the cheeks, resembling acne. (Courtesy of Dr AM Chancellor, Tauranga, New Zealand.)

Carbamazepine (Tegretol) (*continued*)

- Available as 100 mg and 200 mg tablets, or 200 and 400 mg controlled-release tablets that are helpful for avoiding peak-dose adverse effects.
- Plasma half-life: 24–45 hours initially but after continued long term use it falls to about 9 (8–24) hours.
- The drug must be introduced in a low dose to offset mild neurotoxicity (sedation, vertigo, ataxia, diplopia, nausea, headache). The usual starting dose in adults is 100 mg three times daily, or preferably, half a 200 mg or 400 mg controlled-release tablet twice daily for 2 days, followed by half a tablet in the morning and a whole tablet at night, and further increases if necessary, aiming to maintain the plasma level within the therapeutic range and control seizures (rather than waiting for another seizure to occur). Even with this cautious approach and the development of tolerance some patients are unable to remain on carbamazepine because of neurotoxicity. In addition a morbilliform skin rash limits its usefulness in 5–8% of patients.
- Adverse effects:
- Dose-related: neurotoxicity (dizziness, double vision, unsteadiness), nausea, vomiting, cardiac arrhythmia and orofacial dyskinesia.
- Idiosyncratic: skin rash (5–8% of patients), agranulocytosis, aplastic anemia, syndrome of antidiuretic hormone secretion (leading to fluid retention and hyponatremia) hepatotoxicity, photosensitivity, Stevens–Johnson syndrome, lupus-like syndrome, thrombocytopenia and pseudolymphoma.
- A major inducer of hepatic cytochrome P450 activity. Variable autoinduction of metabolism accounts for the wide range of doses and for the substantial interindividual variation in concentration found with the same dose.
- Drug interactions: carbamazepine accelerates the clearance of itself (i.e. it induces its own metabolism), ethosuximide, clonazepam, clobazam, corticosteroids, theophylline, haloperidol, warfarin and hormones. So, most women taking the oral contraceptive pill require daily estrogen in a dose of 50 µg. Mutual enzyme induction or inhibition with phenobarbitone (phenobarbital), phenytoin, or primidone can result in a small rise or fall in steady-state concentrations of either of both drugs. The metabolism of carbamazepine is inhibited, causing neurotoxicity, by sodium valproate, cimetidine, danazol, dextropropoxyphene (propoxyphene), diltiazem, erythromycin, isoniazid, and verapamil.

Phenytoin (Dilantin)

- First used as an antiepileptic drug in 1938.
- Effective for generalized tonic-clonic and partial seizures.
- No longer a drug of first choice, particularly in young women, because it may cause cosmetic changes (gum hyperplasia, acne, hirsutism, and facial coarsening), as well as sedation and unfavorable effects on cognitive function (e.g. attention, memory).
- Available as a 6 mg/ml suspension, as chewable 50 mg tablets, and as capsules of 30 mg and 100 mg.
- Plasma half-life: about 24 (9–40) hours.
- One of only a few drugs with zero order kinetics at therapeutic dosage – as the concentration rises, the capacity of the hepatic cytochrome P-450 enzyme system to metabolize the drug becomes saturated (usually at around 300 mg/day), and so a small increment in dose can produce a large rise in serum level. Conversely, the circulating concentration may fall precipitously when the dose is modestly reduced.

- Starting dose for children: 5 mg/kg daily, for adults starting and maintenance dose: 300 mg daily, given as a single dose or in divided doses. (Note, this is not the loading dose that is required for status epilepticus.)
- If seizures continue, an increment of 30 mg is appropriate, particularly if the serum concentration is above 12 mg/l (60 µmol/l).
- Adverse effects: mental slowing, unsteadiness of gait, slurred speech and tremor, and physical examination reveals gaze-evoked nystagmus and tandem gait ataxia. Other predictable adverse effects include nausea, anorexia, vomiting, dyspepsia, cognitive impairment, depression, aggression, drowsiness, headache, paradoxical seizures, megaloblastic anemia, hyperglycemia, hypocalcemia, osteomalacia and neonatal hemorrhage. Prolonged use is associated with coarsening of facial features, gum hyperplasia (**98**), acne and hirsutism.
- Idiosyncratic effects include blood dyscrasia, lupus-like syndrome, reduced serum IgA, pseudolymphoma (lymphadenopathy), rash, Stevens–Johnson syndrome, Dupuytren's contracture, hepatomegaly and hepatotoxicity and teratogenicity. Long term use may cause peripheral neuropathy, cerebellar degeneration due to Purkinje cell loss and osteomalacia.
- Drug interactions: an enzyme inducer and may reduce the efficacy of many lipid-soluble drugs such as other anti-epileptic drugs, anticoagulants, corticosteroids, cyclosporine, oral contraceptives, and theophylline. Its metabolism may be inhibited, causing neurotoxicity by enzyme inhibitors such as allopurinol, amiodarone, chloramphenicol, cimetidine, imipramine, isoniazid, metronidazole, phenothiazines and sulfonamides.

Barbiturates

Phenobarbitone (phenobarbital)

Has been used an anti-epileptic drug since 1912.

- Inexpensive, widely available and as good as carbamazepine and phenytoin in controlling generalized tonic-clonic and partial seizures.
- Main drawback: its effect on cognition and behavior: fatigue, listlessness and tiredness in adults and insomnia, hyperkinesia and aggression in children (and sometimes in elderly patients). Subtle impairments of mood, memory and learning can occur in all age groups.
- Usual dose varies from 90 to 300 mg/day.

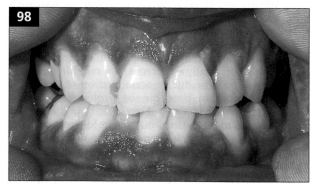

98 Gum hypertrophy in a 20 year old female caused by many years' ingestion of phenytoin for epilepsy.

- Long plasma half life of 3–4 days; can therefore be taken as a single daily dose.
- In adults, it should be restricted to patients who cannot tolerate first-line anti-epileptic drugs or as an adjunct to first line therapy in refractory epilepsy.
- Withdrawal can lead to a temporary increase in seizure frequency.

Methylphenobarbitone (Prominal) (mephobarbital)
Methylphenobarbitone (mephobarbital) is metabolized to phenobarbitone (phenobarbital), and is given in twice the dose of phenobarbitone but confers no special advantage.

Primidone (Mysoline)
Primidone is metabolized to phenobarbitone (phenobarbital) and phenylethylmalonamide, both of which are pharmacologically active. Efficacy is similar to that of phenobarbitone.

Clonazepam (Rivotril)
- A 1,4 benzodiazepine (like diazepam).
- Effective for generalized tonic-clonic and myoclonic seizures, and generalized absence (petit mal) epilepsy and partial seizures.
- Has more sustained and effective anti-epileptic activity than diazepam (Valium) but tolerance develops.
- Available as 0.5 mg and 2.0 mg tablets.
- Dose varies from 0.5–4.0 mg three times daily.
- Long plasma half life of 20–40 hours.
- Adverse effects include sedation, irritability, and aggression.
- Few patients benefit from long term treatment and nearly half have an exacerbation of seizures when the drug is withdrawn, particularly if pre-existing brain damage.

Clobazam (Frisium)
- A 1,5 benzodiazepine.
- Less sedative than clonazepam and diazepam but still commonly cause tiredness as well as depression and irritability.
- Has a limited role as a long term anti-epileptic drug (like clonazepam) but can be effective as a short term treatment to 'cover' for special events such as holidays, weddings and surgery and for catamenial exacerbations.
- A single dose of 10–30 mg can also be helpful if taken immediately after the first seizure in patients who have regular clusters of generalized tonic-clonic and partial seizures.

Vigabatrin (gamma-vinyl GABA) (Sabril)
- A specific, irreversible inhibitor of GABA transaminase, leading to elevated GABA levels and enhanced inhibitory GABAergic transmission.
- Available in 500 mg tablets for use in partial seizures.
- Dose: one 500 mg tablet twice daily, increasing weekly as required to a dose of 2–3 g/day.
- Effective as a first line or add-on therapy in reducing partial seizure frequency by more than half in 30–60% of patients with drug-refractory complex partial seizures.
- Well tolerated; adverse effects mainly constitute drowsiness, agitation, irritability, weight gain, depression and psychotic behavior.
- Microvacuolation had been seen in the brains of dogs (but not humans) after vigabatrin treatment.

- Visual field defects are the most common serious adverse effect, which limits the use of this drug.

Lamotrigine (Lamictal)
- Inhibits voltage-gated sodium channels and reduces the release of glutamate, an excitatory amino acid neurotransmitter implicated in the pathophysiology of epilepsy.
- Effective in both partial and generalized tonic-clonic and absence seizures in adults and children.
- A weak inhibitor of dihydrofolate reductase, so long term therapy may disturb folate metabolism.
- Does not significantly induce or inhibit hepatic oxidative drug-metabolizing enzymes, nor affect the plasma concentrations of concomitant anti-epileptic drugs.
- Metabolism induced by anti-epileptic drugs that induce liver enzymes such as carbamazepine, phenytoin and phenobarbitone (phenobarbital) (half-life about 15 hours).
- Metabolism inhibited by sodium valproate (half-life about 60 hours).
- Plasma half-life: about 29 hours (mean).
- Eliminated largely as an N-glucuronide conjugate.
- Available as 5 mg dispersible, 25 mg, 50 mg, 100 mg and 200 mg standard tablets.
- Starting dose in patients not taking sodium valproate is 25 mg once a day for 2 weeks, followed by 100 mg per day given in two divided doses for 2 weeks. Thereafter, the dose should be increased to achieve the optimal response. The usual maintenance dose is 200–400 mg per day in two divided doses.
- Starting dose in patients taking sodium valproate is 25 mg every alternate day for 2 weeks, followed by 25 mg once a day for 2 weeks. The usual maintenance dose is 100–200 mg a day, given once a day or in two divided doses.
- Adverse effects: a generalized maculopapular skin rash appears within 4 weeks of gradually starting treatment in about 2–5% of patients. The incidence of rash is proportional to the rapidity with which the drug is commenced. It usually resolves after immediate withdrawal of lamotrigine, after which the drug can be re-introduced slowly. Rarely, serious skin rashes such as Stevens-Johnson syndrome and angioedema have been reported. Some patients complain of insomnia which can be minimized by giving the second dose in the afternoon. Dose-related adverse effects include dizziness, headache, diplopia, ataxia, somnolence, nausea, asthenia, blurred vision and vomiting.

Gabapentin (Neurontin)
- A GABA-related amino acid.
- Mechanism of action: uncertain; it may affect L-type voltage-dependent calcium channels.
- Effective when used in doses of 1800 mg/day and as an 'add-on' treatment in reducing the frequency of seizures by more than half in about 40% of patients with complex partial seizures and 60% with secondarily generalized tonic-clonic seizures.
- Not effective for absence seizures.
- Available as 300 mg and 400 mg capsules.
- Usual maintenance dose: 1200–2400 mg/day, but higher doses may be more effective.
- Does not seem to interact with other anti-epileptic drugs.
- Adverse effects on cognitive function may arise with higher doses.

Ethosuximide

- Used only for absence seizures; not effective against generalized tonic–clonic seizures.
- Infants require a dose of 20–40 mg/kg per day but lower weight-related doses are used in adults. In children over 6 years of age, it is started with a dose of 250 mg capsules twice daily, increasing if necessary to three of four capsules daily.
- Adverse effects include drowsiness and bone marrow depression.

Topiramate (Topamax)

- A sulfamate derivative structurally unique among anti-epileptic drugs.
- Reversibly decreases the number of action potentials in spontaneous epileptiform bursts and reduces burst duration in cultured hippocampal neurons, suppressing intrinsic bursting of proximal subiculum neurons, and reducing voltage-gated sodium currents in cultured cerebellar granule cells.
- Reduces elevated levels of excitatory amino acids, glutamate and aspartate.
- Reversibly enhances post-synaptic GABA receptor currents.
- Effective as adjunctive therapy for partial seizures, in Lennox–Gastaut syndrome and possibly some primary generalized epilepsies such as drop attacks. It is not helpful for, and may aggravate, absence seizures.
- Needs to be commenced gradually, with 25 mg alternate days at night or daily at night, otherwise adverse cognitive effects may be prohibitive. Cognitive disturbances may manifest as slowed speech (and even mimic dysphasia and dysnomia) and a vulnerability to behavioral disturbances (i.e. cranky, not the same person). Other adverse effects include weight loss, renal stones in 1% of patients and a theoretical risk of teratogenicity.

Tiagabine

- A derivative of nipecotic acid that potently and selectively inhibits neuronal and glial GABA uptake. It specifically inhibits the GABA transporter GAT-1 and interacts only weakly with GABA receptors.
- Effective against partial and generalized convulsive seizures.
- May be contraindicated in generalized absence epilepsy.

Failed monotherapy

A single agent (monotherapy) generally achieves satisfactory seizure control without significant adverse effects in about half of patients. Although another 15–20% attain better control with the addition of a second anti-epileptic drug, it is often better to strive for seizure control with monotherapy by gradually introducing another agent and then gradually withdrawing the initial agent. Overall, about 70% of patients can be controlled with monotherapy.

Withdrawal of antiepileptic medication

- Anti-epileptic drug withdrawal should be considered in patients who have been free of seizures for 2 years or longer; taking anti-epileptic drugs long term is inconvenient and costly, and associated with adverse cognitive and behavioral effects, so it is essential to ascertain whether they are still necessary or not.
- Drug withdrawal is not likely to be successful (i.e. seizures recur) if:

  – Late age at onset (>16 years of age).
  – Mental retardation.
  – Symptomatic epilepsy (i.e. underlying untreated cause).
  – Certain epileptic syndromes, such as juvenile myoclonic epilepsy, when unprovoked seizures have occurred.
  – Family history of epilepsy.
  – Slow wave activity or focal epileptiform activity on EEG prior to medication withdrawal.
  – History of atypical febrile seizures.
- There are no definite predictors of recurrence but EEG findings of epileptiform activity prior to, or during, drug withdrawal are highly predictive of a further seizure if anti-epileptic medication is ceased. Relapses may also occur in patients with normal EEGs however.
- Withdrawal of any anti-epileptic drug must always be gradual in a step-wise fashion, over at least 6 weeks (and probably months for barbiturates) because abrupt withdrawal may provoke rebound seizures.

Status epilepticus (see p.82)

Surgical treatment of epilepsy

Practised for more than a century, but improved understanding of the pathogenesis of epilepsy and the recent advent of high resolution MRI brain imaging and improved surgical expertise have made it an effective treatment for refractory seizures. Once undertaken, it is irreversible.

Pre-requisites

- The patient has epilepsy and it is resistant to anti-epileptic drugs in maximally tolerated doses.
- No realistic hope of spontaneous remission of the epilepsy.
- All diagnostic tests point to a single common epileptogenic focus (see below).
- The seizures are causing medical, social and educational handicap and the patient's quality of life is likely to improve after successful surgery.
- The risk–benefit ratio for the proposed surgery is acceptable.
- A nationally recognized epilepsy surgery programme with comprehensive pre-and post-surgical evaluation and support facilities is available.

Pre-surgical evaluation

- Clinical history and seizure pattern.
- Scalp EEG (background, interictal and ictal features).
- MRI brain.
- Neuropsychometry.
- Visual field examination.
- Intracarotid amytal or 'WADA' test: determines the dominant hemisphere for speech and whether memory can be sustained without the function of the temporal lobe that is to be removed. In some centers, this is only performed in left handed patients.

If the above tests are concordant and identify a single focus and a visible structural lesion (e.g. focal cortical dysplasia, mesial temporal sclerosis, Sturge–Weber syndrome), then no further investigation may be required. However, most centers still perform video-EEG to capture at least a couple of seizures to be absolutely sure that the lesion that is to be resected is the lesion responsible for the seizures.

If the scalp EEG is not clearly lateralizing or the MRI shows no definite lesion, then further studies are required:

- Video-telemetry with scalp (and, in some centers, foramen ovale-sphenoidal) EEG recording (video-EEG).
- Interictal and ictal SPECT (may be helpful in some but not all cases), and interictal PET (if available) (**99, 100**).
- Intracranial/subdural electrode recording (usually to differentiate between temporal and extratemporal foci, but again not in all cases).

Surgical procedures
- Removal of a mass of epileptogenic tissue:
- Amygdalo-hippocampectomy: intractable partial epilepsy and seizure onset in mesial temporal lobe.

     N.B. Anterior temporal lobectomy used to be undertaken in cases of intractable partial epilepsy with seizure onset in temporal lobe and normal memory function in remaining brain, but is no longer done because the seizure focus is often the amygdala/hippocampus, even in the presence of a temporal lobe structural lesion.
- Removal of structurally abnormal tissue:
- Lesionectomy (usually frontal lobe): refractory seizures due to a focal pathology in resectable cortex.
- Hemispherectomy: intractable focal +/− generalized seizures with unilateral hemispheric pathology and contralateral non-functional hemiparesis.
- Disconnection procedures (separation of epileptogenic cortex from rest of brain):
- Multiple subpial transections (usually in areas of eloquent cortex): intractable partial seizures emanating from unresectable foci in primary cortices.
- Corpus callosotomy (the anterior two-thirds is sectioned initially, and the posterior one-third about 6–12 months later): usually for drop attacks.

Outcome
- Seizure-freedom:
- Anterior temporal lobectomy and amygdalo-hippocampectomy: >80% of patients. If concordant video-EEG and MRI brain.
- Lesionectomy: 30–40% of patients (poorer localization of a single focus, and obvious pathology is less common).
- Hemispherectomy: 75–85% of patients.
- Corpus callosotomy: 30–40% of patients; best response with atonic and tonic seizures.
- Other favorable outcomes include improved physical functioning, psychosocial behavior and learning.

PROGNOSIS

Risk of a second seizure after a first seizure
- 31–71%, depending on other risk factors:
- EEG: epileptiform discharges: 80% risk; non-specific abnormalities: 40% risk; normal: 12% risk.

Risk of seizure recurrence after >2 years remission
About 30% of children with epilepsy who are free of seizures for 2 years or longer will experience a recurrence of seizures when their medications are withdrawn and about 70% will remain free of seizures. As epilepsy is a heterogeneous entity (like TIA and stroke, see pp.186, 192), the chance of recurrence varies among individual patients and depends on several factors such as the epilepsy syndrome and other factors listed below.

As stated above (p.80), predictors of an increased risk of recurrence are:

- Late age at onset.
- Mental retardation.
- Epilepsy syndrome (e.g. juvenile myoclonic epilepsy).
- Etiology (symptomatic epilepsies tend to recur whereas idiopathic and cryptogenic epilepsies do not).
- A family history of epilepsy.
- Slow wave activity on EEG prior to medication withdrawal.
- A history of atypical febrile seizures.

However, there are no definite predictors of recurrence. For example, although EEG findings of paroxysmal discharges certainly increase the risk of a relapse after anti-epileptic drug withdrawal, they don't indicate a 100% risk, and relapses also occur in patients with normal EEGs. So, the EEG findings alone are not a sufficient guide for anti-epileptic drug withdrawal. Anti-epileptic drug withdrawal should be considered in all patients, even those with risk factors for recurrence, but other factors can be crucial in coming to a decision (such as whether the patient is going to drive a motor vehicle or not).

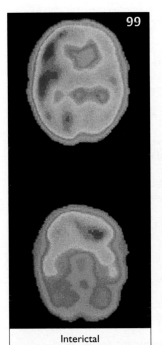 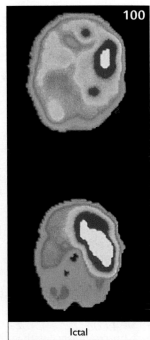

| Interictal | Ictal |

99, 100 Positron emission tomography (PET) scan of metabolism of 18-fluorodeoxyglucose (fludeoxyglucose F 18) (a physiologic radionuclide) that is injected intravenously and its uptake and distribution is measured and imaged. The kinetics of brain uptake of 18-FDG reflect the kinetics of glucose brain uptake and therefore provide an index of brain metabolism. Interictally (**99**) there is evidence of diminished glucose metabolism in the region of the epileptic focus in the left fronto-temporal lobes (a blue or green or yellow 'cold spot') but during the ictus (**100**) there is increased metabolism (a white or red 'hot spot')

Prediction equation for recurrence of seizures

Increased risk

Age >16 years at onset of seizures	add 45
Taking >1 anti-epileptic drug	add 50
Seizures occurred after starting anti-epileptic drug treatment	add 35
History of primary or secondarily generalized tonic-clonic seizures	add 35
History of myoclonic seizures	add 50
Abnormal EEG in past year	add 20

Decreased risk

Increasing time (number of years, t) without seizures	add 200/t
	subtract 175

	Total score T
Divide total score (T) by 100 and exponentiate	$z = e^{T/100}$

Probability of recurrence of seizures:
* Continued treatment

By 1 year	$1-0.89^z$
By 2 years	$1-0.79^z$

* Slow withdrawal

By 1 year	$1-0.69^z$
By 2 years	$1-0.60^z$

(Medical Research Council Anti-epileptic Drug Withdrawal Study Group [1993] Prognostic index for recurrence of seizures after remission of epilepsy. *BMJ*, **306**: 1374–1378.)

Mortality

The standardized mortality ratio for epilepsy is high. About 25% of deaths may be related directly to seizures: status epilepticus, accidental injury and sudden unexplained death in epilepsy (SUDEP).

Risk factors in children
* Onset of epilepsy in the first 12 months of life.
* Severe developmental delay present at the onset of epilepsy.
* Symptomatic epilepsy (e.g. brain malformation).
* Severe myoclonic epilepsies of infancy and early childhood.
* Infantile spasms (deaths mainly due to the treatment of spasms – with steroids and ACTH).

Risk factors in adults
* Young age.
* Male sex.
* Generalized convulsive seizures.
* Underlying structural brain lesions.
* Sleep.
* Non-compliance with anti-epileptic medication.

STATUS EPILEPTICUS (SE)

DEFINITION
A continuous seizure lasting at least 30 minutes, or two or more discrete seizures without interictal recovery (i.e. between which the patient does not recover consciousness) and lasting more that 30 minutes. SE is a medical emergency.

CLASSIFICATION
Convulsive
* Generalized tonic-clonic status epilepticus (SE).
* Partial SE (e.g. somatomotor [epilepsia partialis continua], somatosensory, aphasic).

Non-convulsive
* Generalized SE:
- Absence SE (other names: petit mal SE, epilepsia minor continua, spike wave stupor, prolonged petit mal automatisms).
- Atypical absence SE.
* Partial SE (confusional state, coma.)

EPIDEMIOLOGY
* Incidence: 15–30 per 100 000 per year.
* Age: any age.

ETIOLOGY
Epilepsy (two-thirds of convulsive SE, the vast majority of non-convulsive SE)
* Poor anti-epileptic drug compliance.
* Recent reduction in dose or discontinuation of anti-epileptic drug.
* Drug (alcohol, phenobarbitone [phenobarbital]) withdrawal.

Symptomatic (one-third of convulsive SE have no history of epilepsy)
* Traumatic brain injury.
* Stroke: the most frequent cause of simple partial status.
* Hypoxic encephalopathy.
* Fever/infection.
* Meningoencephalitis.
* Brain abscess.
* Brain tumor.
* Metabolic disturbance: hyponatremia, uremia, hypoglycemia, hepatic encephalopathy, hypocalcemia, hypomagnesemia, mitochondrial encephalopathy.
* Toxins.
* Drug overdose: tricyclic antidepressant, phenothiazine, theophylline, cocaine, isoniazid, chemotherapy drugs.

PATHOPHYSIOLOGY
Delayed control of SE is associated with prolonged epileptic activity which may outstrip metabolic capacity and glucose delivery, and lead to metabolic and hypoxic-ischemic brain and systemic injury. The seizures compromise cerebral vascular autoregulation, which in turn compromises hypothalamic autonomic regulation, and raised intracranial pressure may supervene.

Complications such as cardiovascular collapse, arrhythmias, aspiration pneumonia, acute lung injury, and pulmonary hypertension may compromise cerebral oxygen delivery further. Metabolic derangement and cerebral and systemic acidosis with hyperpyrexia, rhabdomyolysis, and disseminated intravascular coagulation may cause multiple organ failure.

CLINICAL FEATURES

The clinical presentation of SE can be categorized into:

- Prolonged seizures.
- Convulsive generalized status characterized by unconsciousness, cyanosis and repeated generalized tonic-clonic convulsive movements of the limbs with no interictal recovery.
- Convulsive partial status characterized by repeated partial seizures manifesting as focal motor convulsion or neurologic deficits (e.g. somatosensory, visual, auditory) not associated with altered consciousness or secondary generalization. The most common forms are: somatomotor simple partial SE (a succession of simple partial seizures with Jacksonian march, without persistent segmental myoclonus) and epilepsia partialis continua (persistent myoclonus in a limited area of the body, present for weeks or months and sometimes in combination with somatomotor or tonic-clonic seizures).
- Non-convulsive SE presenting with continuous or fluctuating clouding of consciousness, confusion, automatisms, fluttering of the eyelids or other involuntary orofacial dyskinetic movements and amnesia. Fluctuating conscious level is more frequent in absence status whereas focal neurologic signs point to complex partial SE.

History from a witness, examination of the patient, and investigations must proceed concurrently with instituting appropriate treatment.

DIFFERENTIAL DIAGNOSIS

Pseudostatus epilepticus should be suspected if there is aberrant motor activity, an on/off pattern of seizure activity, poor response to treatment and lack of metabolic consequences.

INVESTIGATIONS

- Electroencephalogram (EEG) (**101–103**).
- Full blood count and ESR.
- Urea and electrolytes.
- Plasma glucose.
- Liver function tests.
- Plasma calcium, phosphate and magnesium.
- Anti-epileptic drug levels.
- Toxicology screen.
- Arterial blood gases.
- EEG.
- CT brain scan: exclude structural intracranial lesion.
- Lumbar puncture: if CNS infection possible.
- Serum lactate: may be useful to help exclude pseudoseizures.

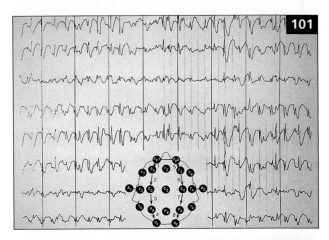

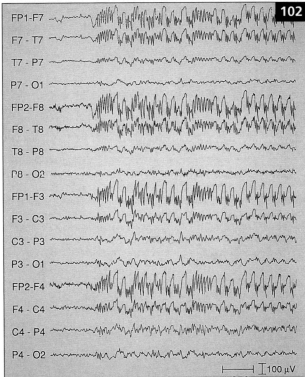

101, 102 EEGs (**101**, 8 channel; **102**, 16 channel) of two young adolescents each in a state of prolonged clouding of consciousness due to non-convulsive generalized absence status epilepticus.

103 EEG (21 channel) showing generalized non-convulsive status epilepticus on the left hand side of the recording which is terminated in the middle of the recording by the i.v. injection of clonazepam 1 mg.

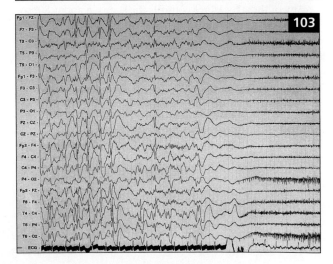

DIAGNOSIS

- Repetitive epileptic seizures without interictal recovery and epileptiform activity on the EEG.
- Diagnosis may require EEG monitoring because some patients have seizure discharge without detectable motor activity and may be difficult to diagnose.
- If the EEG is normal without evidence of even interictal slowing of the background rhythm then the diagnosis should be reconsidered.
- If the diagnosis is in doubt (e.g. ?pseudostatus epilepticus), observe one tonic-clonic attack and assess the level of consciousness post-ictally. If further doubt, attempt to capture at least one episode whilst monitoring the patient and the EEG.

TREATMENT

All forms of convulsive SE are neurologic emergencies that must be treated promptly and aggressively to prevent adverse sequelae. In non-convulsive status, other medical factors such as the age and respiratory status may need to be taken into consideration. The aims are to stop the seizures as soon as possible and identify and treat the cause.

Immediate treatment for premonitory SE

- Ensure protected airway, remove false teeth if present.
- Oxygen 10 l/min via high-flow mask. Be prepared for a rapid sequence induction and endotracheal intubation because all anti-epileptic drugs except phenytoin can cause neurologic depression and depress respiratory drive even in the face of metabolic acidosis.
- Insert an i.v. line and take 30 ml venous blood for urea and electrolytes, glucose, liver function tests, calcium, magnesium, full blood count, anti-epileptic drug concentrations and toxicology screen.
- Administer a benzodiazepine, either:
- i.v. diazepam 2 mg boluses per minute up to 20 mg (10 mg if older than 60 years of age or hypotensive), or
- i.v. clonazepam 0.2 mg boluses per minute up to 1 mg, or
- i.v. midazolam up to 5mg, or
- i.v. lorazepam over 1–2 minutes (or rectal if no venous access), or
- intramuscular midazolam if difficulties with venous access.

Lorazepam is often preferred as it has a long duration of anti-epileptic effect and the best parenchymal distribution.

Any of these measures controls the status in about 80% of cases but may take minutes to work. In the 20% of cases who do not respond, this regime can be repeated in 5–10 minutes time or another benzodiazepine can be given. Beware of adverse events which include respiratory and CNS depression causing respiratory arrest, hypotension and impaired consciousness. N.B. Benzodiazepines are not a substitute for a long term parenteral anti-epileptic drug (see below).

- Dextrostix (glucose test): if low dextrostix reading or known diabetic, give glucose 50 ml of 50% i.v., and thiamine 100 mg i.v.
- Arterial puncture (usually femoral artery) for arterial blood gases.

- Correct metabolic abnormalities, such as hypoxia and hypoglycemia, and treat the underlying cause if known: i.e. dexamethasone 16 mg if a brain tumor, arteritis or parasitic brain infection, and thiamine 100 mg if the patient is alcoholic. It is not usually necessary, and may be harmful, to give bicarbonate to correct acidosis.

Early SE

- Decide promptly whether to use a long term parenteral anti-epileptic drug, the aim of which is to prevent seizure recurrence. Most patients are treated with phenytoin, and some are now treated with fosphenytoin.
- Intravenous phenytoin loading dose of 18 mg/kg in 100–150 ml of 0.9% normal saline given no faster than 50 mg/min by infusion pump, and while monitoring the pulse, blood pressure, respirations and cardiac rhythm with EKG.
- Brain concentrations of phenytoin peak at 10 minutes and are three to four times those in plasma after injection.
- If the patient is currently prescribed phenytoin, blood levels are usually low due to poor compliance.
- Never give phenytoin intramuscularly because phenytoin has a pH of 12.
- Phenytoin, when coadministered with diazepam, will abolish at least 80% of episodes of convulsive SE.
- Systemic and local reactions to i.v. phenytoin are common. Respiratory and CNS depression, and cardiac arrhythmias can be life threatening. Thrombophlebitis necessitates frequent changes of cannulas and makes central administration the preferred route.
- Fosphenytoin is a disodium phosphate ester of phenytoin, which has been licensed recently because it offers several advantages over phenytoin (which has to be given i.v. and major adverse effects are common). Fosphenytoin is freely soluble in aqueous solutions and can be administered i.v. or intramuscularly. Intravenous fosphenytoin is tolerated at infusion rates up to three times faster than those for phenytoin, therapeutic levels are established within 10 minutes, it is rapidly metabolized (conversion half-life of 8–15 minutes) into phenytoin by endogenous phosphatases in the body, and it is as effective as phenytoin in treating SE. Intramuscular administration of fosphenytoin is characterized by rapid and complete absorption, no requirement for cardiac monitoring, and a low incidence of adverse effects which are similar to those of parenteral phenytoin (nystagmus, dizziness pruritus, paresthesias, headache, somnolence, and ataxia). It has the promise to be suitable for administration in the ambulance because it causes few local adverse effects (e.g. pain, burning and itching at the injection site) and does not cause respiratory and CNS depression.

N.B. Avoid neuromuscular blockade initially because it masks ongoing ictal activity.

Absence status

- Clonazepam i.v. (see above).
- Valproic acid: via nasogastric or rectal route.

Resistant SE

- Reconsider the diagnosis (particularly if you are saying to yourself 'I have never seen anything like this before': consider pseudostatus and seek EEG confirmation, if possible).
- Review the patient's ventilatory status and consider intubation.

- Intravenous phenobarbitone (phenobarbital) 15–20 mg/kg, no faster than 100 mg/min (preferably 50 mg/min), or until seizures stop (e.g. additional 10 mg/kg doses even up to 100 mg/kg; phenobarbitone is a very effective drug and is generally better to pursue than chopping and changing with the alternatives below). Monitor for respiratory depression and hypotension, or
- Benzodiazepine infusion (e.g. clonazepam 3 mg in 500 ml 5% dextrose at 20 ml/hour and titrate). Not a substitute for phenytoin. Monitor for respiratory depression,
  Or
- Intravenous chlormethiazole 0.8% 40–100 ml over 10 minutes.
  If seizures stop, continue the infusion at 0.5 to 1.0 ml/min and monitor respiration.
  Or,
- Intramuscular paraldehyde 5–10 ml, or dilute 10 ml paraldehyde in 100 ml 0.9% normal saline and infuse over 10–15 minutes or until seizures stop.
- However, in Australia chlormethiazole is no longer used, and paraldehyde is no longer available.
- For patients in partial status epilepticus, despite phenytoin and clonazepam, consider administering vigabatrin, which is very water-soluble, via nasogastric tube in a dose of 1 g stat, which is repeated 8–12 hours later and then continued 8–12 hourly.

Refractory SE
Seizure activity for about an hour in which the patient has not responded to therapy.

- Reconsider the diagnosis.
- Transfer to an intensive care unit.
- Monitor vital signs closely and treat hyperthermia.
- Initiate therapy for the underlying etiology as soon as possible.
- Further doses of phenobarbitone (phenobarbital) or a continuous infusion of the older anesthetic agent thiopentone (thiopental) or the newer agent propofol will usually control the seizures. (N.B. it is unwise to paralyse the patient, because clinical signs will be lost, unless continuous EEG activity is being monitored.)
- Monitor EEG.
- If the EEG suggests ongoing seizures or if the patient has overt convulsions, and the patient has received full loading doses of phenytoin and phenobarbital (phenobarbital), an i.v. infusion of midazolam or clonazepam may help. Midazolam has the advantage of a shorter half-life and so the patient wakes up sooner after the infusion has ceased. Midazolam is given i.v. with a loading dose of 200 μg/kg as a slow i.v. bolus, followed by 0.75–10 μg/kg/min continuous infusion. Higher doses may be necessary, especially with prolonged infusion, due to possible tachyphylaxis. Adjust the maintenance dose to stop electrographic seizures based on EEG monitoring. EEG should be recorded continuously for the first 1–2 hours during and after the initiation of midazolam loading and infusion, and then monitored either continuously or for 30–60 minute intervals every 2 hours during the maintenance phase. The primary aim of therapy is suppression of electrographic seizures.

- Continue maintenance doses of phenytoin and phenobarbital (phenobarbital), and follow levels to determine optimal doses.
- Use i.v. fluids and dopamine (up to 10 μg/kg/min) to treat hypotension. Decrease the dosage of thiopentone (thiopental) or midazolam if any signs of cardiovascular compromise.
- Discontinue the midazolam infusion at 12 hours while monitoring the EEG and observe for further clinical or electrographic seizure activity. If seizures recur, reinstate the infusion and repeat this step at 12–24 hour intervals or longer if the patient's seizures remain refractory.

N.B. Although barbiturate coma is extremely effective in terminating refractory generalized SE, it frequently causes hemodynamic instability due to myocardial depression and vasodilatation (and thus requires invasive hemodynamic monitoring and the use of pressor agents) and patients may take days to wake up after it has ceased and so they require prolonged intubation. Continuous i.v. infusion of midazolam can be as effective and less toxic. Midazolam is a water-soluble benzodiazepine with rapid CNS penetration and a short elimination half-life of 1.5–3.5 hours.

Maintenance treatment
When seizures have been abolished, an appropriate oral regimen is required:

- Regular anti-epileptic medication should be recommenced.
- For previously untreated patients, continue with phenytoin. An oral loading dose of 300 mg should be given 6–12 hours after the initial i.v. injection. Thereafter the dose can be altered according to clinical response, adverse effects and serum concentrations.
- If the seizure type can be characterized, or if the patient is a young woman, preference may be given to commencing an oral regimen of carbamazepine or sodium valproate. If the patient is unconscious or cannot swallow, both can be given via a nasogastric tube.

PROGNOSIS
Convulsive SE
- High mortality (up to 10–12%): more often due to the underlying cause than direct neurologic damage caused by the status.
- Morbidity: determined by the underlying cause and duration of SE. The longer the duration, the more refractory it becomes to treatment and the higher the morbidity and mortality.

Non-convulsive SE
- Generalized absence SE: good outcome if treated appropriately.
- Complex partial SE: prognosis depends on the underlying cause and the quality of treatment.

Familial hemiplegic migraine (FHM)

A rare autosomal dominant subtype of migraine with aura. Genes for FHM map to chromosomes 19p13 and 1q but some families with FHM do not link to either locus, indicating genetic heterogeneity of FHM. The CACNa1A gene at 19p13 encodes the α_{1A} subunit (the ion conducting part) of a brain specific P/Q type voltage-dependent calcium channel, suggesting that migraine may be a 'cerebral calcium channelopathy'.

PATHOPHYSIOLOGY

Triggered by the action of a multitude of environmental and biochemical factors on the cerebral cortex or hypothalamus (the latter of which, in turn, is modulated by seasonal patterns, diurnal and biologic clocks, and hormonal factors and coitus); the premonitory symptoms of elation, yawning or a craving for sweet foods, experienced by about 25% of patients, suggest hypothalamic activation.

Triggers

- Emotional stress and tension.
- Relaxation after stress.
- Fatigue.
- Hormonal changes: fall in estradiol levels at menstruation and midcycle.
- High dose estrogen-containing contraceptives.
- Strong sensory stimulation: bright or flickering light; loud noise; strong smells; occipital nerve compression (e.g. 'swim-goggle migraine').
- Head trauma, such as heading the ball in soccer ('footballer's migraine').
- Food idiosyncrasies/allergies: rich foods (e.g. chocolate, fatty foods), red wines, specific dietary amines (cheese).
- Missing meals.
- Sleeping late in the morning.
- Meteorologic changes.
- Vasodilators, such as alcohol, monosodium glutamate, and anti-anginal agents.
- Substance misuse.
- Physical activity (footballer's migraine, coital cephalgia).

Trigeminovascular reflex (115)

The activated cerebral cortex and hypothalamus stimulate brainstem nuclei, dorsal raphe nuclei (which contain serotonin) and locus coeruleus (containing noradrenaline) and trigger the trigeminovascular reflex which constitutes serotonergic and noradrenergic pathways that project from the brainstem to the cortical microcirculation and the spinal trigeminal nucleus and spinal cord.

Axons of the first division of the trigeminal nerve, which innervate the pain-sensitive intracranial structures, depolarize as a result of direct neuronal activation or vasodilatation of dural and cerebral arteries, or both, leading to central transmission of nociceptive pain signals to bipolar neurons in the trigeminal ganglion and on to the trigeminal nucleus in its most caudal extent in the caudal medulla and the dorsal horn of the spinal cord at C1 and C2 (accounting for the commonly reported neck pain with migraine). Impulses are then transmitted to the ventroposteriomedial nucleus of the thalamus via the quintothalamic tract, from where they are relayed to the cortex.

Stimulation of the trigeminal ganglion leads to the release of powerful vasodilator neuropeptides such as calcitonin gene-related peptide (CGRP) from trigeminal neurons that innervate the cranial circulation. This peptide is not only a vasodilator but it also mediates a sterile neurogenic inflammation (vasodilatation and edema) within the dura mater.

Migraine aura and headache

At the onset of aura, regional cerebral blood flow to the clinically involved part of the brain is reduced by about 20%, and reduced neuronal activity spreads in a wave across the cerebral cortex, usually beginning in the occipital region and slowly moving forward (spreading depression of Laeo).

Migraine headache begins while regional cerebral blood flow is reduced. Platelets in the blood release serotonin (5-hydroxytryptamine, 5-HT), and this leads to platelet aggregation. During the headache, the level of a vasodilator peptide, CGRP increases in the external jugular venous blood, and some intracranial arteries (particularly those of the dura mater) become dilated and inflamed. Vascular dilatation and neurogenic inflammation is believed to be responsible for the pulsatile nature of the headache.

Migraine attacks can be ameliorated by activating 5-hydroxytryptamine 1D (5-HT1D) presynaptic receptors within the vessel wall, thus blocking release of vasoactive neuropeptides, causing vasoconstriction of certain cerebral and dural arteries, and inhibiting depolarization of trigeminal axons, functionally blocking activation of trigeminal perivascular nerve terminals.

CLINICAL FEATURES

Precipitating factors

See Triggers, above.

Phase one: prodrome

- Occurs in 25–50% of migraineurs.
- Gradual onset and evolution over up to 24 hours.
- Lightheadedness, dulled perception, irritability, withdrawal, cravings for particular foods (particularly sweet foods), frequent yawning, elation and speech difficulties.

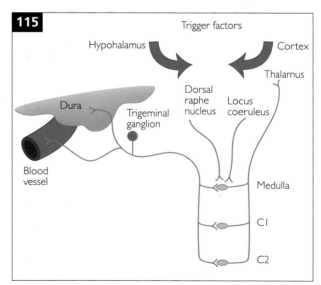

115 Diagram showing how the trigeminovascular pathway may be activated to produce migraine headache.

Phase two: aura
- 15–25% of migraine attacks are associated with aura.
- Visual symptoms most commonly: blurred vision, flashing lights (photopsia) or shimmering zigzag lines of light (fortification spectra), sometimes around an area of impaired vision or blindness (scintillating scotoma) in a part of the visual field of one or both eyes (**116**).
- Somatosensory: tingling or pins and needles, or less commonly numbness, in the face, arm, hand or leg.
- Dysphasia: difficulty understanding and expressing speech.
- Gradual onset, symptoms 'build up' or progress over 5–10 minutes, then subside within 5–60 minutes.
- Followed within 60 minutes by headache; the aura may continue into the headache phase.

Phase three: headache
Present in most, but not all migraine attacks (cf. 'migraine without headache' or 'acephalgic migraine').

Site
- Unilateral in two-thirds of patients, and bilateral in one-third.
- Frontotemporal region commonly, spreading to occipital region.

Quality
- Throbbing/pulsatile.
- Moderate to severe.

Aggravating factors
- Physical activity/movement.
- Bright light (photophobia, 80%).
- Loud noise (phonophobia).

Associated features
- Scalp tenderness on the affected side (about two-thirds of cases).
- Nausea (90% of patients).
- Vomiting (60%).
- Diarrhea (20%).
- Heightened awareness of sensations such as smell and noise.
- Fluid retention at onset, and polyuria as headache subsides.

Duration
- 4–72 hours.
- Commonly 2–6 hours in children, and 6–24 hours in adults.

Phase four: postdrome
For up to 24 hours after the headache has subsided, most migraineurs feel tired and 'drained' or 'washed-out', with aching muscles. Others however, become euphoric for a period of time.

Periodicity with recurrence
Migraine is paroxysmal; clearly defined episodes recur as often as 4–6 times each month.

Family history
Family history of migraine is present in more than half of patients.

SPECIAL FORMS
Migraine variants
Less than 5% of migraineurs.

Retinal migraine
Monocular, rather than binocular hemianopic visual disturbance.

Ophthalmoplegic migraine:
- Paralysis of ≥1 of the ocular cranial nerves, usually the IIIrd nerve, at the height of a migraine headache.
- The paralysis usually resolves but may persist after recurrent episodes.
- This entity does not embrace a transient dilatation or constriction (Horner's syndrome) of one pupil as this is quite commonly seen during severe migraine attacks.
- The cause of the cranial neuropathy in ophthalmoplegic migraine is probably transient ischemia of the cranial nerve.

Vertebrobasilar migraine
Gradual onset and evolution over several minutes of brainstem, cerebellar and visual disturbances, often accompanied or followed by headache and syncope.

Hemiplegic migraine
- Hemiparesis preceding or occurring with a migraine headache.
- A family history of hemiplegic migraine is often present and the gene is located on chromosome 19 or 1.

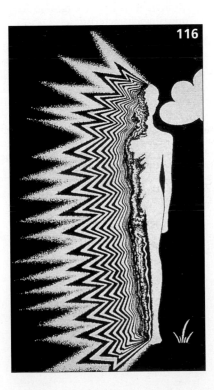

116 Illustration of the type of visual aura a migraineur may describe; in this case shimmering zigzag lines of light (fortification spectra).

Migrainous infarction

- Permanent focal neurologic symptoms persisting beyond 24 hours after the cessation of migraine headache. Cranial CT or MRI scan shows features consistent with cerebral infarction.
- The cause is probably arterial thrombosis, provoked by arterial spasm and a procoagulant state (e.g. cigarette smoking and the oral contraceptive pill).

Menstrual migraine

Just before menstruation, plasma estradiol (rather than progesterone) levels fall rapidly below about 20 ng/ml which sets in motion a series of changes (perhaps through prostaglandins) that culminate in the onset of migraine in about 60% of women migraineurs and exclusively at that time in about 14%. Migraine is relieved by pregnancy in about 60% of women, many, but not all, of whom have a history of menstrual migraine.

Migraine in childhood

- Headache and vomiting are common but the child may be unable to describe the symptoms and may simply appear pale, ill, limp, and inert, complaining of poorly localized abdominal pain.
- Fever up to 38.5°C (101.3°F) may be present so that the suspicion of appendicitis or mesenteric adenitis often arises.
- Rather than accept a label of 'bilious attacks' or 'periodic syndrome', recurrent headaches or vomiting attacks in children which may develop at times of excitement or stress should be considered as possibly migrainous and not psychosomatic.

DIFFERENTIAL DIAGNOSIS
Abrupt onset of headache ('thunderclap headache')
Primary

- Cluster headache.
- Benign exertional or sex headache.
- Idiopathic stabbing headache.

Secondary

- Subarachnoid hemorrhage.
- 'Sentinel headache' (enlargement of a cerebral aneurysm without rupture).
- Intracerebral hemorrhage.
- A precipitous rise in blood pressure: drug induced headache.
- Head injury.
- Acute obstruction of the CSF pathways.

Unilateral headache

- Cluster headache.
- Temporal arteritis.
- Glaucoma.
- Temperomandibular joint disease.
- Internal carotid or vertebral artery dissection.
- Structural intracranial lesion.

Continuous or daily headache
Primary

- Tension headache: just headache, and sometimes mild photophobia and phonophobia but no other features of sensory sensitivity.
- Mixed migraine/tension headache.

Secondary

- Drug-rebound headache: a periodic daily bilateral headache that has gradually increased in frequency, and changed in character from the typical migraine headaches, in concurrence with increasing consumption and misuse of analgesic drugs, particularly those which also contain caffeine.
- Systemic infection.
- Giant cell arteritis.
- Raised intracranial pressure: idiopathic intracranial hypertension, brain tumor.

Vertebrobasilar migraine
Neurocardiogenic syncope.

Migraine aura without headache (acephalgic migraine)

- TIA.
- Epileptic seizure.
- Arteriovenous malformation.
- Mitochondrial DNA disorders (e.g. MELAS, see p.162).
- Cerebral autosomal dominant arteriopathy with subcortical infarction and leukoencephalopathy (CADASIL) (see p.261).

INVESTIGATIONS

- Should only be necessary if headache is suspected to be secondary to another disorder.
- 'Alarm symptoms' include:
- Onset above age 50 years.
- Aura without headache.
- Aura symptoms of acute onset without spread.
- Aura symptoms that are very brief (<5 mins) or unusually long (>60 min).
- Aura symptoms that are stereotyped (i.e. always at the same body site).
- Sudden increase in migraine frequency or change in migraine characteristics.
- High fever.
- Abnormal neurologic examination.
- The role of imaging in patients with suspected migraine is to exclude structural causes for the headache such as AVMs or tumors. A contrast-enhanced CT scan is satisfactory for this, and is usually normal (unless there is an AVM or tumor). If MRI is performed, the T2W image occasionally shows areas of altered signal in the white matter which may be residual ischemic changes following a recent or prolonged attack, or may rarely be due to CADASIL. The appearance is non-specific however.

DIAGNOSIS
Clinical

- At least 5 attacks.
- Attacks last 4–72 hours if untreated or unsuccessfully treated.
- At least two of:
- Unilateral headache.
- Pulsating headache.
- Moderate or severe headache.
- Headache aggravated by routine physical activity.
- At least one of:
- Nausea, with or without vomiting.
- Photophobia.
- Phonophobia.

TREATMENT
Avoid precipitating/triggering factors
Identify these by keeping a diary if necessary.

Treatment of the acute migraine attack
Ancillary measures
- Rest in a quiet dark room.
- Intravenous fluids if severely dehydrated.

Non-specific analgesics and antiemetic/prokinetic compounds
- Treat as early as possible (e.g. aspirin 600–900 mg or ibuprofen 400–800 mg, together with metoclopramide 10 mg), and wait 40 minutes. If headache persists, try a specific treatment such as ergotamine 1 mg capsule or sumatriptan 50 mg tablet, and wait >1 hour. If headache persists, repeat. (See below.)
- Anti-emetic and prokinetic compounds (e.g. metoclopramide 10 mg or domperidone 10–20 mg) if nausea and vomiting are a problem. Metoclopramide is preferable because it improves the oral absorption of other drugs (which is impaired in migraine attacks) and may have a favorable central effect. If vomiting is severe, suppositories of domperidone, prochlorperazine, or chlorpromazine may be helpful.
- Simple analgesic drugs:
- Aspirin 2 or 3 × 300 mg chewable tablets (600–900 mg) orally.
- Paracetamol (acetaminophen) 2 × 500 mg tablets (1g) orally.
- Compound codeine-containing analgesic (e.g. codeine 15–30 mg) but may cause or exacerbate nausea.
- Non-steroidal anti-inflammatory drugs:
- Ibuprofen.
- Naproxen: oral, rectal.
- Diclofenac: oral (potassium salt-rapid absorption), intramuscular.
- Ketorolac: intramuscular.
- Other non-specific drugs:
- Chlorpromazine: intramuscular, but long term considerations (e.g. tardive dyskinesia).
- Narcotic analgesic use is highly controversial, not evidence-based, and is associated with prominent adverse effects and a high risk of dependency. Most patients who require narcotics are misusing analgesics or ergots.
- Lignocaine infusion: may be indicated for prolonged severe migraine unresponsive to other therapy or for rebound headache (for the latter, all analgesics are withheld during the infusion). Procedure: a 12-lead EKG is obtained and examined before and 30–60 minutes after starting the infusion. Lignocaine is delivered by a pump device at a rate of 2 mg/min (no bolus is given). The patient is attached to a bedside cardiac monitor, and a rhythm strip is obtained every 5 minutes for the first 30 minutes, then every 15 minutes for 3 hours, and thereafter every 2 hours. Pulse rate and blood pressure are measured every 5 minutes for the first 30 minutes, then every 15 minutes for 3 hours, and thereafter every 2 hours while the patient is awake. The infusion is maintained until the patient has been headache free for at least 12 hours. The duration of infusion should not exceed 14 days. Contraindications include significant heart disease (e.g. severe sinoatrial, atrioventricular, or intraventricular heart block), epileptic seizures, or allergic reaction to lignocaine.

Specific antimigraine agents
Ergot alkaloids:
- Alpha adrenergic agonists with potent 5-HT1 receptor affinity. Also stimulants of dopamine D2 receptors in brainstem and gut (vomiting and diarrhea), and vascular adrenergic and 5-HT2 receptors (vasoconstriction).
- Ergotamine exists in several forms:
- 1 mg capsule of ergotamine tartrate, or combined with caffeine.
- 2 mg suppository of ergotamine tartrate combined with caffeine 100 mg.
- 2 mg tablet of ergotamine tartrate combined with caffeine and an antiemetic.
- Dihydroergotamine mesylate can also be given orally (absorbed erratically), or more effectively, by suppository (1–2 mg), inhalation (0.36 mg), sublingual (1–2 mg), intramuscular (0.5–1 mg) and intravenous (0.5–1 mg) routes.
- Effective in about half of cases.
- If two doses at intervals of 2–6 hours are ineffective, no more should be given for that attack.
- Limitations include poor oral and rectal bioavailability (<3%); frequent, long-lasting adverse effects (nausea, vomiting, diarrhea, muscle cramps, malaise, cold/tingling fingers and toes); and risk of headache and ergotism (generalized vasospasm, causing acral cyanosis, digital necrosis, intermittent claudication, and tissue infarction) with chronic recurrent use (>1 day per week).
- The drug of choice in a limited number of migraine sufferers who have infrequent or long duration headaches and are likely to comply with dosing restrictions. For most migraine sufferers requiring specific migraine treatment, a triptan is generally a better option from both an efficacy and side-effect perspective.

Triptans:
Selective and potent agonists of 5-HT1B, 1D, 1F, and to some extent 5-HT1A receptors. Antimigraine effects are mediated by:
- Inhibition of firing of cells in trigeminal nuclei (5-HT1B or D receptors in the brainstem: second generation triptans).
- Inhibition of dural neurogenic inflammation and plasma extravasation (presynaptic 5-HT1D receptor stimulation on trigeminal neurons).
- Vasoconstriction of meningeal, dural, cerebral or pial vessels (stimulation of presynaptic vascular 5-HT1B receptors).

First-generation triptans: sumatriptan:
- A specific and selective agonist of 5-HT1D presynaptic receptors on cranial blood vessels, inhibiting trigeminal neuronal firing at the trigeminal nerve ending.
- Available as subcutaneous injection (6 mg), oral tablets (25, 50 and 100 mg), nasal spray (20 mg), and rectal preparations.
- Subcutaneous sumatriptan injection (6 mg):
- Bioavailability: 96%.
- Therapeutic plasma levels: within 10 minutes.
- 79% of patients improved at 2 hours after injection ('therapeutic gain' [TG]: active minus placebo = 52%); 71% (TG: 51%) improved within 1 hour.
- 60% of patients pain-free at 2 hours after injection (TG: 42%); 43% (TG: 35%) pain-free after 1 hour.

(Continued overleaf)

First-generation triptans: sumatriptan (*continued*):
- Oral sumatriptan tablets (100 mg):
- Bioavailability: 14%.
- Therapeutic plasma levels: within 30–90 minutes.
- 59% (95% CI: 57–60%) of patients improved at 2 hours after tablets(TG: 33%).
- 29% (27–30%) of patients pain-free at 2 hours (TG 26%).
- Oral sumatriptan is more effective than conventional treatment with aspirin and metoclopramide or oral ergotamine plus caffeine, particularly in the second and third attacks, suggesting greater consistency for sumatriptan.
- Recurrence of headache occurs within 24–48 hours in about one-third of responders to sumatriptan (and any other acute antimigraine drug). Repeated drug administration is usually effective, but the headache may recur again.
- Adverse effects of sumatriptan are common but are usually mild and short-lived. The most frequent are tingling, paresthesias, and warm sensations in the head, neck, chest, and limbs; less frequent are dizziness, flushing, and neck pain or stiffness. The risk and intensity is greater with the fixed subcutaneous formulation. 'Chest-related symptoms' include short-lived heaviness or pressure in the arms and chest, shortness of breath, chest discomfort, anxiety, palpitations, and, very rarely, chest pain. The mechanism is unknown. The risk of sumatriptan-induced myocardial ischemia in the absence of coronary artery disease appears to be acceptable (e.g. no greater than the risk of exercise-induced myocardial ischemia in sportsmen).

Second-generation triptans:
- Zolmitriptan 2.5 mg, 5 mg: similar to oral sumatriptan.
- Naratriptan 2.5 mg: slower action and perhaps fewer and less severe adverse effects, but lower efficacy.
- Rizatriptan 10 mg, 40 mg: better efficacy and consistency, and similar tolerability.
- Almotriptan 12.5 mg: similar efficacy, better consistency and tolerability.
- Eletriptan 20 mg, 40 mg and 80 mg: 80 mg orally is more effective than sumatriptan 100 mg orally with similar consistency but lower tolerability.
- Frovatriptan: possibly lower efficacy than oral sumatriptan.

Advantages over oral sumatriptan:
- Higher bioavailability: 45–75%.
- More rapid therapeutic plasma levels: within 30–60 minutes.
- Greater potency at 5-HT1B/D receptor sites.
- Increased lipophilicity and brain penetration (hence, direct attenuation of excitability of cells within the trigeminal nuclei of the brainstem, as well as vasoconstriction and peripheral inhibition of trigeminal perivascular terminals).
- Cheaper alternatives for patients who do not respond to oral sumatriptan.

None of these agents is consistently effective in all patients and all attacks, and some cause disturbing adverse effects. Rizatriptan 10 mg, eletriptan 80 mg, and almotriptan 12.5 mg provide the highest likelihood of success. Ergotamine and sumatriptan should not be prescribed for patients with suspected coronary artery disease, Prinzmetal variant angina, or uncontrolled hypertension.

Prevention
Non-pharmacologic
- Avoid precipitating factors (e.g. dietary-chocolate, oranges, monosodium glutamate).
- Stress reduction through relaxation exercises and tapes, meditation, yoga, swimming and similar strategies will reduce migraine frequency in many patients.
- Regular exercise such as swimming.
- Acupuncture in short courses by an experienced therapist can be a useful adjunct to other strategies in some patients.

Pharmacologic
- The indication for prophylactic therapy is when the patient needs it. This is usually when the migraine attacks are frequently interfering with their life and recurring every 2 weeks or so and not responding quickly and adequately to acute treatment.
- Efficacy is limited: at most about half of patients will have a reduction in attack frequency of half or more.
- Adverse effects occur commonly.
- The choice of prophylactic agent is primarily determined by the patient and which potential adverse effects are most acceptable (see *Table 15*).
- Discuss the adverse effect profile of each drug with the patient and determine their preference. Asthma (beta blockers) and weight gain (pizotifen [pizotyline] and valproate) are by far the major concerns.
- Establish realistic expectations with the patient before starting: the medication may reduce the frequency of attacks but uncommonly abolishes attacks, and so occasional breakthrough attacks requiring acute treatment will occur.
- Start slowly, with dosage increments every 7–10 days to minimize adverse effects.
- Encourage patients to persist for at least 3 months to adequately trial the drug and because most adverse effects become less prominent with time.
- Follow on with a drug free interval to reassess the frequency and severity of migraine attacks.

Menstrual migraine
- Try standard prophylactic (interval) therapy, as above, before hormone manipulation.
- Continuous bromocriptine therapy, 2.5 mg tds, added to the existing prophylactic regime may be beneficial. Adverse effects, such as light-headedness and nausea can be minimized by gradual introduction of medication, beginning with 1.25 mg daily and followed by daily incremental 1.25 mg increases over 1 week to full dosage (i.e. 25 mg tds).
- Non-steroidal anti-inflammatory drug, such as diclofenac (enteric coated) 50 mg bd commencing 24 hours before anticipated menstruation (to attempt to counteract the overflow of prostaglandin from the contracting uterus).
- Application of a gel containing 1.5 mg estradiol to the skin 48 hours before the expected onset of menstruation.
- Subcutaneous implantation of estradiol pellets, starting with 100 mg, inhibits ovulation and maintains estradiol levels, while regular monthly periods can by induced by cyclical oral progestogens. Depoprovera, a different oral contraceptive pill, or 3 monthly cycles of the oral contraceptive pill are alternative strategies.

- Tamoxifen citrate, 10–20 mg daily preceding and during menstruation may help; tamoxifen competes at estrogen and anti-estrogen binding sites and is a calcium channel blocker. However, the anti-estrogenic effect in young women, such as osteoporosis, is an obvious problem with this strategy.

CLINICAL COURSE

- Migraine is paroxysmal. Clearly defined episodes of migraine recur as often as three or six times each month but sufferers remain symptom-free between attacks.
- The frequency of migraine attacks may increase until it develops into chronic daily headache (transformed migraine), often as the result of stress or the over-use of ergotamine or analgesics.
- Migraine symptoms frequently change over time.
- The severity of the attacks often diminish with time and in some patients the attacks cease in latter years, particularly after the menopause in women.
- In some women however, attacks increase in frequency at the menopause.
- Remission occurs in 70% of pregnancies.
- For young women, below the age of 25 years, the relative risk of ischemic stroke among migraineurs is increased (compared with age-matched controls), particularly among those taking the oral contraceptive pill, but the absolute risk is extremely small (17–50 per 100 000 per year).

MUSCLE CONTRACTION/TENSION-TYPE HEADACHE

DEFINITION
An episodic or chronic continuous headache due to sustained muscle contraction.

EPIDEMIOLOGY
- *Prevalence*:
- Episodic tension-type headache: 38% 1 year period prevalence.
- Chronic tension-type headache: 2.2% 1 year period prevalence.
- *Age*:
- Any age.
- Onset before 10 years of age in 15%.
- Peak prevalence 30–39 years of age.
- *Gender*: F > M: 1.2:1.

ETIOLOGY
Unknown. Perhaps, at least in part, a disorder of the CNS with probable trigeminal activation and sensitization of second-order trigeminal neurons and some peripheral component. Generation of nitric oxide may have a role in central sensitization.

Table 15 Adverse effects of prophylactic agents in migraine

Agent	Dose	Adverse effects
β-adrenoreceptor blockers		
Propranolol	40–240 mg/day	Tiredness, exercise intolerance, postural hypotension, vivid dreams,
Metoprolol	100–200 mg/day	probably contraindicated in asthmatic patients
Anti-epileptic drugs		
Sodium valproate	400–800 mg/day	Drowsiness, tremor, weight gain, abnormal liver enzymes, risk of teratogenicity in pregnant women
5-HT receptor antagonists		
Pizotifen (pizotyline)	0.5–3 mg nocte	Drowsiness, sedation, weight gain
Methysergide	1–4 mg/day	Drowsiness, leg cramps, small (0.5%) risk of retroperitoneal or pleural fibrosis if treatment is not stopped for 1 month every 4–6 months and screened with physical examination, CXR, and renal function
Non-selective calcium channel blockers		
Flunarizine		Constipation; rare extrapyramidal adverse effects with flunarizine
Verapamil	40–120 mg tds	Effective in preventing cluster headache
Vitamins		
Riboflavin (vitamin B$_2$)	400 mg/day	Diarrhea, polyuria
Herbal medicines		
Feverfew		
Non-steroidal anti-inflammatory drugs		
Naproxen		Small risk of peptic ulceration
Hormonal manipulation		
Antidepressants		
Amitriptyline	50–150 mg/day	Drowsiness, dry mouth, blurred vision
Dothiepin		Useful for concurrent tension-type headaches

Predisposing factors

Genetic factors

First degree relatives of probands with chronic tension headache have about three times the risk of chronic tension headache than the general population, suggesting the importance of genetic factors in chronic tension headache.

Physical abnormalities:

- Imbalance of bite: some patients have an uneven bite that throws strain on one temperomandibular joint and leads to the development of a clicking noise in the joint and pain radiating from the affected joint over the face and head (Costen's syndrome). Dental attention is required to correct the bite and it is necessary to reduce excessive jaw clenching (bruxism) and the underlying anxiety state.
- Cervical spondylosis: degenerative changes in the cervical spine may lead to spasm of cervical muscles which may respond to manipulative or other therapy for the neck problem.
- Eye strain: refractive errors or ocular imbalance may be a source of tension and should be corrected. At school or at work, the patient should sit in a comfortable chair which is adjusted to the height appropriate for the desk (to ensure good posture) with light adjusted to the correct angle for comfort.
- Prolonged fasting, as occurs for the traditional Jewish Day of Atonement fast (Yom Kippur), is a strong precipitator of a nonpulsating, bilateral, frontal headache of mild to moderate intensity, particularly among chronic headache sufferers. The mechanism may include metabolic changes, such as hypoglycemia or the accumulation of certain metabolites but the headache tends to occur within 18 hours of fasting.

Psychologic factors

- Stress may be clearly associated with exacerbations of headache in some patients and may be helped by readjustment of stresses, alteration of life-style or psychologic counselling.
- Sleep disturbance is a major perpetuating factor in patients with intermittent muscle contraction headache, which contributes to it becoming chronic.
- Chronic tension-type headache is usually, but not always, related to or exacerbated by anxiety or depression (as well as sleep disturbance).

PATHOPHYSIOLOGY

- Constant involuntary tightening or overcontraction of the frontal, temporal and occipital muscles, induced mentally or physically, may be the cause in some patients who experience some relief by learning to relax the appropriate muscles.
- Psychogenic mechanisms are relevant in other patients.
- Some form of sensitization with second-order trigeminal neurons is likely to be involved.

CLINICAL FEATURES

- Site: usually bilateral, and diffuse or at the vertex of the head, around the head, or in the neck or occiput. Occasionally unilateral.
- Nature: non-pulsatile, tight, pressing, heavy or band-like sensation.
- Onset: may occur during times of fatigue, stress, or anxiety.
- Timing: episodic, but may become constant, occurring all day every day, for months and even years.
- Exacerbating and relieving factors: episodic headache may be relieved by relaxation or analgesics. Chronic daily headache is not relieved by analgesics and excessive medication may itself induce or exacerbate headache.

- Associated symptoms: nausea may be present, but not vomiting or sensory sensitivity to head movement, light or sound (although one of the latter pair is acceptable). Patients are commonly polysymptomatic and may have a fear of an underlying brain tumor or other medical ailment.

DIFFERENTIAL DIAGNOSIS

- Migraine: muscle contraction/tension-type headaches occur in about half of migraine sufferers, often as a background pain, but are not usually unilateral and are not accompanied by sensitivity to light, noise or physical motion, nor vomiting or visual disturbance (as migraines are). Sometimes migraine is gradually transformed into chronic muscle contraction/tension-type headache, but more frequently it is episodic muscle contraction/tension-type headache which becomes chronic. In both instances overuse of drugs frequently plays a role in aggravating the disorder. Discontinuation of daily drug intake often results in improvement.
- Cervicogenic pain: muscle contraction/tension-type headache may also occur as a result of pain referred from the neck.
- Chronic drug-induced (analgesics or ergotamine) headache (often in a migraineur).
- Raised intracranial pressure.

INVESTIGATIONS

Not necessary unless a secondary headache is suspected.

DIAGNOSIS

Based on the history.

Episodic tension-type headache:

A At least 10 previous headaches episodes fulfilling criteria B–D listed below. Number of days with such headache <180/year (<15/month).

B Headache lasting from 30 minutes to 7 days.

C At least 2 of the following pain characteristics:
- Pressing/tightening (non-pulsating) quality.
- Mild or moderate intensity (may inhibit, but does not prohibit activities).
- Bilateral location.
- No aggravation by walking stairs or similar routine physical activity.

D Both of the following:
- No nausea or vomiting (anorexia may occur).
- Photophobia and phonophobia are absent, or one but not the other is present.

E At least one of the following:
- History, physical and neurologic examinations, and appropriate investigations do not suggest headache associated with head trauma, vascular disorders, non-vascular intracranial disorder, substances or their withdrawal, non-cephalic infection, metabolic disorder, or disorders of the cranium, neck, eyes, ears, nose, sinuses, teeth, mouth, or other facial or cranial structures.
- One of the disorders mentioned in E above is present, but tension-type headache does not occur for the first time in close temporal relation to the disorder.

Chronic tension-type headache

A Average headache frequency >15 days/month (180 days/year) for >6 months fulfilling criteria B–D listed below.

B At least 2 of the following pain characteristics:
– Pressing/tightening (non-pulsating) quality.
– Mild or moderate severity (may inhibit, but does not prohibit activities).
– Bilateral location.
– No aggravation by walking stairs or similar routine physical activity.
C Both of the following:
– No vomiting.
– No more than one of the following: nausea, photophobia or phonophobia.
D As for E above.

TREATMENT
Reassurance
Prompt and convincing.

Consider discontinuing or minimizing heavy analgesic intake
For patients in whom episodic tension-type headache or, less frequently, migraine become transformed into chronic tension-type headache, overuse of analgesic drugs frequently plays a role in aggravating the disorder, and discontinuation of daily drug intake often results in improvement.

Relaxation exercises, psychotherapy and biofeedback training
A course in relaxation training may be highly beneficial in a well motivated patient. They are now conducted by psychologists, physiotherapists, and many hospitals and community health centers. Various forms of biofeedback may assist relaxation but do not make a substantial impact.

Pharmacotherapy
• Tricyclic antidepressants: amitriptyline, in particular, may be very helpful, commencing with one-half of a 25 mg tablet at night and gradually increasing to three tablets (75 mg) as a single nocturnal dose, provided there are no adverse effects such as drowsiness and confusion. If effective, an improvement will usually be noticed within 2 weeks. Treatment should be continued for about 6 months and then gradually phased out to see whether it is still necessary or whether improvement can be maintained with relaxation alone.
• Anxiolytics, such as the benzodiazepines, have a limited role. They should be used for short periods only, and under supervision, because of the risk of habituation, dependency and drug-induced headache.
• Sodium valproate, 200–400 mg three times daily, may help control chronic tension-type headache.

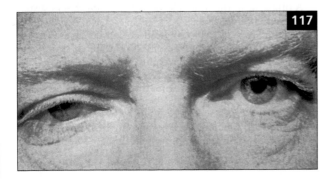

117

CLUSTER HEADACHE (MIGRAINOUS NEURALGIA)

DEFINITION
A rare form of primary headache marked by recurrent episodes, lasting 15–180 minutes, of excruciating unilateral periorbital pain and associated autonomic features, that tend to occur once or twice a day in bouts or clusters, lasting from weeks to months at a time, separated by remission periods of months or 1–2 years.

EPIDEMIOLOGY
• Incidence: 6 (3–10)/100 000/year.
• Lifetime prevalence: 0.3 (95% CI: 0.2–0.6)/1000.
• Age: any age, but unusual in children and most common 20–50 years of age.
• Gender: mainly men (ratio 10:1).

ETIOLOGY AND PATHOPHYSIOLOGY
• A neurovascular disorder, which is hypothesized to be generated in the CNS in pacemaker or circadian regions of the hypothalamic gray matter. The trigeminal/cervical nuclear overlap is also central to the pathogenesis (see Migraine, p.95). Activation of the trigeminovascular system (i.e. release of calcitonin gene-related peptide [CGRP] from peripheral terminals of trigeminal nociceptive neurons, which supply cephalic blood vessels) underlies symptoms of cluster headache. Increases in neuropeptide markers of this system rapidly return to normal after treatment with sumatriptan.
• The mechanism by which nitroglycerine can induce a headache attack in cluster headache patients which is indistinguishable from a spontaneous attack is at least partly due to activation of the trigeminovascular system.

CLINICAL FEATURES
• Severe, boring, unilateral periorbital pain that may radiate upwards over the frontotemporal region and downwards to the face, jaw, neck and shoulder.
• Edema of the ipsilateral eyelid.
• Redness of the ipsilateral eye (conjunctival injection).
• Watering of the ipsilateral eye (lacrimation).
• Miosis with or without ptosis ipsilaterally in about 20% of cases (117); permanent partial Horner's syndrome (ptosis and miosis) ipsilaterally in about 5% of patients.
• Swelling, dilatation, and tenderness of the superficial temporal vessels occasionally.
• Rhinorrhea and a blocked nostril ipsilaterally.
• Temporal spacing of attacks: the pain usually lasts 15 minutes to 2 hours and recurs once or twice a day, often at night at the same time, for several weeks (active periods), followed by an attack-free period (remission period).
• Vasodilators, notably alcohol, nitrates and calcium channel blockers, may precipitate attacks during the active period, but not in remission periods.

117 Facial photograph during an attack of cluster headache showing unilateral eyelid edema, ptosis, miosis and conjunctival injection of the right eye.

FURTHER READING

HEADACHE

Goadsby PJ (1999) Short-lasting primary headaches: focus on trigeminal autonomic cephalgias and indomethacin-sensitive headaches. *Curr. Opin. Neurol.*, **12**: 273–277.

Lance JW (2000) Headache and face pain. *Med. J. Aust.*, **172**: 450–455.

Van Gijn J (1999) Pitfalls in the diagnosis of sudden headache. *Proc. R. Coll. Physicians. Edin.* **29**: 21–31.

MIGRAINE

Bahra, Matharu MS, Buchel C *et al.* (2001) Brainstem activation specific to migraine headache. *Lancet*, **357**: 1016–1017.

Bateman DN (2000) Triptans and migraine. *Lancet*, **355**: 860–861.

Boyle CAJ (1999) Management of menstrual migraine. *Neurology*, **53** (Suppl 1): S14–S18.

Ducros A, Denier C, Joutel A, *et al.* (2001) The clinical spectrum of familial hemiplegic migraine associated with mutations in a neuronal calcium channel. *N. Engl. J. Med.*, **345**: 17–24.

Ferrari MD (1998) Migraine. *Lancet*, **351**: 1043–1051.

Ferrari MD, Roon KI, Lipton RB, Goadsby PJ (2001) Oral triptans (serotonin 5-HT$_{1B/1D}$ agonists) in acute migraine treatment: a meta-analysis of 53 trials. *Lancet*, **358**: 1668–1675.

Gervil M, Ulrich V, Kyvik KO, *et al.* (1999) Migraine without aura: a population-based twin study. *Ann. Neurol.*, **46**: 606–611.

Goadsby PJ, Ferrari MD, Olesen J, *et al.* for the Eletriptan Steering Committee (2000) Eletriptan in acute migraine: A double-blind, placebo-controlled comparison to sumatriptan. *Neurology*, **54**: 156–163.

Goldstein DJ, Roon KI, Offen WW, *et al.* (2001) Selective seratonin 1F (5-HT 1F) receptor agonist LY334370 for acute migraine: a randomized controlled trial. *Lancet*, **358**: 1230–1234.

Hand PJ, Stark RJ (2000) Intravenous lignocaine infusions for severe chronic daily headache. *Med. J. Aust.*, **172**: 157–159.

Hoffman EP (2001) Hemiplegic migraine – downstream of a single-base change. *N. Engl. J. Med.*, **345**: 57–59.

Launer LJ, Terwindt GM, Ferrari MD (1999) The prevalence and characteristics of migraine in a population-based cohort. The GEM study. *Neurology*, **53**: 537–542.

Montagna P (2000) Molecular genetics of migraine headaches: A review. *Cephalgia*, **20**: 3–14.

Silberstein SD, for the US Headache Consortium (2000) Practice parameter: Evidence-based guidelines for migraine headache (and evidence-based review). *Neurology*, **55**: 754–763.

Tfelt-Hansen P, Saxena PR, Dahlof C, *et al.* (2000) Ergotamine in the acute treatment of migraine. A review and European consensus. *Brain*, **123**: 9–18.

Ulrich V, Gervil M, Kyvik KO, *et al.* (1999) Evidence of a genetic factor in migraine with aura: A population-based Danish twin study. *Ann. Neurol.*, **45**: 242–246.

MUSCLE CONTRACTION/TENSION-TYPE HEADACHE

Goadsby PJ (1999) Chronic tension-type headache: where are we? *Brain*, **122**: 1611–1612.

Hand PJ, Stark RJ (2000) Intravenous lignocaine infusions for severe chronic daily headache. *Med. J. Aust.*, **172**: 157–159.

Holroyd KA, O'Donnell FJ, Stensland M, *et al.* (2001) Management of chronic tension-type headache with tricyclic antidepressant medication, stress management therapy and their combination. A randomized controlled trial. *JAMA*, **285**: 2208–2215.

Ostergaard S, Russell MB, Bendtsen L, Olesen J (1997) Comparison of first degree relatives and spouses of people with chronic tension headache. *BMJ*, 314: 1092–1093.

Russell MB, Ostergaard S, Bendsten L, Olesen J (1999) Familial occurrence of chronic tension-type headache. *Cephalgia*, **19**: 207–210.

Schwartz BS, Stewart WF, Simon D, Lipton RB (1998) Epidemiology of tension-type headache. *JAMA*, 279: 381–383.

Tomkins GE, Jackson JL, O'Malley PG, *et al.* (2001) Treatment of chronic headache with antidepressants: a meta-analysis. *Am. J. Med.*, **III**: 54–63.

Welch KMA (2001) A 47-year-old woman with tension-type headaches. *JAMA*, **286**: 960–966.

CLUSTER HEADACHE

Ekbom K (1991) Treatment of acute cluster headache with sumatriptan. *N. Engl. J. Med.*, **325**: 322–326.

Goadsby PJ, Edvinsson L (1994) Human in vivo evidence for trigeminovascular activation in cluster headache. *Brain*, **117**: 427–434.

Goadsby PJ, Lipton RB (1997) A review of paroxysmal hemicranias, SUNCT syndrome and other short-lasting headaches with autonomic feature, including new cases. *Brain*, **120**: 193–209.

Leone M, D'Amico D, Frediani F, *et al.* (2000) Verapamil in the prophylaxis of episodic cluster headache: A double-blind study versus placebo. *Neurology*, **54**: 1382–1385.

May A, Bahra A, Büchel C, Frackowiak RSJ, Goadsby PJ (1998) Hypothalamic activation in cluster headache attacks. *Lancet*, **352**: 275–278.

Vertigo

VERTIGO

DEFINITION
An illusion of movement.

EPIDEMIOLOGY
Incidence: very common.

ETIOLOGY AND PATHOPHYSIOLOGY
Peripheral (most common)
Inner ear (semicircular canals, utricle, saccule)
- Benign paroxysmal positional vertigo (25% of cases).
- Vestibular neuronitis ('viral' labyrinthitis).
- Ménière's disease.
- Benign recurrent vertigo.
- Trauma (including perilymph fistula): head injury.
- Infection: otitis media, syphilis.
- Vascular lesions.

Vestibular nerve
- Meningitis.
- Acoustic neuroma and other cerebello-pontine angle tumors (usually cause unsteady gait and rarely cause vertigo, particularly if there is no deafness).
- Ototoxins: aminoglycosides, frusemide (furosemide) (cause imbalance rather than vertigo).

Central
- Tumors (usually posterior fossa).
- Vertebro-basilar ischemia (but may also cause infarction of the labyrinth): cerebellar or brainstem infarction.
- Vascular malformation in brainstem (VIII nucleus)
- Multiple sclerosis involving brainstem.
- Trauma to brainstem.
- Basilar migraine (may also cause end organ or peripheral involvement).
- Arnold–Chiari malformation.
- Syringobulbia.
- Drugs (alcohol, anti-epileptic drugs, barbiturates).
- Complex partial seizures can cause vertigo but almost always with other more typical symptoms.
- Vertigo is rarely, if ever, due to cervical spondylosis.

CLINICAL FEATURES AND DIAGNOSIS
'Doctor, I'm dizzy' is one of the most common symptoms in neurologic practice.

Is it vertigo or another cause of dizziness such as pre-syncope?
- Encourage the patient to describe the dizzy sensation in their own words.
- A symptom of relative movement, whether it is one of self or of the environment, is usually indicative of vertigo and of an underlying vestibular pathology. A sensation of spinning is the most commonly described vertiginous symptom, and is attributed to semicircular canal involvement. Linear sensations of rocking, tilting and sudden dropping are also valid descriptors of vertigo and probably reflect involvement of the otolith organs (utricle and saccule) which sense linear motion.
- Vertigo due to a vestibular disorder tends to be episodic, and triggered or aggravated by head movements, rather than postural changes alone. Conversely, constant dizziness, persisting for months and years, that is not associated with or aggravated by head movements does not usually have a primary vestibular cause; more commonly it has a psychiatric basis. Moving or large field visual stimuli, such as large cinema screens and supermarket aisles, may induce visual vertigo. Sometimes this leads to secondary agoraphobia (e.g. avoidance of large shopping complexes) and a misdiagnosis of a primary psychiatric disorder.
- Associated symptoms include nausea, vomiting and ataxia, due to the vertigo. The risk of psychologic complications, such as panic disorder and depression increases in proportion to the chronicity of vestibular symptoms. This makes assessment difficult as an underlying vestibular disorder may be overlooked in patients with prominent psychiatric complaints.
- If doubt remains after taking the history, reproduce in the patient the sensations of physiologic vertigo (rotation on the spot with eyes closed) and lightheadedness (hyperventilation) which can be compared with the patient's presenting symptoms.

Is the vertigo due to a peripheral (labyrinthine) or central (CNS) lesion?
A neurologic examination targeted to an assessment of standing and walking balance, eye movements, hearing, otoscopy, and the Dix–Hallpike maneuver is important to elicit focal neurologic signs and exclude central pathology.

Labyrinthine
- Vertigo generally more prominent than ataxia and nystagmus (exception: bilateral vestibular failure).
- Auditory symptoms common.
- Nystagmus, typically a mixed torsional (ocular motion in the frontal plane, sometimes incorrectly referred to as rotatory) and horizontal nystagmus that beats away from the side of the lesion, is readily suppressed by visual fixation and abates quickly as the acute vertigo settles.
- No focal neurologic features.
- Positive Dix–Hallpike maneuver in patients with benign positional vertigo (see p.110): mixed torsional and upbeating nystagmus begins after a short latent period, is accompanied by moderately severe vertigo, fatigues after up to 30 seconds, and is often less marked with repeated maneuvers (habituation).

Infections
- Viral encephalitis.
- Cerebral toxoplasmosis.

Focal basal ganglia lesions
- Stroke.
- Brain tumor.
- Arteriovenous malformation.
- Toxins (exposure to manganese, carbon disulfide).

Toxins
- Manganese.
- Carbon disulfide.
- Wasp sting.

The chances of identifying an underlying pathologic cause for dystonia depends on the age of onset and the distribution of the dystonia (see below).

CLINICAL FEATURES
Dystonia
Muscle contractions that are prolonged (often twisting a part of the body into characteristic postures), and commonly intermittent (causing repetitive, often rhythmic jerks into dystonic postures) but are sometimes continuous, causing constant twisted postures.

Initially, movements and postures appear only during specific movements (action dystonia) and subside with rest. Voluntary movements are accompanied by 'overflow' of muscle spasms and dystonic postures spreading to adjacent muscle groups not normally recruited in the task. If the syndrome progresses (as is common with children but rare in adults), the initial action dystonia becomes evident at rest and then spreads to affect other parts of the body. Dystonia is therefore usually considered a 'mobile' movement disorder because fixed postures and persistence of dystonia at rest occur only in severe, advanced dystonia and hemiplegic dystonia.

Associated rhythmic postural tremors and myoclonus (jerky movements), at about 3 Hz or at faster rates, similar to those of benign essential tremor, are superimposed on the dystonic postures in many patients. Combinations of these movements frequently lead to misdiagnosis.

Spasms are relieved by 'sensory tricks' or 'gestes antagonistique', in which tactile stimuli applied to or near the affected body part relieve the muscle spasm. Movements also disappear during rapid eye movement sleep and deep (stage three and four) sleep.

HISTORY
The clinical features (and course) are determined by the patient's age, anatomic distribution of the dystonia and its cause.

Age of onset
- Childhood-onset: commonly inherited and usually autosomal dominant; an underlying pathologic cause can be identified in up to about 40% of cases; dystonia usually starts in the feet and legs, with a disorder of gait, and progresses to become generalized or multifocal; speech tends to be involved early. It progresses slowly over about 10 years from a focal action dystonia to a generalized dystonia.
- Adolescent-onset: an underlying cause in 30% of patients; intermediate progression.

- Adult-onset dystonia: usually sporadic; an underlying cause in about 10% of patients; dystonia usually starts in body parts other than the legs and frequently remains focal or segmental; rapid progression.

Distribution of dystonia
- Typically, dystonia begins in one part of the body as a focal action dystonia. The legs are commonly affected first in children (onset before 13 years of age), less commonly in adolescents (onset 13–20 years of age), and very rarely in adults (onset after age 20 years). The dystonia progresses to a multifocal or generalized dystonia in about 60% of children, 35% of adolescents, and 3% of adults.
- Hemidystonia: any age; an underlying pathologic cause can be identified in over 80% of cases (usually a structural basal ganglia lesion such as stroke, tumor or AVM).
- Segmental, multifocal or generalized dystonia: commonly inherited; an underlying cause in about 45% of patients.
- Focal dystonia: underlying cause found in less than 10%.

Etiology of dystonia
Drug-induced dystonia
Neuroleptic antipsychotics and anti-emetics produce two types of dystonic reaction: acute dystonic reactions and tardive dystonias.
- Acute dystonic reactions or oculogyric crises (see below) follow exposure to D2 receptor antagonists (half of cases occurring within 48 hours, and 90% within 5 days of exposure) and most commonly in young men. The dystonia particularly affects the eyes, jaws, neck and trunk. Pre-treatment with anticholinergics reduces the risk of oculogyric crises. Oculogyric crises resolve with anticholinergics and withdrawal or reduction of the offending drug.
- Tardive ('delayed') dystonia occurs in 1.5–2% of patients receiving long term neuroleptic therapy. Less frequently, levodopa, dopamine antagonists and selective serotonin reuptake inhibitors may also produce dystonia. The latency between drug exposure and onset of dystonia ranges from 3 weeks to 40 years, with 20% occurring in the first year. Tardive dystonia most commonly affects the cranial, neck and trunk muscles. Paradoxical dystonia (worse at rest and relieved by movement) may occur. Treatment is based on withdrawal of the offending drug if possible. Remission rates are low (10–20%) and may take up to 5 years after drug withdrawal. Treatment with tetrabenazine and anticholinergics is helpful in about half of cases.

Past history of relevance
- Abnormal perinatal history.
- Delayed milestones.
- Precipitating illness.
- Seizures.

Family history of dystonia

PHYSICAL EXAMINATION
Physical signs which may be a clue to an underlying cause of secondary dystonia:
- Intellectual impairment.
- Defects of vision, hearing, or sensation.
- Kayser–Fleischer rings (**118**).

- Abnormalities of optic fundi or eye movements.
- Loss of postural reflexes.
- Pyramidal, cerebellar, or sensory signs.
- Hepato-splenomegaly.

SPECIAL SYNDROMES
Early onset primary torsion dystonia (generalized)
- Autosomal dominant inheritance.
- GAG deletion in DYT1 gene on chromosome 9 (9q34) which codes for the ATP-binding protein torsin A.
- Penetrance: about 30-40%.
- Expression of dystonia in relatives: highly variable.
- Age of onset: 12.5 years (mean), 4–44 years (range).
- Onset: in one limb in 90% of patients; it is rare to begin in the neck or larynx unless the onset is in adulthood. The dystonia spreads to the trunk but rarely affects cranial muscles. A past or family history of an action tremor is common.

Adult-onset focal dystonia syndromes
Spasmodic torticollis (cervical dystonia)
- Torsion or tilting of the head due to sustained contraction of neck muscles (**119**).
- Associated tremulous or jerky head movements are common.
- Neck pain is common, affected muscles may hypertrophy.
- Arm or oromandibular dystonia and blepharospasm occur in a small percentage of patients.

Cranial dystonia
Blepharospasm:
- Bilateral orbicularis oculi muscle spasm results in inability to maintain eye opening.
- Sometimes associated with cervical or oromandibular dystonia.

Oromandibulfacial dystonia (Meige syndrome)
- Forceful opening, closure or lateral deviation of the jaw.
- Closure, pursing or retraction of lips.
- Protrusion of tongue.

Spasmodic dysphonia (laryngeal dystonia)
- Adductor spasm or vocal cords: strained speech, glottal stops and variation of voice pitch.

- Abductor spasm of vocal cords: whispering dysphonia (rare).
- Spasm false vocal cords: inspiratory breathing dystonia.

Writer's cramp (arm dystonia)
- Writing provokes stiffness, spasm or tremor of digits and hand, with overflow of muscle activity to proximal arm muscles.
- Resolves completely with cessation of writing.
- May affect other fine manual tasks in 25% of cases.

Dopa-responsive dystonia with diurnal variation (Segawa's disease)
- Autosomal dominant inheritance (5–10% of inherited childhood dystonias) with reduced penetrance.
- Gene defects: several autosomal dominant mutations involving the gene *GCH1* coding for the enzyme guanine triphosphate (GTP) cyclohydrolase I on chromosome 14q. The enzyme is involved in the synthesis of tetrahydrobiopterin (BH4) in the metabolic pathway manufacturing dopamine and serotonin. The clinical picture results from dopamine deficiency. Other genetic defects include autosomal recessive mutations in the gene for tyrosine hydroxylase, which also interrupts dopamine synthesis.
- Children and adolescents affected.
- F>M: 3:1.
- Lower limb dystonia: usually starts in the legs as an equinovarus deformity causing walking difficulties.
- Fluctuates diurnally, being less in the morning and becomes worse as the day goes on, or becomes noticeable in the afternoon and evening, particularly with exercise.
- Other features: postural instability; later progression to a parkinsonian syndrome.
- Responds to small doses of levodopa.
- Many cases are misdiagnosed as 'cerebral palsy'.

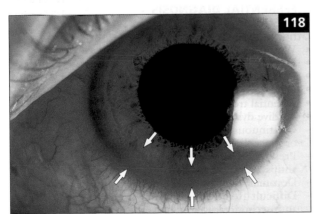

118 Typical appearance of a corneal Kayser–Fleischer ring in Wilson's disease (arrows).

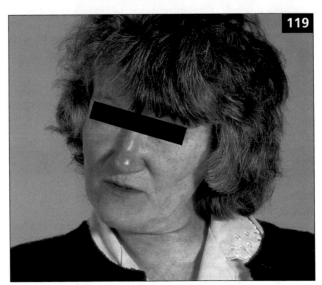

119 Photograph of a patient with focal cervical dystonia (spasmodic torticollis). (Courtesy of Dr AM Chancellor, Tauranga, New Zealand.)

DIAGNOSIS
- Is it dystonia? Clinical (see above).
- Is there a cause for the dystonia? Etiology, clinical and laboratory investigations (see *Table 16*, above).

TREATMENT
Most dystonias can be controlled to some extent, often after a trial of several medications (as with the treatment of migraine), but their underlying cause cannot often be cured.

General
- Physiotherapy: helps prevent dystonic muscles developing contractures.
- Speech and occupational therapy: provide aids to communication and mobility. Mechanical braces are usually not helpful and may lead to problems such as skin ulceration as the dystonic spasms fight the constraint.
- Psychotherapy (supportive): often useful for this distressing condition.
- Psychiatric assessment and intervention: if secondary depression occurs.

Specific
Childhood- and adolescent-onset segmental, multifocal and generalized dystonia
- Levodopa 100 mg and carbidopa 25 mg, one tablet twice daily. Build up to two tablets three times daily for 3 months. If responsive, continue long term. N.B. Adverse effects of long term levodopa that are seen in Parkinson's disease do not occur.
- Anticholinergic agents: if no response to levodopa, start benzhexol (trihexyphenidyl) in low dose (2.5 mg twice daily) and increase slowly (by 2.5 mg a day every 7–14 days) up to a dose that is effective or causes intolerable adverse effects such as dry mouth, blurred vision, urinary hesitancy, anorexia, weight loss, forgetfulness, confusion, behavioral change, hallucinations and chorea. Young people may tolerate doses up to 180 mg a day. About half of patients benefit from anticholinergics.
- Benzodiazepines (e.g. diazepam), often in high dose, seem to relax dystonic spasms.
- Baclofen, orally in high dose, or intrathecally in much lower doses.
- Carbamazepine.
- Dopamine receptor antagonists and neuropletics such as phenothiazines, haloperidol (2–6 mg/day), tetrabenazine and pimozide (alone or in combination with anticholinergic drugs or benzodiazepines) may dampen down excessive movements by causing a degree of drug-induced parkinsonism but they may also lead to tardive dyskinesia. Tetrabenazine, which depletes the brain of dopamine, carries less risk of inducing tardive dyskinesia but it may cause depression.
- Risperidone (1.5–3 mg/day), a neuroleptic with high affinity for 5-HT2 receptors, may be effective in patients with idiopathic segmental dystonia partly insensitive to haloperidol.
- Combination of low dose tetrabenazine (25 mg three times daily), pimozide (gradually increasing the dose up to 12 mg daily) and benzhexol (trihexyphenidyl) (gradually increasing to the maximum tolerable dose).

Adult-onset focal dystonia
- Anticholinergic agents: effective in about one in five people. Large doses (40–120 mg benzhexol [trihexyphenidyl] daily) may be required and a long latent interval of weeks to months may elapse before improvement occurs.
- Botulinum toxin A (BTX-A), injected in small doses into the dystonic muscle(s), with or without EMG guidance, is effective within 7–10 days in 80–90% of patients with focal dystonias such as blepharospasm, spasmodic torticollis, and spasmodic dysphonia. It is taken up by peripheral nerve terminals and prevents calcium-dependent release of acetylcholine, resulting in chemical denervation and paralysis of the injected muscle, and reduction or abolition of the dystonic spasms. The effect lasts for about 2–4 months when terminal sprouting restores muscle end plate neurotransmission. Up to 5% of initially responsive patients may subsequently not respond, due to incorrect storage of the toxin, underdosing, injection of inappropriate muscles, a worsening or change in the pattern of dystonia (possibly with involvement of deep, inaccessible muscles), development of contractures, altered perception of response, and the development of immunity. Immunity is associated with very frequent injections, 'booster' injections, and higher doses. Higher doses of BTX-F may be effective with few adverse effects.
- Facial nerve section is a possible treatment of last resort for blepharospasm in those in whom anticholinergic drugs and botulinum toxin are ineffective and who are prepared to have a permanent facial palsy, but it is fortunately hardly ever done. Chemical myotomy is another alternative.
- Peripheral nerve or root section for torticollis is rarely indicated.
- Thalamotomy for stable hemidystonia can be useful but bilateral thalamotomy for generalized dystonia is rarely contemplated, mainly because of the risk of compromising speech.
- Pallidotomy and pallidal stimulation are currently being evaluated in the treatment of dystonia with encouraging results.

Curative
Identify, treat and eliminate the underlying cause.

NATURAL HISTORY
- Primary (idiopathic) dystonia of childhood- or adolescent-onset tends to progress in the first 5 years of the illness, more slowly over the next 5 years and very slightly, if at all, in adulthood.
- Idiopathic adult-onset focal dystonia does not tend to progress.
- About 1 in 20 (5%) patients with any form of idiopathic dystonia may experience a spontaneous improvement or even resolution. This is most likely in the first 5 years of the illness. Although subsequent relapses are common, some patients experience remissions lasting years or decades.
- The estimated risk for children or siblings of familial cases developing clinical dystonia is about 20%; the risk for sporadic cases is lower at about 8–14%.

ESSENTIAL TREMOR (ET)

DEFINITION
A low frequency (4–9 Hz) postural tremor which is absent at rest and not associated with the clinical signs of parkinsonism or other neurologic deficits.

EPIDEMIOLOGY
- Incidence: 8 (95% CI: 4–14)/100 000/year.
- Prevalence (lifetime): 0.3–1.7%.
- Age of onset: bimodal: young adults (median about 15 years) and elderly.
- Gender: M=F.

PATHOLOGY
No characteristic pathological or biochemical findings.

ETIOLOGY
- Hereditary: autosomal dominant inheritance (50% of patients) via a penetrant autosomal dominant gene. The responsible gene(s) remain unknown.
- Sporadic: probably the same entity as hereditary ET.

PATHOPHYSIOLOGY
- Unknown.
- A central source of oscillation that is influenced by somatosensory reflex pathways.
- Enhanced olivocerebellar oscillation and activation of cerebellothalamocortical pathways probably have an important role in the generation and transmission of the tremor because:
- Functional imaging studies (PET and functional MRI) reveal increased olivary glucose metabolism and increased blood flow bilaterally in the cerebellum and red nuclei and contralaterally in the globus pallidus, thalamus and primary sensorimotor cortex of patients with essential tremor.
- Lesions of the ipsilateral cerebellum diminish essential tremor.
- Ventrointermediate thalamotomy or microstimulation reduce tremor.

- It is thought that the cerebellum introduces an error in the timing of muscle bursts during voluntary movement, and repeated corrective movements lead to tremor.

CLINICAL FEATURES
Tremor
- Postural or action tremor of the finger, hands and forearms when they are held outstretched against gravity, or used for specific, usually visually-guided, manual tasks ('position-specific postural tremor').
- Variable kinetic component (tremor during any form of movement).
- 4–12 cycles per second.
- Bilateral, but may be asymmetric.
- Other body parts involved in about half of cases: the head (40%), tongue, lips, voice (15–20%), face, and trunk; and postural tremor of lower limbs (15%).
- Visible.
- Persistent, but the amplitude may fluctuate.
- Exacerbated by emotional upset such as excitement and anger.
- Improved temporarily by alcohol, in small quantities, in about half of patients.
- Relatively longstanding (i.e. longer than 5 years).
- Froment's sign (a rhythmic resistance to passive movements of a limb about a joint when there is a voluntary action of another body part).

DIFFERENTIAL DIAGNOSIS (see *Tables 17, 18*)
Intention or 'terminal' tremor due to cerebellar disease
- Slower (3–5 cycles per second).
- Principally in a horizontal plane.
- Not present at rest.
- Increases with action and progressively increases during a voluntary movement (terminal or intention tremor).
- Unlike kinetic tremor, which is tremor during any form of movement; 'intention' or 'terminal' tremor is the pronounced exacerbation of kinetic tremor toward the end of goal-directed movement.
- The head may be affected, but usually as titubation (repetitive nodding or 'yes-yes').
- May be incapacitating.
- Responds to propranolol and diazepam.

Table 17 Common tremors classified according to frequency and behavior

Frequency (Hz)	Behavioral characteristics	Disease locus	Disease processes
2.5–3.5	Postural/kinetic	Cerebellar/brainstem	Alcoholic degeneration, multiple sclerosis, trauma
4–5	Rest	Substantia nigra/striatum	Parkinson's disease, drugs (neuroleptics, ?MPTP)
	Rest/postural/movement/kinetic	Red nucleus	
	Postural/kinetic	Cerebellum	
5.5–7.5	Postural/kinetic	?Cerebellum	Essential tremor, Parkinson's disease,
		?Cerebrum–cerebellum	drugs (valproate, lithium, antidepressants)
8–12	Postural/kinetic	?Cerebellum	Enhanced physiologic tremor, essential tremor, drug intoxications

INVESTIGATIONS
First line
- Electrolytes.
- Glucose.
- Renal function.
- Hepatic function.
- Drug and toxin screen.
- Brain imaging: CT or MRI scan.
- EEG (**123**): generalized spike wave discharges, photo-sensitivity, focal (particularly posterior) epileptiform discharges, vertex spikes in REM sleep, may be found in most of the disorders that cause the progressive myoclonic epilepsy syndrome. Slowing of background activity occur in all forms of PME but is usually much more prominent and early in those diseases with diffuse neuronal damage and storage compared with those diseases with restricted neuronal degeneration.

Second line
- Polygraphic EEG–EMG monitoring and back-averaging: the most essential and useful electrophysiologic technique to try and show a relationship between a cortical spike and a muscle contraction. EEG-EMG backaveraging techniques can be used to detect EEG potentials that are not present in routine EEG recordings. This technique increases the signal-to-noise ratio and records preceding EEG waveforms that are time-locked to the myoclonus.
- Somatosensory-evoked potentials (SEP): useful for further investigating the pathophysiology of myoclonus. Giant somatosensory-evoked potentials may be found in stimulus-sensitive, cortical reflex myoclonus caused by most of the disorders that cause the progressive myoclonic epilepsy syndrome.
- Copper studies: Wilson's disease.
- Enzyme activities: storage diseases.
- Genetic testing: mitochondrial disease, Huntington's disease, spinocerebellar ataxias.
- Chromosomal fragility: ataxia-telangiectasia.
- Spinal imaging: segmental pathologic condition.
- Tissue biopsy: storage disease, mitochondrial disease.

DIAGNOSIS
Clinical and electrophysiologic.

TREATMENT
The myoclonus may not be severe enough to warrant symptomatic treatment. Treatment of the underlying cause (e.g. renal failure) may obviate the need for specific treatment. Anti-epileptic treatment for seizures may reduce the myoclonus.

Specific medication for myoclonus
- Sodium valproate, benzodiazepines (clonazepam) and lamotrigine are the most effective conventional drugs. Valproate use may be limited by gastrointestinal effects, sedation and liver toxicity. Clonazepam can be limited by sedation, imbalance, behavioral changes, and tolerance.
- Piracetam may be useful.
- Serotonin precursors may be used for post-hypoxic myoclonus or progressive myoclonic epilepsy.
- Phenytoin has a deleterious effect.
- In contrast to the general principle of monotherapy in epilepsy, polytherapy may produce additional benefit in the treatment of severe myoclonus, although drug toxicity needs to be avoided.

Physical therapy

Social rehabilitation

PROGNOSIS
Depends on the cause; myoclonus may occur as a transient or persistent phenomenon in many conditions such as viral encephalitis, suppurative meningitis, intoxications with strychnine and tetanus, and metabolic disorders such as uremia and anoxic encephalopathy.

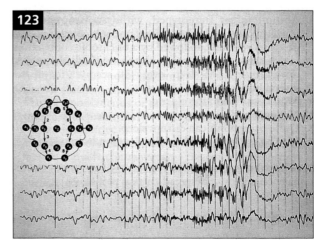

123 EEG, 8 channel, sleep recording, in a young adult with myoclonic seizures, showing trains of fast spikes followed by a single slow wave (multispike and wave).

DYSKINESIAS

DEFINITION
Abnormal dystonic and choreoathetoid involuntary movements that may occur spontaneously, after a sudden voluntary movement, after prolonged physical exertion, or during sleep, which occur during full consciousness, and are of variable duration.

EPIDEMIOLOGY
Prevalence
- Tardive dyskinesia: about 20% of patients on long-term antipsychotic medication.
- Paroxysmal dyskinesia: rare, except when associated with late stage Parkinson's disease.

Age of onset
- 21 years (mean); range 1–60 years (paroxysmal kinesogenic dyskinesia [PKD]).
- 30 years (mean); range 1–77 years (paroxysmal non-kinesogenic dyskinesia [PNKD]).
- 13 years (mean); range 1–29 years (paroxysmal exertion-induced dyskinesia [PED]).
- Idiopathic paroxysmal dyskinesias have a younger age of onset compared with secondary dyskinesias.
- Gender: F<M = 3:5 (i.e. about 60% as common in women than men).

CLASSIFICATION
Continuous dyskinesias
Tardive dyskinesia.

Paroxysmal dyskinesias
Kinesigenic (Paroxysmal kinesigenic dyskinesia)
Abrupt onset of episodes of abnormal involuntary movements after a sudden voluntary movement.

Non-kinesigenic (Paroxysmal non-kinesigenic dyskinesia)
Spontaneous onset of attacks of abnormal involuntary movements.

Exertion-induced dyskinesia
Attacks of abnormal involuntary movements precipitated by prolonged physical exertion.

Hypnogenic dyskinesia
Attacks of abnormal involuntary movements occurring only during sleep.

ETIOLOGY
Tardive dyskinesia
Long term antipsychotic medication.

Paroxysmal kinesigenic dyskinesia
Familial: 65% of cases, usually autosomal dominant inheritance with complete or incomplete penetrance. Linked to the pericentromeric region of chromosome 16.

PATHOPHYSIOLOGY
Tardive dyskinesia
Dopamine receptor hypersensitivity.

Paroxysmal kinesigenic dyskinesia
- Decreased inhibitory influences of the medial globus pallidus and substantia nigra on the thalamus, or
- Damage to the thalamic reticular nucleus itself, thus making the thalamus more sensitive to superficial or deep sensory input.

Paroxysmal hypnogenic dyskinesia (PHD)
May be associated with frontal epilepsy.

CLINICAL FEATURES
Tardive dyskinesia
Continuous involuntary movements of the orobuccolingual and masticatory muscles of a choreiform nature.

Paroxysmal dyskinesis
Precipitating factors
Paroxysmal kinesigenic dyskinesia (PKD):
- Sudden voluntary movement of a limb; orofacial movements such as yawning and talking; movements associated with startle or hyperventilation.

Paroxysmal exertion-induced dyskinesia (PED):
- Walking, running for 5–15 minutes.

Paroxysmal hypnogenic dyskinesia (PHD):
- Sleep.

Prodromal symptoms immediately prior to onset of attack
Muscle tension; tingling; numbness; dizziness.

Site of involvement
Limbs, often unilaterally; oromandibular and facial muscles: dysarthria or anarthria.

Nature of involvement
Dystonia and/or choreoathetosis or athetosis.

Associated symptoms
Pain in the affected body part sometimes; perhaps sleep disorders (e.g. sleep apnea, narcolepsy).

Exacerbating factors
Paroxysmal kinesigenic dyskinesia (PKD):
- Stress; fatigue; menses; alcohol; cold; heat.

Duration of attacks
From seconds up to several hours to days. Attacks may become shorter or longer with time.

SPECIAL FORMS
Superior oblique myokymia, causing paroxysmal diplopia or 'shimmering of vision'.

DIFFERENTIAL DIAGNOSIS
- Epileptic seizures (movement-induced seizures, reflex epilepsy or subcortical epilepsy): paroxysmal dyskinesias are dystonic or choreoathetoid with preserved consciousness, a normal EEG during attacks, and absence of a post ictal state.
- Psychogenic: attacks associated with or triggered by hyperventilation and odors.

INVESTIGATIONS
Cranial CT and MRI scan: often normal.

TREATMENT
The precipitating circumstance is the most important factor in determining the underlying mechanism of the paroxysmal movement disorder, the natural history and response to treatment. Long lasting attacks suggest a good response to medication.

Tardive dyskinesia
- Difficult to treat.
- Withdrawal of the responsible antipsychotic drug may induce a remission, but this can take months or even years, and may be impractical if the patient has a serious underlying psychiatric disorder.
- Increased doses of dopamine antagonists (e.g. tetrabenazine) paradoxically may lead to improvement, presumably by depleting presynaptic dopamine, but may also cause depression.
- Baclofen, benzodiazepines, and calcium-channel blockers may be effective; anticholinergics make tardive dyskinesia worse.

Paroxysmal dyskinesias
Almost all patients with PKD improve with anti-epileptic drugs in contrast to only one-quarter of patients with PNKD. Short-lasting (and non-kinesigenic) attacks generally fail to improve with medication. Carbamazepine and phenytoin seem more effective than other anti-epileptic drugs in PKD and clonazepam in PNKD. Drugs that enhance GABAergic neurotransmission, such as benzodiazepines, valproic acid, and phenobarbitone (phenobarbital), increase the latency to the onset of attacks and reduce the severity, while drugs that impair GABAergic transmission decrease the latency.
- Clonazepam (PNKD).
- Tetrabenazine (PKD).
- Lorazepam (PHD).
- Chronic stimulation of the ventro intermediate (Vim) thalamus may impove dystonic paroxysmal non-kinesigenic dyskinesia.

TOURETTE SYNDROME (TS)

DEFINITION
A genetically determined chronic neuropsychiatric disorder that develops in children and adolescents and is characterized by multiple motor and vocal tics (quick, involuntary movements that occur repeatedly and non-rhythmically in the same way) which last more than 1 year and cause considerable social, vocational and functional impairment. It is commonly associated with obsessive–compulsive behavior, attentional and executive dysfunction, and aggressive behavior. The syndrome was first described in 1825 by Dr Georges Gilles de la Tourette.

EPIDEMIOLOGY
- Prevalence: 3–10/1000; much more common than previously appreciated; many cases are mild and do not come to medical attention or are not recognized.
- Tics: common during childhood development (4–12% of children aged 6–12 years), and possibly more common in children with learning problems. The relationship between such tics and the disorder of TS remains unclear. Commonly, tics are transient and disappear.
- Age of onset: before age 21, usually 2–15 years.
- Gender: M>F (3:1); as yet unexplained.

PATHOLOGY
Limited histopathologic data have failed to identify any definitive pathologic changes in the striatum (**124**).

ETIOLOGY AND PATHOPHYSIOLOGY
- Commonly familial and inherited as an autosomal dominant trait with reduced penetrance and variable expression.
- A linkage has been found to chromosome 18 in some families.
- No evidence for genetic linkage at the dopamine D2 or D3 receptor loci has been found.
- It is hypothesized by some that the TS genetic locus is common and is involved in normal brain development, and that the occurrence of the clinical disorder TS represents an excessive expression or abnormal persistence of normal developmental characteristics. The appearance of the typically associated clinical features of TS (i.e. tics, obsessive–compulsive behavior, inattention, and hyperactivity) commonly occurs during normal childhood development (as a form of 'developmental' or 'physiological' TS) and reflects normal synaptogenesis in basal ganglia and limbic regions. The medical disorder TS differs only quantitatively from this process.
- Other hypotheses are that:
  – TS is a basal ganglia disorder characterized by striatal dopamine receptor hypersensitivity.
  – TS is a cingulate and orbitofrontal cortex disorder characterized by dysfunction of the central endogenous opioid system in limbic and orbitofrontal basal ganglia/thalamic loops.
- Reports of TS following head trauma, carbon monoxide poisoning, neuroleptic drugs, other toxic and metabolic encephalopathies, Creutzfeldt–Jakob disease, Huntington's disease, and encephalitis lethargica are more likely to be coincidental than causal.

CLINICAL FEATURES
Chronic, multiple motor and vocal tics

Tics involving the face or neck (e.g. repeated eye blinking and throat clearing) is the most common initial feature. Other common initial symptoms include complex movements such as touching, striking or hitting, and jumping.

Tics are brief stereotyped movements (motor tics) or sounds produced by moving air through the nose, mouth or throat (vocal tics). They are classified as motor and vocal, and simple and complex, although the boundaries of these are not well defined:

- Simple motor tics: eye blinking, facial grimacing, neck jerking, shoulder shrugging.
- Complex motor tics: facial gestures, smelling, groaning behaviors, touching, stamping, hitting or biting oneself, jumping.
- Simple vocal tics: sniffing, coughing, throat clearing, grunting, snorting, barking.
- Complex vocal tics: repeating words or phrases out of context, palilalia (increasingly rapid repetition of a word or phrase), echolalia (repetition of words), and coprolalia (foul language).

With time, the tics become more prominent and involve the shoulders and arms, followed by the legs. Involvement of the muscles of respiration causes vocal tics such as grunting, barking or coughing noises which interrupt conversation. The expulsion of air imparts an explosive quality to the speech and occasional associated hissing sounds.

Some patients develop repetitive involuntary explosive stereotyped verbal utterances during compulsive expiration, which may consist of obscene expletives (coprolalia). Patients may also repeat the last word or sentence of others' (echolalia) or their own speech (palilalia), repeat motor acts (echopraxia) and sometimes obscene (copropraxia) and other gestures.

The tics occur many times a day (usually in bouts) nearly every day, or on again, off again for more than a year. There are periodic changes in the type, number, frequency, and location of the tics, and in the waxing (increasing) and waning (decreasing) of their severity. Symptoms will sometimes mysteriously disappear for weeks or months at a time.

Although tics are described as being quick, involuntary movements that occur repeatedly and non-rhythmically in the same way, they are not strictly 'involuntary'. Most people with TS have some control over their symptoms. However, this control, which can be exerted from seconds to hours at a time, tends to delay more severe tics. They become irresistible and must eventually be executed; some people wait until they are in private before doing so.

Associated disorders, behaviors and consequences
Coexist in about half of all patients.

Obsessive–compulsive disorder (about 50% of cases)
The presence of obsessions or compulsions causing marked distress or interfering with normal functioning. Obsessions are recurrent persistent ideas, thoughts, impulses or images that are intrusive and inappropriate and cause anxiety or distress. They are a product of the person's own mind and are not simply excessive worries about real-life problems. Examples include fear of contamination, need for symmetry, and pathologic doubt. Compulsions are repetitive behaviors or mental acts that a person feels driven to perform, often in response to an obsession. The aim of them is to prevent or reduce anxiety or distress, not to provide pleasure or gratification. Examples include checking, washing, counting, needing to ask or confess, and symmetrizing or being precise.

Attention deficit disorder (ADD)
Characterized by five or more of the following: failure to give attention to details or making careless mistakes in schoolwork, work, or other activities; frequent difficulty organizing tasks and activities; easy distractibility by extraneous stimuli; failure to follow through on instructions and finish work or duties; often leaving seat in classroom or in other situations in which remaining seated is expected; difficulty playing or engaging in leisure activities quietly; talking excessively.

Sleep disorders
Sleep talking, insomnia, nightmares, enuresis, and somnambulism.

Other types of behavior
- Learning difficulties.
- Hyperactivity.
- Self-injury.
- Antisocial behavior.
- Aggressive behavior.
- Inappropriate sexual activity.
- Lack of discipline.

These disorders and behaviors may wax and wane and may persist even after the tics have largely disappeared. Many patients are left-handed or ambidextrous and have minor neurologic abnormalities. A family history of tics, obsessive–compulsive behavior, or ADD is commonly present.

124 Brain of a drug addict showing basal ganglia (globus pallidus) disease bilaterally due to the use of illicit drugs. Tics are occasionally due to organic basal ganglia disease.

DIFFERENTIAL DIAGNOSIS
Normal variants (i.e. physiologic)
- Tics are common in children between the ages of 2–6 years but most are transient and disappear.
- 'Colds' or 'allergies': some of the most common tics, such as eye blinking, sniffing, throat clearing, and coughing are commonly ascribed to 'colds' and 'allergies'.
- 'Nervous habits': tics such as facial grimaces or head jerks are often considered to be 'nervous habits'.

Developmental basal ganglia syndrome
Primary (hereditary)
Primary tic disorders:
- Tourette syndrome.
- Chronic motor tic disorder.
- Chronic vocal tic disorder.
- Transient tic disorder.

Related primary neuropsychiatric disorders:
- Primary obsessive–compulsive disorder.
- Primary ADD.
- Developmental stuttering.

Inherited neurologic disorders
- Huntington disease.
- Neuroacanthocytosis.
- Torsion dystonia.

Secondary (symptomatic)
- Autisms, pervasive developmental disorder.
- Mental retardation.
- Fetal alcohol syndrome.
- Intrauterine infection or exposure to illicit drugs (**124**).
- Perinatal asphyxia.
- Carbon monoxide toxicity.
- Encephalitis.
- Head trauma.
- Stroke.
- Post-infectious (immune-mediated).
- Sydenham's chorea.

Tic-inducing drugs
- Neuroleptic agents.
- Stimulants.

INVESTIGATIONS
- Blood: DNA analysis.
- EEG: abnormal in many cases although non-specifically.

DIAGNOSIS
Tourette syndrome (TS)
1 Multiple (two or more) motor and/or vocal tics.
2 Onset in the first two decades of life.
3 Tics present for more than 1 year.
4 Tics are not caused by tic-inducing drugs (e.g. stimulants or neuroleptic agents), other environmental insults to the brain (e.g. perinatal hypoxia, intrauterine infection, or exposure to alcohol), or to hereditary neurologic disorders that may produce tics (e.g. neuroacanthocytosis or Huntington's disease).
5 There is no evidence of significant brain dysfunction (e.g. mental retardation, pyramidal tract signs, or seizures) other than tics.

Tourette disorder (TD)
1 Criteria 1–5 for Tourette syndrome are satisfied.
2 Tics cause distress or significant impairment in social, academic, occupational, or other important areas of functioning.

Clinical features increasing confidence for the diagnosis of TS or TD
1 Multiple tic types that vary over time.
2 Tics wax and wane in severity.
3 Coprolalia.
4 A positive family history of TS or TD.

N.B. The type or severity of tic is not considered in the diagnosis of TS. For example, coprolalia is not required for the diagnosis; it occurs in less than one-third of clinic populations and in less than 5% of affected members of studied TS pedigrees.

TREATMENT
Education and counselling of the patient and family.

Psychologic support
Promote the child's self-esteem and competency and provide support in the challenges of school or work and in social relationships.

Pharmacologic intervention
Symptomatic treatment of TS with drugs can be helpful but improvements are usually incomplete and short-lasting.

Tics
Neuroleptics with dopamine-blocking activity are most widely used. Those with a greater selectivity for the dopamine D2 receptor subtype, such as haloperidol, pimozide and sulpiride can be effective in reducing the frequency and severity of tics for patients with severe symptoms. Medication needs to be administered carefully and in small doses to obtain the maximum benefit and the minimum number and degree of adverse effects; tardive dyskinesia often develops with prolonged usage. Other effective treatments include tetrabenazine, a dopamine-depleting agent, and clonidine, which is a central α_2 adrenergic receptor antagonist and is thought to reduce presynaptic release of noradrenaline.
- Pimozide, beginning with 0.5 mg daily and increasing by 0.5 mg increments to as high as 10 mg daily if necessary, is effective in up to 80% of cases. Adverse effects include sedation, weight gain, depression, and restless legs.
- Haloperidol, for patients who fail to respond to pimozide because the risk of long term adverse effects such as tardive dyskinesia is greater with haloperidol than pimozide. Starting dose 0.5 mg three times daily by mouth, increasing to as much as 10 mg three times daily if necessary.
- Trifluoperazine or thiothixene can be effective in refractory cases.
- Clonidine may help a few: increasing up to 6 micrograms per kg daily, oral, in three divided doses, but sedation can occur. Withdrawal must be slow to avoid rebound hypertension.
- A combination of neuroleptics may be required.

- Naltrexone, an opiate antagonist, has improved attention and reduced the number of tics in a double-blind randomized trial.
- Botulinum toxin reduces urge and tic frequency.

Obsessive–compulsive disorder
Obsessive–compulsive disorder can be controlled with anti-depressant medication, and drugs with serotonin reuptake blocking activity, such as clomipramine and fluvoxamine, appear to be the most effective.

Attention deficit disorder
ADD can be treated with psychostimulant medications, but when patients have combined features of ADD and TS, stimulant drugs tend to worsen the tics. Desipramine has been shown in a recent double-blind controlled trial to be useful in the treatment of ADD in TS without a deterioration in tic severity.

PROGNOSIS

- TS is a lifelong illness.
- Many people experience remissions of symptoms (particularly tics), commonly in the late teens and early twenties, which may be complete, or incomplete and followed by subsequent relapses.
- Lifelong medical treatment with pimozide or haloperidol is often required but many patients can be restored to a full active life in the community, without any compromise to life expectancy.
- A person with TS has about a 50% chance of passing the gene to his or her children. However, only about 10% of children who inherit the TS gene will have symptoms severe enough to seek medical attention.

NEUROLEPTIC MALIGNANT SYNDROME (NMS)

DEFINITION
A rare but potentially life-threatening complication of neuroleptic drug treatment.

EPIDEMIOLOGY
- Incidence: 0.2% of patients treated with neuroleptics.
- Age: all ages, particularly young and middle-aged adults; mean age 40 years.
- Gender: M=F.

ETIOLOGY
D$_2$ dopamine receptor antagonists
Neuroleptic drugs
- Phenothiazines: chlorpromazine;
- Butyrophenones: haloperidol – most common.

Non-neuroleptic antiemetic, anesthetic and sedative drugs
- Metoclopramide.
- Prochlorperazine.
- Droperidol.
- Promethazine.

Withdrawal of dopamine agonists (anti-parkinsonian medication)
Infrequent.

Risk factors
- Previous episodes (one-third develop subsequent episodes on re-challenge).
- Dehydration.
- Agitation.
- Rapid rate and parenteral route of neuroleptic administration.
- Pre-existing organic brain disease or mood disorders, particularly if taking lithium.

PATHOPHYSIOLOGY
- An acute reduction in brain dopamine activity; probably dopamine receptor blockade in the hypothalamus, caudate and pallidum primarily.
- Commonly due to an increase in dose of neuroleptic drugs within the therapeutic range, rather than a toxic manifestation.
- Infrequently, withdrawal of anti-parkinsonian medication precipitates NMS.

CLINICAL FEATURES
Rapid onset, usually within a few days of starting treatment with a dopamine receptor antagonist (16% within 24 hours, 66% within 1 week, 96% within 30 days), but sometimes after stopping treatment.

History
Often there is a history of psychiatric illness, requiring treatment with a neuroleptic. Occasionally, recent withdrawal of anti-parkinsonian medication has taken place.

Developmental Diseases of the Nervous System

ARNOLD–CHIARI MALFORMATION

DEFINITION
A number of developmental anomalies of the hindbrain, base of skull, and upper cervical canal characterized by caudal displacement of the cerebellar tonsils, and sometimes more of the cerebellum and lower brainstem, through the foramen magnum into the cervical spinal canal.

CLASSIFICATION OF CHIARI MALFORMATIONS
Type I
Cerebello-medullary malformation
Herniation of the cerebellar tonsils below the foramen magnum into the cervical spinal canal with elongation of the medulla (**126, 127**). Meningomyelocele is rare. Hydrocephalus (see p.468) and syringomyelia (see p.541) may develop, the latter in up to 50% of cases (**128–130**).

Type II
Cerebello-medullary malformation with meningomyelocele
Cerebellum and medulla are displaced inferiorly and are deformed (**131**). The medulla is elongated and often folded upon itself in an S-shaped pattern or overlies the cervical cord, which may be small with upward directed roots. Meningomyelocele (protrusion of spinal cord/cauda equina, dura and arachnoid through a defect in the vertebral lamina, forming a cystic swelling) is invariably present (see p.140).

Type III
Cerebellar herniation with a high cervical or occipito-cervical meningomyelocele
Includes cervical spina bifida, cerebellar herniation through the defect, and an open, dystrophic posterior fossa. Rarely compatible with post-natal life.

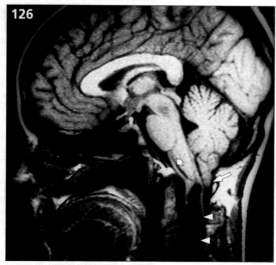

126 MRI brain sagittal T1W image of a 40 year old lady with altered sensation to pain and temperature over the right chest from T4 to T9, showing Chiari malformation with herniated cerebellar tonsils (arrow) within the foramen magnum and reaching the midlevel of the posterior arch of C1, cervical syrinx (arrowheads), and syringobulbia (short arrow) with the tract extending upwards in the midline of the ventral medulla to the pontomedullary junction.

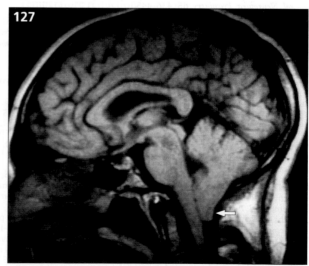

127 Chiari type I malformation: midline sagittal MR T1W imaging (TR=500 ms, TE=15 ms) showing caudal displacement of cerebellar tissue, with herniation of the cerebellar tonsils below the foramen magnum (arrow).

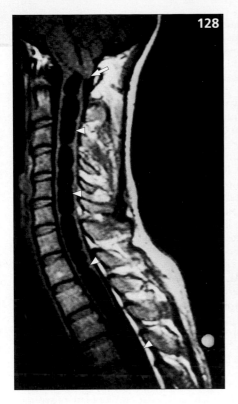

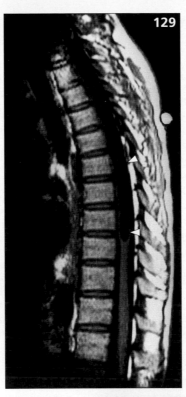

128, 129 MRI cervical and upper thoracic spine, sagittal T1W images, showing herniated cerebellar tonsils (arrow) and a large syringo-hydro-myelia (arrowheads) extending down to the upper end plate of T9.

130 MRI thoracic spine, axial gradient echo image, showing large hyperintense (white, arrows) central syringo-hydro-myelia occupying most of the thoracic spinal cord in cross-section.

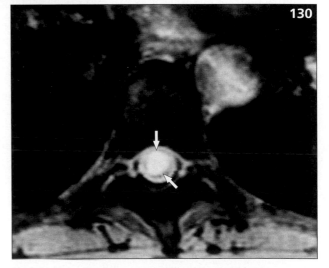

Type IV
Cerebellar hypoplasia only
May be related to or equivalent to Dandy–Walker malformation.

EPIDEMIOLOGY
- Incidence: uncommon.
- Age of onset of symptoms: type II: infancy, type I: teens or young adulthood.
- Gender: M=F.

PATHOLOGY
- Caudal descent of the cerebellar tonsils.
- Medulla and pons elongated.
- Medulla and cerebellum occlude foramen magnum.
- Remainder of cerebellum, which is small, is also displaced, obliterating the cisterna magna.
- Fibrosis of arachnoid tissue around herniated brainstem and cerebellum.
- A kink or spur in the upper cervical spinal cord, pushed posteriorly by the lower end of the fourth ventricle. In this type of malformation, a meningomyelocele is nearly always found, and hydromyelia of the cervical cord is common.

Associations
Bony abnormalities
- Posterior fossa: small.
- Foramen magnum: enlarged and grooved posteriorly.
- Base of skull: flattened or infolded by the cervical spine.
- Fused cervical vertebrae (Klippel–Feil syndrome).
- Spinal dysraphism (see p.139).

CNS abnormalities
- Developmental abnormalities of the cerebrum: poly-microgyria.

- Aqueduct stenosis.
- Hydrocephalus (due to aqueduct stenosis or CSF outflow obstruction at base of the brain).
- Syringomyelia and syringobulbia (**126, 128–130**).
- Lumbosacral meningocele or meningomyelocele (see p.140).
- Filum terminale: lower spinal cord may extend to the sacrum.
- Others, such as fusion of the corpora quadrigemina, cysts of the foramen of Magendie, upward herniation of the cerebellum through an abnormally large tentorial notch, enlargement of the mass intermedia, fusion of the thalami, and hydromyelia.

ETIOLOGY AND PATHOPHYSIOLOGY
- Unknown.
- Probably a failure of coordinated development of the brainstem, cerebellum and upper cervical spinal cord.
- Arnold–Chiari malformations are traditionally viewed as a congenital anomaly but may be acquired. One hypothesis is that the CSF pressure difference between the spinal and cranial compartments causes tonsillar herniation. Others suggest that a mismatch between the volume of the posterior fossa and its tissue contents may produce downward herniation of the cerebellar tonsils.

CLINICAL FEATURES
Chiari type 1 malformation
May be asymptomatic or cause symptoms and signs of progressive dysfunction of the:
- Cerebellum (progressive cerebellar ataxia),
- Medulla (spastic quadriparesis), or
- Lower cranial nerves (dysphagia),

at any time during life, sometimes being delayed until adult life.

Other progressive symptoms include those of:
- Raised intracranial pressure (e.g. headache) due to hydrocephalus (see p.468), and
- Syringomyelia (see p.541).

Symptoms occasionally arise acutely, such as headache or vertigo and ataxia following neck extension (e.g. dental extraction and chiropractic manipulation), coughing, sneezing and Valsalva maneuver (inducing hindbrain herniation); and syncope on exertion.

Examination findings include:
- A short 'bull' neck in about 25% of cases.
- Low hairline.
- Torsional or downbeating nystagmus with neck extension.
- Permanent signs of cerebellar, medulla, high cervical cord or lower cranial nerve dysfunction.

Downbeat nystagmus is usually in the primary position of gaze, and increases in gaze slightly below horizontal, especially in gaze down and laterally. It is due to a disturbance of the vestibulo-cerebellar pathways and is highly suggestive of a craniocervical junction disorder such as Arnold–Chiari malformation, basilar invagination or ankylosing spondylitis. However, it may also be seen in cerebellar disease (when other cerebellar eye signs are usually present), drug intoxication (phenytoin, carbamazepine, lithium), brainstem encephalitis, magnesium depletion, communicating hydrocephalus, Wernicke's encephalopathy, multiple sclerosis, vascular disease and as a paraneoplastic phenomenon. It may coexist with periodic alternating nystagmus.

Chiari type II malformation
Usually presents in infancy with:
- Progressive enlargement of the head, due to hydrocephalus, and
- Spinal meningomyelocele.

Diagnosis may be delayed until the spinal cord is compressed at the cranio-cervical junction causing:
- Spastic quadriparesis (limb spasticity, hyperreflexia and extensor plantar responses).

- Cerebellar ataxia (predominantly affecting the legs and later the arms).
- Downbeat nystagmus.
- Weakness and wasting of the tongue, sternomastoid and trapezius muscles due to lower cranial nerve palsies (XI and XII).
- Recurrent vocal cord paralysis, laryngeal stridor, or respiratory obstruction during physical activity, due to periodic venous congestion in the medulla.

Some remain asymptomatic well into adult life and present later with pain in the back of the head, neck, shoulders and upper limbs, exacerbated by head movement and cough, sneeze or strain ('hindbrain hernia headache'). This may be followed by the evolution of weakness and spasticity in the limbs, gait ataxia and difficulty swallowing. Clinical features of syringomyelia (see p.541) may also coexist.

DIFFERENTIAL DIAGNOSIS
- Multiple sclerosis.
- Tumor of the high cervical cord or lower medulla (foramen magnum).
- Motor neuron disease (Chiari I may present with progressive severe bulbar palsy and generalized hyperreflexia due to severe stretch injury to lower cranial nerves [caused by caudal displacement of medulla] and/or direct brainstem compression).
- Autosomal dominant cerebellar ataxia of late onset.
- Dandy–Walker syndrome: a developmental anomaly with cystic dilatation of, or near, the fourth ventricle. It causes obstructive hydrocephalus, cerebellar and/or brainstem signs.

INVESTIGATIONS
MR scan of the brain and cervical spinal cord is the investigation of choice

Chiari I malformation
- T1W midline sagittal MRI (or myelography) shows the inferior displacement of the cerebellar tonsils, the tips lying in the C1–C2 region (**126, 127**).
- The tonsils may lie up to 5 mm below the foramen magnum in normal individuals – this is a fairly frequent finding.
- The tonsils usually appear 'pointed' rather than rounded as in the normal.
- The position of the brainstem and fourth ventricle and the rest of the brain should appear normal in uncomplicated type 1.
- Syringomyelia may be present in 20–73% of cases (**126, 128–130**).
- May be associated with C2 and C3 fusion (Klippel–Feil syndrome), short clivus or odontoid or C1 abnormalities.

Chiari II (the Arnold–Chiari malformation)
Midline sagittal and axial images of the brain and spinal cord are required.

Brain:
- The cerebellar tonsils, vermis and brainstem are herniated through the foramen magnum and the fourth ventricle outlets are obstructed causing hydrocephalus (**131**).
- The cervicomedullary junction may be kinked.

- The frontal horns of the lateral ventricles are squared-off.
- The fourth ventricle is compressed.
- The aqueduct is stretched.
- The superior aspect of the cerebellum is herniated superiorly through the tentorial hiatus (which is enlarged), i.e. the whole posterior fossa is too small.
- Corpus callosum agenesis or partial abnormalities are frequent.
- Heterotopias and abnormal gyral patterns are common.

Spinal cord:
- A lumbosacral myelomeningocele is nearly always present (see p.140).
- The cord is nearly always tethered.
- A lipoma of the filum terminale may be present.

Less optimal imaging techniques:
- Plain skull and cervical spine x-rays may show cranial enlargement, a small posterior fossa with low tentorial insertion and dural sinuses, basilar impression (platybasia), enlargement of the foramen magnum, elongation of cervical arches, widened cervical canal, fusion of cervical vertebrae, and Klippel–Feil anomaly.
- Myelography followed by CT scanning of the craniocervical junction (the contrast material in the subarachnoid space helps to reveal the abnormality).
- Vertebral angiography.

TREATMENT
- The meningomyelocele and hydrocephalus should be treated promptly in an affected infant.
- When signs of progressive neurologic deficit appear in later life, hydrocephalus (if present) should be treated surgically by shunting and suboccipital craniectomy and upper cervical (C1) decompression laminectomy may help decompress the region.
- If clinical progression is slight or uncertain, a conservative approach is recommended, with ongoing observation and reassessment.

RACHISCHISIS (DYSRAPHISM)

DEFINITION
Defective closure of the neural groove (dysraphism).

EPIDEMIOLOGY
- Incidence: the incidence varies widely from one country to another and is about 1 per 1000. The disorder is more likely to occur in a second child if one child has already been affected (the incidence rises from 1 per 1000 to 40–50 per 1000). Abnormalities of closure of the cranium are more frequent than defects of closure of the vertebral arches. Even so, spina bifida occulta is found in 5% of the normal population. Meningomyelocele is 10 times more frequent than meningocele.
- Age: infants and children predominantly.

ETIOLOGY AND PATHOPHYSIOLOGY
Some degree of failure occurs during the first 3 weeks of fetal development of the folding and fusion of the dorsal midline structures of the primitive neural tube with its normal covering of meninges, bone and skin. Genetic and environmental factors are thought to interact. A genetically-determined variant of the 5,10- methylenetetrahydrofolate reductase gene that specifies a product with reduced enzyme activity is associated with NTDs. Folic acid reduces the risk of NTDs, not by correcting a simple nutritional deficiency but by overcoming the reduced activity in the conversion of 5,10-methylenetetrahydrofolate to 5 methyltetrahydrofolate.

PATHOLOGY
Brain
Anencephaly
Absence of cranial vault and its contents (**132**). The undeveloped brain lies in the base of the skull as a small vascular mass without recognizable nervous tissue. It is the most frequent of the rachischises. It has many associations with other conditions in which the vertebral laminae fail to fuse. It is incompatible with life.

131 Chiari II malformation. T1W midline sagittal view of the brain and upper cervical cord shows marked abnormality of the brainstem and cerebellum with downwards displacement of the cerebellum and no true fourth ventricle.

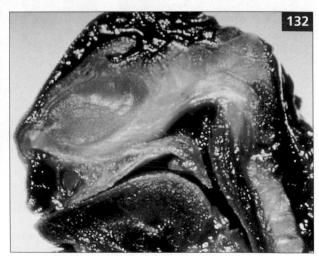

132 Pathologic specimen, sagittal section, of a dead fetus with anencephaly, showing absence of the cranial vault and its contents.

Cranial meningocele
Meninges protrude through a defect in the skull.

Meningoencephalocele
Meninges and brain parenchyma protrude through a defect in the skull.

Dandy–Walker syndrome
A failure of development of the midline portion of the cerebellum. A cyst-like structure, representing the greatly dilated fourth ventricle, expands in the midline, causing the occipital bone to bulge posteriorly and to displace the tentorium and torcula upward. In addition, the corpus callosum may be deficient or absent, and there is dilatation of the aqueduct, third and lateral ventricles.

Spinal cord
In the spine, dysraphism is most common in the lumbosacral area.

Spina bifida occulta
- Closure defect, due to failure of fusion, of one or more vertebral arches.
- The spinal cord remains inside the vertebral canal and there is no external sac.
- A congenital dural sinus tract occasionally communicates the skin with the lumbar CSF sac via the incompletely closed vertebral arch, and predisposes to recurrent bacterial meningitis.
- Lipomas or dermoids in the cauda equina region may be present and may not become symptomatic until later life.
- A skin dimple, vascular anomaly or tuft of hair may be present over the site of the lesion in the low back in the midline (**133**).
- Tethering of the spinal cord: may become symptomatic in children and sometimes adolescents (see p.142).

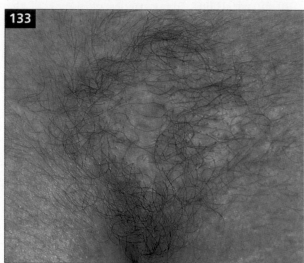

133 Photograph of the low back of a patient with spina bifida occulta showing a tuft of hair over the site of the spina bifida occulta, and a vertical midline scar following surgical resection of a cauda equina lipoma that was causing neurologic symptoms and signs.

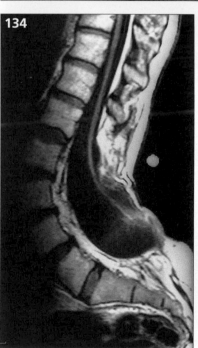

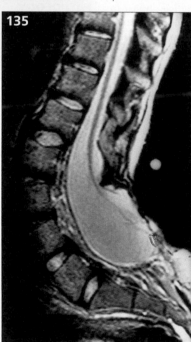

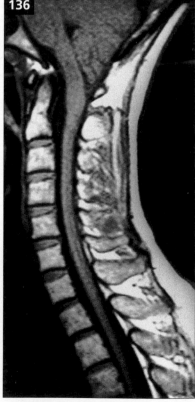

134, 135 MRI lumbosacral spine, sagittal T1 (**134**) and dual echo T2W (**135**) images showing a lumbosacral meningomyelocele and narrowing of the elongated lumbar cord with cord tethering. There is no lipomatous or other soft tissue mass related to the spinal dysraphism. Disc degeneration is noted incidentally at L2/3 and L3/4.

136 MRI cervical spine, sagittal T1W image, of the same patient in **134, 135**, showing inferior displacement of the medulla and cerebellum and elongation of the medulla (Chiari II malformation).

Meningocele
Meninges (dura and arachnoid) protrude through a defect in the vertebral arch as a cystic CSF-filled dural sac. The cord remains in the canal. Seldom are there any neurologic consequences.

Meningomyelocele
Meninges and spinal cord or (more commonly the cauda equina) roots protrude through the defect in the neural arch as a dural sac containing spinal cord or roots closely applied to the fundus of the cystic swelling (**134, 135**) . It may be associated with overlying dermal defects, Arnold–Chiari malformation (**136**), or hydrocephalus. Motor, sensory and bladder disturbances are common.

Spina bifida aperta (myeloaraphia/rachischisis)
Exposed neural tube without overlying leptomeninges, vertebral arch or dermis. The dural sac is open and neural tissue is exposed on the back. Severe neurologic deficits are always present.

Diastematomyelia
A septum (bony spicule or fibrous band) protrudes into the spinal canal from the body of one of the thoracic or upper lumbar vertebrae and through the spinal cord in an anterior–posterior direction, thus dividing the spinal cord into two for a variable vertical extent (**137, 138**). The division of the cord may be complete, each half with its own dural sac and set of nerve roots. This longitudinal fissuring and doubleness of the cord is referred to as diplomyelia. With growth this leads to a traction myelopathy. Often associated with spina bifida.

Associations
- Hydrocephalus as a result of aqueduct stenosis.
- Posterior fossa abnormalities.
- Syringomyelia.
- Klippel–Feil syndrome (fusion of cervical vertebrae or of atlas and occiput).

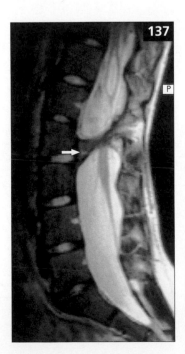

137, 138 Diastematomyelia. T2W midline sagittal (**137**), and T1W axial (**138**) MRI of the lumbar spine show a bony bar (arrow) across the center of the spinal canal with neural tissue (arrowheads) passing round it. Note also the spinal canal is abnormally wide and the visible vertebral bodies and posterior elements are misshapen.

- Congenital dislocation of the odontoid process and atlas.
- Platybasia and basilar impression.

Complications
- Recurrent ascending bacterial meningitis due to the presence of a sinus tract from skin to lumbar CSF.
- Progressive hydrocephalus from an often associated Chiari malformation.

CLINICAL FEATURES
Cranial meningoencephalocele
Small encephaloceles protruding into the nasal cavity may cause no neurologic signs unless innocently snipped off, when CSF rhinorrhea may result. Larger occipital encephaloceles may be associated with blindness, ataxia, and mental retardation.

Lumbosacral meningomyelocele
Lumbosacral polyradiculopathy
The child is typically born with a lumbosacral meningo-myelocele covered by delicate, weeping skin; sometimes it may have ruptured *in utero* or during birth. If the sac contains elements of spinal cord or cauda equina, there is neurologic dysfunction appropriate to the level of the lesion. If lumbosacral, the legs do not move unless the sac is stroked, which may elicit involuntary movements of the legs. The deep tendon reflexes are absent, there is no response to pinprick over the lumbosacral dermatomes and urine constantly dribbles. If entirely sacral, bladder and bowel sphincters are affected but the legs are not.

Progressive spastic weakness of the leg muscles
Stretching of the spinal cord, which is securely attached to the lumbar vertebrae, during the period of rapid lengthening of the vertebral column (see Tethered cord syndrome, p.142).

Acute or progressive cauda equina syndrome
Sudden or repeated stretching of the implicated sensory and motor nerve roots.

Syringomyelia (see p.541)

Spina bifida occulta
No clinical symptoms. May have overlying tuft of hair (**133**), discoloration, dimple or dermal sinus.

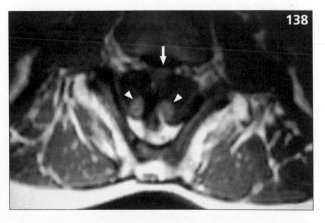

Tethered cord syndrome

- Derives from adhesion of the conus to one of the lower lumbar vertebrae resulting in malascent of the conus medullaris.
- Causes:
- Intradural fibrous adhesions.
- Diastematomyelia.
- Intradural lipomas.
- Dermal sinus tracts.
- Tight filum terminale.
- Clinical features:
- Onset: may be delayed until adolescence or even later if low traction on conus; may require additional mechanical triggers if low traction on conus.
- Progressive sensorimotor (segmental) deficits in the lower limbs (in about three-quarters of cases).
- Severe pain: perineogluteal region and non-dermatomal leg pain (three-quarters).
- Cutaneous stigmata of spinal dysraphism, such as subcutaneous lipoma, midline hypertrichosis, sacral nevus (two-thirds).
- Bowel and bladder dysfunction (two-thirds).
- Mild upper motor neuron signs coexisting with symptoms of conus dysfunction (one-sixth).

Associated hydrocephalus

- Rapid increase in head size.
- Downward deviation of the eyes ('setting sun' eyes) due to upgaze paresis as a result of pressure on the posterior commissure in the rostral midbrain.

INVESTIGATIONS

Meningoceles/meningomyeloceles

- Plain x-rays of the relevant part of the spine are useful to delineate the vertebral abnormalities (e.g. lumbosacral spine x-rays may show failure of fusion of one or more vertebral arches, hemivertebrae, block vertebrae, diastematomyelia).
- CT brain scan (+/− intrathecal contrast) may further delineate bony elements and soft tissues (ideally with 2D and 3D reconstructions) and may reveal enlarged ventricles due to hydrocephalus.
- MRI spine (midline sagittal T1 and T2W plus axials of the relevant part) is the investigation of choice for imaging the cord, meningocele contents (cord elements or just CSF) and associated abnormalities such as tethering of the cord, lipomas of the filum terminale, or dermoids in the cauda equina region (**134, 135**).
- Beware of the dangers of lumbar puncture: iatrogenic damage to the spinal cord by a needle inserted into a spinal cord that is tethered to the margin of one of the low lumbar or sacral vertebral bodies.

Diastematomyelia

- Plain x-rays may demonstrate the bony spur plus associated anomalies.
- CT with intrathecal contrast will demonstrate the relationship of the bony spur to the cord, nerve roots and thecal sac.
- MRI is really the investigation of choice (see Meningocele). It will demonstrate the position of the cord-tethering and splitting (**137, 138**).

DIAGNOSIS

Pre-natal

- Amniotic fluid alpha-fetoprotein and acetylcholinesterase immunoassay (removed at 15–16 weeks of pregnancy); blood contamination is a source of error.
- Uterine ultrasound.

Post-natal

Clinical ± radiologic (see Features, above).

TREATMENT

Prevention

- Genetic screening could identify women who will require folic acid supplements to reduce their risk of having a child with a NTD.
- Folic acid supplementation during pregnancy.
- Termination of pregnancy if the diagnosis is established at 16 weeks pregnancy and parents agree to a termination.

Conservative

If high spinal lesions and total paraplegia, kyphosis, hydrocephalus, and other major congenital anomalies, because of poor prognosis (see below).

Meningomyelocele

Excise in the first few days of life if the objective is to prevent fatal meningitis.

Hydrocephalus

Ventriculoperitoneal or ventriculoatrial shunt is used if hydrocephalus needs to be decompressed.

PROGNOSIS

Less than 30% of patients with high spinal lesions and total paraplegia, kyphosis, hydrocephalus and other major congenital anomalies survive beyond 1 year. 80–90% of the survivors are totally dependent on others for their care because of some degree of intellectual handicap and paraplegia.

TUBEROUS SCLEROSIS

DEFINITION

Tuberous sclerosis complex (TSC) is a neurocutaneous syndrome characterized by intellectual handicap, epileptic seizures, and hamartomas affecting multiple organs systems, including skin, kidney, brain and heart.

EPIDEMIOLOGY

- Prevalence: 3.7 per 100 000 population in Scotland, but may be as high as 8–9 per 100 000.
- Age: infancy and childhood.
- The disease may be present clinically and radiologically at birth but is usually not recognized until 2–3 years of age when delay in reaching milestones of natural maturation, mental retardation, or epileptic seizures become evident. Adenoma sebaceum appear later, usually between 4–10 years of age, and progress thereafter.
- Gender: M=F.

PATHOLOGY

The TSC affects all tissues, including the lymphatic system, with the possible exceptions of the peripheral nervous system, meninges, skeletal muscle and pineal gland.

Brain

Cortical tubers and subependymal nodules

Macroscopically, the brain is normal in size but may show areas (5 mm–3 cm [0.2–1.2 in]) of broadening, unnatural whiteness, and firmness on the surface of the cerebral cortex ('cortical tubers'). Their cut surface reveals a lack of demarcation of cortex from white matter and the presence of white flecks of calcium ('brain stones'). The surface of the lateral ventricles may be encrusted with white or pink-white masses ('subependymal nodules') resembling candle gutterings. Rarely, nodules of abnormal tissue are seen in the basal ganglia, thalamus, brainstem, cerebellum and spinal cord.

Microscopically, the tubers are composed of interlacing rows of plump fibrous astrocytes (like an astrocytoma but lacking in glial fibrillar protein). The structure of the cerebral cortex and ganglionic structures is diffusely disturbed with gliosis and the presence of atypical monstrous neurons and giant glial cell forms. Nodules composed of masses of subependymal glial cells intermixed with distorted neurons or giant glial cells protrude into the ventricles. These gliomatous deposits may obstruct the foramina of Monro or the aqueduct or floor of the fourth ventricle, causing hydrocephalus.

The cortical tubers and subependymal nodules both show histologic evidence of abnormal growth and migration, and occasionally they give rise to subependymal giant-cell astrocytomas. Neoplastic transformation of abnormal glial cells usually takes the form of a large-cell astrocytoma, but may, less commonly, give rise to a glioblastoma or a meningioma. Calcification may occur.

Skin

- Hypomelanotic macules are the first skin lesions to appear in about 90% of cases of TSC. They vary from a few millimeters to several centimeters in size, have an oval ash leaf shape with one end round and the other pointed, are arranged in a linear fashion over the trunk or limbs, contain sweat glands, and become pink when rubbed. Because of the reduced number and function of melanoblasts, which normally absorb light in the ultraviolet range, these lesions are more readily seen with a Wood's lamp, which transmits only ultraviolet rays.
- Adenoma sebaceum are small, red-pinkish-yellow, wart-like skin lesions with a smooth glistening surface, about 2 mm in size, which tend to be limited to the nasolabial folds, cheeks, and chin; sometimes also involving the forehead and scalp. They are angiofibromas characterized by hyperplasia of connective and vascular tissue.
- Shagreen patches are thick, slightly elevated, flesh-colored yellowish skin, 1–10 cm (0.4–4 in) in diameter, with a 'pigskin', 'orange peel', or 'elephant hide' appearance, over the lower trunk, most often in the lumbosacral region. These are plaques of subepidermal fibrosis.
- Subungual fibromas are fibromatous involvement of the nail bed, which usually appear at puberty and continue to develop with age. Other skin changes include café-au-lait spots, fibroepithelial tags (soft fibromas), and port wine hemangiomas.

Other

There is an increased incidence of:
- Glial tumors.
- Hydrocephalus.
- Spina bifida.
- Rhabdomyomas of the skeletal muscle and heart.
- Endocrine tumors.
- Cyst formation in the kidneys, pancreas, and liver.
- A honeycomb appearance of the lung.
- Phakomas of the retina: composed mainly of neuronal and glial components.

ETIOLOGY AND PATHOPHYSIOLOGY

- Familial (i.e. inherited as an autosomal dominant or recessive trait) in about 40% of cases, and sporadic (i.e. new mutations) in at least 60% of cases.
- Genetic heterogeneity: mutations in two genes. One gene, TSC1, is located on the long arm of chromosome 9 (9q34), and a second gene, TSC2, on chromosome 16p13.3.
- About 50% of TSC families show genetic linkage to TSC1 and 50% to TSC2.
- Among sporadic cases, mutations in TSC2 are more frequent and often accompanied by more severe neurologic deficits.
- Multiple mutational subtypes have been identified in the TSC1 and TSC2 genes.
- The TSC1 (chromosome 9) and TSC2 (chromosome 16) genes encode distinct proteins, hamartin and tuberin, respectively, which are widely expressed in the brain and may interact as part of a cascade pathway that modulates cellular differentiation, tumor suppression, and intracellular signalling. Tuberin has a GTPase activating protein-related domain that may contribute to a role in cell cycle passage and intracellular vesicular trafficking.

CLINICAL FEATURES

Clinically extremely variable with manifestations ranging from very severe illness to absence of symptoms (i.e. the *forme fruste*). Considerable variation is also observed within families.

- The usual presenting features in childhood are delay in reaching milestones, progressive intellectual handicap and epileptic seizures that are difficult to control, but only one aspect may be prominent. Over half of affected individuals have normal intelligence and a quarter do not have seizures.
- The seizures initially take the form of salaam spasms (i.e. flexion myoclonus with hypsarrhythmia [irregular dysrhythmic bursts of high-amplitude spikes and slow waves in the EEG]), later becoming atypical absence or more typical generalized seizures.
- Focal neurologic deficits and seizures may arise as a result of brain tumors.
- Dystonia and athetosis may also occur.
- Behavioral and affective disorders are present in about half of patients.
- Hypomelanotic macules may be visible on the skin using a Wood's light.
- Adenoma sebaceum typically occurs in childhood over the cheeks and bridge of the nose in a butterfly distribution (**139**). In some patients it may be more subtle and restricted to a few lesions in the nasolabial folds.
- Gingival and subungual (beneath the fingernails) fibromas begin to appear in adolescence (**140**).
- Phakomata (white nodules) appear in the retina on ophthalmoscopy.
- Other congenital abnormalities such as spina bifida and hydrocephalus may be present.
- Family history may be revealing.

DIFFERENTIAL DIAGNOSIS

- Mental retardation:
- Acquired destructive lesions: obstructive hydrocephalus.
- Chromosomal abnormalities.
- Multiple congenital anomalies: rubella.
- Developmental abnormality of the brain.
- Metabolic and endocrine disease: cretinism.
- Progressive neurodegenerative disease: lipidoses.
- Psychosis.
- Epilepsy (see p.65).
- Adenoma sebaceum: acne vulgaris.
- Other neurocutaneous syndromes:
- Sturge–Weber syndrome (see p.151).
- Von Hippel–Lindau disease (see p.392).
- Neurofibromatosis (see p.147).
- Ataxia telangiectasia (see p.444)

INVESTIGATIONS

CT scan or MRI scan

CT scan (**141–144**) or, preferably, MRI scan (**145**) of the brain may reveal:

- Cortical and subcortical tubers (50% calcified on CT, 3% enhance on MR).
- Subependymal nodules (80% calcified on CT, 30% enhance on MR).
- White matter lesions: seen on MRI as curvilinear or wedge-shaped bands radiating from the ventricles; 12% enhance.
- Atrophy and enlarged ventricles.
- Giant cell astrocytoma: usually near the foramen of Monro (**145**). These are larger than the other subependymal nodules and grow and obstruct the foramina. On CT or MR a prominent enhancing nodule near the foramen of Monro is likely to be a giant cell astrocytoma.

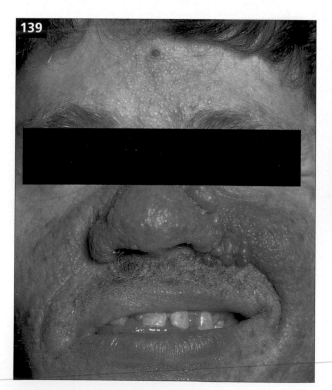

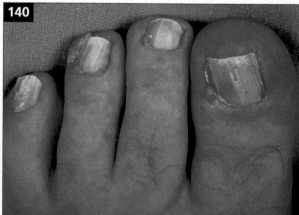

140 Ungual fibroma adjacent to the lateral border of the nail bed of the left great toe and third toe in a patient with tuberous sclerosis. (Courtesy of Dr AM Chancellor, Tauranga, New Zealand.)

139 Photograph of the face of a patient with tuberous sclerosis showing diffuse small adenoma sebaceum (pink, wart-like angiofibromas) throughout the cheeks, chin and forehead, and larger lesions in the nasolabial fold on the left. (Courtesy of Dr AM Chancellor, Tauranga, New Zealand.)

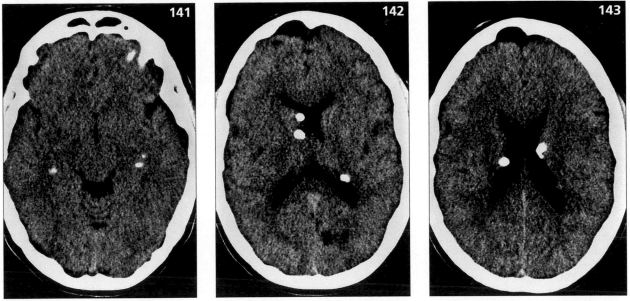

141–143 CT scan of the brain, non-contrast, axial slices, showing small white calcified subependymal nodules in the temporal horns bilaterally (**141**), frontal horn of the right lateral ventricle and posterior horn of the left lateral ventricle (**142**), and the lateral ventricles bilaterally (**143**) in a patient with tuberous sclerosis.

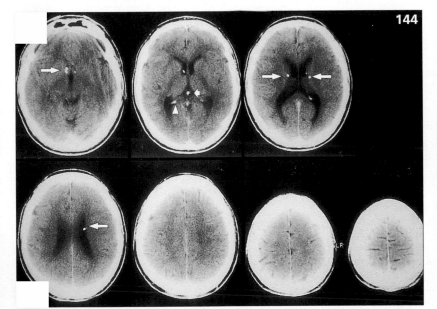

144 CT scan of the brain, non-contrast, axial slices, showing small white calcified subependymal nodules in the frontal horn of the right lateral ventricle, and the lateral ventricles bilaterally (arrows), not to be confused with the calcified pineal gland centrally (short arrow) and calcified choroid plexus laterally (arrowheads). (Courtesy of Dr AM Chancellor, Tauranga, New Zealand.)

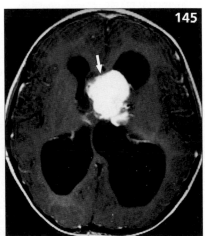

145 T1W axial MRI post-contrast showing a mass at the foramen of Monro (arrow) with marked contrast enhancement and mixed signal features in a patient with tuberous sclerosis. There is secondary hydrocephalus (the lateral ventricles are very large).

EKG

Echocardiograph
?Cardiac rhabdomyoma.

Abdominal ultrasound
Liver, kidneys.

Blood
DNA analysis for mutations in the TS genes located on chromosomes 9 (TSC1) and 16 (TSC2).

DIAGNOSIS
Definite TSC
Two major diagnostic features or one major plus two minor features.

Probable TSC
One major plus one minor feature.

Possible TSC
One major or two or more minor features.

Major diagnostic features
- Facial angiofibromas (adenoma sebaceum).
- Ungual fibromas.
- Retinal hamartomas.
- Hypomelanotic macules (three or more).
- Shagreen patch.
- Renal angiomyolipoma.
- Cardiac rhabdomyoma.
- Pulmonary lymphangiomatosis.
- Subependymal nodules.
- Subependymal giant cell astrocytomas.
- Tubers.

Minor diagnostic features
- Dental enamel pits in deciduous or permanent teeth.
- Bone cysts.
- Renal cysts.
- Gingival fibromas.
- Hamartomatous rectal polyps.

The diagnosis of people with minimal disease expression (the forme fruste) can be very difficult. In children the phenotype is often incomplete or not fully assessable. Hence mildly affected subjects, at risk for severely affected offspring, may remain undiagnosed. The detection of (small) mutations in the TS genes located on chromosomes 9 (TSC1) and 16 (TSC2) has recently become possible and may be helpful in the diagnosis of ambiguous cases.

TREATMENT
Symptomatic
- Epilepsy: anti-epileptic medication. It is rarely helpful to attempt tumor excision, particularly in severely affected individuals.
- Raised intracranial pressure: partial tumor excision or ventricular decompression.
- Adenoma sebaceum: dermabrasion of facial lesions may benefit patients who are not mentally impaired but they regrow slowly.

PREVENTION
Counselling of affected individuals against childbearing.

PROGNOSIS
- Slow progression, mainly in cognitive function, ultimately leading to death in adolescence or early adult life.
- Status epilepticus is now a less common cause of death, with better control of epilepsy.
- Malignant gliomas cause a significant minority of deaths.
- Incomplete forms of TS may have a better prognosis.

NEUROFIBROMATOSIS

DEFINITION
The neurofibromatoses are a group of neurocutaneous syndromes primarily affecting tissues derived from the neural crest. They consist primarily of two distinct neuroectodermal disorders (phakomatoses) which are inherited as autosomal dominant traits and characterized by localized overgrowths of ectodermal and mesodermal elements in the nervous system and skin.

CLASSIFICATION
- Neurofibromatosis 1 (NF-1): the more common type, also previously called peripheral and von Recklinghausen's neurofibromatosis. The responsible gene is located on chromosome 17q11.2, and is believed to function as a tumor suppressor gene. The protein product of the NF1 gene is called neurofibromin, a protein that negatively regulates signals transduced by Ras proteins.
- Neurofibromatosis 2 (NF-2): the less common type, also previously called central neurofibromatosis. The gene is located on chromosome 22q12.

EPIDEMIOLOGY
- Incidence:
- NF-1: 1 in 2500 live births.
- NF-2: 1 in 33 000 live births.
- Prevalence:
- NF-1: 1 in 5000.
- NF-2: 1 in 210 000.
- Age:
- NF-1: pigmentary lesions are nearly always present at birth but neurofibromas are infrequent then. Both lesions increase in number during late childhood and adolescence.
- NF-2: symptoms usually begin in the 'teens or early twenties', but occasionally as early as the first and as late as the seventh decade of life.
- Gender: M=F.

PATHOLOGY
Skin
- Hyperpigmented lesions (café-au-lait patches) which are characterized by an excess of melanosomes in the malpighian cells, which accounts for the dark color (there is no excess of melanocytes) and abnormally large melanosomes in some of the basal cells of the epidermis.
- Skin tumors: the collagen and elastin of the dermis is replaced by a loose arrangement of elongated connective tissue cells.

Nervous system
- Nerve tumors: composed of a mixture of fibroblasts and Schwann cells, except optic gliomas which contain a combination of astrocytes and fibroblasts.
- There is an increased incidence of brain tumors such as gliomas, meningiomas, and acoustic neuromas.
- Malignant degeneration of tumors occurs in 2–5% of cases, peripherally they become sarcomas and centrally, astrocytomas or glioblastomas.

ETIOLOGY AND PATHOPHYSIOLOGY
Autosomal dominant inheritance or spontaneous mutation. About 50% of cases have no family history.

NF-1
NF-1 is caused by a mutation of the NF-1 gene located on chromosome 17q11.2; 50–70% of patients inherit the mutation as an autosomal dominant trait and 30–50% (i.e. the remainder) of patients represent a new mutation. Full penetrance is exhibited.

The NF-1 gene codes for a large cytoplasmic protein of 2818 acids. The NF-1 gene product, neurofibromin, contains a small region in the central part of the protein that bears sequence similarity with a family of proteins that regulate the proto-oncogene p21-ras. These p21-ras regulatory proteins are collectively termed guanosine triphosphatase (GTPase)-activating proteins (GAPs). Since p21-ras can transform cells, neurofibromin (which downregulates/inhibits p21-ras activity) suppresses the growth of cells. The identification of somatic mutations in NF-1 from tumor tissue suggests that NF-1 is probably a tumor suppressor gene. The mutation probably results in a loss of NF-1 gene expression, which leads to a loss of neurofibromin.

Neurofibromin is hypothesized to function as a tumor suppressor (negative growth regulator) by:
- Inactivating the p21-ras proto-oncogene, thus reducing cell proliferation in some cell types, such as Schwann cells and astrocytes (in astrocytomas).
- Regulating microtubule signal transduction in the cytoskeleton.
- Influencing progression through the cell cycle and promoting growth arrest at the 'commitment' stage of the cell cycle, causing cells to exit from the cell cycle and remain in G_0/G_1.

The loss of neurofibromin causes a loss of suppression of cell growth, predisposing to particular benign and malignant neoplasms, which arise primarily from cells of neural crest origin (e.g. neurofibromas, neurofibrosarcomas, optic gliomas, and pheochromocytoma) and also immature myeloid cells (e.g. juvenile myelomonocytic leukemia, and the monosomy 7 syndrome, a childhood variant of myelodysplasia). The exact mechanism remains uncertain however.

NF-2
Inactivating mutations of both alleles of the NF-2 gene on chromosome 22q12.1, consistent with the tumor suppressor gene hypothesis. The gene product is merlin.

CLINICAL FEATURES
Clinical expression is very variable.

NF-1 type
Skin pigmentation
Multiple (more than 5) brown skin macules appear shortly after birth, usually on the trunk, but can occur any place on the body, and vary in size from a millimeter or two to several centimeters, and in color from a light to a dark brown (café-au-lait spots). Axillary and inguinal freckles or diffuse pigmentation also occur.

Skin neurofibromas

These appear in late childhood or early adolescence. They are situated in the dermis and form discrete, soft or firm papules which are flesh-colored or violaceous, vary in size from a few millimeters to 1 or more centimeters, and come in all shapes: flattened, sessile, pedunculated, conical and lobulated. When pressed, the soft tumors tend to invaginate through a small opening in the skin: 'buttonholing'.

Plexiform neuromas

Overgrowth of subcutaneous tissue, often in the face, scalp, neck and chest, which feel like a bag of worms or strings to palpation. The underlying bone may enlarge. If there is overlying hyperpigmentation which extends to the midline, suspect an intraspinal tumor at that level.

More deeply located neurofibromas

Firm discrete nodules may attach to a nerve which may compress the spinal cord, nerve roots, brachial or lumbosacral plexus, and peripheral nerves and cause pain and muscle weakness in the distribution of innervation of the relevant nerves. For example, neurofibromas developing on spinal nerve roots may extend through the intervertebral foramen in dumb bell fashion and compress the spinal cord (**146–149**). If not, they may attain considerable size in the posterior mediastinum or retroperitoneal space.

Vestibulocochlear (VIIIth cranial) nerve sheath neurofibroma

Nerve deafness, dizziness, headache, staggering.

Meningioma (see p.374)

Glioma (see p.364)

Optic nerve glioma (see p.372)

Progressive monocular blindness, optic atrophy, nystagmus, enlargement of the optic foramen, abnormal contour of sella turcica, and failure to thrive (if the hypothalamus is invaded).

Lisch nodules

Nodules appear as small whitish pigmented iris hamartomas.

Choroidal abnormalities

Bright, multiple, patchy regions at and around the entire posterior pole of most, if not all, eyes when viewed by infrared monochromatic light examination (but are not seen under conventional ophthalmoscopic examination or fluorescein angiography). These regions correspond to hypofluorescent areas on indocyanine-green angiography.

Other tumors
- Ganglioneuromas.
- Pheochromocytomas.
- Carcinoid tumor of the intestine.

Other features or associations
- Macrocephaly.
- Cortical dysplasias.
- Heterotopias.
- Aqueduct stenosis.
- Learning disabilities.
- Intellectual decline.
- Speech impediments.

- Headache.
- Epileptic seizures.
- Short stature.
- Cranial bone defects with pulsating exophthalmos.
- Bone cysts.
- Bone hypertrophy.
- Pathologic fractures (pseudoarthrosis).
- Bony malformations of the spine.
- Kyphoscoliosis.
- Syringomyelia.
- Stroke (ischemic).

Patients with NF-1 may have Schwann cell tumors on any nerve, but bilateral acoustic neuromas are virtually non-existent in families with this disorder.

NF-2 type

Bilateral or multiple acoustic neurilemmomas
- The hallmark.
- The first symptom is usually unilateral loss of hearing, which is often first noticed when using a telephone. There may be a history of intermittent ringing or roaring in one or both ears or some unsteadiness, particularly when walking at night on uneven ground (when visual cues are eliminated).
- Other symptoms include vertigo, facial weakness, sensory change, headache, seizures, or a change in vision.
- Symptoms are usually caused by pressure on the vestibulocochlear and facial nerve complex.

Other features
- Multiple CNS tumors:
- Neurilemmomas on cranial and spinal nerves.
- Intracranial and intraspinal meningiomas.
- Astrocytoma of the optic nerve, brainstem, spinal cord.
- One or more café-au-lait spots; skin changes are less common than in type 1.
- Subcutaneous neurofibromas.
- Lens opacity or cataracts.

TERMINOLOGY

Because NF-1 and NF-2 may have both central and peripheral nervous system manifestations, the terms used previously – 'peripheral neurofibromatosis' (for von Recklinghausen's form) and 'central neurofibromatosis' (for bilateral acoustic neuroma) – have been discarded as misleading and confusing.

DIFFERENTIAL DIAGNOSIS
- Normal patches of skin pigmentation: 10% of the population have one or more café-au-lait spots, but not more than six spots, particularly exceeding 1.5 cm (0.6 in) in diameter.
- Multiple lipomas.
- Sporadically occurring tumors of the nervous system: meningiomas, schwannomas, neurofibromas and gliomas.

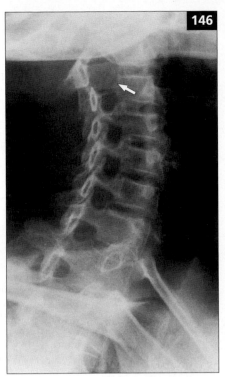

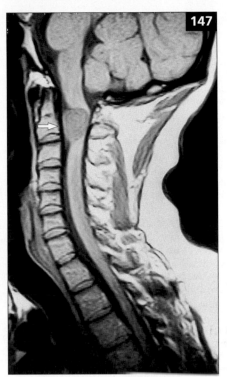

146 Cervical spine x-ray, oblique lateral view, showing enlargement of the C2/3 intervertebral foramen (arrow) caused by a neurofibroma developing on the C3 spinal nerve root and extending through the intervertebral foramen.

147 MRI cervical spine, sagittal T1W image showing a well circumscribed, low-density, neurofibroma (arrow) measuring 2 cm (0.8 in) in diameter in the anterior-posterior plane and 2.5 cm (1 in) in the rostral-caudal plane which is compressing the upper cervical spinal cord at C2.

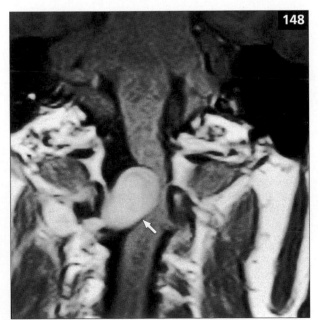

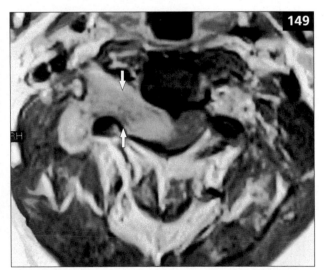

148 MRI cervical spine, coronal T1W image, after gadolinium contrast injection, showing the same lesion in **147** as a well circumscribed, dumb bell-shaped, high intensity, contrast-enhancing neurofibroma (arrow) measuring 4 cm (1.6 in) laterally in the coronal plane, extending from the upper cervical spinal cord at C2 through the C2/3 intervertebral foramen. The upper cervical spinal cord is displaced to the left (to the right in the image) and compressed to a crescentic shape.

149 MRI cervical spine, axial T1W image at the level of C2/3, after gadolinium contrast injection, showing the same lesion as in **147, 148** as a well circumscribed, high intensity, contrast-enhancing neurofibroma (arrows) extending from the upper cervical spinal cord at C2 (which is displaced to the left [to the right in the image]) through the C2/3 intervertebral foramen.

INVESTIGATIONS
NF-1

- Slit lamp examination of irides.
- Neuropsychologic assessment of IQ.
- Visual evoked potentials.
- Molecular DNA analysis.
- 24-hour urinary catecholamines if pheochromocytoma suspected.
- Imaging:
- Bone dysplasias and pseudarthroses of the long bones are best shown on plain radiography occasionally combined with CT.
- MRI is the investigation of choice for brain and optic nerve abnormalities though CT can be used (contrast enhanced).
- Optic gliomas (pilocystic astrocytomas pathologically) are seen in 15–40% of patients with NF-1. MRI (or CT) shows thickening and increased signal (on T2W image) of the optic nerves (usually bilaterally) or chiasm with variable enhancement. The signal alterations may extend posteriorly along the optic pathways (see p.372).
- Areas of increased signal on T2W image are often seen in the basal ganglia, cerebral peduncles, and hemispheric white matter. The exact cause of these is debated, but growth or new enhancement after adolescence may indicate malignant gliomatous change and requires short time interval follow-up scans.
- De novo cerebellar, brain stem and cerebral astrocytomas are also seen in NF-1.
- Plexiform neurofibromas favor the Vth nerve and orbit, are soft and elastic, and appear as enlarged nerves. These may undergo sarcomatous change.
- Astrocytomas of the spinal cord also occur (MRI demonstrates these best).

NF-2

- Audiometry.
- Molecular DNA analysis.
- Imaging:
- MRI is the investigation of choice for brain and spinal lesions.
- Enhanced T1W MRI is the best technique to demonstrate bilateral acoustic schwannomas. Any coincidental meningiomas or schwannomas elsewhere in the brain (Vth nerve is the next most common site) will be seen as strongly enhancing (white) masses, and gliomas (e.g. ependymomas) may also be seen.
- Other brain abnormalities include aqueduct stenosis, polymicrogyria and pachygyria.
- In the spine, multiple nerve sheath tumors occur on the nerve roots usually in the cauda equina. These may be intra or extra dural.
- Other spinal abnormalities include dural ectasia (lateral thoracic outpouchings of dura and scalloping of the posterior surfaces of the vertebral bodies) and syringomyelia.

DIAGNOSIS
NF-1
Clinical

Two or more of the following clinical criteria:
- Six or more café-au-lait macules whose greatest diameter is:
- >5 mm (>0.2 in) in prepubertal individuals, and
- >15 mm (>0.6 in) in postpubertal individuals.
- Two or more neurofibromas of any type or one plexiform neurofibroma.

- Freckling in the axillary or inguinal regions.
- Optic glioma (see p.372).
- Two or more Lisch nodules (iris hamartomas).
- A distinctive osseous lesion such as sphenoid dysplasia or thinning of long-bone cortex with or without pseudoarthrosis.
- A first-degree relative (parent, sibling, or child) with NF-1 by the above criteria.

Molecular DNA analysis

NF-2
Clinical

One of the following clinical criteria:
- Bilateral vestibulocochlear (VIIIth cranial) nerve tumors imaged by CT or gadolinium-enhanced MRI scan.
- A first-degree relative (parent sibling or child) with NF-2 and either a unilateral VIIIth nerve tumor, or any two of the following: neurofibroma, meningioma, glioma, schwannoma, or early- (juvenile) onset posterior subcapsular lenticular opacity.

Molecular DNA analysis

Mild and severe phenotypic subtypes of NF-2 can be defined using age at onset of symptoms ($\geq$20 years vs. <20 years), number of associated intracranial tumors (<2 tumors vs. $\geq$2 tumors), and spinal tumors (absent vs. present).

It is important to distinguish between NF-1 and NF-2 because the genetic basis and natural history are distinct. It is also important to differentiate between NF-2 and the sporadic unilateral acoustic neuroma, the latter of which is not inherited, it tends to develop later in life, and raises far fewer problems in management (see p.383).

TREATMENT

- Most people do not experience any functionally disabling complications.
- Surgical resection or decompression of tumors is indicated for gliomas and meningiomas and when neurofibromas compress cranial and peripheral nerves or spinal cord. The skin tumors should not be excised unless they are cosmetically objectionable or increase in size, suggesting malignant change. Plexiform neuromas of the face should be dealt with by an experienced plastic surgeon because they may involve cranial nerves superficially or affect the underlying bone by eroding it (a pressure effect) or causing it to hypertrophy from increased blood supply.
- Treatment of acoustic neuroma (see p.383).
- Genetic counselling for patient and family, including presymptomatic diagnosis of family members.

PROGNOSIS
NF-1

A progressive disease but the prognosis varies with the grade of severity, being more favorable in those with only a few lesions.

NF-2

- Bilateral acoustic neuromas are inherited in an autosomal dominant pattern with penetrance of over 95%, so that for any offspring of an affected parent the risk that these tumors will develop is about 50%. There are marked inter-family differences in tumor susceptibility and disease severity.
- The mean age at death is about 35 years. Almost all deaths are a result of a complication of neurofibromatosis.

STURGE–WEBER DISEASE (ENCEPHALOTRIGEMINAL VASCULAR SYNDROME)

DEFINITION
A rare, congenital and sporadic neuroectodermal degeneration (phakomatosis) characterized by:
- A cavernous or capillary cutaneous hemangioma (port wine stain) on one side of the face, but sometimes asymmetrically bilateral, in the distribution of the ophthalmic division of the trigeminal nerve, together with,
- A venous hemangioma of the meninges, usually ipsilateral to the skin lesion, and
- Atrophy, gliosis and calcification of the underlying cerebral cortex.

In 1879, W Allen Sturge described a child with sensorimotor seizures contralateral to a facial 'port wine mark', and in 1922 and 1929, Parkes Weber radiographically demonstrated the atrophy and calcification of the cerebral hemisphere homolateral to the skin lesion.

EPIDEMIOLOGY
- Incidence: uncommon. Isolated facial port wine stains without neurologic complications occur in about 1 in 5000 births.
- Age: present from birth.
- Gender: M=F.

PATHOLOGY
- Capillary or cavernous hemangiomatous malformation within but not always limited to the ophthalmic division of the trigeminal nerve; in some cases, additional divisions of the trigeminal nerve and other body parts are involved (**150**).
- Venous hemangioma of the leptomeninges in the parieto-occipital region. When the skin lesion involves the ophthalmic division of the trigeminal nerve, the venous hemangioma is usually present in the occipital lobes, whereas a facial nevus is more often associated with involvement of the parietal and frontal lobes.
- Atrophy of the subcortex of the brain on the side of the facial lesion, beneath the large number of abnormal blood vessels in the meninges, probably due to stagnation of blood flow and consequent hypoxia. In some cases, a band of calcification develops within the lesion in the second and third layers of the cerebral cortex.

ETIOLOGY AND PATHOPHYSIOLOGY
- Unknown.
- Sporadic usually; familial occurrence is exceptional.
- Intrauterine developmental malformation.
- There seems to be a close correlation between the maldevelopment of the embryonic vasculature of the eyelid and forehead and that of the parieto-occipital parts of the brain.

CLINICAL FEATURES
- Cutaneous angiomatosis (vascular nevus) on one side of the face and scalp involving the first (ophthalmic) division of the trigeminal nerve.
- Present at birth.
- Deep red (port wine nevus).
- Varies in its extent (**150**): it may be limited to only the upper eyelid and forehead or may extensively involve the entire head and even other parts of the body.
- Involvement of the upper eyelid nearly always indicates an associated brain lesion. Nevi lying entirely below the upper eyelid or high on the scalp are not usually associated with a brain lesion, but can occasionally be associated with a vascular malformation of the meninges overlying the brainstem and cerebellum.
- Margins may be flat or raised.
- Surface may elevated or irregular due to soft or firm papules, composed of vessels.
- Epileptic seizures (partial and secondary generalized), which usually begin in infancy or early childhood, sometimes followed by transient postictal (Todd's) or permanent paralysis, are usually the first neurologic symptom.
- Intellectual handicap in some cases.
- Hemiparesis, hemisensory defect, and homonymous hemianopia contralateral to facial nevus in severe cases, may arise abruptly or insidiously. The arm and leg may be small.
- Angiomatosis of choroid of eye with abnormal distension and enlargement of the eyeball (buphthalmos) ipsilateral to the lesion, sometimes with later glaucoma, causing blindness.
- Megalencephaly due to impaired cerebral venous return has been reported.
- Hypertrophy of the face in some cases: increased cutaneous vascularity may result in an overgrowth of connective tissue and underlying bone.

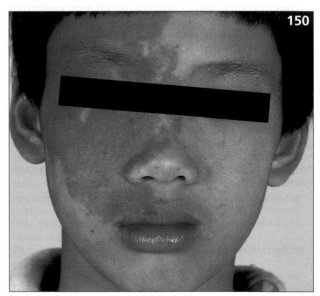

150 Facial photograph showing a cutaneous capillary hemangioma (port wine stain) on one side of the face in the distribution of the ophthalmic and maxillary divisions of the trigeminal nerve.

CLINICAL FEATURES
- Severe or recurrent episodes of:
- Epistaxis.
- Upper or lower gastrointestinal hemorrhage.
- Hematuria.
- Sudden focal neurologic dysfunction: stroke syndrome due to intracranial or intraspinal hemorrhage, or arterial obstruction by paradoxical embolism of thrombus from the systemic venous circulation or right heart to the brain.
- Iron deficiency anemia.
- Progressive focal neurologic dysfunction: enlargement of the intracranial or intraspinal vascular lesions, or occurrence of brain abscess due to embolism of septic material to brain via pulmonary fistulae.
- Epileptic seizures: arteriovenous malformation.
- Family history.
- Dyspnea, fatigue, cyanosis, polycythemia, clubbing, chest bruit.
- Telangiectases on lips, tongue, palate, nasal mucosa, face, conjunctivae, trunk, nail beds, finger pulps (**154, 155**).
- Cerebral and spinal telangiectases are usually asymptomatic.

INVESTIGATIONS
- Full blood count.
- Iron studies if microcytic, hypochromic anemia.

Brain arteriovenous malformation
- CT brain scan.
- MRI brain scan.
- MR angiography.

Pulmonary arteriovenous malformation
- Chest x-ray (**156–158**).
- Arterial blood gases and finger oximetry.
- High resolution helical CT (**159, 160**).
- Pulmonary angiography.

Gastrointestinal arteriovenous malformations, telangiectases, angiodysplasias
- Endoscopy.
- Angiography.
- CT for liver lesions.

DIAGNOSIS
Clinical
Any two of the following:
- Recurrent epistaxis.
- Telangiectases elsewhere than in the nasal mucosa.
- Evidence of autosomal dominant inheritance (the disease is found in heterozygotes but penetrance may be incomplete).
- Visceral involvement.

Molecular DNA
Mutation of the endoglin gene on chromosome 9q3, in some cases.

TREATMENT
Nasal telangiectases
- Humidification.
- Packing.
- Transfusion.
- Estrogen therapy.
- Septal dermoplasty.
- Laser ablation.
- Cautery eradicates a bleeding lesion, but satellite ones tend to form.

Skin telangiectases
- Topical agents: oxidized cellulose (Oxycel or Gelfoam) applied to the lesion.
- Laser ablation.

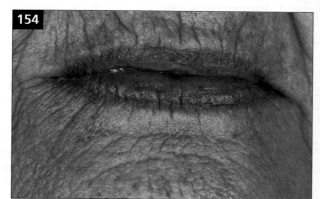

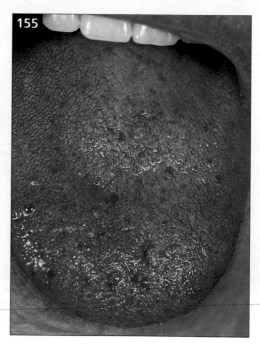

154, 155 Telangiectases of the upper and lower lips (**154**) and tongue (**155**) in a patient with hereditary hemorrhagic telangiectasia.

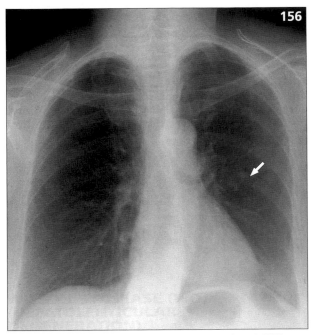

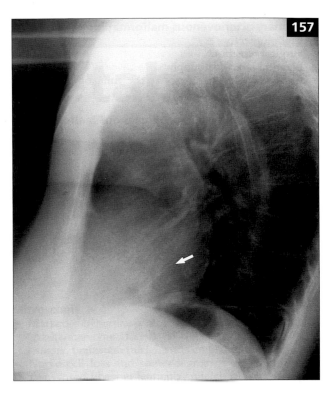

156, 157 Chest x-ray. Posterior–anterior (**156**) and lateral (**157**) views showing a pulmonary arteriovenous malformation in the left anterior mid zone (arrow, **156**) and the anterior aspect of the left lower lobe (arrow, **157**).

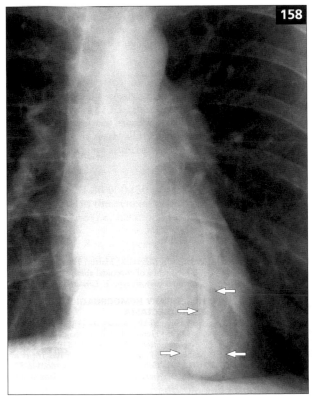

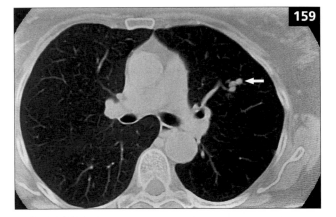

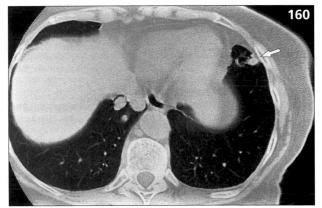

158 Chest x-ray posterior–anterior showing a pulmonary arteriovenous fistula (arrows). (Reproduced with permission from Hankey GJ, Warlow CP [1994] *Transient Ischaemic Attacks of the Brain and Eye*. WB Saunders, London.)

159, 160 Chest CT scan, images in the axial plane, at the level of the mid thorax (**159**) and the right hemidiaphragm (**160**) showing a pulmonary arteriovenous malformation in the left anterior mid zone (arrow, **159**) and the anterior aspect of the left lower lobe (arrow, **160**).

DIAGNOSIS

Clinical and laboratory evidence of:

- K–F rings.
- Low serum ceruloplasmin and copper.
- High urine copper excretion over 24 hours.
- High hepatic copper content on liver biopsy.

The abundance of specific mutations of the gene on chromosome 13 and their location at multiple sites across the genome have limited molecular genetic diagnosis to kindreds of known patients. The DNA-based diagnostic test can be done only in siblings of an index patient whose diagnosis was made according to phenotypic criteria and only if DNA from both patients is available.

Presymptomatic risk

Siblings of WD patients have a 25% chance of having the disease. Since both of a sibling's parents are carriers, 1/4 have the disease, 2/4 will be carriers, and 1/4 will have no WD gene.

Children of WD patients have a 1/200 chance of having the disease: from the patient, their children will definitely inherit the abnormal gene; for the patient's spouse, a normal person, the chance of carrying the gene is 1/100 and the chance they will pass it on is 1/2.

Grandchildren of WD patients have a 1/400 chance of having the disease: all children of the patient are carriers; from the patient's child, grandchildren have a 50% chance of inheriting a gene (1/2); from the other parent, a normal person, they have a 1/200 chance of inheriting the gene $(1/2 \times 100)$.

Presymptomatic screening

All siblings, aunts, uncles, children, nieces, nephews and cousins should be screened for WD, because those with even mild or non-apparent WD will ultimately become seriously ill if not treated.

The most appropriate screening test is 24-hour urine measurement of copper, which should be performed in asymptomatic individuals at about age 5 years and again at age 15 years. Blood ceruloplasmin is helpful but is normal in 5–10% of WD patients. Screening can begin for low ceruloplasmin and abnormal liver function tests at age 2 years. Ophthalmologic assessment for K–F rings can be diagnostic but they do not have to be present to have WD.

TREATMENT (see *Table 22*)

WD is a manifestation of copper toxicosis and, in most cases, symptoms can be prevented or reversed by achieving and maintaining a negative copper balance.

Table 22 Recommended treatment of, and pharmacologic agents for, Wilson's disease

Recommended treatment

Clinical status	Recommended treatment
Asymptomatic	Maintenance therapy
	Penicillamine
	Trientine
	Zn salts
Neurologic/psychiatric symptoms	Penicillamine
	Trientine
	BAL (can use in conjunction with oral therapy)
	Tetrathiomolybdate (experimental)
Chronic active hepatitis, or Hepatic insufficiency	Penicillamine
	Trientine
Fulminant hepatic failure	Orthotopic liver transplantation
	Chelation therapy and plasmapheresis pendingtransplantation

Pharmacologic agents

Agent	Daily adult dose	Mode of action
Penicillamine*	1–2 g orally in 2–4 divided doses	Chelator Possible inducer of metallothionein (MT)
Trientine hydrochloride	1.2–2.4 g orally in 2–4 divided doses	Chelator
Zinc salts	600 mg of metallic zinc orally in three divided doses	Prevents copper absorption by inducing intestinal MT; may also induce hepatic MT
British antilewisite (BAL) (dimercaprol)	3 ml of 10% BAL in peanut oil i.m.	Chelator
Tetrathiomolybdate**	Up to 2 mg/kg orally in divided doses	Chelator

* Administered with supplemental pyridoxine 25 mg orally daily   **Experimental

Presymptomatic

- Reduction of dietary copper to less than 1 mg/day: avoid copper-rich foods (liver, mushrooms, cocoa, chocolate, nuts and shellfish).
- Zinc sulfate, 200 mg orally, three times daily, blocks copper absorption from the gut. Adverse effects: epigastric pain, nausea, vomiting, and sideroblastic anemia.

Symptomatic

Medical

Limit dietary copper to less than 1 mg/day (see above).

Chelating agents:

Penicillamine (a copper chelator) can be taken orally. Begin with 250 mg orally twice a day before food and increase slowly over a few weeks to 1.0–2.0 g daily in 2–4 divided doses. Add pyridoxine 25 mg daily, particularly during pregnancy, a growth spurt, malnutrition or prolonged intercurrent illness. Pyridoxine deficiency, due to d-penicillamine, can be detected early by the presence of abnormal tryptophan metabolites in the urine. About 10% develop penicillamine sensitivity (rash, arthralgia, fever, leukopenia): temporarily reduce the dose or try a course of cortisone. Reinstitute in low dose (250 mg daily) with small, widely spaced increases. If the penicillamine sensitivity persists or if severe immune-mediated reactions (lupus-like or nephrotic syndromes) occur, the drug should be discontinued and zinc acetate (50 mg elemental zinc 5 times daily) or trientene substituted.

Triethylene tetramine dihydrochloride (trientine, TETA) is as effective as penicillamine and has fewer adverse effects, but is expensive. It is taken orally, 1.2–2.4 g daily in 2–4 divided doses before food. It is poorly absorbed from the gut. TETA reduces intestinal copper absorption and increases urinary copper excretion. Add zinc acetate 50–150 mg as a single dose at night (separate from the ingestion of trientene tablets) to prevent zinc deficiency. Toxic reactions are rare: sideroblastic anemia, reactivation of penicillamine-induced lupus, colitis and duodenitis.

Metal to metal antagonists:

Zinc sulfate or acetate can be used if penicillamine or trientene toxicity occurs. Doses are taken orally, 200 mg three times daily. It blocks copper absorption from the gut. Toxic reactions are rare: nausea, epigastric pain, vomiting, sideroblastic anemia. It is useful for maintenance therapy, treatment of the pregnant patient, and the initial as well as maintenance treatment of the presymptomatic patient. It does not seem to be optimal for initial treatment because it is somewhat slow acting and may take several months to control copper toxicity.

Ammonium tetrathiomolybdate blocks intestinal absorption of copper and binds copper present in tissues. Early studies suggested it may depress bone marrow and cause serious epiphyseal deformities in growing animals (and presumably children). A safe and effective initial treatment in a recent open study of 33 patients.

Metal-binding agent:

British antilewisite (BAL) (dimercaprol): if advanced neurologic lesions which have failed to respond to other treatments. Crosses the blood–brain barrier better than chelating agents.

- Monitor clinical response, full blood count, proteinuria, and urine copper excretion.
- A further 8% or so show no response to treatment.
- The appropriate drug needs to be continued for the patient's lifetime.

In about 20% of patients, chelation treatment results in an initial worsening of neurologic symptoms before improvement begins, and a few (1–2%) may deteriorate rapidly once treatment is started. This is thought to reflect the mobilization of copper from tissues, e.g. liver, and its redistribution in the brain, and for the redistribution of copper within neurons themselves.

Chelating agents have been used during pregnancy in WD patients without teratogenic effects.

Surgical

Liver transplantation: cures WD by removing the site of the metabolic lesion; chelation therapy need not be continued. If there is irreversible liver damage due to acute and chronic liver failure its place in the management of advanced neurologic disease is less clear.

CLINICAL COURSE AND PROGNOSIS

Course and prognosis vary greatly. Untreated, the course is invariably progressive and fatal. Most patients reach a terminal stage with severe dystonia and contractures, though a few may become akinetic. The disease may last from a few months (it tends to run a more acute course in younger patients) to many years with occasional periods of relative remission. With treatment, most patients improve or recover completely, but some do not. Some get worse before they get better (about 25%), some get worse and do not get better, remaining permanently disabled, and some die, fortunately very few. Pseudosclerotic patients have a better prognosis than the dystonic.

PREVENTION

Younger siblings can now be identified by means of molecular DNA techniques as normal, heterozygous or presymptomatic carriers of the WD gene. For the latter and relatives detected by screening (see above), prophylactic treatment can be started. Experience to date shows that such patients remain in good health so long as they take their medication.

INVESTIGATIONS

- Urea and electrolytes: most patients have clinical or biochemical evidence of impaired adrenal function and reserves: low sodium and chloride levels and elevated potassium levels.
- Adrenal function tests: serum cortisol levels decreased, urinary excretion of corticosteroids reduced, plasma ACTH increased, ACTH stimulation test negative: lack of rise in 17-hydroxyketosteroids after ACTH stimulation.
- Plasma VLCFAs (C26:0): increased several fold. The plasma VLCFA ratio C26:0/C22:0 is also increased several-fold compared with values for control.
- Skin fibroblast concentrations of VLCFAs: increased.
- CT brain scan: shows symmetric areas of low density in the parieto-occipital white matter, with later involvement of the temporal, parietal and frontal lobes. This can extend across the splenium of the corpus callosum and into the cerebellum. Contrast enhancement may occur around the periphery of the lesions. Occasionally there may be calcification and mass effect in the white matter lesions.
- MRI brain scan (**170**) in ALD shows increased signal on T2W image, decreased on T1W image in the areas outlined above, and loss of gray/white matter differentiation. MRI is more sensitive than CT and may also show extension into the long motor tracts and visual pathways. Enhancement may occur at the edges of the white matter lesions. Magnetic resonance spectroscopy shows a diminution in the N-acetylaspartate peak and an increase in the choline peak. In AMN, MRI brain is often normal, but shows involvement of the spinal cord and peripheral nerves.
- CSF protein may be elevated.
- Nerve conduction studies: often abnormal in AMN and suggest a mixture of axonal loss and multifocal demyelination.
- Molecular genetic analysis: for possible sequence variations in the ALD gene by polymerase chain reaction (PCR) amplification and single strand conformation polymorphism (SSCP) analysis.

DIAGNOSIS

- Demonstration of excessive VLCFAs in plasma or skin fibroblasts (a ketogenic diet can cause raised levels in normals) in a patient with appropriate clinical and neuroimaging findings and family history.
- The progressive childhood form of X-ALD may be accompanied by 'non-diagnostic' concentrations of plasma VLCFAs.

Presymptomatic screening

DNA analysis is the most reliable method for establishing the carrier status in X-ALD kindred; about 10% of heterozygous women have normal plasma VLCFA levels using current assays. However, the distribution of mutations over the whole coding region complicates such detection. Study of the ALP-P expression in white blood cells or fibroblasts may help circumvent this problem and identify heterozygous women, particularly when the mutation is not identified.

TREATMENT
Adrenal insufficiency

Adrenal steroid replacement therapy: may prolong life, increase general strength, and improve school performance but does not alter neurologic disability.

Neurologic disability

Three therapeutic approaches are under current investigation.

Dietary therapy

Attempts to lower the levels of saturated VLCFAs have included diets enriched in monounsaturated fatty acids (oleic acid), devoid of VLCFAs, supplemented with glycerol (glyceryl) trioleate oil (GTO) and glycerol (glyceryl) trierucate (GTE) (the 4:1 mixture of GTO and GTE oil is popularly referred to as Lorenzo's oil), and containing erucic acid (an omega 9 mono-unsaturated 22-carbon fatty acid), which competes with saturated fatty acids for the microsomal fatty acid elongating enzyme system. Although marked reduction of plasma levels of lignoceric (C24:0) and hexacosanoic acid (C26:0) have been achieved, there has been little or no effect on neurologic progression in patients who are already neurologically affected. One explanation is that little erucic acid crosses the blood–brain barrier and enters the brain. At present, dietary therapy is of limited value in correcting the accumulation of saturated VLCFAs in the brains of patients with ADL.

Bone marrow transplantation

When undertaken at an early stage of the disease in childhood, long term benefits have been described in small series.

Immunosuppression

Experimental.

PROGNOSIS

- ADL: rapidly progressive and fatal disorder within 3–5 years after clinical symptoms are detected.
- AMN: slowly progressive course over years. About 35% of patients will have substantial neurologic progression during a 3 year period, and cerebral involvement may develop in up to half at some point. The presence and severity of adrenal insufficiency has no bearing on the severity of the neurologic disease.
- Male siblings of the patient have a 50% risk of receiving the ALD gene from their mother but because the disorder is so clinically heterogeneous with various phenotypes, the risk of a male sibling developing AMN is less than 50%.

METACHROMATIC LEUKODYSTROPHY (MLD)

DEFINITION
An autosomal recessive lysosomal disorder characterized by demyelination of the white matter in the CNS and the peripheral nerves.

EPIDEMIOLOGY
- Incidence: rare (only 50 or so cases of adult form described in the literature).
- Age: late infantile form (age at onset, 1–2 years); juvenile form (age at onset, 3–15 years); adult form (age at onset, older than 16 years): mean age of onset 23 years; range 16–62 years.
- Gender: M=F.

PATHOLOGY
- Accumulation of sulfatides in the brain, peripheral nerves, and non-neural organs.
- Demyelination of the periventricular white matter (**171**) and peripheral nerves, with reduction of myelin sheath thickness in peripheral nerve.

ETIOLOGY AND PATHOPHYSIOLOGY
- Deficiency of the enzyme arylsulfatase A (ASA), which hydrolyses various sulfatides, including galactosyl sulfatide and lactosyl sulfatide, the major sulfate-containing lipids of the nervous system.
- Autosomal recessive inheritance.
- The gene is located on chromosome 22q13.
- Eight different MLD alleles:
- Type 0 alleles without residual activity of arylsulfatase;.
- Type R alleles with some residual activity of arylsulfatase.
- Late infantile form (age at onset, 1–2 years): homozygosity for type 0 alleles.
- Juvenile form (age at onset, 3–15 years): compound heterozygosity for type 0/type R alleles.
- Adult form (age at onset, older than 16 years): homozygosity for type R alleles.

CLINICAL FEATURES
Late infantile form (age at onset, 1–2 years)
Gait and behavioral disturbance.

Juvenile form (age at onset, 3–15 years)
Gait and behavioral disturbance.

Adult form (age at onset, older than 16 years)
Progressive neurologic or psychiatric symptoms and signs, which include any of:
- Dementia.
- Behavioral abnormalities: aggressiveness, irritability, impaired social awareness, and inappropriate behavior.
- Ataxia.
- Paraparesis.
- Polyneuropathy.

DIFFERENTIAL DIAGNOSIS
- Pseudodeficiency of arylsulfatase:
- A common genetic polymorphism, with an estimated gene frequency of 7.3%.
- Caused by a mutation affecting the polyadenylation of the arylsulfatase mRNA.
- Low arylsulfatase is not accompanied by accumulation of sulfatides in the organs, because the residual activity is supposedly sufficient to ensure normal sulfatide metabolism.
- Memory disturbances, ataxia, fatigue, tremor or loss of vision are present.
- Blood DNA analysis reveals homozygosity for the pseudodeficiency allele.
- Multiple sclerosis.
- Huntington's disease.
- Parkinson's disease.

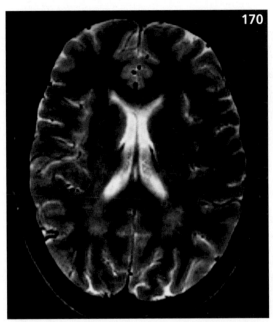

170 T2W axial MRI showing diffuse bilateral increased signal mainly in the parieto-occipital white matter in adrenoleukodystrophy. The more anterior white matter is beginning to look affected.

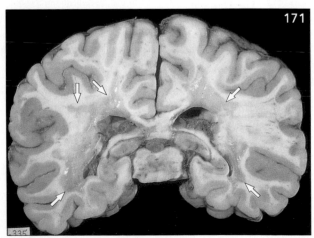

171 Brain, coronal section, showing extensive demyelination of the periventricular white matter (arrows).

INVESTIGATIONS
Blood
- Arylsulfatase activity in leukocytes: decreased (less than 35–110 nmol/h per mg of protein).
- DNA analysis.

Urine
Accumulation of sulfatides in urinary sediment.

EMG
Slowing of nerve conduction velocities (NCV): mean peroneal NCV: 25 m/s (range: 0–30 m/s [late infantile], 10–28 m/s [juvenile], 15–39 m/s [adult]; normal 44–57 m/s).

CT scan of the brain
Extensive areas of hypodensity in the white matter, especially in the frontal lobes, which does not enhance (**172**, left).

MRI brain
Extensive increased signal in the white matter on T2W image (**172**, right) due to diffuse demyelination of the periventricular white matter. The imaging features on CT and MRI are non-specific.

CSF
Normal or slightly elevated protein concentration.

Skin biopsy
Decreased arylsulfatase activity in fibroblasts (<270–770 nmol/h per mg of protein).

Peripheral (e.g. sural) nerve biopsy with acidic cresyl violet staining
- Accumulation of sulfatides as brown metachromatic deposits in Schwann cells and in large perivascular macrophages.
- Segmental demyelination and remyelination with slight onion bulb formation (less active in adult than late infantile and juvenile forms).
- Reduced myelinated fiber density and myelin sheath thickness.
- Ultrastructural examination reveals various types of inclusion, mainly lamellar zebra-like bodies and tuffstone bodies.

DIAGNOSIS
- Progressive symptoms of mental deterioration, behavioral abnormalities, or ataxia in combination with hypomyelination of the CNS and slowing of NCV.
- Decreased arylsulfatase activity in leukocytes or fibroblasts (not specific).
- Increased amounts of sulfatides in urinary sediment.
- Morphologic demonstration of accumulation of sulfatides in various tissues, e.g. sural nerve or brain.
- DNA analysis: to confirm or exclude a pseudodeficiency state of arylsulfatase activity.

TREATMENT
Late infantile
Bone marrow transplantation: conflicting results.

CLINICAL COURSE AND PROGNOSIS
Late infantile form (age at onset 1–2 years)
- Rapid course.
- Fatal outcome.

Juvenile form (age at onset 3–15 years)
More protracted course.

Adult form (age at onset, older than 16 years)
- Slowly progressive.
- The interval between the onset of one symptom (e.g. behavioral abnormality or ataxia) and the occurrence of the second symptom is about 3.7 years (range 1–20 years). The third symptom occurs, on average, 2 years (range 0–7 years) later.
- In the final stages , most are demented, severely ataxic, and have behavioral abnormalities. Psychosis is very rare.
- Death occurs 10 years (range 3–24 years) after onset of symptoms.

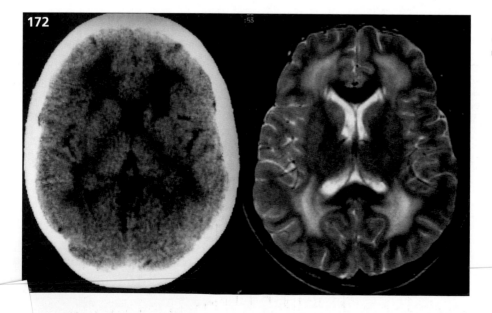

172 CT brain scan (left); T2W MRI (right) shows increased white matter signal.

ADULT-ONSET GLOBOID CELL LEUKODYSTROPHY (KRABBE DISEASE)

DEFINITION
A rare autosomal recessive disorder caused by deficiency of the lysosomal enzyme galactosylceramide β-galactosidase (β-galactocerebrosidase), resulting in accumulation of galacto-cerebroside in the central and peripheral nervous systems, particularly the white matter of the brain and causing demyelination.

One of the leukodystrophies, a group of inheritable diseases in which the abnormal metabolism of myelin components leads to progressive demyelination.

EPIDEMIOLOGY
- Incidence: rare.
- Age: adult-onset: a rare variant of the more common infantile-onset form of Krabbe disease.
- Gender: M=F.

ETIOLOGY AND PATHOPHYSIOLOGY
- Autosomal recessive inheritance.
- A variety of mutations of the human galactocerebrosidase gene on chromosome 14q24.3-q32.1 have been identified.
- Deficiency of the lysosomal enzyme galactosylceramide β-galactosidase (β-galactocerebrosidase), which catalyses lysosomal hydrolysis of myelin-specific galactolipids including galactosylceramide (galactocerebroside) and galactosylshingosine (psychosine), leads to the accumu-lation of galactosylsphingosine (galactocerebroside) or psychosine, which is neurotoxic to both the central and peripheral nervous systems, resulting in demyelination of the white matter of the brain and peripheral nerves.

PATHOLOGY
Macroscopic
A marked reduction in the cerebral white matter, which feels firm and rubbery.

Microscopic
- Widespread demyelination and astrocytic gliosis in brain, spinal cord, and nerves.
- Perivascular infiltration of large multinucleated macro-phages containing accumulated galactocerebroside (globoid cells) (**173**).
- Tubular or crystalloid inclusions in Schwann cell cytoplasm seen on electron microscopy.
- Large-fiber, demyelinating, sensorimotor polyneuropathy.

CLINICAL FEATURES
- Asymmetric spastic quadriparesis or hemiparesis, with brisk or absent/depressed reflexes.
- Visual failure with optic atrophy.
- Cognitive decline/dementia in some patients.
- Cerebellar ataxia.
- Peripheral neuropathy.
- Developmental delay, deafness, rigidity and seizures with infantile onset.

DIFFERENTIAL DIAGNOSIS
- Other lysosomal storage diseases: MLD, ALD, GM2 gangliosidosis.
- Multiple sclerosis.
- LHON.
- Wilson's disease.
- Mitochondrial disease: Leigh disease.

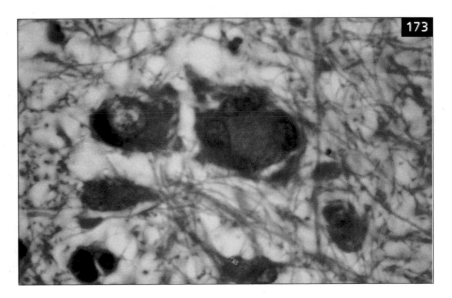

173 Microscopic section, high power, of brain white matter showing large histiocytes containing galactocerebroside (globoid cells) in a patient with Krabbe disease. (Courtesy of Professor BA Kakulas, Royal Perth Hospital, Australia.)

Table 23 *(continued)*

Arterial territory	Area supplied	Typical syndrome if total territory involved
Basilar artery		
Top of basilar artery	Rostral midbrain Part of thalamus Inferior temporal, occipital lobes	Variable pupillary abnormalities Ptosis or lid retraction Supranuclear vertical gaze paresis Somnolence Hemiballismus Amnesia Cortical blindness
Superior cerebellar artery	Midbrain (dorso-lateral), superior cerebellar peduncle, superior cerebellum	Ipsilateral Horner's syndrome Ipsilateral limb ataxia and tremor Contralateral spinothalamic sensory loss Contralateral central facial weakness Contralateral IVth nerve palsy sometimes
Anterior inferior cerebellar artery	Base of pons Rostral medulla Rostral cerebellum Cochlea Vestibule	Ipsilateral Horner's syndrome Ipsilateral facial sensory loss (pain, temperature) Ipsilateral nuclear facial and abducens palsy Ipsilateral deafness and tinnitus Vertigo, nausea, vomiting and nystagmus Ipsilateral ataxia of limbs and dysarthia
Posterior inferior cerebellar artery	Lateral medulla, inferior cerebellum	Ipsilateral Horner's syndrome Ipsilateral facial sensory loss (pain, temperature) Vertigo, nausea, vomiting and nystagmus Ipsilateral paralysis of palate (dysphagia) Ipsilateral paralysis of larynx (dysphonia) Ipsilateral ataxia of limbs Contralateral hemisensory loss below neck

Paramedian branches	Paramedian pons	Any of the lacunar syndromes:
		    Pure motor hemiparesis
		    Ataxic hemiparesis
		    Pure hemisensory loss
		    Hemiparesis-hemisensory loss
		Internuclear ophthalmoplegia
		Locked-in syndrome, if bilateral

Posterior cerebral artery	Occipital lobe Inferior temporal lobe	Contralateral homonymous hemianopia Cortical blindness if bilateral Amnesia (especially if bilateral)
Paramedian mesencephalic arteries	Rostral medial midbrain	Hemisensory-motor loss
Thalamic-subthalamic (thalamoperforating)	Postero-medial thalamus inferiorly	Hemisensory loss, amnesia
Posterior communicating artery		
Polar arteries (tuberothalamic)	Anterior lateral thalamus	Hemisensory loss, amnesia
Thalamo-geniculate	Ventrolateral thalamus	Pure hemisensory loss
Posterior choroidal arteries	Anterior and posterior thalamus	Hemisensory loss, amnesia

* Complete internal carotid artery occlusion, if symptomatic, usually produces symptoms in the MCA territory, but the ophthalmic and anterior cerebral artery territories can also be involved alone, or in combination with the MCA, depending on collateral supply.
** Basilar artery occlusion may also involve the territory of one or both posterior cerebral arteries.
N.B. Incomplete syndromes are common, and the symptoms of infarction and hemorrhage are similar.

182 T2W axial MRI of an infarct in the right hemisphere (arrow), obtained at 12 hours after symptom onset, in a patient with a left hemiparesis, visual-spatial-perceptual dysfunction and a left homonymous hemianopia (a total anterior circulation syndrome). Note the altered signal in gray and white matter and the mass effect.

Table 24 Clinical features, anatomy, pathology, etiology, and prognosis of the four clinical stroke syndromes

	Total anterior circulation syndrome (TACS) (*182, 183*)	Partial anterior circulation syndrome (PACS) (*184–186*)	Lacunar syndrome (LACS) (*187*)	Posterior circulation syndrome (POCS) (*188–194*)
Clinical features	1 Hemiparesis and hemisensory loss and 2 Homonymous hemianopia and 3 Cortical dysfunction (dysphasia or visual-spatial-perceptual dysfunction)	Any combination of two of preceding three in TACS or (3) alone, or monoparesis	1 Hemiparesis or 2 Hemisensory loss or 3 Hemisensorimotor loss or 4 Ataxic hemiparesis No hemianopia or cortical dysfunction	Brainstem symptoms and signs (e.g. diplopia, vertigo, dysphagia, ataxia, bilateral limb deficits, hemianopia or cortical blindness)
Anatomy	Fronto-temporal-parietal lobes or Thalamus/internal capsule/occipital lobe	Lobar	Small deep lesion in either corona radiata, internal capsule, thalamus or ventral pons	Brainstem and/or cerebellum
Pathology	Infarction (85%) or Hemorrhage (15%)	Infarction (85%) or Hemorrhage (15%)	Infarction (95–98%) or Hemorrhage (2–5%)	Infarction (85%) or Hemorrhage (15%)
Etiology	Infarction: occlusion of ipsilateral ICA or MCA, and occasionally PCA; by embolism from heart, aortic arch or carotid or vertebrobasilar arteries, or in situ thrombosis	Infarction: occlusion of branch of MCA or PCA; by embolism from heart, aortic arch, or carotid or vertebrobasilar arteries	Infarction: usually perforating artery microatheroma/lipohyalinosis or rarely arteritis or embolism	Infarction: occlusion of VBA or PCA, or branches; by in situ thrombosis or embolism from heart, aortic arch or VBA
	Hemorrhage: any of possible causes (see p.238)	Hemorrhage: any of possible causes (see p.238),	Hemorrhage: any, but usually hypertensive small vessel disease	Hemorrhage: any of possible causes (see p.238)
Recurrence rates	Low	High in first 3 months	Low but steady over 12 months	High in first 2 months and steady over 12 months
Prognosis at 1 year	Poor	Fair	Fair	Fair
Dead	60%	15%	10%	20%
Dependent	35%	30%	30%	20%
Independent	5%	55%	60%	60%

ICA: internal carotid artery; MCA: middle cerebral artery; PCA: posterior cerebral artery; VBA: vertebrobasilar artery

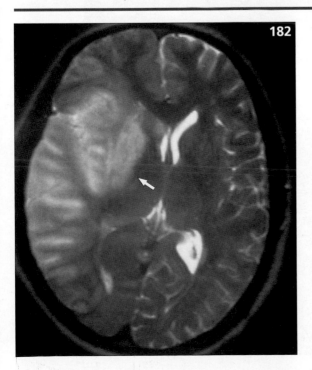

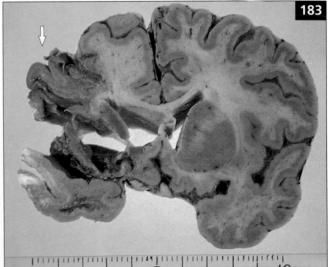

183 Brain, coronal section showing necrosis of the right parietal and temporal lobes, basal ganglia and internal capsule (arrow) due to an old infarct in the right middle cerebral artery territory causing a total anterior circulation syndrome. (Courtesy of Professor BA Kakulas, Department of Neuropathology, Royal Perth Hospital, Australia.)

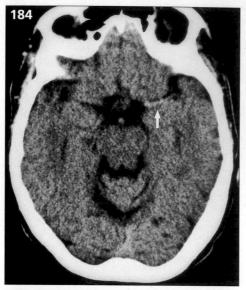

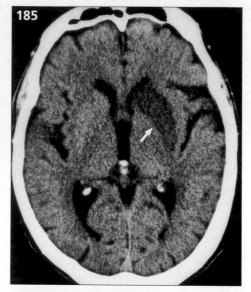

184,185 Plain cranial CT scan showing hyperdensity (due to blood clot) in the origin of the left middle cerebral artery (**184**, arrow), and left striatocapsular infarction in a patient who presented with a partial anterior circulation syndrome (right hemiparesis and dysphasia/cognitive deficit) (**185**, arrow).

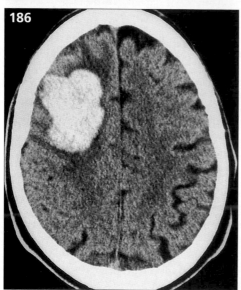

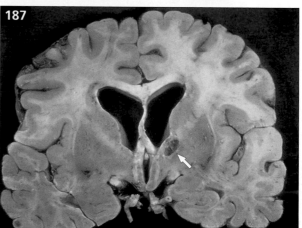

187 Brain at autopsy showing a lacunar infarct (arrow) in the internal capsule of a patient with a previous lacunar syndrome. (Courtesy of Professor BA Kakulas, Department of Neuropathology, Royal Perth Hospital, Australia.)

186 Plain cranial CT scan showing a homogenous area of high density due to hemorrhage in the right frontal lobe of an elderly man with amyloid angiopathy and a partial anterior circulation syndrome (left hemiparesis and cognitive/visual-spatial-perceptual dysfunction).

188,189 Eye signs of a patient with a posterior circulation syndrome due to an embolus to the top of the basilar artery causing midbrain infarction (**188**). Note the lid retraction, skew deviation, right internuclear ophthalmoplegia, and upgaze palsy (**189**).

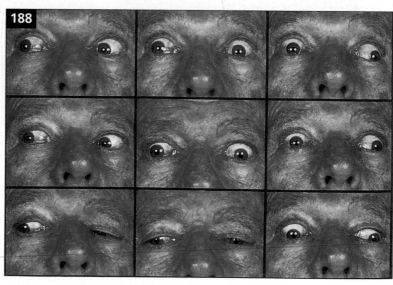

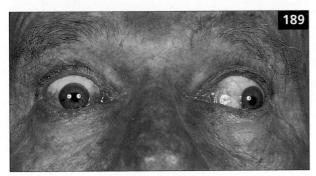

189 Lid retraction, skew deviation, right internuclear ophthalmoplegia, and upgaze palsy in a patient with a posterior circulation syndrome due to an embolus to the top of the basilar artery causing midbrain infarction (see also **188**).

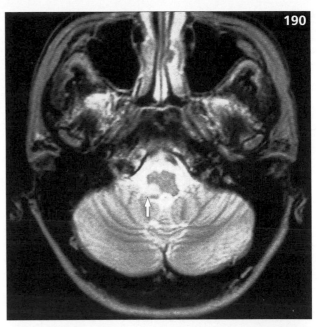

190 MRI brain scan, T2W image, showing an area of high attenuation, consistent with recent infarction in the right lateral medulla (arrow).

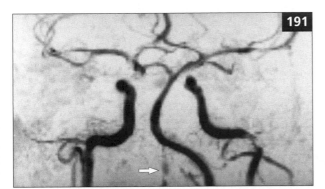

191 MR angiogram showing patchy signal in the right vertebral artery consistent with dissection of the right vertebral artery (arrow).

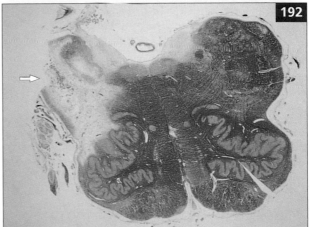

192 Autopsy specimen of brain, horizontal slice through the medulla at the level of the olives, showing pallor in the right lateral medulla (arrow).

193, 194 MRI scan, T2W image (**193**), and ventral surface of the cerebellum and medulla at autopsy (**194**) showing infarction in the right posterior inferior cerebellum (arrows) due to occlusion of the posterior inferior cerebellar artery.

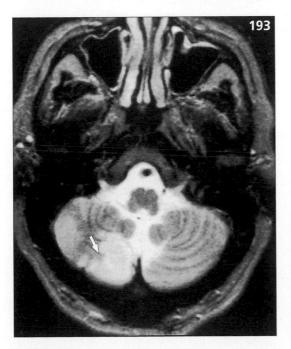

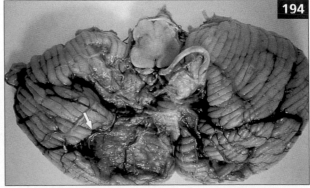

TRANSIENT ISCHEMIC ATTACKS (TIA) OF THE BRAIN AND EYE

DEFINITION
A clinical syndrome characterized by:
- Sudden onset of loss of focal brain or monocular function.
- Symptoms are thought to be due to inadequate brain or ocular blood supply as a result of arterial thrombosis or embolism associated with disease of the arteries, heart or blood.
- Symptoms last less than 24 hours. The 24 hour time limit for the duration of symptoms is purely arbitrary, having more to do with the earth's rotation than biology; there is no qualitative difference between patients with TIA and mild ischemic stroke in terms of etiology and prognosis, only a quantitative difference in terms of duration of symptoms.

EPIDEMIOLOGY
- Incidence: about 50 per 100 000 per year (crude incidence).
- Age: middle-aged and elderly; incidence increases with increasing age.
- Gender: M=F (age <55 years), M>F (age 55–75 years), F>M (age >75 years).

ETIOLOGY
A TIA is not a disease but a symptom of disease of the arteries, heart or blood.

Arterial disease (embolism/low flow) 75–80%
- Extracranial large artery (aorta, carotid, vertebral) atherothromboembolism 40–45%.
- Intracranial large (e.g. middle cerebral, vertebrobasilar) artery atheroma 5–10%.
- Intracranial small (perforating) artery lipohyalinosis/ microatheroma 25% ('lacunar' TIA).
- Non-atheromatous arterial disease (e.g. congenital, arteritis, dissection) <5%.

Cardiac disease (embolism) (see p.209) 20%

Hematologic disease (thrombo-embolism) (see p.218) <5%

CLINICAL FEATURES
Is it a TIA?
- Sudden onset.
- Loss of focal neurologic or monocular function.
- Symptoms maximal at onset: they do not spread or intensify.
- Symptoms resolve within 24 hours.

Focal neurologic symptoms and signs
Motor symptoms
- Weakness or clumsiness of one side of the body, in whole or in part.
- Simultaneous bilateral weakness*.
- Difficulty swallowing*.

Speech/language disturbances
- Difficulty understanding or expressing spoken language.
- Difficulty reading or writing.
- Slurred speech*.
- Difficulty calculating.

Somatosensory
Altered feeling on one side of the body, in whole or in part.

Visual
- Loss of vision in one eye, in whole or in part.
- Loss of vision in the left or the right half of the visual field.
- Bilateral blindness.
- Double vision*.

Vestibular
A spinning sensation*.

* In isolation these symptoms do not necessarily indicate transient focal cerebral ischemia.

Non-focal neurologic symptoms
Non-focal neurologic symptoms are not neuroanatomically localizing and are not due to TIAs unless accompanied by additional focal neurologic symptoms.
- Generalized weakness and/or sensory disturbance.
- Faintness and/or imbalance.
- Altered consciousness or fainting, in isolation or with impaired vision in both eyes.
- Incontinence of urine or feces.
- Confusion or memory disturbance.
- A spinning sensation*.
- Difficulty swallowing*.
- Slurred speech*.
- Double vision*.
- Loss of balance*.

* If these symptoms occur in combination, or with focal neurologic symptoms, they may indicate transient focal cerebral ischemia.

Where is the TIA? (see *Table 25*)

What is the cause of the TIA? (see Etiology [above] and Stroke [p.192])

Table 25 Where is the TIA?

Symptom	Arterial Territory		
	Carotid	Either	Vertebro-basilar
Dysphasia	+		
Monocular visual loss	+		
Unilateral weakness*		+	
Unilateral sensory disturbance*		+	
Dysarthria**		+	
Homonymous hemianopia		+	
Unsteadiness/ataxia**		+	
Dysphagia**		+	
Diplopia**			+
Vertigo**			+
Bilateral simultaneous visual loss			+
Bilateral simultaneous weakness			+
Bilateral simultaneous sensory disturbance			+
Crossed sensory / motor loss			+

* Usually regarded as carotid distribution
** Not necessarily a TIA if an isolated symptom, only if associated with >1 other symptom on the list

DIFFERENTIAL DIAGNOSIS
TIA of the brain
- Migraine aura (with or without headache): younger patients, positive symptoms (visual scintillations, tingling), spread or march of symptoms over minutes.
- Partial (focal) epileptic seizures: symptoms are positive (jerking, tingling), march over seconds, stereotyped recurrences, usually respond to anti-epileptic drugs.
- Transient global amnesia: abrupt onset of loss of anterograde episodic memory for verbal and non-verbal material, usually accompanied by repetitive questioning, which resolves within 24 hours. There is no clouding of consciousness, loss of personal identity, focal neurologic symptoms or epileptic features.
- Labyrinthine disorders: benign recurrent vertigo, benign paroxysmal positional vertigo, acute labyrinthitis, Ménière's disease.
- Metabolic disorders: hypoglycemia, hyperglycemia, hypercalcemia, (hyponatremia).
- Hyperventilation or panic attacks, somatization disorder.
- Intracranial structural lesion: meningioma, tumor, giant aneurysm, arteriovenous malformation, chronic subdural hematoma.
- Acute demyelination: multiple sclerosis.
- Syncope.
  - Drop attacks.
  - Mononeuropathy/radiculopathy.
  - Myasthenia gravis.
  - Cataplexy.

TIA of the eye
Retina
Vascular:
- Low retinal artery perfusion :
  - Internal carotid artery atherothromboembolism or other arterial disorders (**195–197**).
  - Embolism from the heart.
  - Retinal migraine.
- High resistance to retinal perfusion:
  - Intracranial arteriovenous malformation.
  - Central or branch retinal vein thrombosis.
  - Raised intraocular pressure (glaucoma).
  - Raised intracranial pressure (blowing the nose).
  - Increased blood viscosity.
  - Retinal hemorrhage (**198**).

Non-vascular:
- Paraneoplastic retinopathy.
- Phosphenes.
- Lightning streaks of Moore.
- Chorioretinitis.

Optic nerve
Vascular (anterior ischemic optic neuropathy):
- Systemic hypotension.
- Arteritis (e.g. giant cell).
- Malignant arterial hypertension.

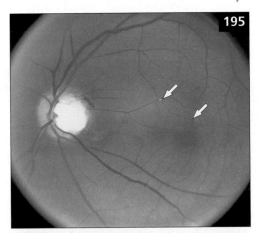

195 Ocular fundus showing golden-orange cholesterol crystals (Hollenhorst plaques) in the cilioretinal artery (arrows). (Reproduced from Warlow, Dennis, van Gijn, Hankey, Sandercock, Bamford, Wardlaw [2000] *Stroke: A Practical Guide to Management,* 2nd edn. Blackwell Scientific, Oxford, UK.)

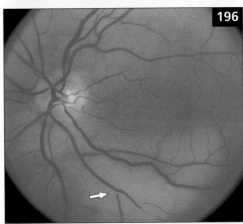

196 Ocular fundus showing an embolus in a peripheral branch of the inferior temporal arteriole (arrow).

197 Ocular fundus photograph of a patient with inferior temporal branch retinal artery occlusion showing pallor of the inferior half of the retina due to cloudy swelling of the retinal ganglion cells caused by retinal infarction. The inferior temporal branch arteriole is attenuated and contains embolic material.

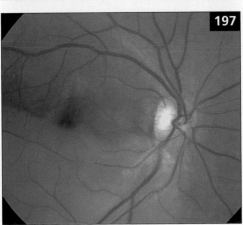

198 Ocular fundus showing a small retinal hemorrhage in a patient complaining of transient monocular visual disturbance.

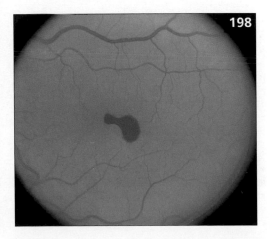

Non-vascular:
- Papilledema.
- Optic neuritis and Uhthoff's phenomenon.
- Dysplastic coloboma.

Eye/orbit
- Vitreous hemorrhage.
- Reversible diabetic cataract.
- Lens subluxation.
- Orbital tumor (e.g. optic nerve sheath meningioma): gaze-evoked loss of vision.

INVESTIGATIONS
All patients
- Full blood count: polycythemia, anemia, thrombocytosis/cytopenia.
- ESR: arteritis, infective endocarditis, myxoma, infections.
- Plasma glucose: diabetes, hypoglycemia.
- Plasma cholesterol: hypercholesterolemia.
- EKG: atrial fibrillation, left ventricular hypertrophy, silent MI.
- Urinalysis: diabetes, renal disease, infective endocarditis, arteritis.

Selected patients
Depending on patient's symptoms, age, general physical condition and willingness to be investigated and treated.

CT brain scan
CT is used to exclude a non-vascular cause of symptoms of TIA of the brain (e.g. meningioma, arteriovenous malformation) that may present like a TIA about 1% of the time (**199**). Not all patients with TIA need a CT brain scan, such as those with TIAs of the eye and perhaps single carotid territory TIAs. Patients with posterior circulation TIA or multiple carotid territory TIAs, particularly if stereotyped, are more likely to have a symptomatic intracranial structural lesion and should undergo CT brain scan.

Duplex ultrasound of the neck vessels (200, 201)
If a carotid territory TIA is present and the patient is fit and willing for carotid artery surgery or stenting (should imaging reveal a severe carotid stenosis on symptomatic side).

Magnetic resonance angiography (MRA) or intra-arterial digital subtraction angiography (IA-DSA) (202–207)
Used if duplex ultrasound evidence of >70% stenosis of symptomatic carotid artery (perhaps lower threshold to >50% stenosis if the duplex is unreliable and a true 70% stenosis could be underestimated as 50% stenosis), and the patient is fit and willing for carotid surgery/stent (**205–207**). Dynamic CT angiography is also under evaluation (**208**). N.B. Practice varies with some surgeons performing carotid endarterectomy on the result of ultrasound alone.

Transthoracic echocardiography (TTE)
Used if there is any abnormality of the heart clinically, on EKG or chest x-ray, followed by transesophageal echocardiography (TOE) if necessary.

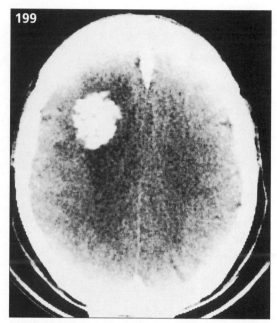

199 Cranial CT scan of a patient presenting with symptoms suggestive, but atypical of a transient ischemic attack which were due to this right frontal arteriovenous malformation.

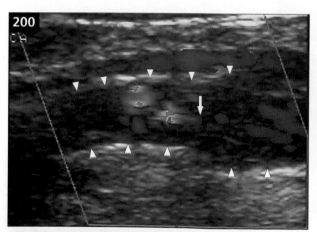

200 Color doppler ultrasound of a tight internal carotid artery stenosis. Note the black outline of the arterial wall (arrowheads) with a thin color jet in the center indicating the stenosis (arrow).

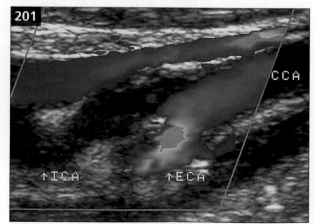

201 Color doppler ultrasound of an internal carotid artery occlusion. The outline of the internal carotid artery is visible but there is no color signal within it, whereas the external carotid is clearly patent.

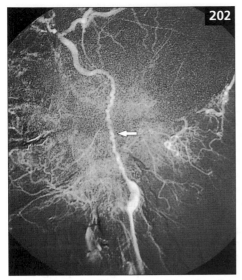

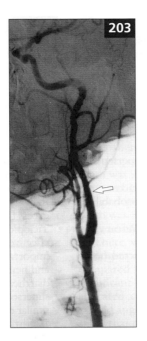

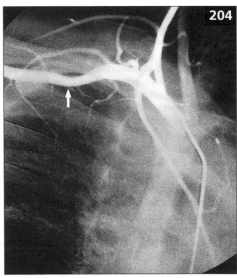

202, 203 Intra-arterial angiograms of fibromuscular hyperplasia. Note the narrowed and beaded appearance of the internal carotid artery (arrow).

204 Angiogram of a patient with painful arm and hand and intermittent blue fingers. It shows a cervical rib and subclavian artery compression (arrow).

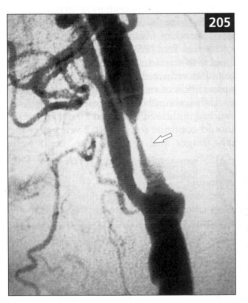

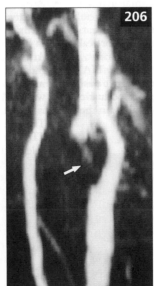

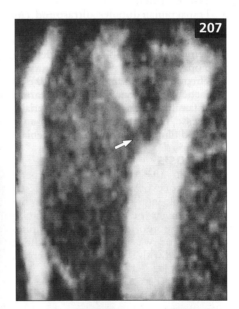

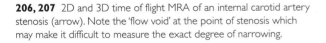

205 Intra-arterial DSA of a tight internal carotid artery stenosis (arrow).

206, 207 2D and 3D time of flight MRA of an internal carotid artery stenosis (arrow). Note the 'flow void' at the point of stenosis which may make it difficult to measure the exact degree of narrowing.

208 Spiral CT angiogram of an internal carotid artery stenosis (arrow). Note the anatomic detail is good, but lots of calcification (there is only a little in this example) may obscure the detail of the lesion.

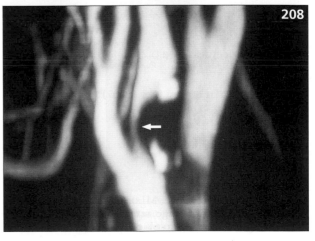

Cardiogenic embolism (see p.209)

Anticoagulation: warfarin (target INR 2.0–3.0), if major cardiac source of embolism:

- Atrial fibrillation (non-rheumatic): reduces annual stroke risk by two-thirds from about 12% to 4%.
- Recent (<3 months) myocardial infarction: treat for at least 3 months, and continue longer if chronic AF or other risk factor: large anterior MI or apex involvement; mural thrombus; high risk (AF, heart failure, previous embolic event).
- Dilated cardiomyopathy.
- Cardiac failure.
- Valvular heart disease: mitral stenosis or regurgitation; mechanical prosthetic aortic or mitral valve.
- Complicated patent foramen ovale not closed surgically (associated with atrial septal aneurysm or mitral valve prolapse) – anticoagulation is controversial/unproven.

PROGNOSIS

As a group, TIA patients have an increased risk of stroke and other serious vascular events of about 8–10% per year. The risk of stroke is about 4–5% in the first month, 12% in the first year, 29% over 5 years. The risk of a coronary event is about 3% per year.

As individuals, TIA patients have a variable prognosis. Independent predictors of an increased risk of stroke and other cardiovascular events are:

- TIAs of the brain (compared with TIAs of the eye).
- Increasing age.
- Increasing number of TIAs in the previous 3 months (i.e. multiple attacks).
- Peripheral vascular disease.
- Carotid stenosis >80%.

Other adverse prognostic factors may include: past history of any TIA, left ventricular hypertrophy, carotid plaque morphology (e.g. ulceration), impaired cerebrovascular reserve.

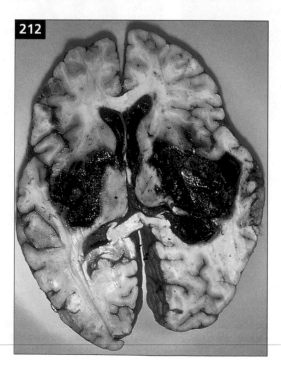

212 Axial slice of the brain at autopsy showing bilateral basal ganglia hemorrhage with rupture into the ventricles in a patient with severe hypertension.

STROKE

DEFINITION

A generic term describing a clinical syndrome characterized by the sudden onset of a focal neurologic deficit (or coma) due to infarction of, or hemorrhage into or over, a part of the brain. The deficit persists for longer than 24 hours or leads to earlier death.

EPIDEMIOLOGY

- Incidence: 2 per 1000 per year.
- Age: any age but the incidence of stroke increases steeply with age.
- Gender: M>F in middle age, F>M in old age.
- Burden: stroke is the third most common cause of death (10–12% of all deaths) in developed countries and a major cause of adult physical disability.

PATHOGENESIS
Cerebral infarction (75–80%)

- Large artery atherothromboembolism (50%):
- Extracranial (aorta, carotid, vertebral arteries) (40–45%).
- Intracranial (ICA, MCA, ACA, Vertebral, Basilar, PCA) (5–10%).
- Small artery microatheroma/lipohyalinosis (lacunar syndromes) (25%).
- Embolism from the heart (20%).
- Blood disease (thrombophilia) (<5%).
- Non-atheromatous arterial disease (e.g. dissection, arteritis) (<5%).

Intracerebral hemorrhage (10–15%) (212)

- Hypertensive lipohyalinosis and microaneurysms (40%).
- Bleeding diatheses (e.g. antithrombotic drugs, thrombocytopenia) (10%).
- Arteriovenous malformation (10%).
- Amyloid angiopathy (10%).
- Hemorrhagic transformation of cerebral infarct (10%).
- Aneurysm (8%).
- Intracerebral tumor (5%).
- Arteritis (<5%).
- Drugs: sympathomimetics (e.g. amphetamines, cocaine) (<5%).
- Arterial dissection (<5%).
- Intracranial venous thrombosis (<5%).

Subarachnoid hemorrhage (5%)

- Aneurysm.
- Arteriovenous malformation.

Unknown (5%)

Vascular risk factors and diseases in first-ever ischemic stroke*

- Hypertension (BP >21.3/12 kPa [160/90 mmHg] on two occasions pre-stroke): 52%.
- Angina and/or past myocardial infarction: 38%.

- Current smoker: 27%.
- Claudication and/or absent foot pulses: 25%.
- Major cardiac embolic source: 20%.
- Transient ischemic attack (TIA): 14%.
- Cervical arterial bruit: 14%.
- Diabetes mellitus: 10%.
- Any of the above: 80%.

* Sandercock PAG, Warlow CP, Jones LN, Starkey IR (1989) Predisposing factors for cerebral infarction: The Oxfordshire Community Stroke Project. *BMJ*, **298**: 75–80.

CLINICAL FEATURES
Is it a stroke?
- Sudden onset.
- Loss of focal neurologic function (see TIA, p.186).
- Symptoms and signs are maximal within a few seconds or minutes, but sometimes evolve over a few hours or progress in a stepwise fashion due to propagation of thrombus, recurrent embolization, or hemorrhagic transformation of the infarct. Progression over more than a few hours or failure to improve after a few days, suggests complications (e.g. brain edema, hydrocephalus) and an alternative diagnosis (e.g. tumor).
- Symptoms persist beyond 24 hours (by arbitrary definition).

Where is the stroke? (see Neurovascular syndromes, p.181)

What is the cause of the stroke?
Infarction or hemorrhage?
There are no clinical features that reliably distinguish intracerebral hemorrhage from infarction. Headache, coma at onset, vomiting and rapid deterioration are more common with hemorrhage but may also occur with infarction. The sudden onset of severe headache associated with neck stiffness or coma distinguishes subarachnoid hemorrhage (SAH) from other causes (see SAH, p.249).

Clues to the cause of the ischemic and hemorrhagic stroke, or alternative diagnosis
Clinical history:
- Age, sex and race.
- Presenting complaint:
- Onset, if gradual: consider low flow (hemodynamic) ischemic stroke; migraine; structural intracranial lesion; multiple sclerosis.
- Precipitating factors: standing up quickly, heavy meal, hot weather, hot bath, warming the face, exercise, valsalva maneuver, chest symptoms such as pain or palpitations, starting or changing blood pressure-lowering drugs, head turning – all suggest low flow; hypoglycemia.
- Injury to head or neck: vertebral/carotid artery dissection, chronic subdural hematoma.
- Associated symptoms:
- Recent headache: carotid/vertebral dissection; giant cell arteritis (or other vasculitis); migrainous stroke/TIA; intracranial venous thrombosis; structural intracranial lesion.
- Epileptic seizures: cortical infarction or hemorrhage; intracranial venous thrombosis; mitochondrial cytopathy; non-vascular intracranial lesion.
- Malaise: inflammatory arterial disorders; infective endocarditis; cardiac myxoma; cancer; thrombotic thrombocytopenic purpura; sarcoidosis.

- Self-audible bruits: internal carotid artery stenosis (distal); dural arteriovenous fistula; glomus tumor; carotico-cavernous fistula.
- Medications/drugs:
- Blood pressure-lowering/vasodilators.
- Hypoglycemic drugs.
- Cocaine, amphetamines, ephedrine, phenylpropanolamine, ecstasy (methylenedioxyamphetamine).
- Oral contraceptives; estrogens in men.
- Allopurinol.
- Interleukin 2.
- Deoxycoformycin (pentostatin).
- L-asparaginase (asparaginase).
- Past medical history:
- Previous stroke or TIA.
- Vascular risk factors (see above).
- Recent myocardial infarction.
- Rheumatic fever.
- Inflammatory bowel disease.
- Celiac disease.
- Irradiation of the head or neck.
- Recurrent deep venous thrombosis.
- Recurrent miscarriages.
- Family history: (gene/chromosome location, if known)
- Connective tissue disorders:
  Ehlers–Danlos syndrome type IV: (collagen 3A1).
  Pseudoxanthoma elasticum.
  Marfan's syndrome: (fibrillin).
  Fibromuscular dysplasia.
  Familial mitral valve prolapse.
- Hematologic disorders:
  Sickle cell (SC) disease/trait.
  Antithrombin III deficiency.
  Protein C deficiency.
  Protein S deficiency.
  Plasminogen abnormality/deficiency.
  Dysfibrinogenemia.
  Hemophilia and other inherited coagulation factor deficiencies.
- Others:
  Familial hypercholesterolemia.
  Neurofibromatosis.
  Homocystinuria.
  Fabry's disease.
  Hereditary cerebral amyloid angiopathy: Dutch type, (amyloid precursor protein).
  Hereditary cerebral amyloid angiopathy: Icelandic type, (cystatin C).
  Migraine.
  Familial cardiac myxoma.
  Familial cardiomyopathies.
  Mitochondrial cytopathy: (mitochondrial tRNA-leu).
  CADASIL (cerebral autosomal dominant arteriopathy with subcortical infarcts and leukoencephalopathy): (notch3 mutations, 19q12).
  Sneddon's syndrome.
  Arteriovenous malformations.
  Cerebral cavernous malformation: (7q22; genetic heterogeneity).
  Intracranial saccular aneurysms.
  Polycystic kidney disease: (polycystin).
  Hereditary hemorrhagic telangiectasia-1: (endoglin).
  Hereditary hemorrhagic telangiectasia-2: (activin receptor-like kinase 1).

Examination:
- Body weight.
- Pulses:
- Present or absent (peripheral vascular disease).
- Tenderness (giant cell arteritis).
- Rhythm (atrial fibrillation).
- Blood pressure:
- Supine and erect (hypertension, postural hypotension).
- Both arms (subclavian steal or aortic dissection).
- Neck bruits*.
- Neck stiffness.
- Heart: murmurs (valvular heart disease).
- Eye:
- Conjunctival injection and rubeosis iridis (ischemic oculopathy) (**8, 9**).
- Horner's syndrome (carotid dissection).
- Ocular fundi: retinal emboli; hypertensive, diabetic or ischemic retinopathy.
- Neurologic examination: impairments (see Neurovascular syndromes, p.181), disabilities and handicaps. Observe the patient attempting functional tasks such as those required for everyday activities of daily living. These are vital in assessing and monitoring the patient's prognosis and structuring an appropriate rehabilitation program.

*N.B. Listening for carotid bruits is not particularly helpful as their absence does not exclude tight carotid stenosis and their presence does not mean that the patient has tight common or internal carotid artery stenosis; a carotid bruit can be a normal finding in young adults; it can be due to external carotid stenosis (which is irrelevant to the patient's symptoms); it can be transmitted from the heart and great vessels in patients with aortic or mitral valve disease, a patent ductus arteriosus or coarctation of the aorta; and it can be part of a diffuse neck bruit in patients with thyrotoxicosis or a hyperdynamic circulation associated with pregnancy, anemia, fever and hemodialysis.

Skin signs of underlying causes of TIA or stroke
- Finger clubbing(**14**): cancer; right to left intracardiac shunt; pulmonary arterial venous malformation; infective endocarditis; inflammatory bowel disease.
- Splinter hemorrhages: infective endocarditis; cholesterol embolization syndrome; vasculitis.
- Scleroderma: systemic sclerosis.
- Livedo reticularis: Sneddon's syndrome; systemic lupus erythematosus; polyarteritis nodosa; cholesterol emboliz-ation syndrome.
- Lax skin: Ehlers–Danlos syndrome; pseudoxanthoma elasticum.
- Skin color: anemia; polycythemia; cyanosis (right to left intracardiac or pulmonary shunt).
- Porcelain white papules/scars: Kohlmeier–Degos' disease.
- Skin scars: Ehlers–Danlos syndrome.
- Petechiae/purpura/bruising: thrombotic thrombocyto-penic purpura; fat embolism; cholesterol embolization syndrome; Ehlers–Danlos syndrome.
- Oro-genital ulceration: Behçet's disease.
- Rash: Fabry's disease.
- Epidermal nevi: epidermal nevus syndrome.
- Café-au-lait patches: neurofibromatosis.
- Thrombosed veins, needle marks: i.v. drug abuse.

DIFFERENTIAL DIAGNOSIS OF STROKE (IN ORDER OF FREQUENCY OF OCCURRENCE IN GENERAL PRACTICE)
- Metabolic/toxic encephalopathy (hypoglycemia, non-ketotic hyperglycemia, hyponatremia, Wernicke–Korsa-koff syndrome, hepatic encephalopathy, alcohol and drug intoxication).
- Functional/non-neurologic (e.g. hysteria).
- Epileptic seizure (postictal Todd's paresis).
- Structural intracranial lesions (subdural hematoma, tumor, arteriovenous malformation).
- Encephalitis (e.g. herpes simplex virus)/brain abscess.
- Head injury.
- Peripheral nerve lesion(s).
- Hypertensive encephalopathy.
- Multiple sclerosis.
- Creutzfeldt–Jakob disease.

INVESTIGATIONS
All patients
Immediate CT brain scan(213–217)
- To exclude non-stroke pathology (**213–215**):
- Unclear history of sudden onset of focal neurologic symptoms (i.e. because of coma, dysphasia, confusion, no witness);
- Atypical clinical features (i.e. gradual onset, seizures, no clear focal neurologic signs); young patient (age <50 years) with no vascular risk factors.
- To distinguish intracranial hemorrhage (**216**) from cerebral infarction (CT must be done within about 10 days of stroke).

Intracranial hemorrhage is seen immediately as a homogeneous area of high density; infarction, if seen, as an area of low density. Within the first few hours of infarction, there is loss of gray/white matter differentiation, slight hypodensity and a little swelling (loss of visibility of the sulci). The lesion is wedge-shaped if cortical and rounded if subcortical. The occluded artery may appear hyperdense (whiter) due to the presence of thrombus (this sign is reliable if present, but its absence means little as far as whether or not the artery is patent).

Within the first few days the infarct margins become clearly demarcated, the infarct more hypodense (darker), and the swelling increases (large infarcts may produce considerable mass effect with midline shift and uncal herniation). After the first week, the swelling subsides and the infarct becomes of similar density to normal brain making it difficult to see (fogging). Fogging lasts for a week or so. After several months, the infarct is a shrunken black area ('hole').

Up to 50% of all infarcts will not be positively identified by CT; larger and older infarcts are more likely to be visible (but see above, fogging). Hemorrhagic transformation of the infarct (HTI) can occur any time within the first few weeks, but is most frequent within the first week and in patients with large infarcts, high blood pressure, or who are given antithrombotic and thrombolytic drugs. HTI may be massive or minor (petechial); massive HTI may be indistinguishable from a de novo primary intracerebral hemorrhage (PICH) (**217–219**).

- To ascertain the likely cause of ischemic or hemorrhagic stroke.
- Otherwise as for TIA patients (see p.186).

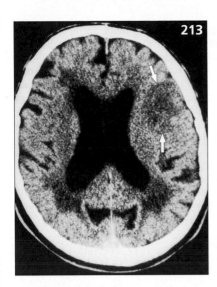

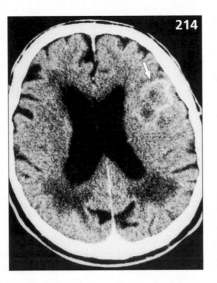

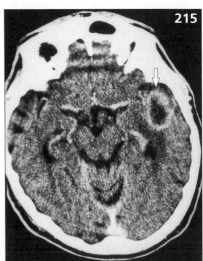

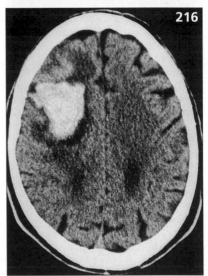

213 Plain cranial CT scan showing low density in the cortex and subcortex of the left frontal lobe (arrows) and also in the periventricular regions of a patient who presented with sudden onset of dysphasia and right hemiparesis and was diagnosed as having suffered an ischemic stroke (but see **214, 215**).

214, 215 Post contrast CT scan in the same patient as **213** showing ring enhancement of the left frontal cortical/subcortical lesion (arrow) (**214**) and another ring enhancing lesion in the left anterior temporal lobe (arrow) due to metastatic carcinoma (**215**).

216 Non-contrast cranial CT scan showing a focal area of high density in the frontal lobe on the right due to hemorrhage secondary to amyloid angiopathy.

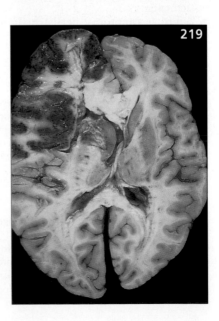

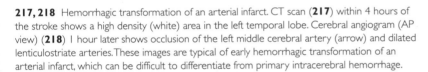

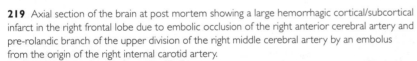

217, 218 Hemorrhagic transformation of an arterial infarct. CT scan (**217**) within 4 hours of the stroke shows a high density (white) area in the left temporal lobe. Cerebral angiogram (AP view) (**218**) 1 hour later shows occlusion of the left middle cerebral artery (arrow) and dilated lenticulostriate arteries. These images are typical of early hemorrhagic transformation of an arterial infarct, which can be difficult to differentiate from primary intracerebral hemorrhage.

219 Axial section of the brain at post mortem showing a large hemorrhagic cortical/subcortical infarct in the right frontal lobe due to embolic occlusion of the right anterior cerebral artery and pre-rolandic branch of the upper division of the right middle cerebral artery by an embolus from the origin of the right internal carotid artery.

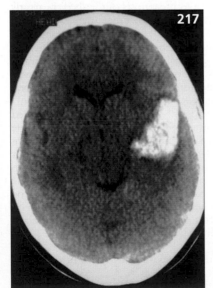

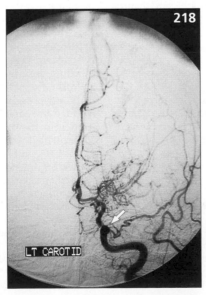

Selected patients
As for TIA patients (see p.188).

MRI brain scan
With or without diffusion and perfusion weighted imaging, if:
- A CT scan performed >10 days after stroke shows a low-density area that could be infarction or resolving hemorrhage and it is essential to distinguish them.
- CT scan is negative and it is crucial to be able to localize the infarct. MRI is more sensitive in detecting infarcts than CT (particularly brainstem and small subcortical infarcts), but can be difficult to use in very sick, confused patients and may show so many 'holes' in some patients that it is just confusing. The evolution of the appearance of infarction is similar to CT (including fogging). A recent infarct is bright on T2W imaging (T2WI) and dark on T1WI. An occluded artery shows up as an absent 'flow void', sometimes with a bright blob in it on T2WI (the clot). Special sequences can show very early changes of infarction (within minutes of the interruption of blood flow) such as diffusion- or perfusion-weighted imaging or spectroscopic imaging, but these are still being evaluated.
- Arterial dissection suspected (N.B. catheter angiography remains the gold standard).
- Trying to identify the response to thrombolytic therapy (e.g. perhaps the greatest benefit is obtained with a large diffusion/perfusion mismatch).

CSF examination
Useful if SAH is still suspected despite a normal CT scan (must wait until at least 12 hours have elapsed since the onset of stroke symptoms before doing the CSF examination) or if positive blood VDRL or TPHA.

DIAGNOSIS
A clinical diagnosis, based on the sudden onset of a focal neurologic deficit, which is correct about 95% of the time. Factors that may reduce the reliability of the clinical diagnosis of stroke include:
- Unclear history: impaired conscious level; dysphasia; dementia.
- Unusual symptoms: persistent headache; personality change.
- Unusual signs: fever; papilledema.
- Young age: less likely to have degenerative vascular disease.
- Progressing neurologic signs.

The diagnosis of stroke can sometimes be confirmed by CT or MRI brain scan, or at autopsy. The CT scan can be normal in stroke, provided other causes of an apparent focal neurologic deficit, such as multiple sclerosis and psychogenic behavior, have been excluded.

TREATMENT

Organized and coordinated multidisciplinary care (Stroke Unit)
Compared with conventional care in a general ward, organized and coordinated care by an interested and trained multidisciplinary team in a stroke unit reduces death and dependency at 1 year after stroke from about 62.0% to 56.4%. This is an odds reduction of about 29% (odds ratio (OR) 0.71), a relative risk reduction (RRR) of 9% (95% CI: 4% –14%) and absolute risk reduction (ARR) of 5.6%. Therefore, treating 1000 patients in a stroke unit prevents about 56 patients from dying or becoming dependent compared to treating 1000 in a general ward. The number of patients needed to treat (NNT) in a stroke unit to prevent one from death or dependency is about 18. Although preferable, a geographically dedicated stroke unit is not necessary. There are insufficient data on the cost of stroke unit care but it does not increase length of stay. Patients with TIA and mild non-disabling stroke do not need admission if facilities are available for rapid, appropriate investigation and follow-up as an outpatient.

General
Assess, manage and monitor:
- Airway: care must be taken to maintain a patent airway in patients with depressed consciousness or bulbar dysfunction.
- Oxygen therapy: if the patient is hypoxic (oxygen saturation <95%); of no benefit if hemoglobin is fully saturated.
- Vital systemic signs: temperature, heart rate, blood pressure, respiration, fluid input and output. Maintaining fluid balance and preventing dehydration is essential.
- Vital neurologic signs: Glasgow coma scale, pupils, body postures.
- Fever: should be investigated (MSU, CXR, blood cultures, sputum culture and so on) and treated appropriately; elevated temperature is an adverse prognostic factor.
- Blood pressure (BP) rises transiently after stroke, especially hemorrhagic stroke, and falls during the first 7 days.

Current empirical policy is not to initiate new antihypertensive therapy for the first 7 days after stroke because a reduction in blood pressure may substantially lower cerebral blood flow in the ischemic penumbra surrounding an infarct (because of loss of autoregulation in ischemic brain) and lead to further ischemic brain damage, particularly if there is a tight stenosis of the feeding artery. Blood pressure should only be lowered, and cautiously at that (by about 15% over 24 hours), in the presence of hypertensive crises such as hypertensive encephalopathy, left ventricular failure, aortic dissection, or intracerebral bleeding, or if the blood pressure is very high and poses a real risk of cerebral hemorrhage. We don't know what level of blood pressure is 'too high' but treatment is recommended if: systolic BP >26.7–29.3 kPa (200–220 mmHg) (ischemic stroke) or >24–26.7 kPa (180–200 mmHg) (hemorrhagic stroke); or diastolic BP >16–17.3 kPa (120–130 mmHg) (ischemic stroke) or >13.3–14.7 kPa (100–110 mmHg) (hemorrhagic stroke).

Oral antihypertensive agents are recommended, such as a diuretic, beta-blocker, ACE inhibitor (low dose) or calcium-channel blocker; nifedipine capsules, and parenteral medications should be avoided because of the rapid and sometimes precipitous fall in blood pressure.

- Low blood pressure may reflect hypovolemia due to excessive losses by sweating and insufficient intake by mouth or tube, and should be corrected by raising the foot of the bed and by fluid replacement via a safe route.
- Swallowing function: maintain fluid and electrolyte balance and nutrition initially with i.v. saline and/or nasogastric tube until swallowing function is assessed by a trained nurse or speech pathologist and dietary requirements by a dietician. Percutaneous endoscopic gastrostomy tube is preferred for patients who require feeding by tube for more than about 2 weeks.
- Bladder function: after attempted voiding, residual bladder volume of urine is estimated by a nurse trained in the use of bladder ultrasound. If the residual urine volume is more than 100 ml, the bladder should be emptied by catheter every 6–8 hours.
- Immobile patients: should be turned frequently (e.g. every 2 hours) to prevent pressure sores. Proper positioning and early mobilization by nurses and physiotherapists help to prevent complications of immobility such as joint contractures, pneumonia and painful 'frozen' shoulder. Deep venous thrombosis and pulmonary embolism can be prevented by regular passive and active joint movement, early mobilization, graduated compression support stockings, aspirin and subcutaneous heparin.
- Blood glucose should be maintained within normal limits; elevated blood glucose is an adverse prognostic factor and may be harmful.
- Depression should be treated with psychosocial support and antidepressants if necessary. Early socialization may help.
- Brain edema: cytotoxic edema, which does not cause much brain swelling (i.e. no net change in brain volume, just a shift of fluid from extracellular to intracellular space) is followed by vasogenic edema (which does cause brain swelling). Specific treatments for brain edema (see below) do not reduce the edema but shrink the surrounding normal brain. The onset, degree and duration of the effect of each agent on intracranial pressure (ICP) is quite variable.
- General: restrict fluids, elevate head of bed, treat fever; avoid hypoxia and hypercapnia; avoid hypo-osmolar fluids.
- Specific: osmotic diuretics, providing BBB intact. A bolus of mannitol (1g/kg i.v. as a 20% solution over 1 hour), usually decreases ICP by about 50% after about 90 minutes but returns to the pre-treatment levels after about 210 minutes.
- Steroids: should be effective for vasogenic edema, but have not been shown to be effective in acute stroke.
- Hyperventilation if patient is deteriorating: quick onset of effect on ICP (within 2–30 minutes) but it lasts only for about 30 minutes.
- Barbiturates: useful because they reduce ICP more than they reduce BP, so cerebral perfusion pressure increases.
- CSF drainage, e.g. ventricular drain.
- Surgical decompression (hemicraniectomy): when the ICP is rising despite the above measures, and before signs of herniation (ipsilateral pupillary loss of reactivity followed by dilatation, periodic breathing [even in conscious patient], contralateral Babinski sign).

Specific
Acute ischemic stroke
- Aspirin 160–300 mg daily for acute ischemic stroke reduces death and dependency from 47.0% to 45.8%, a RRR of 3% (95% CI: 1–5%) and an ARR of 1.2%. Therefore, treating 1000 patients prevents about 12 dying or becoming dependent. The NNT is 83. All patients with acute ischemic stroke should be given aspirin immediately (unless allergic/intolerant of aspirin or entering a trial of thrombolysis).
- Intravenous thrombolysis with streptokinase or tissue plasminogen activator (tPA) within 6 hours of ischemic stroke reduces death and dependency from 59.6% to 55.2%, an odds reduction of 17% (95% CI: 6–27%), a RRR of 9% (95% CI: 4–14%) and ARR of 4.4%. Treating 1000 patients prevents 44 from death or dependency. The NNT is 23. For patients presenting within 3 hours, i.v. tPA reduces death and dependency from 67.8% to 55.2%, an odds reduction of 42% (95% CI: 26–54%) and ARR of 12.6%. Treating 1000 patients prevents 126 from death or dependency. The NNT is 8. However, thrombolysis is also hazardous. The risk of early death (within 14 days of stroke) is increased from 15.4% (control) to 19.0% (thrombolysis), a 3.6% absolute excess (OR: 1.3, 95% CI: 1.13–1.5). This is because of an excess of early symptomatic intracranial hemorrhage (2.5% [control] vs. 9.4% [thrombolysis]; OR: 3.5, 95% CI: 2.8–4.4), and fatal intracranial hemorrhage (1.0% [control] vs. 5.4% [thrombolysis]; OR: 4.15, 95% CI: 3.0–5.8) (see *Table 27*, p.199).

Thrombolytic therapy for acute ischemic stroke is therefore very much like carotid endarterectomy for symptomatic severe carotid stenosis (see TIA, p.186); both are associated with an early hazard yet a greater longer term net benefit. The burning question is no longer whether thrombolysis (and carotid endarterectomy) is effective, but in whom it is effective, in whom it is ineffective, and in whom it is dangerous. At present it is not known exactly which combination of clinical and imaging features reliably identify patients who will benefit or be harmed by thrombolysis. Nor is it clear what is the optimal thrombolytic agent, dose, half-life, and route of administration. Furthermore, the most effective concomitant neuroprotective, antithrombotic and antihypertensive regime, if any, remains to be established. What it known from current data is that the clinical features of the patient and the findings of early brain imaging have considerable potential for refining patient selection for thrombolysis.

Plain CT brain scan signs of major infarction which involves more than one-third of the middle cerebral artery territory predicts an increased risk of symptomatic intracranial hemorrhage after thrombolysis. However, it is neither sensitive nor specific, and the interrater reliability among physicians involved in acute stroke care is less than ideal. A new CT scoring system (ASPECTS) is reported to be a simple and reliable method of quantifying early ischemic changes on CT scan, like an 'ECG of the brain', and which accurately predicts risk of symptomatic intracranial hemorrhage and functional outcome in ischemic stroke patients treated with intravenous thrombolytic therapy (Barber *et al.*, 2000). However, its external validity and reliability remains to be established.

Magnetic resonance (MR) imaging can provide a perfusion-weighted image (PWI) which reveals the region of brain which is underperfused and 'at risk', and a diffusion-weighted image (DWI) which identifies the core of early infarction. A mismatch between the acute PWI lesion and the (smaller) DWI lesion may represent the ischemic penumbra of potentially salvageable brain. Clinical trials are evaluating whether patients with a PWI/DWI mismatch are likely to benefit clinically from early reperfusion. If confirmed, a further challenge will be to optimize the availability and feasibility of undertaking MRI brain scans within the first few hours of stroke onset in sick, dysphasic, disorientated and claustrophobic patients with acute stroke. Finally, patient selection for thrombolysis may also be improved by proof of arterial occlusion by means of non-invasive imaging (e.g. magnetic resonance angiography, transcranial doppler).

Clearly, further studies are required, and are in progress (e.g. International Stroke Trial – 3) to refine patient selection, and establish the balance of risks and benefits of thrombolysis in a broader range of patients presenting at different stages, with differing types and severities of stroke, different risk factors, and different brain imaging findings. Whilst awaiting the results of these studies, rt-PA has been licenced for use in the United States (1997), Canada (1999) and Germany (August 2000) for patients presenting within 3 hours of acute ischemic stroke who are similar to the patients included in the trials and provided there is a stroke service which can ensure its safe administration.

rt-PA remains to be licenced for use in other parts of Europe and America, and in Australasia and Asia. One lesson learnt from the North American experience is that treating patients who violate the guidelines outlined in *Table 28* is associated with excess risk and poor patient outcome. If rt-PA is to be licenced in other countries, it is essential that its use is restricted, at least initially, to dedicated stroke units which are appropriately equipped, prepared to respond to demand and adhere strictly to current guidelines (see *Table 28*), and prepared to undertake prospective, systematic and rigorous audit as part of a national register (if not as part of an approved randomized trial). This will ensure that stroke patients have access to this effective (yet risky) treatment, that stroke physicians gain experience and expertise in its use, and that quality control and patient selection continues to be optimized by correlation of baseline demographic, clinical, imaging and treatment data with early and long term patient outcome.

- Heparin and heparinoid in acute ischemic stroke have no net effect on death or dependency (RRR: 1%, 95% CI: –5 to 6% or (–5 – +6), despite significantly reducing the odds of deep vein thrombosis by about 79% (OR: 0.21, 95% CI: 0.15–0.39) and pulmonary embolism by about 39% (OR: 0.61, 95% CI: 0.45–0.83).
- Trials of neuroprotective agents (e.g. selfotel, aptiganel, chlormethiazole, tirilazad, lubeluzole) have failed to identify a favorable treatment effect, and some have revealed dose-limiting intolerance and systemic adverse effects, such as excessive sedation and hypertension. Trials of other agents (e.g. magnesium) are in progress.
- Other medical treatments such as hemodilution, corticosteroids, and glycerol (glycerin) have not been proven effective.

Primary intracerebral hemorrhage (PICH) (see p.238)
Surgery for PICH is associated with a non-significant increase in odds of death and dependency at 6 months (OR: 1.23, 95% CI: 0.77–1.98). Further evidence from ongoing trials is awaited.

Subarachnoid hemorrhage (see p.249)
Early aneurysm surgery is now usual practice for patients in good clinical condition but this has not been supported by a randomized controlled trial. Antifibrinolytic drugs prevent re-bleeding but increase the risk of cerebral ischemia and have no net effect on overall outcome. Oral nimodipine helps to prevent delayed cerebral ischemia and significantly reduces the risk of a poor outcome by about 31% (RR: 0.69, 95% CI: 0.58–0.84).

Minimizing complications
Complications after stroke (see *Table 29*, p.200) are common yet preventable. The key is to anticipate them in high risk patients, implement appropriate prevention strategies, and regularly (at least daily) assess patients. Patients at particular risk are the elderly, those with pre-existing handicap or diabetes, a total anterior circulation syndrome (TACS), urinary incontinence and hospitalized for more than 30 days.

Rehabilitation
Rehabilitation begins on day 1 as an integral part of acute treatment and aims to maximize survival free of handicap by facilitating normal recovery and minimizing complications. It involves an organized, coordinated multi-disciplinary team undertaking regular patient assessment, short and long term goal setting with the patient and family/carer (including discharge planning), intervention, re-assessment, and re-intervention. Failure to achieve pre-specified goals usually reflects inaccurate assessment, unrealistic expectations, progression of comorbid conditions (e.g. angina, arthritis), or the intercurrence of a complication (see *Table 29*, p.200) or another stroke.

Table 27 Risks and benefits of thrombolytic therapy for acute ischemic stroke

Outcome events	Thrombolysis (%)	Control (%)	OR	95% CI of OR	Absolute risk per 1000 patients treated (95% CI)
Within 6 hours					
Early (<10 days)					
• Death	16.6%	9.8%	1.85	1.48–2.32	+68 (44–93)
• Fatal Intracranial hemorrhage	5.4%	1.0%	4.15	2.96–5.84	+44
• Symptomatic Intracranial hemorrhage	9.4%	2.5%	3.53	2.79–4.45	+70 (58–83)
*At final follow-up (3–6 months)**					
• Death	19.0%	15.4%	1.31	1.13–1.52	+36 (17–56)
• Death or dependency	55.2%	59.6%	0.83	0.73–0.94 -	-44 (-15 to -73)
Within 3 hours					
*At final follow-up (3–6 months)**					
• Death	22.0%	20.7%	1.11	0.84–1.47	+17 (-28 to +62)
• Death or dependency	55.2%	67.8%	0.58	0.46–0.74	-126 (-71 to -181)

*The final follow up varied among the different studies – some completed the study after 3 months, some after 6 months

Table 28 Suggested guidelines for the use of Intravenous rt-PA in ischemic stroke

- Thrombolysis with intravenous r-tPA should be considered in all patients with a definite ischemic stroke who present within 3 hours of onset.
- Thrombolytic therapy should only be administered by physicians with expertise in stroke medicine, who have access to a suitable stroke service, with facilities for immediately identifying and managing hemorrhagic complications.
- Thrombolysis should be avoided in cases where the CT brain scan suggests early changes of major infarction (e.g. edema, sulcal effacement, mass effect).

Other exclusion criteria

Past history:
- Any intracranial hemorrhage.
- Stroke, serious head injury or myocardial infarction in previous 3 months.
- Gastrointestinal or urinary bleeding within previous 21 days.
- Major surgery within previous 14 days.
- Arterial puncture or noncompressible site within previous 7 days.
- Heparin exposure in preceding 48 hours and partial thromboplastin time not normal.

Current (i.e. pre-treatment):
- Seizure at stroke onset.
- Neurologic deficits are mild.
- Neurologic condition is improving rapidly.
- Systolic blood pressure >24.7 kPa (185 mmHg) or diastolic blood pressure >14.7 kPa (110 mmHg).
- Oral anticoagulant use or INR >1.7.
- Platelet count <100 × 10^9/l.
- Prolonged partial thromboplastin time.
- Blood glucose <2.8 mmol/l (50 mg/dl) or >22 mmol/l (400 mg/dl).
- Caution in patients with severe stroke (NIH stroke scale score >22).

- Discuss potential benefits and adverse effects of treatment with patient and family before treatment.
- Recommended dose of r-tPA is 0.9 mg/kg up to a maximum of 90 mg, the first 10% of the dose as a bolus over 1 minute, the rest as an infusion over 60 minutes.
- Perform neurologic assessments every 15 minutes during infusion of rt-PA, every 30 min for the next 6 hours, and every 60 minutes for the next 16 hours. If severe headache, acute hypertension, or nausea and vomiting occur, discontinue the infusion and obtain an emergency CT brain scan.
- Measure blood pressure every 15 min for 2 hours, every 30 minutes for 6 hours, and every 60 minutes for 16 hours; repeat measurements more frequently if systolic blood pressure is >24 kPa (180 mmHg) or diastolic blood pressure is >14 kPa (105 mmHg), and administer antihypertensive drugs as needed to maintain blood pressure at or below those levels.

ATHEROSCLEROTIC ISCHEMIC STROKE

DEFINITION

Arteriosclerosis is a generic term embracing all varieties of structural changes that result in hardening (and thickening) of the wall of large and small, and elastic and muscular arteries and arterioles ('arteriolosclerosis').

Atherosclerosis is one form of arteriosclerosis, characterized by an intimal pool of necrotic, proteinaceous and fatty substances in the hardened arterial wall (*athere* = porridge or gruel in Greek).

Atherosclerotic ischemic stroke is cerebral infarction caused by low blood flow to a part of the brain as a result of the complications of atherosclerosis: acute *in situ* thrombotic arterial occlusion, low flow distal to a severely narrowed or occluded artery, or embolism of atherosclerotic plaque or thrombus to the brain.

EPIDEMIOLOGY

- Atherosclerosis is the most common, but not the only, cause of cerebral ischemia and infarction, accounting for up to 75% of cases.
- Age: atherosclerosis begins in children and young adults and is almost universal in the elderly.
- Gender: both sexes, slight excess in men during middle age.

PATHOLOGY
Cerebral infarction
Ischemic necrosis of brain tissue
Pale infarction
Devoid of blood. After 8–48 hours of ischemia, the infarcted gray and white matter swells, the line of demarcation between gray and white matter becomes indistinct, the white matter loses its smooth 'grain', becoming uneven and granular, and the swollen tissue feels softer. Histologically, there is evidence of necrosis: a hematoxylin and eosin stain reveals neurons with a brightly eosinophilic cytoplasm and a darker nucleus, oligodendrocytes and glial cells with homogeneously pale or dark nuclei that have serrated borders and a collapsed or retracted nuclear membrane, astrocytes which are swollen with fragmented processes, axis cylinders which are fragmented and myelin sheaths which swell and disintegrate after 8 hours (**220**).

After 2 days, the infarcted brain becomes mushy and friable. Polymorphonuclear neutrophilic leukocytes, macrophages and other phagocytic cells infiltrate the necrotic tissue, and are particularly prominent around small vessels, where they phagocytose degradation products and become transformed into fatty macrophages. After 10 days, the swelling subsides, the necrotic tissue becomes liquefied and, if the infarct is small, early cavitation takes place as early as 3 weeks (**221**).

Hemorrhagic infarction
Extravasation of blood from many small vessels in the infarcted area. It is usually due to embolic occlusion of a cerebral artery, which causes ischemic necrosis of the brain tissue supplied by the artery and necrosis of the artery itself (due to lack of blood supply to the artery via the vasa vasorum). If the embolus lyses or fragments distally, blood flows into the necrotic artery and penetrates that arterial wall, resulting in hemorrhagic infarction.

Sites
- Wedge-shaped cortical/subcortical infarcts: usually due to large or medium-sized cerebral artery occlusion (e.g. MCA or its branches) by *in situ* thrombosis or embolus.
- Elongated sickle-shaped strips of infarction of variable width from the frontal to the occipital lobes due to infarction in the borderzone between the most distal parts of the anterior and middle cerebral arteries, often due to severe carotid occlusive disease.
- Small, deep lacunar infarcts, commonly in the internal capsule, thalamus and ventral pons due to disease affecting the small (40–800 microns diameter) perforating arteries of the brain (**222**); i.e. the lenticulostriate perforating branches of the middle cerebral artery (MCA), the thalamoperforating branches of the proximal posterior cerebral artery, and the perforating branches of the basilar artery to the brainstem. These usually manifest as a 'lacunar' clinical syndrome and make up about 25% of ischemic strokes and TIAs.

Large and medium artery atherosclerosis
- Fatty streaks: focal accumulations of subendothelial smooth muscle cells and macrophages containing lipid (cholesterol and cholesterol ester).
- Fibrous plaque: a central core of lipid and cell debris surrounded by smooth muscle cells, collagen, elastic fibers and proteoglycans. A band of fibrous tissue (the fibrous cap) separates the lipid core (the atheroma) from the lumen of the vessel.
- Mature atheroma: three main constituents: proliferated cells, predominantly smooth muscle cells; lipids (cholesterol esters) and lipid-laden macrophages ('foam cells'); connective tissue elements such as elastins and glycosaminoglycans.
- Complicated lesions: mature fibrous plaque with various types of degenerative changes such as calcification (due to precipitation of calcium salts in the tissues), intraplaque hemorrhage, intimal ulceration, rupture and mural thrombosis.

Sites
- Large- and medium-sized arteries (e.g. aortic arch), particularly at places of arterial branching (e.g. the carotid bifurcation [**223, 224**]), tortuosity (e.g. the carotid siphon), and confluence (e.g. the basilar artery [**225, 226**]).
- Individuals with atheroma affecting one artery almost always have atheroma affecting several other arteries, either with or without clinical manifestations.
- Some sites are remarkably free of atheroma (e.g. ICA between its origin and the siphon, and the main cerebral arteries distal to the circle of Willis). Consequently, occlusion of a branch of the MCA is more likely to be due to embolism than local thrombosis on an atheromatous plaque.

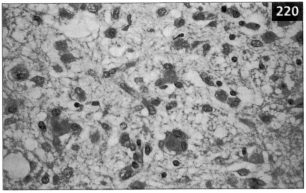

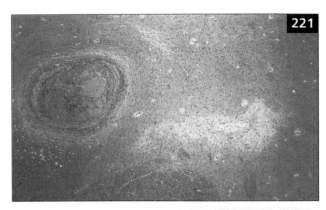

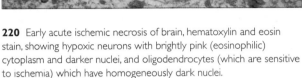

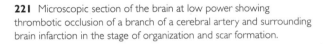

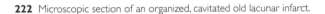

220 Early acute ischemic necrosis of brain, hematoxylin and eosin stain, showing hypoxic neurons with brightly pink (eosinophilic) cytoplasm and darker nuclei, and oligodendrocytes (which are sensitive to ischemia) which have homogeneously dark nuclei.

221 Microscopic section of the brain at low power showing thrombotic occlusion of a branch of a cerebral artery and surrounding brain infarction in the stage of organization and scar formation.

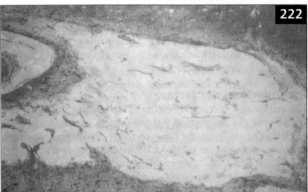

222 Microscopic section of an organized, cavitated old lacunar infarct.

223 Longitudinal section of the common carotid artery and proximal internal carotid artery at autopsy showing atheroma of the origin of the internal carotid artery. (Reproduced with permission from Hankey GJ, Warlow CP [1994] *Transient Ischaemic Attacks of the Brain and Eye*, WB Saunders.)

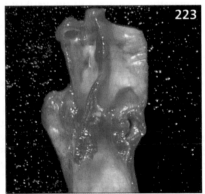

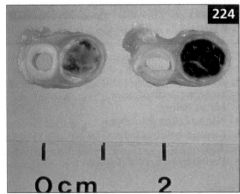

224 Autopsy specimen of a cross-section of the internal and external carotid arteries in the axial plane showing a patent external carotid artery and complete occlusion of the internal carotid artery due to *in situ* atherothrombosis.

225 CT brain scan with contrast showing a very ectatic basilar artery (arrows).

226 Photograph of the base of the brain at post mortem showing atheromatous aneurysmal dilatation and tortuosity of the basilar artery. (Reproduced with permission from Hankey GJ, Warlow CP [1994] *Transient Ischaemic Attacks of the Brain and Eye*, WB Saunders.)

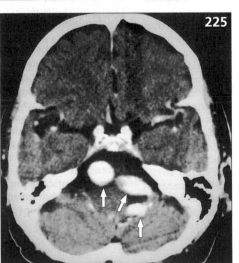

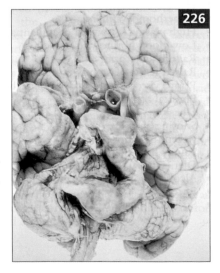

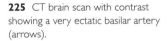

Mitral valve
- Rheumatic endocarditis (stenosis* or regurgitation).
- Infective endocarditis*.
- Mitral annulus calcification.
- Mitral valve prolapse.
- Non-bacterial thrombotic (marantic) endocarditis.
- Libmann–Sacks endocarditis.
- Antiphospholipid antibody syndrome.
- Prosthetic heart valve*.
- Papillary fibroelastoma.

Left ventricle
- Mural thrombus:
- – Acute myocardial infarction (within previous few weeks)* (**236, 237**).
- – Left ventricular aneurysm or akinetic segment.
- – Dilated cardiomyopathy*.
- – Mechanical 'artificial' heart*.
- – Blunt chest injury (myocardial contusion).
- Myxoma and other tumors*.
- Hydatid cyst.
- Primary oxalosis.

Aortic valve
- Rheumatic endocarditis (stenosis or regurgitation).
- Infective endocarditis*.
- Syphilis.
- Non-infective thrombotic (marantic) endocarditis.
- Libman–Sacks endocarditis.
- Antiphospholipid antibody syndrome.
- Prosthetic heart valve*.
- Calcific stenosis/sclerosis/calcification.

Congenital heart disease (particularly with right to left shunt)

Cardiac manipulation/surgery/catheterization/valvulo-plasty/angioplasty

*Substantial risk of embolism.

Prevalence of potential cardiac sources of embolism in patients with first-ever ischemic stroke*
- Any AF (**238**): 13%.
- – Without rheumatic heart disease: 12%.
- – With rheumatic heart disease: 1%.
- Mitral regurgitation: 6%.
- Recent (<6 weeks) myocardial infarction: 5%.
- Prosthetic valve: 1%.
- Mitral stenosis: 1%.
- Paradoxical embolism: 1%.
- Any of the above: 20%.
- Other sources of uncertain significance: aortic stenosis/sclerosis; mitral annulus calcification, mitral valve prolapse and so on: 11%.

*Sandercock PAG, Warlow CP, Jones LN, Starkey IR (1989) Predisposing factors for cerebral infarction: The Oxfordshire Community Stroke Project. *BMJ*, **298**: 75–80.

Note:
- Not all cardiac sources of embolism pose equal threats (see Diagnosis).
- Not all emboli are of the same size or the same material (fibrin, platelets, calcium, infected vegetations, tumor and so on).

Atrial fibrillation
The most common cause of cardioembolic stroke, accounting for up to 12% of all ischemic strokes, and an even greater proportion of ischemic strokes in the *very* elderly where its frequency in the population is highest. Atrial fibrillation is the cause of stroke in many of these patients but it is not always the cause because:
- Other possible causes of stroke, which may also be the cause of the AF, such as ischemic heart disease and hypertension (e.g. carotid atheroma, intracerebral hemorrhage), are present in about 20% of fibrillating stroke patients.
- Some AF patients have lacunar (presumed non-embolic) syndromes.
- 'Only' about 13% of non-rheumatic fibrillating patients have detectable (by TOE) thrombus in the left atrium (although some thrombi may have embolized or be too small to be detected) and it is unknown if these patients have a higher stroke risk than those without detectable thrombi.
- In a few cases the AF is caused by the stroke.

The average absolute risk of stroke in unanticoagulated non-rheumatic AF patients is about 5% per annum (six times greater than in those in sinus rhythm) and about 12% per annum in

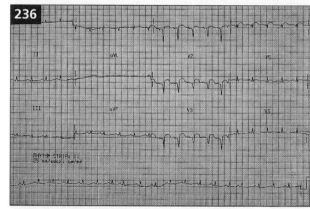

236 Electrocardiograph of a patient with a recent acute anteroseptal myocardial infarction showing sinus tachycardia, and Q waves and ST segment elevation in leads V1–V3.

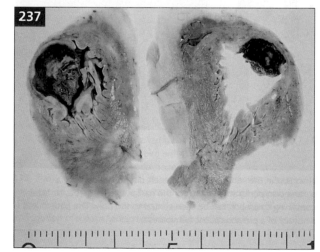

237 Cross-section of the left ventricle showing mural thrombus adjacent to an area of myocardial infarction.

unanticoagulated fibrillating TIA/stroke patients. The risk of stroke among patients in AF is variable; some are at particularly high risk and others at particularly low risk of embolization.

Risk factors for embolization in AF patients
Low risk: no other detectable heart disease (so-called lone AF).
High risk:
- Rheumatic mitral valve disease.
- Previous cerebral or systemic embolic event.
- Increasing age.
- Hypertension.
- Diabetes.
- Left ventricular systolic dysfunction.
- Enlarged left atrium defined by echocardiography.
- Spontaneous echo contrast in the left atrium, probably a consequence of blood stasis.
- Left atrial thrombi, left atrial appendage size and dysfunction, and various hemostatic variables are perhaps adverse risk factors also.

Uncertain risk:
- Recent onset AF.
- Paroxysmal AF: probably depends on frequency and duration of episodes of AF.
- Thyrotoxic AF.

Coronary heart disease

Coronary heart disease is common in patients with TIA and ischemic stroke: about 20–40% have a past history of MI or current angina. Stroke may occur in up to 5% of patients with recent acute myocardial infarction, due to:
- Embolism of left ventricular mural thrombus.
- Systemic hypotension.
- Intracerebral hemorrhage secondary to thrombolysis, anticoagulants or aspirin.
- Embolism of catheter thrombus during coronary angioplasty/stenting.
- Concurrent non-cardiac cause of stroke.

After the acute period, the risk of stroke is much lower, about 1% in the first year, perhaps higher if there is persisting left ventricular thrombus. Chronic left ventricular aneurysm after MI often contains thrombus but embolization is uncommon.

Prosthetic heart valves
- The risk of embolism is about 2% per annum for all prosthetic valves, provided patients with mechanical valves are on anticoagulants.

- Mechanical valves have a higher risk of embolism than tissue valves, but there is no difference in stroke risk between the different types of mechanical valve.
- Some Bjork–Shiley tilting disc valves have disintegrated and embolized pieces to the brain.
- Prosthetic mitral valves are more prone to thrombosis than aortic valves.
- Infective endocarditis is a potential risk for any type of prosthetic valve.

Rheumatic valvular disease
- Rheumatic mitral stenosis/regurgitation is a well recognized cause of left atrial dilatation causing thrombus formation and embolism to the brain.
- The valves also degenerate so even patients in sinus rhythm who have no thrombus in the left atrium are at risk of embolism of degenerate and sometimes calcific fragments of valve into the circulation.
- Stroke may also occur as a result of infective endocarditis (see p.215) and intracerebral hemorrhage due to anticoagulation in these patients.

Non-rheumatic sclerosis/calcification of the aortic and mitral valves
These may also be a source of embolism in some patients but unless calcific emboli are seen in the retina or on CT it is difficult to attribute confidently the TIA or ischemic stroke to this condition, which is very common in normal elderly people.

Mitral valve (or leaflet) prolapse
Uncomplicated mitral valve prolapse is not a cause of embolism from the heart to the brain. It is only likely to be relevant to the etiology of an ischemic stroke or TIA if it is complicating infective endocarditis, AF, gross mitral regurgitation, or thrombus in the left atrium. Prolapse may be familial and associated with various inherited disorders of connective tissue.

Infective endocarditis (see p.215)

Non-bacterial thrombotic (marantic) endocarditis (see Infective endocarditis, p.215)

Non-ischemic 'primary' cardiomyopathies
Primary cardiomyopathies are well recognized causes of intracardiac thrombus, particularly the dilated type rather than hypertrophic subaortic stenosis. Many are familial.

Sinoatrial disease (sick sinus syndrome)
- May be associated with intracardiac thrombus and embolism, particularly if bradycardia alternates with tachycardia, or the patient is in AF.
- May be familial.

Atrial septal aneurysm
- Uncommon.
- May be complicated by thrombus and embolism to the brain.
- Often associated with a patent foramen ovale and so has the potential for paradoxical embolism from the venous system. The presence of both atrial septal aneurysm and patent foramen ovale increases the risk of recurrent stroke (hazard ratio 4.2, 95% CI: 1.5–12).

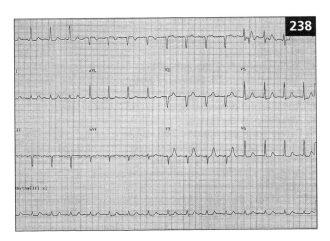

238 Electrocardiograph showing atrial fibrillation.

Disseminated intravascular coagulation
- Manifests as an acute or subacute global encephalopathy, rather than stroke-like episodes, in a very sick patient.
- CT brain scan reveals widespread hemorrhagic infarcts and hemorrhages.
- Low platelet count, low plasma fibrinogen, raised fibrin degradation products and raised D-dimer point to the diagnosis.

Pregnancy and the puerperium
The relative risk of stroke in the pregnant woman is 13 times the risk in the non-pregnant woman of the same age, but the absolute risk of stroke in the last trimester of pregnancy and the puerperium is no more than 30 per 100 000 deliveries (i.e. about 1 in every 3000 deliveries). About three-quarters of ischemic strokes are due to arterial occlusion and one-quarter venous occlusion. Causes include:
- Paradoxical embolism from the venous system of the pelvis or legs.
- Valvular heart disease.
- Cardiomyopathy of pregnancy.
- Arterial dissection during labor.
- Hematologic disorders.

Less commonly:
- Amniotic fluid embolism.
- Air or fat embolism.
- Metastatic choriocarcinoma.

Estrogens/oral contraceptives
- High estrogen dose oral contraceptive use is associated with a threefold increased risk of TIAs and stroke. But the absolute risk is very small.
- The risk is greater in women who are older, who smoke and who have other vascular risk factors such as hypertension.
- Exogenous high doses of estrogens given to elderly men for treatment of prostatic cancer and male survivors of MI increase their risk of vascular death.

Heparin-induced thrombocytopenia
Heparin may paradoxically lead to thrombus formation and thrombocytopenia by two mechanisms:
- Type I consists of a transient decrease in platelet count 1–5 days after heparin is started and is thought to be due to reversible clumping of platelets.
- Type II is a persistent depression of the platelet count beginning 3–22 days after the introduction of heparin which is thought to be mediated by IgG antibodies against a heparin–platelet membrane complex.

Nephrotic syndrome
Can be complicated by ischemic stroke, perhaps due to 'hypercoagulability': loss of antithrombotic proteins in the urine.

Desmopressin and intravenous immunoglobulin
May cause hypercoagulability and ischemic stroke, perhaps by altering blood viscosity, hemorrheology, platelet aggregability or clotting factor levels.

Snake bite
May cause ischemic stroke but is more likely to cause defibrination and bleeding.

DISSECTION OF THE CAROTID AND VERTEBRAL ARTERIES

DEFINITION
Tearing of the intima and/or media of arteries.

EPIDEMIOLOGY
- Incidence: symptomatic ICA dissection: >2.6 per 100 000; probably higher as may cause transient minor symptoms (or be asymptomatic). Vertebral artery dissection: 1–1.5 per 100 000 per year. One of the commonest causes of stroke in young people, and 2% of all ischemic strokes.
- Age: any age; can occur in the very young.
- Gender: M=F.

PATHOLOGY
Tear in the intima or media, leading to bleeding within the arterial wall, which tracks or dissects longitudinally and circumferentially between the intima and media, or media and adventitia of the arterial wall. The dissection can tear through the intima allowing the partially coagulated intramural blood to enter the lumen of the artery.

Site
Predominantly extracranial:
- Carotid dissections: the vast majority occur just above the bifurcation of the common carotid artery into the internal and external carotid arteries; common carotid artery and intracranial carotid dissections are rare. Multiple dissections in 25% of patients.
- Vertebrobasilar dissections: at the C2 level in more than 80% of cases, possibly reflecting increased susceptibility to mechanical torsion and stretch at this location. Extracranial dissections are commonly bilateral (60% of cases).

Complications
Pseudoaneurysms may form if the dissection spreads through the media of the artery; intracranial dissections may rarely present as a mass lesion or may rupture and present with subarachnoid and intracerebral hemorrhage; extracranial pseudoaneurysms rarely rupture because the artery wall is much thicker.

ETIOLOGY AND PATHOPHYSIOLOGY
Spontaneous
Predisposing conditions
- Point mutation in one allele of the COL1A1 gene that encodes the proα1(I) chains of type I procollagen, resulting in substitution of alanine for glycine (G13A) in about half of the α1(I) chains of type I collagen.
- Family history: 5% of cases.
- Genetic disorders of collagen.
- Marfan's syndrome.
- Ehlers-Danlos syndrome types IV and VI.
- Cystic medial necrosis.
- Osteogenesis imperfecta.
- Pseudoxanthoma elasticum.
- Polycystic kidney disease.
- Fibromuscular dysplasia.
- Reticular fiber deficiency.
- Accumulation of mucopolysaccharides.
- Possibly atheromatous risk factors (hypertension, diabetes, smoking, high cholesterol).
- Possibly hyperhomocystinemia.

Trauma

- Sports.
- Whiplash injury.
- Neck manipulation.
- Activities such as reversing the car or painting the ceiling.
- Iatrogenic: cerebral angiography.

Mechanisms of brain or ocular ischemia

- Occlusion of the dissected artery by the false lumen or by superimposed thrombus.
- Embolism of thrombus that may have formed on the intimal flap or in the wall.

Mechanisms of cranial nerve involvement in ICA dissection

- Compression or stretching of the cranial nerve by the expanded artery. This is likely for lower cranial nerves IX to XII which lie close to the ICA below the jugular foramen in the retrostyloid and posterior retroparotid space and may be compressed or stretched by an expanded or aneurysmal ICA. This is particularly so for cranial nerves X and XII which have the longest anatomic relationship to the ICA.
- Interruption of the blood supply to the cranial nerve via the nutrient vessels, which are small (200–300 microns in diameter) branches of the ICA. Mechanisms include mechanical compromise by dissection, distal embolization, or pressure gradient changes in collateral supply (hemodynamic). There are three vascular systems which play a significant role in nutrient supply to most of the cranial nerves. Accepting that anatomic variations are common, they basically involve:
- The inferolateral trunk: often arises from the ICA, and supplies cranial nerves III, IV, VI, and the first division of V.
- The middle meningeal system: derives from the external carotid artery, and supplies the second and third division of cranial nerve V, and also VII.
- The ascending pharyngeal system derives from the external carotid artery and supplies cranial nerves IX through to XII.

Mechanism of cervical spinal cord or root disturbance in vertebrobasilar dissection

Dissection of the vertebral arteries, which lie very close to the spinal roots, and from which arise the anterior spinal artery, may lead to symptoms of a cervical radiculo-myelopathy due to nerve ischemia or compression by hematoma in vessel wall.

CLINICAL FEATURES

May be asymptomatic; a history of preceding trauma is often present, although it may be trivial and may not be relevant.

History

Any combination of the following symptoms, which may be minor and transient or more persistent.

Carotid dissection

- Pain around the eye or frontal region, sometimes in the neck, and sometimes generalized and non-specific, is common and may be the only feature.
- Acute or delayed focal monocular or carotid territory ischemic symptoms: ipsilateral visual loss; contralateral hemisensori-motor deficit; difficulty speaking; onset of ischemic symptoms usually within a few days of dissection but can be as long as several weeks and even a few months.
- Symptoms of single or multiple cranial nerve palsy: III, IV, V,VI, VII,IX, X, XI, XII.
- Pulsatile tinnitus may occur.
- Dysgeusia (impaired taste sensation due to VII nerve [chorda tympani] palsy) may occur.

Vertebrobasilar dissection

- Pain.
- Focal vertebrobasilar ischemic symptoms: occipital/temporal lobe, brainstem, cerebellum; most commonly a lateral medullary or cerebellar infarct.
- Upper limb peripheral motor deficits: bilateral distal upper limb amyotrophy.

Examination

Carotid dissection

- Focal monocular or carotid territory ischemic symptoms.
- Oculosympathetic palsy (Horner's syndrome) ipsilaterally (**255**).
- Cranial nerve palsy (single or multiple): III, IV, V, VI, VII, IX, X, XI, XII, in at least 10% of patients with extracranial ICA dissection; may occur without symptoms of carotid ischemia.
- Neck bruit.

Vertebrobasilar dissection

- Focal vertebrobasilar territory ischemic symptoms.
- Cervical radiculomyelopathy.

DIFFERENTIAL DIAGNOSIS
Carotid dissection

Brainstem stroke: the combination of unilateral Horner's syndrome and lower cranial nerve palsies with contralateral hemisensori-motor deficit may be due to brainstem dysfunction and draw attention to the vertebrobasilar circulation but may also be a 'false localizing sign' of a unilateral extracranial carotid artery dissection. A history of neck trauma, and pain and a bruit over the carotid artery may be a clue to the diagnosis of carotid dissection.

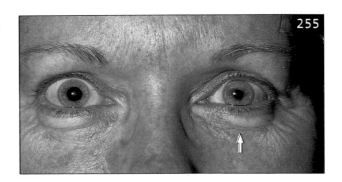

255 Horner's syndrome (left, arrow) due to interruption of the ascending postganglionic pupillodilator oculosympathetic fibers in the wall of the left internal carotid artery by dissecting blood.

Small vessels (arterioles, capillaries, venules)
Hypersensitivity angiitis
- Exogenous stimuli proved or suspected:
- – Drug-induced angiitides.
- – Henoch–Schönlein purpura.
- – Serum sickness and serum sickness-like reactions.
- – Angiitis associated with infectious diseases.
- Endogenous antigens likely to be involved:
- – Angiitis associated with neoplasms (particularly lymphoid malignancies).
- – Angiitis associated with other underlying diseases.
- – Angiitis associated with congenital deficiencies of the complement system (hypocomplementemic angiitis).
- Mixed cryoglobulinemia.
- Cutaneous angiitides.

PATHOLOGY
Acute, subacute or chronic inflammation in the arterial and/or venous wall with or without granuloma formation and necrosis (**260**).

Vascular lesions
Granulomatous angiitis
A distinctive chronic inflammatory reaction of blood vessels characterized by a predominance of modified macrophages (i.e. epithelioid cells) which are aggregated into nodular clumps referred to as granulomas and which respond to foreign bodies by coalescing to form giant cells that often conglomerate around the foreign body.

Necrotizing angiitis
Inflammation and necrosis (usually fibrinoid necrosis) of vessel walls.

Brain lesions
- Focal or multi-focal cerebral infarction.
- Intracerebral hemorrhage.
- Subarachnoid hemorrhage.

ETIOLOGY
A primary manifestation of disease or a secondary component of another disorder such as connective tissue disease, drug abuse, neoplasia or infection (see Classification, above).

PATHOGENESIS
Immunopathogenic
- *In situ* formation or deposition of immune complexes in blood vessel wall leading to activation of the complement-mediated inflammatory response.
- Direct antibody-mediated damage via antibodies directed at endothelial cells or other tissue components.
- Antibody-dependent cellular cytotoxicity directed against blood vessels.
- Cytotoxic T lymphocytes directed at blood vessel components.
- Granuloma formation in blood vessel wall or adjacent to blood vessel.
- Cytokine-induced (i.e. interleukin 1, TNF-alpha) expression of adhesion vehicles for leukocytes on endothelial cells.

Non-immunopathogenic
- Infiltration of blood vessel wall or surrounding tissue by microbiologic agents.
- Direct invasion of blood vessel by neoplastic cells.
- Unidentified mechanisms.

Mechanisms of tissue dysfunction
- Angiitis (causing ischemia or hemorrhage).
- Coagulopathy (cf. antiphospholipid syndrome, p.218).
- Emboli (cf. non-bacterial thrombotic endocarditis, p.216).
- Compression from granulomas.
- Antineuronal antibody effects.

CLINICAL FEATURES
- Variable in onset, nature and duration.
- Features are determined partly by the size and location of the involved vessel(s).
- Most commonly vasculitis presents as an acute or subacute focal or diffuse encephalopathy or meningo-encephalopathy with headache, altered mentation, seizures and cognitive and behavioral abnormalities, with multifocal neurologic signs.
- Less commonly, patients present with a multiple sclerosis-like picture (i.e. relapsing and spontaneously remitting focal neurologic dysfunction), features of a rapidly progressive space-occupying lesion, multiple cranial neuropathies (e.g. Wegener's granulomatosis) and rarely, with a spinal cord syndrome, extrapyramidal syndrome or stroke syndrome.
- Systemic symptoms and signs may be present such as fever, headache, malaise, weight loss, joint aches and pains, facial rash, livido reticularis.

CLINICAL HISTORY
Demographic data
- Age: young: Takayasu's arteritis, SLE; older: GCA.
- Gender: F: Takayasu's arteritis.
- Race: oriental: Takayasu's arteritis.

Symptoms
- Headache: GCA.
- Scalp, face, temporal pain: GCA.
- Blindness: GCA, WG.
- Diplopia: WG.
- Syncope: Takayasu's arteritis.
- Jaw/tongue claudication: GCA, Takayasu's arteritis.
- Arm claudication: Takayasu's arteritis.
- Sinus pain and drainage, nasal discharge: WG.
- Oral ulcers: SLE, Behçet's disease.
- Dry eyes, dry mouth: SS.
- Anxiety, depression: SLE.
- Fever, headache, malaise, fatigue, weight loss, arthralgia, sweats: non-specific.
- Skin rash: PAN, AAG, LG, sarcoid, Behçet's disease, SLE, Sneddon's, hypersensitivity.
- Malar rash: SLE.
- Photosensitivity: SLE.
- Joint aches and pains (arthritis): SLE, RA.
- Stiffness/aches/pains in neck, shoulders, lower back, hips and legs (polymyalgia): GCA.
- Chest pain (pleurisy, pericarditis): SLE, LG, Behçet's.
- Asthma: AAG.
- Cough, shortness of breath: LG, sarcoid, Behçet's.
- Abdominal pain: PAN, inflammatory bowel disease, Kohlmeier–Degos disease.

Past history

- Allergy: AAG.
- Deep vein thrombosis/pulmonary emboli: SLE, APLAb, Behçet's.
- Recurrent spontaneous abortions: SLE, APLAb.
- Epileptic seizures: SLE.
- Anemia: non-specific.
- Thrombocytopenia: SLE, APLAb.
- (False) positive VDRL: APLAb.
- Infection with toxoplasma, aspergillus, varicella-zoster, cytomegalovirus, herpes simplex virus, HIV: infectious arteritis.
- Illicit drug abuse: amphetamine, cocaine: drug-induced arteritis.

Family history

- Collagen vascular diseases or angiitides.
- Multiple spontaneous abortions: APLAb.
- Deep venous thrombosis or pulmonary emboli: APLAb.
- Neonatal heart block in patient's child (woman).

PHYSICAL EXAMINATION

- Malar rash: SLE.
- Skin nodules, purpura: AAG, LG, sarcoid, Kohlmeier–Degos disease, hypersensitivity.
- Skin macules, papules, plaque: LG, Sneddon's syndrome.
- Skin infarcts (**261**).
- Skin fibrosis: scleroderma.
- Oral ulcers: SLE, Behçet's disease.
- Ischemic necrosis of lips, palate, nasal septum: TA, WG.
- Sinus inflammation/nasal mucosal ulceration: WG.

- Chondritis (auricular, nasal, laryngo-tracheal): relapsing polychondritis.
- Altered mental state, dementia, psychosis: SLE.
- Blindness or altitudinal visual field defect: GCA.
- Uveitis: sarcoid, Behçet's disease.
- Optic nerve head swelling (**262**)/pallor/hemorrhage: GCA.
- Retinal periphlebitis, hard exudates: sarcoid.
- Retinal vein occlusion: Behçet's disease.
- Mononeuritis multiplex: PAN, AAG, WG, LG.
- Temporal artery tenderness, thickening, nodularity: GCA.
- Absent peripheral pulses: TA.
- Carotid/chest bruit: TA.
- Hypertension: TA, PAN.
- Blood pressure difficult to record or different between the arms: TA.
- Aortic regurgitation: TA.
- Pleuritic or pericardial friction rub: SLE.
- Chest crackles/wheeze: AAG, LG, SLE.
- Arthritis: sarcoid, SLE, RA.

> *Abbreviations:* TA: Takayasu's arteritis; GCA: giant cell arteritis; PAN: polyarteritis nodosa; AAG: allergic angiitis and granulomatosis of Churg–Strauss; WG: Wegener's granulomatosis; LG: lymphomatoid granulomatosis; SLE: systemic lupus erythematosus; RA: rheumatoid arthritis; APLAb: antiphospholipid antibody syndrome; MCTD: mixed connective tissue disease; SS: Sjögrens syndrome

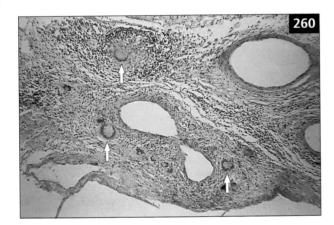

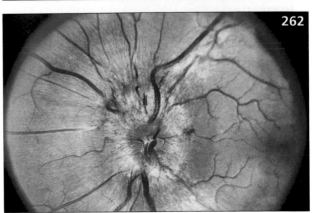

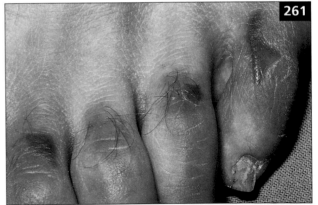

260 Histologic section of basal meninges showing infiltration with mononuclear cells and multinucleate giant cells (arrows) in a patient with infective arteritis of the CNS due to tuberculosis.

261 Vasculitic infarcts of the skin in a patient with polyarteritis nodosa.

262 Ocular fundus of a patient with a left optic neuropathy due to sarcoidosis showing a swollen, congested optic disc with peripapillary hemorrhages (papillitis).

Extent of visceral and other organ involvement
- Urine:
- – Glomerular red cells: PAN, WG, LG, SLE.
- – Casts*.
- – Protein (if positive, 24-hour urine protein)*.
- – Eosinophils.
- Creatinine: PAN, WG, LG, SLE.
- Liver function tests: transaminases*: GCA.
- Hepatitis B surface antigenemia: PAN.
- Chest x-ray* (infiltrates, nodules, cavities) (**266, 267**): WG, LG, SLE, sarcoid.
- Gallium scan: sarcoid.
- Ophthalmologic examination using low dose fluorescein angiography with slit-lamp video microscopy of the anterior segment: slowing of flow, multifocal attenuation of arterioles, erythrocyte aggregates, areas of small vessel infarction, and multifocal segments of intense leakage from post-capillary and collecting venules.

Underlying infection
- Antibodies against borreliosis*, salmonellosis, yersiniosis, toxoplasmosis, aspergillus.
- Viral antibodies (including varicella-zoster virus, cytomegalovirus, HIV, herpes simplex virus).
- Hepatitis screening.
- VDRL, TPHA.
- Cryoglobulins*.
- Paraproteins (serum protein electrophoresis)*.
- CSF*:
- – Cell count, total protein, glucose, quantitative analysis of immunoglobulins, oligoclonal band analysis.
- – Moderate mononuclear CSF pleocytosis (usually 50–80 cells/mm^3; but can be up to 800 cells/mm^3).
- – CSF protein usually elevated to around 1–1.5 g/l (10–15 g/dl), but may be up to 5.8 g/l (58 g/dl).
- – Xanthochromia, hypoglycorrhachia and an elevated CSF gammaglobulin with oligoclonal banding of IgG have been reported.
- – The primary value of CSF studies is to exclude other causes of a meningitis.

Associated coagulation abnormalities
- PT, APTT, dRVVT*: APLAb, SLE (35%).
- Anticardiolipin antibodies*: APLAb, SLE (35%).

Others
- Angiotensin converting enzyme: sarcoidosis.
- Lysozyme and beta2-microglobulin: sarcoidosis.
- Cell-mediated immunity (anergy): sarcoidosis, LG.
- Sinus x-ray/CT: WG.
- Echocardiography: atrial myxoma.
- EEG: frequently abnormal, showing generalized non-specific slow wave activity of variable degree and location.
- Indium-labelled white-cell brain imaging: increased uptake and accumulation in the brain of indium-labelled leukocytes.

Brain biopsy
- Cerebral or spinal cord biopsy establishes the diagnosis in about 70% of cases.
- False-negative biopsies occur in about 30% of autopsy-proven patients.
- The relatively low diagnostic yield from cortical biopsy may be related to the segmental nature of the lesions and the lack of leptomeningeal tissue in the biopsy.

- The risk of serious morbidity from brain biopsy is about 0.5–2.0%.
- The decision to biopsy is made on an individual basis; if an extended period of treatment with potentially hazardous immunosuppressant drugs is being considered, then the need to establish an unequivocal tissue diagnosis becomes of primary importance.

The results of blood and CSF laboratory tests, EEG, brain imaging with CT and MRI, and cerebral angiography are neither sensitive nor specific but are usually essential to rule out infectious or malignant disease, which can mimic CNS angiitis clinically.

DIAGNOSIS
The diagnosis is made histologically. A combined leptomeningeal and wedge cortical tissue biopsy, preferably of the temporal tip of the non-dominant hemisphere and including a longitudinally-orientated surface vessel is required. If organs other than the brain are affected, biopsy specimens should be obtained.

TREATMENT
The decision to treat and how will depend on the clinical condition and course of the patient and the philosophies of the attending clinician. If the patient is well then time is available to allow a period of observation of the natural history of the disease. If the patient is very sick, however, empirical immunosuppressive therapy, may be commenced whilst awaiting biopsy confirmation (see below).

Once the histologic diagnosis is confirmed then anti-inflammatory and immunosuppressive therapy (with corticosteroids and/or cyclophosphamide) should be considered, bearing in mind that the treatment of CNS angiitis is inferred from clinical experience with systemic angiitis or anecdotal, lacking any controlled study. Start with oral or intravenous glucocorticoid (e.g. prednisolone 1–2 mg/kg per day) in divided doses every 8–12 hours. After the disease is controlled, reduce to one morning dose, and thereafter, taper the daily dose as rapidly as clinical disease permits. Ideally, patients should be slowly converted to alternate-day therapy with a single morning dosage of short acting glucocorticoid (prednisone, prednisolone, methyl-prednisolone) so as to minimize adverse effects; prednisone doses of 15 mg daily (or less) given before noon usually do not suppress the hypothalamic pituitary axis. However, the disease may flare on the day off steroids, in which case use the lowest single daily dosage that suppresses disease.

Strategies to minimize adverse effects of steroid include:
- Calcium (1000 mg daily) for most patients to minimize osteoporosis.
- Vitamin D 50 000 units one to three times weekly if 24-h urinary calcium excretion <120 mg, (monitor for hypercalcemia).
- Estrogen replacement therapy if post-menopausal.
- Calcitonin and biphosphonates may also be useful.
- Hyperglycemia, hypertension, edema and hypokalemia should be treated.
- Infections should be identified and treated early.
- Immunizations with influenza and pneumococcal vaccines are safe and should be given if the disease is stable.

The addition of cyclophosphamine (1.5–2.5 mg/kg per day orally) to prednisolone (1 mg/kg per day) may be effective.

Strategies to minimize adverse effects of cyclophosphamide include:

- Monitor the leukocyte count closely, keeping it above 3000 per cubic millimeter and the neutrophil count above 1500 per microlitre.
- If severe neutropenia or bladder toxicity occurs despite low doses of cyclophosphamide and a fluid intake of >3 liters/day, azathioprine 1–2 mg/kg per day or methotrexate can be used successfully with prednisone.
- A pulsed regimen of 10–15 mg/kg intravenously once every 4 weeks has less bladder toxicity that daily oral doses (1.5–2.5 mg/kg per day) but bone marrow suppression can be severe.

When the disease has been controlled for a few months, taper immunosuppressive agents and attempt to discontinue them. The role of antiplatelet agents and anticoagulants is uncertain. Campath-1H humanized monoclonal antibody treatment remains experimental.

Clinical approach to the patient with suspected CNS vasculitis

1 Is it cerebrovascular (i.e. TIA, stroke, vascular meningo-encephalopathy) or not?
2 Where is (are) the lesion(s) neuroanatomically?
3 What is the pathologic nature of the lesion(s): ischemic or hemorrhagic?
4 What is the etiology of the lesion(s): have more common disorders of the arteries (atheroma, dissection), heart and blood been excluded?
5 Are there other clinical features or investigation results to indicate that this is part of a specific vasculitic syndrome (i.e. sinus disease: Wegener's granulomatosis; jaw claudication: temporal arteritis)?

6 If a syndrome is recognized and if it is associated with an underlying disease or an offending antigen, treat the underlying disease or remove the offending antigen where possible.
7 Establish the histologic diagnosis of angiitis by obtaining a tissue biopsy before committing the patient to a long course of immunosuppressive medication.
8 Determine the extent of disease activity.
9 Start treatment with appropriate agents in disorders in which treatment is of proven benefit and is essential (i.e. prednisone in temporal arteritis; cyclophosphamide and prednisone in Wegener's granulomatosis).
10 In patients with systemic angiitis, start with glucocorticoid therapy. Add a cytotoxic agent such as methotrexate or cyclophosphamide if an adequate response does not result of if the disorder is likely to respond only to cytotoxic agents, such as Wegener's granulomatosis.
11 Avoid immunosuppressive therapy (glucocorticoids or cytotoxic agents) in disorders which rarely result in irreversible organ system dysfunction and which usually do not respond to such agents.
12 Closely follow patients for development of toxic adverse effects of treatments.
13 Continually attempt to taper glucocorticoids to an alternate-day regimen and discontinuation when possible, and to taper and discontinue cytotoxic drugs as soon as is feasible upon induction of remission.
14 In the event of unacceptable adverse effects or lack of efficacy, consider alternative agents such as azathioprine.

PROGNOSIS
Variable.

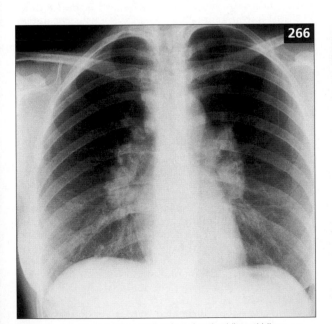

266 Chest x-ray, posterio-anterior view, showing bilateral hilar lymphadenopathy in the patient in **262** with sarcoidosis.

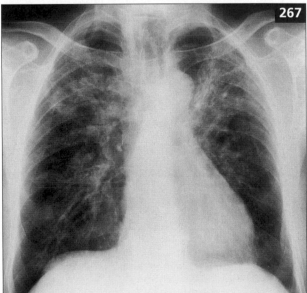

267 Chest x-ray, posterio-anterior view, of a patient with Wegener's granulomatosis showing a loss of volume in the upper zones of the lungs bilaterally and coarse interstitial infiltrate with confluence and cavitation in the upper zones bilaterally.

GIANT CELL ARTERITIS (GCA)

DEFINITION

A systemic angiitis that involves a wide variety of medium and large arteries, and tends to affect older people (over 50 years) causing two main clinical syndromes: temporal (cranial) arteritis and polymyalgia rheumatica, which respond rapidly to corticosteroid therapy.

EPIDEMIOLOGY

- Incidence:
- Temporal arteritis: 18 per 100 000 per annum among people >50 years; higher incidence in northern than southern Europe.
- Polymyalgia rheumatica: 13–68 per 100 000 population aged over 50 years per annum.
- Prevalence: 223 per 100 000 (1 in 500) among people over age of 50 years.
- Race: mainly white people.
- Gender: F>M; 2–3:1.
- Age: elderly; seldom under age 60 years, extraordinarily rarely under 50 years (one case reported at age 35 years).

PATHOLOGY

Macroscopic

Any medium or large artery in the body (aorta, carotid, vertebral, coronary, femoral and so on) may be affected, but most commonly branches of the external carotid (superficial temporal, facial, occipital arteries), ophthalmic, vertebral and posterior ciliary arteries, as well as the aorta and its branches. These are all vessels with substantial quantities of elastin in their walls. Curiously, other vessels with lesser amounts of elastin, such as the proximal central retinal artery, and the petrous and cavernous portions of the internal carotid arteries, and their branches, may also be involved, but the cervical segment of the carotid artery is minimally involved and there is a striking lack of arteritic involvement of the intracranial arteries except in rare cases. Particularly common sites of arterial stenosis in the cerebral circulation are the internal carotid artery just before dural penetration and the extracranial vertebral artery just before entering the skull.

Microscopic

A panarteritis characterized by intimal proliferation and thickening, destruction of the internal elastic lamina, and infiltration of the media by mononuclear cells (predominantly T lymphocytes of the helper/inducer subset), giant cells, and occasional eosinophils with granuloma formation (268–270). The granulomatous changes are considered classical of GCA although the presence of giant cells is not required for the diagnosis.

ETIOLOGY AND PATHOGENESIS

- Unknown.
- Genetic predisposition:
- Increased prevalence in Northern Europeans.
- Reports of multiple family cases.
- Frequency of human leukocyte antigen HLA-DR4 is twice normal.
- Association with DRB1-04 variants, particularly the second hypervariable region of DRB1-04.

- Immunopathogenic mechanisms, especially cell-mediated immunity, are probably involved. An antigen-driven immune response is likely to be the primary event, and arterial damage a secondary effect. There is no direct relationship with other connective tissue diseases.

CLINICAL FEATURES

History

Systemic

Consitutional symptoms: fever, malaise, fatigue, anorexia, weight loss, night sweats, depression, and arthralgias.

Myalgic

Proximal, symmetric muscle pain and stiffness of polymyalgia rheumatica:

- Intense pain and stiffness in the neck, shoulders and buttocks.
- Worse in the morning: patients 'roll out of bed like a log'.

Arteritic

- Headache (92% of cases):
- Due to partial occlusion of an artery.
- The site varies: may be temporal, occipital, or generalized; severe and persistent; patients may sit up in a chair all night.
- Often described as a new type of pain.
- Pain, swelling, erythema and tenderness over the affected arteries (e.g. superficial temporal arteries may stand out and be tender on brushing the hair).
- 'Claudication-like' symptoms of partial arterial occlusion:
- Pain on chewing (jaw and tongue claudication due to maxillary and lingual artery occlusion): up to 65% of cases.
- Pain and blanching of the tongue (lingual artery).
- Intermittent claudication and Raynaud's phenomenon, more common in arms ('aortic arch syndrome').
- Ischemic symptoms of total arterial occlusion:
- Visual impairment (25–50% of cases): usually sudden, painless deterioration of vision in one eye, often on waking in the morning. It may persist.
- Neurologic problems (31% of cases): TIA of the brain or stroke (7%); TIA of the eye (amaurosis fugax): 10%; deafness; peripheral neuropathy.

Examination

- Thickening, tenderness and nodularity of the temporal arteries, sometimes with reduced or absent pulsation (271).
- Bruits over large arteries; tenderness of arteries to palpation occasionally.
- Visual acuity varies from 6/6 to no light perception;.
- Visual field defects; altitudinal visual field defects (loss of either the upper or more commonly the lower half of the field in one eye) are particularly common (in contrast to the central scotoma usually occurring in optic neuritis due to demyelination) and are due to occlusion of the upper or lower division of posterior ciliary artery, which supplies the optic nerve; inferior nasal sectorial defect; central scotoma.
- Ophthalmoscopy: distended veins, a swollen optic disc (may be segmental), and, occasionally, cotton-wool spots (272) and splinter or flame-shaped hemorrhages at or near the disc margin.

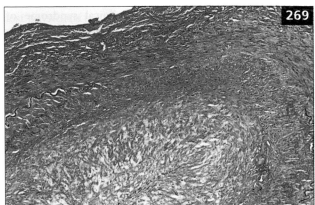

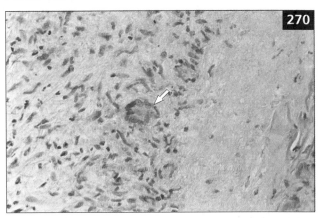

268–270 Cross-section of a temporal artery biopsy. Low power magnification (**268**) showing the lumen is occluded by extensive granulomatous inflammatory reaction involving the total thickness of the vessel. Higher power (**269**) showing the intimal surface is replaced by a fibroblastic proliferation, occluding the lumen; and the sub-intimal zone has extensive fibrinoid necrosis with marked disruption of the internal elastic lamina. There is histiocytic proliferation, and nodules of eosinophil cells and occasional multinucleated giant cells are present. In the outer muscle and adventitial coats there is a light infiltrate of lymphocytes and plasma cells. High power section (**270**) of a temporal artery biopsy from a patient with active giant cell arteritis showing (in the center of the field) a multinucleate giant cell with the nuclei arranged around the periphery of the cell in a horseshoe pattern (arrow).

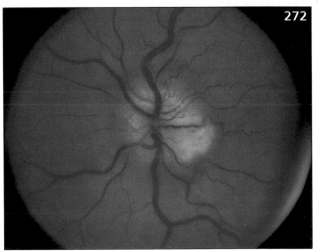

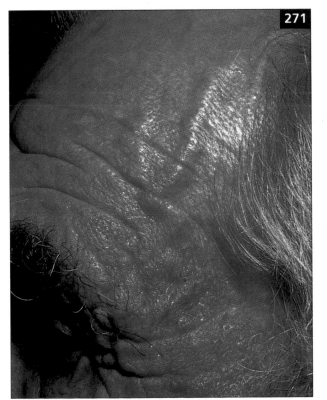

271 Lateral photograph of the forehead of a patient with giant cell arteritis showing a visibly enlarged, tender, temporal artery.

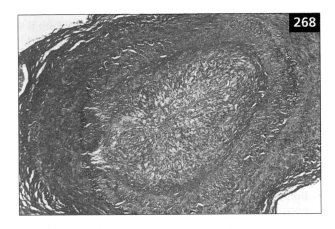

272 Fundus photograph of anterior ischemic optic neuropathy due to giant cell arteritis of the posterior ciliary artery showing a swollen optic disc, cotton-wool spots at the disc margin, and distended veins. (**271, 272** courtesy of Mr M Wade, Department of Medical Illustrations, Royal Perth Hospital, Australia.)

MRA and spiral CT may show the AVM but usually the lesion is visible on MRI (**293, 294**) or contrast CT and neither angiographic technique supplies enough information to replace conventional angiography, so are probably not of much help.

N.B. All forms of imaging may fail to show small, compressed or obliterated vascular malformations.

DIAGNOSIS
Clinical clues to the diagnosis
- Known hereditary hemorrhagic telangiectasia or Sturge–Weber syndrome.
- Subarachnoid hemorrhage with a past history of seizures.
- Carotid, orbital or skull bruit in a patient presenting with headache, seizures or intracranial hemorrhage.

Diagnosis is established by MRI or angiography

PROGNOSIS
- The course is difficult to predict: the AVM may remain static, grow, or even regress.
- The long term crude annual case fatality is 1–1.5%.
- The annual risk of first (incident) bleeding is about 2–3% and is similar in patients with or without a previous hemorrhage.
- The case fatality for a first bleed is about 10–15%, and the overall morbidity is about 50%.
- The annual risk of future re-bleeding is probably higher, particularly in the first year after initial hemorrhage, and one study has suggested that the risk is as high as about 18% per year (among patients who have had a hemorrhage at initial presentation). The risk of re-hemorrhage appears to be greater in patients over 60 years, if there is an associated saccular aneurysm (the risk is about 7% per year), if there is only a single draining vein, or if venous drainage is impaired or confined to the deep venous system.
- For untreated AVMs, the annual risk of developing *de novo* seizures is 1%.

TREATMENT
Treatment decisions are based on the risk of bleeding for each individual AVM and the risks of the proposed treatment. Advances in anesthetic and microsurgical techniques have resulted in substantial reductions in operative morbidity. Operative mortality is now less than 1% in carefully selected patients.

Conservative
- AVMs discovered incidentally in the elderly.
- Large or critically located AVMs:
- Control hypertension.
- Avoid antithrombotic agents, including aspirin.
- Anti-epileptic drugs for symptomatic seizures.
- Elective cesarean section at 38 weeks gestation for pregnant women with AVM.

Surgical excision
Superficial (and thus surgically accessible), small AVMs that link a single cortical arterial branch through a shunt to a cortical vein are the best surgical candidates.

Spetzler and Martin (1986) classification for evaluating the risk of surgery in patients with AVMs:

Graded feature		Points assigned
Size of AVM:		
Small	(maximal diameter <3 cm [<1.2 in])	1
Medium	(maximal diameter 3–6 cm [>1.2–2.4 in])	2
	(maximal diameter >6 cm [>2.4 in])	3
Location:		
Non-eloquent area of brain		0
Eloquent area of brain*		1
Pattern of venous drainage:		
Superficial only		0
Any deep		1

*Sensorimotor, language, or visual cortex; hypothalamus or thalamus; internal capsule; brain stem; cerebellar peduncles; or cerebellar nuclei.

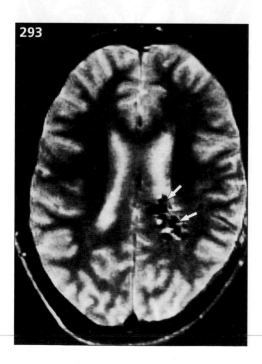

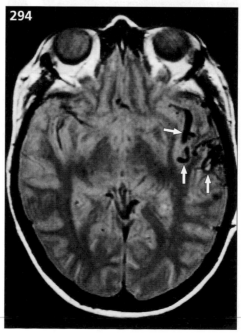

293 T2W MRI of an AVM in the left occipital lobe. Note the dark areas (arrows) which are 'flow voids' marking the abnormal arteries.

294 PDW MRI of a left temporal AVM. Again note the serpiginous dark structures which are flow voids in abnormal arteries (arrows).

The assigned grade of the AVM (1–5) corresponds numerically to the cumulative score. A score of 4 or 5 is associated with the highest risk of persistent neurologic deficits after surgery.

Stereotactic radiosurgery (radiotherapy)

Used for small (<3 cm [<1.2 in] diameter), deep AVMs <2.5–3 cm (1–1.2 in] in diameter. Radiotherapy is effective in obliterating about 80–90% of these AVMs within a latency interval of 2–3 years.

A stereotactic frame is screwed into the skull vault. Cranial CT scan and cerebral angiogram are undertaken with the frame in place. Using the frame and coordinates the location of the nidus can be plotted. It may involve the use of a gamma knife, proton beam, or linear accelerator. A single session therapeutic radiation dose is applied to the nidus and a little of the penumbra, via multiple focused beams to cause vascular injury, subsequent thrombosis, and delayed obliteration of the AVM. This may cause some necrosis of underlying normal brain tissue; the amount depends on how large the penumbra is. The fact that radiotherapy takes months to years to have an effect is unlike other treatments. As a result, the major disadvantage is that patients remain at risk for hemorrhage during the latency interval until the AVM obliterates.

Endovascular embolization with rapidly polymerizing liquid glues

Preferable for deep and large (>3.5 cm [1.4 in]) lesions, often in combination with open surgery.

295 Section of a saccular aneurysm at the base of the brain, taken at autopsy, showing disruption of the internl elastic lamina and hemorrhage.

296 Section of the brain in the axial plane showing subarachnoid hemorrhage in the anterior interhemispheric fissure and intraventricular extension of the hemorrhage due to a ruptured anterior communicating artery aneurysm. (Courtesy of Professor BA Kakulas, Royal Perth Hospital, Western Australia.)

297 Photograph of the base of the brain at autopsy, with the right temporal lobe resected, showing a ruptured aneurysm of the right middle cerebral artery (arrow) and blood in the Sylvian fissure. (Courtesy of Professor BA Kakulas, Royal Perth Hospital, Western Australia.)

SUBARACHNOID HEMORRHAGE (SAH)

DEFINITION

The spontaneous extravasation of blood into the subarachnoid space when a blood vessel near the surface of the brain leaks. It is a condition, not a disease, that can be produced by many causes.

EPIDEMIOLOGY

- Incidence: 6–8 per 100 000 person years outside Finland; almost three times higher in Finland.
- Age: typically over 40 years of age.
- Gender: F>M = 1.6 (1.1–2.3):1.

PATHOLOGY

Blood in the subarachnoid space, which may be diffuse or localized and may have extended into the brain parenchyma. Most commonly, subarachnoid blood is maximal adjacent to a ruptured saccular aneurysm at the base of the brain (**295–297**). In 10% of cases, the center of the hemorrhage is around the midbrain (perimesencephalic), usually ventral to it, but there is no other pathology; the angiogram is

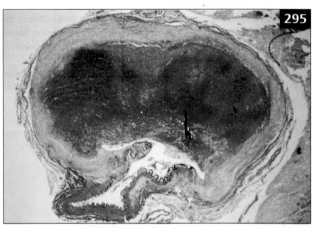

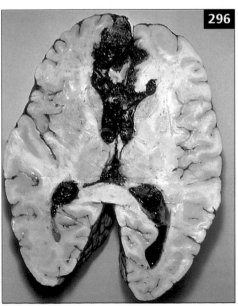

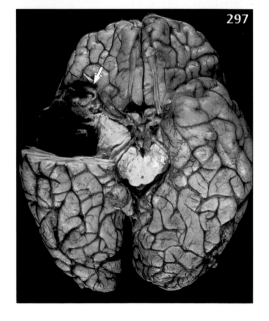

Management
- Repeat the CT scan and compare the bicaudate index with that on any previous scan.
- Spontaneous improvement occurs within 24 hours in half the patients (except those with massive intraventricular hemorrhage); take action if patient further deteriorates or fails to improve within 24 hours.
- Lumbar punctures are reasonably safe if there is no brain shift, and effective in about half the patients who have obstruction in the subarachnoid space and not in the ventricular system.
- External drainage of the ventricles is very effective in restoring the level of consciousness but carries a high risk of re-bleeding (consider emergency clipping or coiling of the aneurysm at the same time), and of infection (this may to some degree be prevented by prophylactic antibiotics or subcutaneous tunnelling).

Hyponatremia
- Almost invariably caused by sodium depletion, not by sodium dilution (SIADH).
- Associated hypovolemia increases risk of delayed cerebral ischemia.

Management
- Give isotonic saline (with or without albumin to expand plasma volume) or a mixture of glucose and saline; no free water.
- If necessary add fludrocortisone acetate, 400 µg/day in two doses, orally or intravenously.
- Keep central venous pressure between 1.1–1.3 kPa (8–10 mmHg), or pulmonary capillary wedge pressure between 1.1–1.6 kPa (8–12 mmHg).

Delayed cerebral ischemia
Up to one-third of patients with a ruptured aneurysm develop cerebral ischemia, mainly between day 5 and day 14 after the initial bleed. Cerebral ischemia or infarction is not confined to the territory of a single cerebral artery or one of its branches. The pathogenesis is complex.

Vasospasm is often implicated because its peak frequency from days 5–14 coincides with that of delayed ischemia and because it is often generalized, like the clinical and radiologic findings, but it is not the only factor in the pathogenesis of cerebral ischemia.

Angiographic evidence of vasospasm occurs in up to 70% of patients with aneurysmal SAH, but neurologic deterioration secondary to vasospasm occurs in about one-third of all patients, and about half of these patients with symptomatic vasospasm die or suffer neurologic disability as a direct result of the ischemia.

Determinants of delayed cerebral ischemia
- SAH caused by a ruptured aneurysm.
- Arterial narrowing.
- Depressed level of consciousness for more than 1 hour after the onset.
- Amount of subarachnoid blood on early CT scanning, not the distribution.
- Acute hydrocephalus.
- Hyponatremia and hypovolemia.
- Detection of emboli on transcranial Doppler monitoring, after surgical clipping.

- Treatment with antihypertensive drugs.
- Treatment with antifibrinolytic drugs.

Management
- Establish diagnosis: clinical and serial brain CT or MRI scans (rule out other causes of deterioration).
- Stop nimodipine.
- Immediately administer a plasma volume expander: 500 ml of a colloid solution such a hetastarch or hemaccel.
- Insert a subclavian vein catheter or pulmonary arterial balloon catheter; maintain central venous pressure between 1.1–1.3 kPa (8–12 mmHg), or pulmonary wedge pressure between 1.9–2.2 kPa (14–18 mmHg).
- Maintain fluid intake with at least 3 l of normal saline (0.9%) per 24 hours.
- Correct hyponatremia.
- Keep hematocrit around 40%.
- Keep arterial pressure 2.7–5.3 kPa (20–40 mmHg) above baseline values; may need inotropic support in intensive care unit.

Cardiac arrhythmias
Rarely need to be treated.

PROGNOSIS
- Half of patients die; sudden death occurs in about 15% of patients: usually ruptured posterior circulation aneurysms and intraventricular hemorrhage.
- Half of survivors remain severely disabled.
- Delayed ischemia is a major cause of death and disability.
- Outcome in patients with familial SAH is worse than in patients with sporadic SAH.
- Non-aneurysmal perimesencephalic SAH: excellent prognosis; re-bleeding and ischemia do not occur.

Adverse prognostic factors

Decreased level of consciousness on admission	++++
Large amount of blood in subarachnoid space on CT scan	+++
Increasing age	++
Loss of consciousness at onset	+
High blood pressure on admission	+
Pre-existing medical condition	+
Aneurysm in posterior rather than anterior circulation	+
Use of anticoagulants	+
Intravenous drug abuse	+
Associated intracranial hematoma	+
Level of creatinine kinase BB in CSF	+

CEREBRAL VENOUS THROMBOSIS

DEFINITION
Occlusion of cortical cerebral veins or dural venous sinuses, or both, by thrombus (phlebothrombosis).

EPIDEMIOLOGY
- Incidence: unknown (previous studies have relied on autopsy data, and more recently cerebral angiography) but uncommon.
- Low prevalence in autopsy series; 0.1–0.9% of autopsies.
- Age: any age, but young and middle-aged women at greatest risk: mean age 40 years.
- Gender: higher incidence in females (1.3:1).

RELEVANT VENOUS ANATOMY
Blood from the brain is drained by cerebral veins which empty into dural sinuses that drain mostly into the internal jugular veins. There is extensive collateral circulation in the cerebral venous system.

Dural sinuses
The most commonly affected by thrombosis are the superior sagittal sinus, lateral sinus, cavernous sinus and straight sinus (**309**).

309 MR venogram, left postero-lateral view, showing the normal appearance of the venous sinuses in the head.

310, 311 Autopsy specimen of brain, vertex of the brain (**310**), and coronal section through the frontal lobes (**311**), showing bilateral parasagittal hemorrhagic infarction due to superior sagittal sinus thrombosis.

Cerebral veins
Three groups of veins drain the blood supply from the brain: superficial cerebral veins (or cortical veins), deep cerebral veins and posterior fossa veins.

PATHOLOGY
- Isolated cortical venous thrombosis is rare, most patients have dural sinus thrombosis with or without cortical vein involvement (**310, 311**).
- The thrombus itself is like other venous thrombi elsewhere in the body. When it is fresh, it is a red thrombus rich in red blood cells and fibrin but poor in platelets; when it is old, it is replaced by fibrous tissue sometimes showing recanalization.
- Hemorrhagic infarction of the brain is common.

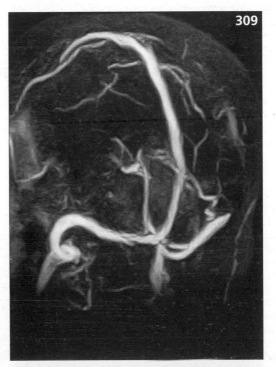

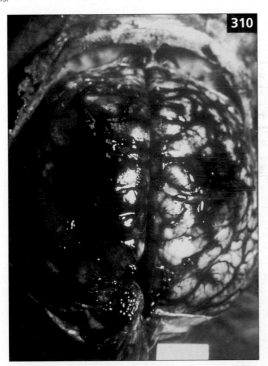

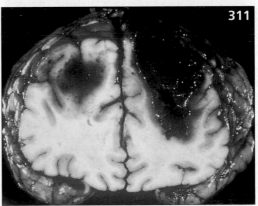

ETIOLOGY

Predisposing factors can be identified in up to 80% of patients.

Local conditions directly affecting the veins and sinuses

Non-infective
- Head trauma (open or closed, with or without fracture).
- Intracranial surgery.
- Brain infarction or hemorrhage.
- Tumor invasion of dural sinuses (meningioma, metastases, glomus tumor).
- Catheterization of, and infusions into, the internal jugular veins (e.g. for parenteral nutrition).

Infective
- Direct septic trauma.
- Local regional infection (scalp, sinuses, ears, mastoids, nasopharynx).
- Intracranial infection:
- Bacterial meningitis.
- Meningovascular syphilis.
- Subdural empyema.
- Bacterial or fungal brain abscess.

Systemic conditions

Non-infective
- Surgery: any surgical procedure, with or without deep venous thrombosis.
- Hormonal:
- Pregnancy or more commonly the puerperium.
- Oral contraceptives (estrogens or progestogens [progestins]) (OCP): age-adjusted odds ratio of 13 for OCP use and risk of CVST; age-adjusted odds ratio of 30 for OCP use combined with prothrombin G20210A gene mutation and risk of CVST.
- Medical:
- Severe dehydration of any cause (including angiography or myelography).
- Hyperviscosity syndrome: multiple myeloma; Waldenstrom's macroglobulinemia.
- Hypercoagulable state:
 Red blood cell disorders: polycythemia; post-hemorrhagic anemia; sickle cell disease/trait; paroxysmal nocturnal hemoglobinuria.
 Platelet disorders: essential thrombocythemia.
- Coagulation disorders (see p.222): deficiency of antithrombin III, protein C, or protein S; circulating lupus anticoagulant; activated protein C resistance (factor V Leiden gene mutation); prothrombin G20210A gene mutation (see p.223); disseminated intravascular coagulation; heparin- or heparinoid-induced thrombocytopenia; antifibrinolytic treatment.
- Extracranial malignancy (non-metastatic effect): any visceral carcinoma, carcinoid, lymphoma, leukemia, L-asparaginase therapy.
- Connective tissue disease: SLE; Wegener's granulomatosis; giant cell arteritis.
- Cardiac: congenital heart disease; congestive heart failure; pacemaker.
- Gastrointestinal: inflammatory bowel disease; cirrhosis.
- Various others: Behçet's disease (**312–314**); sarcoidosis; nephrotic syndrome; androgen therapy; diabetes mellitus; parenteral injections; hyperhomocystinemia.

Infective
- Bacterial: septicemia, endocarditis, typhoid, tuberculosis.
- Viral: measles, hepatitis, encephalitis, herpes, HIV, CMV.
- Parasitic: malaria, trichinosis.
- Fungal: aspergillosis.

Uncertain etiology (20–25%)

PATHOGENESIS

Thrombus formation due to venous stasis, increased clotting tendency, changes in the vessel wall, and less frequently, embolization.

CLINICAL SYNDROMES

Occur in isolation or combination.

Sagittal and/or transverse sinus thrombosis

Syndrome of progressive idiopathic intracranial hypertension
- Headache.
- Obscurations of vision.
- Papilloedema.

Cortical venous thrombosis

Syndrome of subacute or chronic focal or generalized encephalopathy
Evolution over a few days, weeks or months of headache, confusion, drowsiness, epileptic seizures (partial and secondary generalized), raised intracranial pressure, and coma with or without focal neurologic signs.

Stroke-like syndrome (frequently with seizures)
A cortical stroke syndrome (i.e. non-lacunar) occurring in patients suffering from any one of the etiologic conditions should suggest venous thrombosis, particularly if the evolution of the focal neurologic deficit is rather slow, if seizures occur, and if there is hemorrhagic infarction or frank hemorrhage in the territory of drainage of a cortical vein in the cortex/subcortex.

Thunderclap headache
Abrupt onset of very severe pain in the head, perhaps caused by intraparenchymal hemorrhage, venous hemorrhagic infarction, or venous subarachnoid hemorrhage.

Cavernous sinus thrombosis

Syndrome of chemosis, proptosis and painful ophthalmoplegia
Usually due to suppuration spreading from face, orbit or paranasal sinuses (staphylococcal, streptococcal, mucormycosis), causing:
- Pain around the eye and face.
- Conjunctival and eyelid edema, episcleral congestion.
- Proptosis.
- Blindness and papilledema.
- Cranial nerve III, IV, VI, V^1 and perhaps V^2 palsies.

Thrombosis may spread to the contralateral cavernous sinus and other dural sinuses. Suppuration may spread to cause subdural empyema, bacterial meningitis, or infective arteritis and thrombosis of the terminal carotid and middle cerebral artery origin.

Deep cerebral vein thrombosis

Variable clinical features. May have an 'encephalitic' presentation characterized by the gradual onset of headache, confusion, obtundation and vomiting with or without the development of focal neurologic signs such as amnesia or long tract signs due to bilateral thalamic infarction or unilateral temporoparietal infarction (that may become hemorrhagic) depending on the collateral venous circulation and whether the thrombus propagated from the lateral sinus into the vein of Labbé.

DIFFERENTIAL DIAGNOSIS

- Subdural empyema.
- Bacterial meningitis.
- SAH.
- Encephalitis.
- Brain abscess.
- Stroke: arterial occlusion or dissection, SAH.
- Benign thunderclap headache, 'crash' migraine.

INVESTIGATIONS
Cranial CT and MRI imaging

The appearance of the brain in cerebral venous thrombosis depends on whether the venous sinuses or cortical veins (or both) are involved. Thrombosis of the cortical veins usually results in venous infarction (**315**), whereas isolated venous

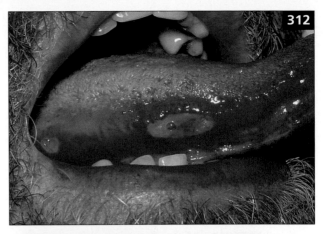

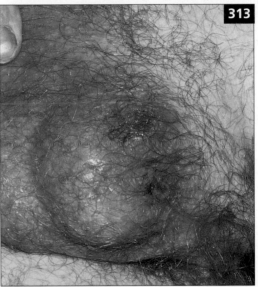

312–314 Tongue (**312**) and and genital (scrotal) (**313**, **314**) ulcers in a young man with Behçet's disease who presented with cerebral venous thrombosis.

315 CT scan without contrast of a 6 hour old venous infarct (compare with the arterial infarct of similar age in **227**). Note the well defined edges, marked swelling, central hemorrhage. There was no sinus involvement.

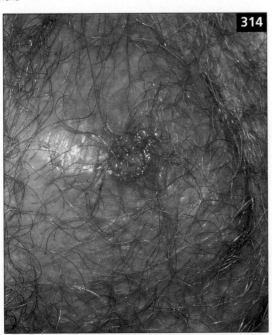

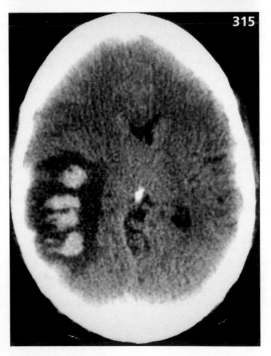

sinus thrombosis may not cause infarction but results in generalized brain swelling and raised ICP (**316, 317**). The imaging of venous thrombosis is therefore directed at:
- Recognizing correctly the venous origin of any parenchymal lesion.
- Diagnosing the extent of any sinus involvement.
- Identifying any predisposing factors (such as tumors pressing on the sinus or local infection).

Venous sinus thrombosis
This may be imaged by CT and MRI and appear as:
- A high density (or altered signal and loss of flow void on MRI) in the sinus (due to the thrombus) (**316–319**).
- A triangular filling defect in the sinus after i.v. contrast ('empty delta' sign (**251, 252**). High splitting of the superior sagittal sinus can mimic a delta sign, as can an adjacent epidural abscess.
- Generalized brain swelling (cerebral edema);
- Local infection such as mastoiditis or sinusitis as a precipitating cause.

Venous infarction
- May be single or multiple.
- Typically more clearly demarcated and of lower density than arterial infarction of the same age (**315**).
- More frequently hemorrhagic than arterial infarcts.
- The hemorrhage typically starts in the center and extends towards the periphery, (whereas in arterial infarcts the hemorrhage is typically around the edge).
- Infarction occupies territories which are not typically arterial, or involve adjacent areas of brain (e.g. occipital lobe and cerebellum) which is difficult to explain from the arterial anatomy.
- More swollen than an arterial infarct of the same age.
- The brain beyond the visible boundaries of the infarct also may appear swollen.
- The cord sign refers to a thrombosed vein, present on pre-contrast views.

Normal scans are more likely when the thrombotic process has been confined to the deep venous system, including the vein of Galen and the straight sinus; and when the patient has presented with signs of intracranial hypertension alone.

MRI of the brain is now the diagnostic procedure of choice because it is non-invasive, sensitive to blood flow, and readily visualizes the thrombus itself.

Four vessel conventional or digitalized intra-arterial cerebral angiography

This technique, which visualizes the entire venous phase on at least two projections (frontal and lateral), has been the gold standard for diagnosis, revealing the partial or complete lack of filling of veins or venous sinuses.

CSF
- Pressure is usually increased.
- May be normal or contain a modest excess of red blood cells, lymphocytes, neutrophils and protein.
- It is usually not necessary to perform a lumbar puncture and CSF examination in patients with suspected cerebral venous sinus thrombosis.

Other investigations
All other investigations are directed towards demonstrating the underlying cause (see Etiology, above).

Coagulation studies (see p.220)
Indicated in all patients, and particularly if family or past history of thrombotic episodes, or unexplained infarction:
- Protein C and S.
- Antithrombin III.
- Prothrombin G20210A gene mutation.
- Factor V Leiden mutation.
- Antiphospholipid antibodies.
- Fibrinogen.
- Plasminogen.

Chest x-ray
Chest x-ray or other imaging, inflammatory markers, autoantibodies, and tissue biopsy if suspected malignancy or connective tissue disease.

DIAGNOSIS
Angiography remains the gold standard for diagnosis but MRI with MR venography allows accurate diagnosis in most cases.

TREATMENT
- Any underlying cause (e.g. infection) should be identified and treated.
- The risks and benefits of anticoagulant therapy with intravenous heparin followed by oral anticoagulation for 3–6 months remain uncertain, based on a systematic review of the only two randomized controlled trials in a total of 70 patients. Anticoagulants may be useful in patients with dural sinus and even cortical venous thrombosis and may not necessarily be harmful, even in the presence of hemorrhagic infarction.
- If patients deteriorate, local thrombolysis with intrasinus urokinase may also have a role but this remains to be evaluated in controlled trials.

PROGNOSIS
Mortality rate <10%. If patients survive, the prognosis for recovery of function is generally favorable and much better than in arterial occlusion.

Prognostic factors
- Topography of thrombosis: deep cerebral vein and cerebellar vein thrombosis carry a much higher risk than cortical vein thrombosis.
- Underlying cause: septic cerebral venous sinus thrombosis still has a mortality rate of 30% in cavernous sinus thrombosis and up to 78% in SSS thrombosis.

VASCULAR DEMENTIA

DEFINITION
An acquired syndrome of cognitive impairment (dementia) that is characterized by the abrupt onset and stepwise progression of deficits of memory and at least two other cognitive functions (e.g. abstract thinking), sufficient to interfere with the person's usual social activities, and caused by vascular diseases of the brain.

EPIDEMIOLOGY
- Incidence: 2.5 per 1000 undemented individuals per year.
- Prevalence: about 22 per 1000 population (up to 40% of cases of dementia: the second most common cause of dementia after Alzheimer's disease); about 62 per 1000 people over the age of 59 years. Estimates of the prevalence of vascular dementia may be unreliable because of different diagnostic and pathologic criteria used in different studies.
- Age: elderly.
- Gender: M=F.

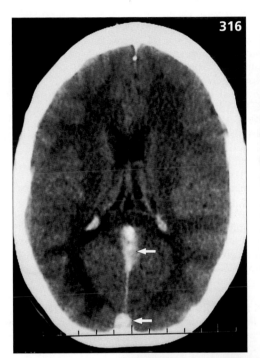

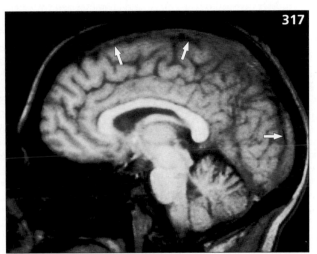

317 Same patient as **316**, T1W midline sagittal MRI shows the thrombus in the sagittal sinus (arrows). There should normally be a flow void in the sagittal sinus.

316 CT scan without contrast shows thrombosed sagittal and straight sinuses (arrows) without any actual infarction complicating meningococcal meningitis.

318, 319 MRI brain scans showing an hypointense (dark) (**318**), and hyperintense (white) (**319**) defect in the venous sinus at the torcula (arrows) due to loss of the flow void as a result of venous sinus thrombosis.

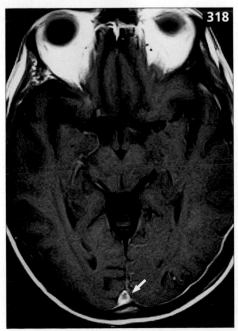

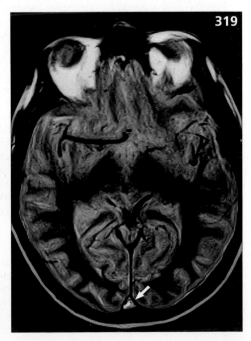

PATHOLOGY AND PATHOGENESIS
Parenchymal pathology
The site of brain tissue loss is a more important determinant of cognitive function than the volume of tissue lost.

Single strategically placed infarcts or hemorrhages
A single infarct or hemorrhage, if located in a strategically important part of the brain, such as the circuits involving the dorsolateral frontal convexity-caudate nucleus-globus pallidus-thalamus, can produce a vascular dementia. Examples include infarction or hemorrhage of the:

- Dominant angular gyrus, situated in the inferior parietal lobule, usually by embolic occlusion of the angular branch of the inferior division of the MCA, and characterized by the acute onset of fluent dysphasia, dysgraphia, memory loss and visuospatial disorientation.
- Thalamus, particularly the dominant dorsomedial thalamus, by occlusion of the paramedian thalamic (thalamoperforate) branches of the posterior cerebral artery, causing memory loss, slowness, apathy, ocular palsies, and drowsiness.
- Caudate nucleus and globus pallidus, usually by thrombotic or embolic occlusion of the penetrating lateral lenticulostriate branches of the middle cerebral artery.
- Basal forebrain and dorsolateral pre-frontal cortex.
- Hippocampus, usually by embolic occlusion of the cortical branches of the posterior cerebral artery, or diffuse cerebral ischemia.

Multiple infarcts or hemorrhages
Cortical/subcortical infarcts or hemorrhages may cause a 'cortical' type dementia with signs of amnesia, aphasia, apraxia, and agnosia. The infarcts are commonly the result of thromboembolism from the heart or a large artery (aortic arch, carotid and vertebrobasilar) to the anterior, middle, or posterior cerebral arteries or their branches, but can also be caused by large vessel disease causing hypoperfusion and infarcts in the borderzones between major arterial territories, and small vessel disease such as microatheroma/lipo-hyalinosis and vasculitis. Multiple cortical/subcortical hemorrhages are most commonly due to amyloid angiopathy but can also be seen with vasculitis, bleeding diatheses, metastases, hemorrhagic infarction and trauma.

Small deep ('lacunar') infarcts may cause a 'subcortical' dementia characterized by signs of psychomotor slowing, poor concentration, indecision and mental apathy. Other features, besides cognitive impairment, include hemiparesis, small stepping gait (*marche á petits pas*), dysarthria, and dysphagia. Typical patients are elderly, ex- or current smokers, with hypertension and diabetes. Rarely, they are part of the syndrome of cerebral autosomal dominant arteriopathy with subcortical infarcts and leuko-encephalopathy (CADASIL), which is a hereditary disease with linkage to chromosome 19, and features of a subcortical dementia, recurrent stroke-like events and visible white matter lesions on brain imaging.

Diffuse white matter infarction
(Subcortical arteriosclerotic leukocencephalopathy, Binswanger's disease). Diffuse or multifocal, often periventricular, areas of demyelination, axonal loss, and reactive gliosis in the white matter probably due to anoxia as a result of arteriosclerotic changes (hyalinization, fibrosis and thickening) in the long penetrating end arteries and arterioles of the periventricular white matter, rather than any atheroma of the large arteries which is variable in extent and severity. White matter lesions are found in about 80% of patients with vascular dementia, about 15% of patients with early-onset Alzheimer's disease and about 75% of patients with late-onset Alzheimer's disease. They are associated with hypertension and, in some studies, with heart disease and diabetes. They are thought to cause dementia by disconnecting the pathways between the cortical and subcortical areas.

Diffuse laminar necrosis (global cerebral ischemia)

Vascular pathology
Hypoxic-ischemic lesions
- Large artery atherosclerosis.
- Small vessel hyaline wall thickening (arteriolosclerosis), microatheroma and lipohyalinosis.
- Embolism from the heart.
- Non-atheromatous angiopathies.
- Granular degeneration of the media of small arteries (CADASIL).
- Cerebral vasculitis
- Neoplastic angioendotheliomatosis (malignant lymphoma of blood vessels).
- Mural dissections.
- Dural arteriovenous malformation.
- Hematologic disease (thrombophilia).

Hemorrhagic lesions
- Subdural hematoma.
- SAH: anterior communicating artery aneurysm.
- Intracerebral hemorrhage (see p.238):
- Amyloid angiopathy.
- Hypertensive small vessel disease.

RISK FACTORS FOR VASCULAR DEMENTIA
Age and stroke are the most important risk factors for developing dementia:
- Increasing age;
- Past history of stroke (symptomatic stroke increases the risk of dementia more than ninefold) or myocardial infarction (one-third of patients).

Other putatitive risk factors include:
- Hypertension (60% of patients).
- Smoking (35%).
- Diabetes (20% of patients).
- Hyperlipidemia (20%).
- Alcohol abuse.
- Family history (CADASIL).
- Lower education level.
- Residing in a rural area.
- Living in an institution.
- Brain atrophy.
- Cortical infarcts.
- Brain white matter lesions.
- Left hemisphere stroke.
- Early urinary incontinence.
- Falls.
- Abnormal EKG (80% of patients compared with 30% of people with Alzheimer's disease).

CLINICAL FEATURES

Slowly progressive intellectual impairment, with recurrent stroke-like events.

History

- Presenting symptoms: sudden onset and stepwise course of cognitive decline with history of transient ischemic attacks, strokes, or both. Epileptic seizures occur in 10% of patients. Incontinence of urine and feces is not uncommon.
- Past history of vascular risk factors: hypertension, diabetes, heart disease, smoking.
- Family history: CADASIL.

Neurologic examination

- Focal neurologic deficits such as pyramidal tract signs (hemiparesis, extensor plantar response, pseudobulbar palsy), extrapyramidal signs, hemisensory loss, hemianopia, and dysarthria.
- Gait abnormality: start and turn hesitation, shuffling, reduced arm swing.
- Grasp reflexes
- Hypertension and hypertensive retinopathy.
- A source of thromboembolism such as AF, valvular heart disease, heart failure, carotid artery disease.

Neuropsychologic examination

- Essential to ascertain the presence or absence of a cognitive deficit, the nature of the deficit (i.e. in what domains) and the degree of the deficit.
- Concentration and executive function: poor learning strategies, impaired word list generation, emotional blunting and lability, poor insight and judgement.
- Memory: impaired learning of verbal and visual information, reduced recall following a delay.
- Verbal output: dysarthria, reduced grammatical complexity of spontaneous speech.
- Depression: present in 25% of patients; depressive symptoms in 60%.
- Anxiety: common.
- Delusions: present in up to one-half of patients.
- Personality alterations: apathetic, listless, lifeless, quiet and labile.

DIFFERENTIAL DIAGNOSIS

Vascular dementia and Alzheimer's disease (mixed or 'double dementia')

Clinical course may be slowly progressive and it may be difficult to interpret the relevance of brain lesions, consistent with infarction, seen on neuroimaging (e.g. white matter lesions).

Alzheimer's disease (see p.407)

- More likely to have retrieval errors and irrelevant intrusions on memory tests and to perform more poorly on a story recall test.
- Less likely to have a history of previous strokes, hypertension, and alcohol abuse, depression, or an abnormal EKG (30% of cases).

Lewy body type dementia (see p.430)

- Marked fluctuations of symptoms.
- Prominent extrapyramidal signs, particularly rigidity and bradykinesia.
- Early and florid visual hallucinations and delusions.
- Poor tolerance of neuroleptic drugs.

Parkinson's disease dementia (see p.420)

- Possibly affects 10–20% of patients with Parkinson's disease.
- Dementia is subcortical (apathy, poor concentration, indecision, slowness of central processing).
- Dementia is usually preceded by parkinsonian features.
- Gait changes of vascular dementia and Parkinson's disease closely resemble each other.
- Dopaminergic medication usually improves the parkinsonian features.

Progressive supranuclear palsy (see p.432)

- Subcortical dementia.
- Preceding parkinsonian features.
- Paralysis of vertical gaze.
- Truncal ataxia.
- Parkinsonian features do not respond to dopaminergic medication.

Multiple systems atrophy (see p.435)

- Dementia is slowly progressive.
- Accompanying signs of dysfunction of any or all of the:
- Pyramidal tract.
- Extrapyramidal system.
- Autonomic system.
- Cerebellum.

Frontal lobe tumors

Early symptoms may be behavioral disturbance (disinhibited and irrational) or mental apathy and indecision. Later signs may be those of raised intracranial pressure (see p.477).

Uncommon but treatable causes of dementia

- Hypothyroidism.
- Vitamin B_{12} deficiency.
- Neurosyphilis.
- Normal pressure hydrocephalus.
- Frontal lobe tumors.
- Cerebral ischemia due to cerebral vasculitis, hyperviscosity syndrome and severe bilateral carotid stenosis.
- HIV dementia (see p.301).

INVESTIGATIONS

CT or MR imaging of the brain

Excludes other causes of dementia (e.g. frontal tumor, hydrocephalus) and almost always identifies one or more vascular lesions. CT brain scan reveals more or less symmetric periventricular and subcortical hypodensity in the cerebral white matter, with or without ventricular dilatation and focal hypodensities and thought to be due to 'small vessel' ischemia and infarction.

MR T2W or proton density imaging demonstrates the same features even better as high signal areas (**320, 321**). These radiologic appearances (leukoaraiosis [leuko=white, araiosis=rarefaction]) are rather non-specific and can be found in apparently normal elderly people. However, they are more commonly associated with gradual dementia, unsteadiness of gait, and recurrent ischemic, particularly lacunar, or occasionally hemorrhagic strokes, and are more frequent in patients with hypertension, other vascular risk factors, atherosclerosis and cerebral atrophy.

Additional features may include multiple small 'holes' in the basal ganglia and pons, and cortical infarcts may also be present.

Blood tests
- Full blood count and ESR.
- Plasma viscosity.
- Serum urea and electrolytes.
- Plasma glucose.
- Serum cholesterol and triglycerides.
- Liver function tests.
- Serum protein electrophoresis.
- Antinuclear antibodies.
- Thyroid function tests.
- Syphilis serology.
- Vitamin B_{12}.
- Coagulation studies (younger patients) (see p.220):
- Antiphospholipid antibodies.
- Proteins C and S.
- Antithrombin III.
- Factor V Leiden mutation.

Other
- EKG.
- Echocardiography: if prosthetic heart valves, rheumatic valvular heart disease, or suspected left atrial myxoma.
- Doppler ultrasonography of the carotid arteries.
- Single photon emission computed tomography (SPECT): asymmetric patchy areas of reduced cerebral blood flow.
- Positron emission tomography (PET): fluorodeoxyglucose PET reveals multifocal regions of reduced cerebral metabolism (due to local infarction or a distant effect of diaschisis) in contrast to symmetric biparietal hypometabolism typically observed in Alzheimer's disease.

DIAGNOSIS
The purpose of the clinical and laboratory assessment is to establish the diagnosis of vascular dementia, the cause of the cerebrovascular disease, and other factors that may be contributing to the cognitive compromise.

The diagnosis of vascular dementia is based on a decline in cognitive function (dementia) that correlates with a clear history of strokes. However, the association between declining cognitive function (dementia) and cerebrovascular disease may not be causal; it may be merely contributory or even coincidental. Various diagnostic criteria exist to aid the diagnosis but many have not been validated.

Hachinski ischemia scale

Item	Score value
Abrupt onset*	2
Stepwise course*	1
Fluctuating course	2
Preservation of personality	1
Nocturnal confusion	1
Depression	1
Somatic complaints*	1
Emotional incontinence*	1
History of hypertension*	1
Evidence of associated atherosclerosis	1
History of stroke*	2
Focal neurologic symptoms*	2
Focal neurologic signs*	2

*Discriminating items after validation at post mortem examination.

A score of 7 or higher is said to be diagnostic of vascular dementia but this scale has poor interrater reliability.

NINDS–AIREN CRITERIA FOR VASCULAR DEMENTIA
Definite vascular dementia
- Clinical criteria for probable vascular dementia.
- Autopsy demonstration of appropriate ischemic brain injury and no other cause of the dementia.

Probable vascular dementia
Dementia
- Decline from a previous higher level of cognitive functioning.
- Impairment of two or more cognitive domains.
- Deficits severe enough to interfere with activities of daily living and are not due to physical effects of stroke alone.
- Patients must not be delirious; must not have psychosis, aphasia or sensory-motor impairment that precludes neuropsychologic testing; and the patient must not have any other disorder capable of producing a dementia syndrome.

Cerebrovascular disease
- Focal neurologic signs consistent with stroke.
- Neuroimaging evidence of extensive vascular lesions.

Relationship between the dementia and the cerebrovascular disease
As evidenced by one or more of the following:
- Onset of dementia within 3 months of a recognized stroke.
- Abrupt deterioration, or fluctuating or stepwise progression of the cognitive deficit.

Possible vascular dementia
- Dementia with focal neurologic signs but without neuroimaging confirmation of definite cerebrovascular disease.
- Dementia with focal neurologic signs but without a clear temporal relationship between dementia and stroke.
- Dementia with focal neurologic signs but with a subtle onset and variable course of cognitive deficits.

TREATMENT

- Treat any underlying causes and risk factors that may be remediable:
  - Cerebral vasculitis: corticosteroids and cyclophosphamide.
  - Hyperviscosity syndrome.
  - Neoplastic angioendotheliomatosis: chemotherapy.
- Control vascular risk factors such as hypertension, smoking, hypercholesterolemia and diabetes.
- Long term antiplatelet therapy such as low dose aspirin.
- Physiotherapy: gait, spasticity.
- Speech therapy: dysarthria, dysphasia, dysphagia.
- Psychologic therapy: visual-spatial neglect.

No benefit is obtained with hemorrheologic agents (pentoxifylline), nootropic compounds (oxiracetam), calcium channel blockers (nimodipine) or neuroprotective agents.

CLINICAL COURSE AND PROGNOSIS

- Characteristically, a progressive stepwise course of cognitive decline but in up to half of patients it can follow a slow progressive course.
- 50% survival: 6.7 years (cf. 8.1 years for Alzheimer's disease).
- Cause of death: heart disease or recurrent stroke.

HYPERTENSIVE ENCEPHALOPATHY

DEFINITION

A relatively rapidly evolving clinicoradiologic syndrome caused by capillary leakage related to abrupt hypertension, and characterized by confusion, cognitive changes, seizures and sometimes cortical blindness; and MRI evidence of diffuse or posterior (parieto-occipital) white matter changes.

EPIDEMIOLOGY

- Incidence: rare.
- Age: any age, mean age: 40 years.
- Gender: M=F.

PATHOLOGY

Macroscopic

The brain appears normal or shows evidence of cerebral swelling or hemorrhages in various sizes. Brain hemorrhage is not a sequela of the encephalopathy but is due to the primary disease causing the encephalopathy or one of the complications of the disease; so it is a complication of uncontrolled hypertension, eclampsia and potential bleeding disorders.

Microscopic

Widespread minute infarcts, with a predilection for the basis pontis, due to fibrinoid necrosis of the walls of arterioles and capillaries, and occlusion of their lumens by fibrin thrombi. Similar vascular changes are found in other organs, particularly the retinae and kidneys.

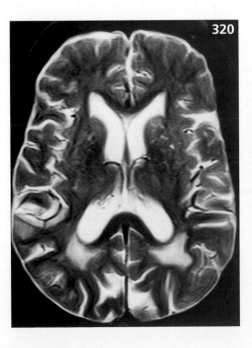

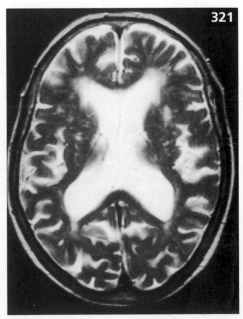

320 T2W MRI in a 78 year old female with vascular dementia due to Binswanger's disease. Note the cerebral atrophy and the diffuse hyperintense areas adjacent to the frontal and posterior horns of the lateral ventricles, representing subcortical ischemic leukoencephalopathy due to 'small vessel disease'.

321 T2W MRI at the level of the lateral ventricles in a 75 year old female with cognitive impairment due to multi-infarct dementia. Note the atrophy and multiple hyperintense areas in the periventricular white matter in keeping with 'small vessel disease'.

ETIOLOGY

- Abrupt increase in blood pressure usually in patients with known hypertension (most common). Encephalopathy is rare in chronic hypertension unless the diastolic blood pressure exceeds 20 kPa (150 mmHg) because the upper limit of anticoagulation is 'set' higher.
- Renovascular hypertension.
- Parenchymal renal disease.
- Acute glomerulonephritis.
- Scleroderma and other connective tissue diseases.
- Vasculitis.
- Drugs: sympathomimetic agents (amphetamines, cocaine, phencyclidine hydrochloride, lysergic acid diethylamide, diet pills), tricyclic antidepressants.
- Ingestion of tyramine in conjunction with a monamine oxidase inhibitor.
- Withdrawal of antihypertensive drugs (centrally acting agents and beta-antagonists).
- Pre-eclampsia, eclampsia.
- Pheochromocytoma.
- Renin-secreting tumor.
- Head injury.
- Autonomic hyperactivity in Guillain–Barré or spinal cord syndromes.
- Bilateral carotid endarterectomy (baroreceptor reflex failure).

PATHOPHYSIOLOGY

Increases in circulating levels of vasoconstrictor substances, such as norepinephrine, angiotensin II, or antinatriuretic hormone lead to an abrupt increase in systemic vascular resistance and blood pressure. Severely elevated blood pressure precipitates endothelial damage, platelet and fibrin deposition, arteriolar fibrinoid necrosis and loss of autoregulatory function with resultant end-organ (brain, retina, kidney, heart) ischemia. Ischemia, in turn, triggers the further release of vasoactive substances, thus initiating a vicious cycle of further vasoconstriction and myointimal proliferation.

Failure of autoregulation of cerebral blood flow leads to a breakdown of the blood–brain barrier with transudation of fluid, causing widespread cerebral edema, and petechial hemorrhages, sometimes culminating in frank, fatal intracranial hemorrhage.

Encephalopathy may occur with a diastolic blood pressure of 13.3 kPa (100 mmHg) or less if autoregulation is normal and easily exceeded by a rapid rise in blood pressure from a normally low level.

RISK FACTORS

- High blood pressure (e.g. poor antihypertensive drug compliance or blood pressure control).
- Pre-existing dysfunction of the vascular endothelium, as may occur in pre-eclampsia and eclampsia or with immunosuppressive therapy, may predispose patients to failure of autoregulation and encephalopathy after relatively slight increases in blood pressure.

CLINICAL HISTORY

- Subacute onset:
- Headache: severe.
- Nausea, vomiting.
- Confusion.
- Declining conscious state.
- Blurred vision or blindness.
- Seizures: partial or generalized.
- Weakness: focal or generalized.
- Past history of hypertension: duration, severity and level of control.
- Extent of pre-existing end-organ damage (heart, brain, retina, kidneys).
- Coexisting acute or chronic illnesses.
- Family history of hypertension.
- Medications: prescription, over-the-counter, illicit; antihypertensive drug compliance.

EXAMINATION

- Disorientation.
- Obtundation.
- Focal neurologic signs (e.g. cortical blindness due to bilateral occipital lobe dysfunction).
- Seizures: generalized or focal.
- Hypertensive retinopathy (including papilledema) (**322, 323**).
- Pulses (if unequal, suspect aortic dissection).
- Blood pressure supine and erect: can be apparently normal, particularly in young or pregnant patients in whom the base-line pressures are normally low. A single blood pressure reading may be deceptive. Blood pressure should be measured frequently and compared with base-line values.
- Cardiac and chest auscultation (suspect congestive heart failure).

DIFFERENTIAL DIAGNOSIS

- Stroke: there may be doubt about the onset of symptoms (i.e. if the patient is confused or obtunded), the blood pressure may be only moderately elevated, and focal or lateralizing neurologic signs may accompany the symptoms of more diffuse brain disturbance (headache, confusion, visual disturbances, and seizures). Even a severely elevated blood pressure is not specific because it can be a consequence of stroke and a cause of stroke.
- SAH.
- Epilepsy.
- Encephalitis.
- Vasculitis of the CNS.
- Brain tumor.
- Reversible posterior multifocal leukoencephalopathy:
- Puerperal eclampsia.
- Renal failure.
- Immunosuppressive agent treatment: cyclosporin: has direct toxic effects on vascular endothelial cells; interferon-alfa; tacrolimus; levamisole; fluorouracil.
- Multiple sclerosis.
- Progressive multifocal leukoencephalopathy.

INVESTIGATIONS

Imaging

CT or MRI brain scan

Scans may show:
- Areas of infarction/ischemia in the distribution of an arterial territory.
- Typical areas of involvement are the posterior parieto-occipital lobes bilaterally.
- The abnormalities may resolve as the patient recovers.
- MRI is more sensitive than CT to these changes, but confused patients tolerate MRI less well than CT.

Causes and consequences of hypertension
- FBP.
- ESR: ?arteritis.
- Serum urea and electrolytes: ?hypernatremia, ?hypokalemia, ?renal impairment.
- Urinalysis: blood, protein, casts, glomerular red blood cells, 24 hour urinary catecholamines.
- EKG: left ventricular hypertrophy.
- Chest x-ray: cardiomegaly, coarctation of the aorta.
- Renal ultrasound.
- Antinuclear antibodies.

DIAGNOSIS

A diagnosis of exclusion, requiring that the differential diagnoses (above) be ruled out.

TREATMENT

The goal of therapy is to reduce systemic vascular resistance and thus reduce the mean arterial pressure gradually by no more than 20–25% or to a diastolic blood pressure of 13.3 kPa (100 mmHg), whichever value is higher, during the first hour. The reason for the cautious reduction is because the lower limit of cerebral bloodflow autoregulation is reached when blood pressure is reduced by about one-quarter and rapid reductions of blood pressure by more than a half can precipitate cerebral ischemia or infarction.

The patient should be placed on a cardiac monitor and intravenous access established.

Hospital admission, preferably to an intensive care unit, should be arranged. An arterial line should be placed as soon as possible to confirm the cuff readings and to guide therapy (along with the clinical response).

Sodium nitroprusside is the drug of choice. It is administered by continuous infusion (0.5–10 µg/kg/min) and therefore the blood pressure demands constant surveillance, preferably intra-arterially. Adverse effects include hypotension, nausea, vomiting, and apprehension.

Effective alternatives include labetalol (20–80 mg i.v. bolus every 5–10 min, up to 300 mg; onset in 5–10 min, duration of action 3–6 hours), diazoxide (50–100 mg i.v. bolus every 5–10 min up to 600 mg; onset in 1–5 min, duration of action 6–12 hours), and nifedipine sublingually, but the latter can cause precipitous falls in blood pressure. Clonidine and methyldopa should be avoided because they depress the CNS, making it difficult to distinguish further CNS deterioration.

Diuretics and fluid restriction should not be prescribed routinely because most patients are volume depleted, presumably due to a pressure-related diuresis.

If neurologic function deteriorates after blood pressure reduction, antihypertensive therapy should be suspended and the blood pressure allowed to increase. Subsequent blood pressure reductions should be effected more slowly. Magnesium sulfate intravenously is effective for eclampsia. A loading dose of phenytoin 15–18 mg/kg (no faster than 50 mg/min) may be required if seizures occur.

PROGNOSIS

Usually reversible within hours of controlling the blood pressure, but the course can be prolonged for days to weeks. If the hypertension cannot be controlled, the outcome is usually fatal.

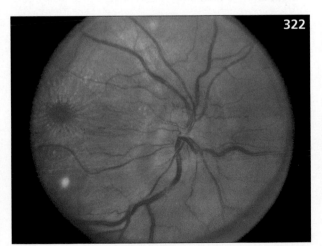

322 Optic fundus showing papilledema, narrow arterioles, and a macular star in a patient with hypertensive encephalopathy.

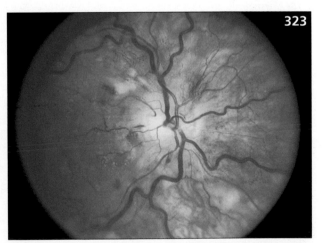

323 Optic fundus showing features of grade IV hypertensive retinopathy (malignant hypertension): superficial flame-shaped retinal hemorrhages near the optic disc, soft exudates, retinal edema and papilledema. (Courtesy of Mr M Wade, Department of Medical Illustrations, Royal Perth Hospital, Western Australia.)

PITUITARY APOPLEXY

DEFINITION
Acute massive infarction or hemorrhage of the pituitary gland.

EPIDEMIOLOGY
• Incidence: rare but probably underestimated because of incomplete non-fatal pituitary infarction. Infarction of more than 25% of the pituitary gland is reported to be present in 1–3% of patients in large unselected autopsy series.
• Age: evenly distributed between 20 and 70 years of age; range 6–83 years.
• Gender: M>F (2:1).

ANATOMY
Arterial blood supply to the pituitary: internal carotid artery via the superior and inferior hypophyseal arteries bilaterally.

PATHOLOGY
• Pituitary infarction (sometimes hemorrhagic) or hemorrhage, most often in an enlarging pituitary adenoma.
• The pituitary may or may not have a pre-existing tumor, and if present, the tumor may be primary or metastatic.
• Primary pituitary tumors are most commonly a pituitary adenoma.
• Chromophobe adenomas predominate over eosinophilic adenomas, merely reflecting the relative prevalence of these tumors. Rarely, basophilic adenomas, craniopharyngiomas, and primary pituitary carcinoma occur.
• Metastatic pituitary tumors are most commonly breast and lung cancers, in patients with widespread disease.
• Most pituitary tumors are endocrinologically silent; a minority are hormone-secreting: acromegaly, Cushing's disease.

ETIOLOGY
Predisposing factors
• Pituitary tumor of any type.
• Pregnancy.
• Diabetes.
• Following obstetric hemorrhage: infarction of non-tumorous pituitary.
• Raised intracranial pressure.
• Bleeding disorders.
• Anticoagulants.
• Upper respiratory infections.
• Radiation therapy of pituitary tumors.
• Trauma.
• Carotid angiography.
• Atherosclerosis.
• Sickle cell trait.
• Acromegaly.
• Cushing's disease (**324**).
• Adrenalectomy.
• Mechanical ventilation.

PATHOPHYSIOLOGY
Infarction of the pituitary with secondary hemorrhage and edema destroys the pituitary and causes rapid expansion of the pituitary lesion, acute compression of adjacent structures (optic chiasm and tracts; cavernous sinus; cranial nerves III, IV, V,

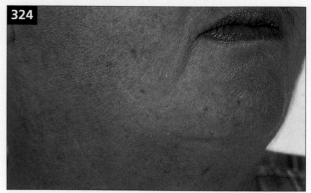

324

324 Facial appearance of a patient with Cushing's disease due to an ACTH-producing pituitary adenoma (which bled) featuring obesity, hirsutism (a fine 'downy' coat), plethora and ecchymoses (due to weakening and rupture of collagenous fibers in the dermis, exposing heavily vascularized subcutaneous tissues).

VI; sympathetic chain; internal carotid and branches; hypothalamus), leakage of blood or necrotic tissue into the subarachnoid space and compromise of neurologic function.

The initial event in post partum pituitary necrosis is probably occlusive arterial spasm of the arteries to the anterior lobe and stalk. After a period of total ischemia, attempts at re-establishment of circulation subsequently lead to vascular congestion and thrombosis of the anterior lobe. The inferior hypophyseal arterial flow is relatively spared accounting for the preservation of the infundibular process in most circumstances.

CLINICAL FEATURES
There are three main clinical syndromes.

Acute apoplexy
• Sudden severe retro-orbital headache.
• Cranial nerve dysfunction:
– II: impaired visual acuity; visual field defects (chiasmal compression).
– III, IV, VI: ophthalmoplegia, diplopia.
– V^1: facial pain.
• Proptosis.
• Eyelid edema.
• Horner's syndrome.
• Nausea and vomiting.
• Altered consciousness, progressing to coma.
• Focal hemispheric dysfunction: hemiparesis, seizures (carotid sinus compression, vasospasm due to SAH).
• Fever.

Subacute meningeal irritation (blood/necrotic tumor in subarachnoid space)
• Fever.
• Neck stiffness.
• Encephalopathy.

Subacute or chronic pituitary insufficiency months or years after the event
• Diabetes insipidus (uncommon).
• Syndrome of inappropriate antidiuretic hormone secretion.
• Anterior hypopituitarism:
– Absence of lactation.
– Persistent amenorrhea.

– Lethargy.
– Acute or delayed adrenal failure.

DIFFERENTIAL DIAGNOSIS
- Meningitis: viral, bacterial.
- Meningoencephalitis: viral, bacterial.
- Brain abscess.
- Cavernous sinus thrombosis.
- Carotid aneurysm.
- SAH: the association of SAH with ocular motor palsies in pituitary apoplexy can be distinguished from SAH due to rupture of an aneurysm by the presence of mixed, and usually, bilateral ophthalmoplegias, multiple cranial nerve palsies, and the presence of an afferent pupillary defect or chiasmal pattern of field loss with pituitary apoplexy, although the latter goes unnoticed in obtunded patients.
- Intracerebral hemorrhage.
- Transtentorial uncal herniation.
- Mesencephalic infarction.
- Parasellar tumor (meningioma or nasopharyngeal tumor).
- Metastatic pituitary tumors.

INVESTIGATIONS
Cranial CT or MRI brain scan
Plain scans often show a midline, hyperdense mass in the pituitary fossa and an expanded sella due to hemorrhagic infarction of the pituitary gland. The mass may compress the cavernous sinus and optic chiasm. Subarachnoid blood may be evident. The CT scan may be normal initially however, in patients with small pituitary tumors in whom radiographs of the pituitary fossa are also normal.

Hypothalamic and pituitary function tests
- Luteinizing hormone.
- Follicle stimulating hormone.
- Thyrotrophin (thyroid stimulating hormone).
- Growth hormone.
- Prolactin: low prolactin is very characteristic.
- Adrenocorticotropin.
- Cortisol.
- Thyroid-releasing and gonadotrophin-releasing hormone stimulation tests.

CSF
- Cells: may contain red and/or white blood cells, and necrotic tumor cells.
- Protein: mildly elevated.
- Gram stain, microscopy for organisms, and culture: negative.

Cerebral angiography
Used if an intracavernous carotid aneurysm needs to be excluded.

TREATMENT
Vigorous support
- Careful evaluation and monitoring of hormonal status.
- Immediate corticosteroid therapy in 'stress dosages' (hydrocortisone 100 mg i.v. every 6–8 hours) due to the high incidence of acute adrenal insufficiency, and other hormone replacement as appropriate.
- Fluid and electrolyte balance (cf. adrenal insufficiency, diabetes insipidus).
- Conservative management if consciousness, vision and endocrine function are maintained.

Surgery
Early transphenoidal neurosurgical decompression of tissues compromised by the rapidly expanding intrasellar mass is indicated if symptoms progress such as deteriorating visual acuity, declining consciousness, or evidence of hypothalamic damage.

PROGNOSIS
- Highly variable and unpredictable clinical course.
- Potentially fatal.
- Ophthalmoplegia often resolves spontaneously but recovery of vision is optimized by early decompression.
- Multiple pituitary hormone deficiencies occur in most patients after pituitary apoplexy and if unrecognized may contribute to morbidity and mortality.

FURTHER READING

NEUROVASCULAR SYNDROMES
Bamford J, Sandercock P, Dennis M, Burn J, Warlow C (1991) Classification and natural history of clinically identifiable subtypes of cerebral infarction. *Lancet*, **337**: 1521–1526.
Tatu L, Moulin T, Bogousslavsky J, Duvernoy H (1996) Arterial territories of the human brain: Brainstem and cerebellum. *Neurology*, **47**: 1125–1135.
Tatu L, Moulin T, Bogousslavsky J, Duvernoy H (1998) Arterial territories of the human brain. Cerebral hemispheres. *Neurology*, **50**: 1699–1708.

TRANSIENT ISCHEMIC ATTACKS (TIA) OF THE BRAIN AND EYE
General
Albers GW, Hart RG, Lutsep HL, *et al.* (1999) Supplement to the guidelines for the management of transient ischemic attacks. A statement from the Ad Hoc Committee on Guidelines for the management of transient ischemic attacks, Stroke Council, American Heart Association. *Stroke*, **30**: 2502–2511.

Hankey GJ (2001) Management of the first-time TIA. *Emergency Medicine*, **13**: 72–84.
Hankey GJ, Warlow CP (1994) *Transient ischaemic attacks of the brain and eye*. WB Saunders/Ballière Tindall, London.
Wolf PA, Clagett P, Easton JD, *et al.* (1999) Preventing ischemic stroke in patients with prior stroke and transient ischemic attack. A statement for healthcare professionals from the Stroke Council of the American Heart Association. *Stroke*, **30**: 1991–1994.

Epidemiology
Brown RD, Petty GW, O'Fallon WM, *et al.* (1998) Incidence of transient ischemic attack in Rochester, Minnesota, 1985–1989. *Stroke*, **29**: 2109–2113.

Diagnosis
Gunatilake S (1998) Rapid resolution of symptoms and signs of intracerebral haemorrhage: case reports. *BMJ*, **316**: 1495–1496.

Prognosis
Johnston SC, Gress DR, Browner WS, Sidney S (2000) Short-term prognosis after emergency department diagnosis of TIA. *JAMA*, **284**: 2901–2906.

Antiplatelet therapy
Algra A, van Gijn J (1996) Aspirin at any dose above 30 mg offers only modest protection after cerebral ischaemia. *J. Neurol. Neurosurg. Psychiatry*, **60**: 197–199.
Algra A, van Gijn J, Koudstaal PJ (1999) Secondary prevention after cerebral ischaemia of presumed arterial origin: is aspirin still the touchstone? *J. Neurol. Neurosurg. Psychiatry*, **66**: 557–559.
Antiplatelet Trialists' Collaboration (1994) Collaborative overview of randomised trials of antiplatelet therapy-I: Prevention of death, myocardial infarction, and stroke by prolonged antiplatelet therapy in various categories of patients. *BMJ*, **308**: 81–106.
Derry S, Loke YK (2000) Risk of gastrointestinal haemorrhage with long term use of aspirin: meta-analysis. *BMJ*, **321**: 1183–1187.
De Schryver ELLM, on behalf of the European/ Australian Stroke Prevention in Reversible Ischaemia Trial (ESPRIT) Group (2000) Design of ESPRIT: An international randomised trial for secondary prevention after non-disabling cerebral ischaemia of arterial origin. *Cerebrovasc. Dis.*, **10**: 147–150.
Hankey GJ, Sudlow CLM, Dunbabin DW (2000) Thienopyridines or aspirin to prevent stroke and other serious vascular events in patients at high risk of vascular disease. *Stroke*, **31**: 1779–1784.

Mohr JP, Thompson JLP, Lazar RM, *et al.* (2001) A comparison of warfarin and aspirin for the prevention of recurrent ischemic stroke. *N. Engl. J. Med.*, **345**: 1444–1451.

The Stroke Prevention in Reversible Ischemia Trial (SPIRIT) Study Group (1997) A randomised trial of anticoagulants versus aspirin after cerebral ischemia of presumed arterial origin. *Ann. Neurol.*, **42**: 857–65.

Wilterdink JL, Easton JD (1999) Dipyridamole plus aspirin in cerebrovascular disease. *Arch. Neurol.*, **56**: 1087–1092.

Carotid revascularization

Alamowitch S, Eliasziw M, Algra A, *et al.* (2001) Risk, causes, and prevention of ischaemic stroke in elderly patients with symptomatic internal-carotid-artery stenosis. *Lancet*, **357**: 1154–1160.

Barnett HJM, Taylor DW, Eliasziw M, *et al.* for the North American Symptomatic Carotid Endarterectomy Trial collaborators (1998) Benefit of carotid endarterectomy in patients with symptomatic moderate or severe carotid stenosis. *N. Engl. J. Med.*, **339**: 1415–1425.

Benavente O, Moher D, Pham B (1998) Carotid endarterectomy for asymptomatic carotid stenosis: a meta-analysis. *BMJ*, **317**: 1477–1480.

Biller J, Feinberg WM, Castaldo JE, *et al.* (1998) Guidelines for carotid endarterectomy. A statement for healthcare professionals from a special writing group of the Stroke Council, American Heart Association. *Stroke*, **29**: 554–562.

CAVATAS Investigators (2001) Endovascular versus surgical treatment in patients with carotid stenosis in the carotid and vertebral transluminal angioplasty study (CAVATAS): a randomized trial. *Lancet*, **357**: 1729–1737.

Cina CS, Clase CM, Haynes RB (2001) Carotid endarterectomy for symptomatic carotid stenosis(Cochrane Review). In: *The Cochrane Library*, Issue **4**, Oxford, Update Software.

European Carotid Surgery Trialists' Collaborative Group (1998) Randomised trial of endarterectomy for recently symptomatic carotid stenosis: final results of the MRC European Carotid Surgery Trial (ECST). *Lancet*, **351**: 1379–1387.

Goldstein LB, Samsa GP, Matchar DB, Oddone EZ (1998) Multicenter review of preoperative risk factors for endarterectomy for asymptomatic carotid artery stenosis. *Stroke*, **29**: 750–753.

Pritz MB (1997) Timing of carotid endarterectomy after stroke. *Stroke*, **28**: 2563–2567.

Rothwell PM (2001) Carotid endarterectomy and prevention of stroke in the very elderly. *Lancet*, **357**: 1142–1143.

Rothwell PM, Slattery JM, Warlow CP (1996) Systematic comparison of the risks of stroke and death due to carotid endarterectomy for symptomatic and asymptomatic carotid stenosis. *Stroke*, **27**: 266–269.

Rothwell PM, Warlow CP (1995) Is self-audit reliable? *Lancet*, **346**: 1623.

Rothwell PM, Warlow CP (1999) Prediction of benefit from carotid endarterectomy in individual patients: a risk-modelling study. *Lancet*, **353**: 2105–2110.

Rothwell PM, Warlow CP, on behalf of the European Carotid Surgery Trialists' Collaborative Group (1999) Interpretation of operative risks of individual surgeons. *Lancet*, **353**: 1325.

Whitty CJM, Sudlow CLM, Warlow CP (1998) Investigating individual subjects and screening populations for asymptomatic carotid stenosis can be harmful. *J. Neurol. Neurosurg. Psychiatry*, **64**: 619–623.

Writing Group (1998) Carotid stenting and angioplasty. *Stroke*, **29**: 336–348.

STROKE
General

Hankey GJ, Warlow CP (1999) Treatment and secondary prevention of stroke: evidence, costs, and effects on individuals and populations. *Lancet*, **354**: 1457–1463.

Hankey GJ (2002) *Stroke: Your Questions Answered.* Churchill Livingstone, Edinburgh, UK.

Keir SL, Lindley RI (1999) Stroke medicine for the geriatrician. *Reviews in Clinical Gerontology*, **9**: 23–38.

Warlow CP, Dennis MS, van Gijn J, Hankey GJ, Sandercock PAG, Bamford J, Wardlaw J (2000) *Stroke: A practical guide to management* 2nd edn. Blackwell Scientific Publications, Oxford, UK.

Epidemiology

Chang CL, Donaghy M, Poulter N, *et al.* (1999) Migraine and stroke in young women: case-control study. *BMJ*, **318**: 13–18.

Gillum LA, Mamidipudi SK, Johnston SC (2000) Ischemic stroke risk with oral contraceptives. A meta-analysis. *JAMA*, **284**: 72–78.

Sudlow CLM, Warlow CP, for the International Stroke Incidence Collaboration (1997) Comparable studies of the incidence of stroke and pathological types. Results from an international collaboration. *Stroke*, **28**: 491–499.

Pathophysiology

Hademenos GJ, Alberts MJ, Awad I, *et al.* (2001) Advances in the genetics of cerebrovascular disease and stroke. *Neurology*, **56**: 997–1008.

Kristián T, Siesjö BK (1998) Calcium in ischemic cell death. *Stroke*, **29**: 705–18.

Imaging

Culebras A, Kase CS, Masdeu JC, *et al.* (1997) Practice guidelines for the use of imaging in transient ischemic attacks and acute stroke. A report of the Stroke Council, American Heart Association. *Stroke*, **28**: 1480–1497.

Keir SL, Wardlaw JM (2000) Systematic review of diffusion and perfusion imaging in acute ischemic stroke. *Stroke*, **31**: 2723–2731.

Markus HS (1999) Transcranial Doppler ultrasound. *J. Neurol. Neurosurg. Psychiatry*, **67**: 135–7.

Wardlaw JM (2001) Radiology of stroke. *J. Neurol. Neurosurg. Psychiatry*, **70** (Suppl 1): i7–i11.

Acute treatment

Barber PA, Demchuk AM, Zhang J, Buchan AM (2000) Validity and reliability of a quantitative computed tomography score in predicting outcome of hyperacute stroke before thrombolytic therapy. *Lancet*, **355**: 1670–1674.

Brott T, Bogousslavsky J (2000) Treatment of acute ischemic stroke. *N. Engl. J. Med.*, **343**: 710–722.

Chen Z, Sandercock P, Pan H, *et al.* (2000) Indications for early aspirin use in acute ischaemic stroke. A combined analysis of 40 000 randomized patients from the Chinese Acute Stroke Trial and the International Stroke Trial. *Stroke*, **31**: 1240–1249.

Davenport R, Dennis M (2000) Neurological emergencies: acute stroke. *J. Neurol. Neurosurg. Psychiatry*, **68**: 277–288.

European Stroke Initiative (2000) European Stroke Inititiative recommendations for stroke management. *Cerebrovasc. Dis.*, **10**: 335–3351.

Gorelick P (2000) Neuroprotection in acute ischaemic stroke: a tale of for whom the bell tolls. *Lancet*, **355**: 1925–1926.

Gubitz G, Counsell C, Sandercock P, Signorini D (2001) Anticoagulants for acute ischaemic stroke (Cochrane Review). In: *The Cochrane Library*, Issue **4**. Oxford: Update Software.

Stroke Unit Trialists' Collaboration (2001) Organised inpatient (stroke unit) care for stroke (Cochrane Review). In: *The Cochrane Library*, Issue **4**. Oxford: Update Software.

Wardlaw JM, del Zoppo G, Yamaguchi T (2001) Thrombolysis for acute ischaemic stroke (Cochrane Review). In: *The Cochrane Library*, Issue **4**. Oxford: Update Software.

Wardlaw JM (2001) Overview of Cochrane thrombolysis meta-analysis. *Neurology*, **57** (Suppl 2): S69–S76.

Complications

Brittain KR, Peet SM, Castleden CM (1998) Stroke and incontinence. *Stroke*, **29**: 524–528.

Carson AJ, MacHale S, Allen K, *et al.* (2000) Depression after stroke and lesion location: a systematic review. *Lancet*, **356**: 122–126.

Davenport RJ, Dennis MS, Wellwood I, Warlow CP (1996) Complications following acute stroke. *Stroke*, **27**: 415–420.

Kim JS (2001) Delayed onset mixed involuntary movements after thalamic stroke. Clinical, radiological and pathophysiological findings. *Brain*, **124**: 299–309.

Koh M, Phan TG, Wijdicks EFM (2000) Management of cerebellar infarction with mass effect. *The Neurologist*, **6**: 172–176.

Korpelainen JT, Nieminen P, Myllylä VV (1999) Sexual functioning among stroke patients and their spouses. *Stroke*, **30**: 715–719.

O'Connell JE, Gray CS (1994) Treating hypertension after stroke. *BMJ*, **308**: 1523–1524.

Smith Hammond CA, Goldstein LB, Zajac DJ, *et al.* (2001). Assessment of aspiration risk in stroke patients with quantification of voluntary cough. *Neurology*, **56**: 502–506.

Vestergaard K, Andersen G, Gottrup H, *et al.* (2001). Lamotrigine for central poststroke pain. A randomised controlled trial. *Neurology*, **56**: 184–190.

Wijdicks EFM (2000) Management of massive hemispheric cerebral infarct. Is there a ray of hope? *Mayo Clin. Proc.*, **75**: 945–952.

Rehabilitation

Bakheit AMO, Thilmann AF, Ward AB, *et al.* (2000) A randomised, double-blind, placebo-controlled, dose-ranging study to compare the efficacy and safety of three doses of botulinum toxin type A (Dysport) with placebo in upper limb spasticity after stroke. *Stroke*, **31**: 2402–2406.

Kwakkel G, Wagenaar C, Koelman TW, *et al.* (1997) Effects of intensity of rehabilitation after stroke. A research synthesis. *Stroke*, **28**: 1550–1556.

Langhorne P, Legg L, on behalf of the Outpatient Therapy Trialists (1999) Therapy for stroke patients living at home. *Lancet*, **354**: 1730–1731.

Community care

Han B, Haley WE (1999) Family caregiving for patients with stroke. Review and analysis. *Stroke*, **30**: 1478–1485.

Mant J, Carter J, Wade DT, Winner S (2000) Family support for stroke: a randomised controlled trial. *Lancet*, **356**: 808–813.

Prognosis and prognostic factors

Bhalla A, Sankaralingam S, Dundas R, *et al.* (2000) Influence of raised plasma osmolality on clinical outcome after acute stroke. *Stroke*, **31**: 2043–2048.

Hajat C, Hajat S, Sharma P (2000) Effects of poststroke pyrexia on stroke outcome. A meta-analysis of studies in patients. *Stroke*, **31**: 410–414.

Hankey GJ, Jamrozik K, Broadhurst RJ, Forbes S, Burvill PW, Anderson CS, Stewart-Wynne EG (1998) Long-term risk of first recurrent stroke in the Perth Community Stroke Study. *Stroke*, **29**: 2491–2500.

Hankey GJ, Jamrozik K, Broadhurst RJ, Forbes S, Burvill PW, Anderson CS, Stewart-Wynne EG (2000) Five-year survival after first-ever stroke and related prognostic factors in the Perth Community Stroke Study. *Stroke*, **31**: 2080–2086.

Langhorne P, Tong BLP, Stott DJ (2000) Association between physiological homeostasis and early recovery after stroke. *Stroke*, **31**: 2526–2527.

Secondary prevention

Blood Pressure Lowering Trialists' Collaboration (2000) Effects of ACE inhibitors, calcium antagonists, and other blood pressure-lowering drugs: results of prospectively designed overviews of randomised trials. *Lancet*, **355**: 1955–1964.

Bucher HC, Griffith LE, Guyatt GH (1998) Effect of HMG CoA reductase inhibitors on stroke: a meta-analysis of randomised, controlled trials. *Ann. Intern. Med.*, **128**: 89–95.

Eastern Stroke and Coronary Heart Disease Collaborative Research Group (1998) Blood pressure, cholesterol, and stroke in eastern Asia. *Lancet*, **352**: 1801–1807.

Gubitz G, Sandercock P (2000) Prevention of ischaemic stroke. *BMJ*, **321**: 1455–1459.

Hankey GJ (1999) Smoking and risk of stroke. *J. Cardiovasc. Risk*, **6**(4): 207–211.

Hankey GJ, Eikelboom JW (1999) Homocysteine and vascular disease. *Lancet*, **354**: 407–413.

The Heart Outcomes Prevention Evaluation Study Investigators (2000) Effects of an angiotensin-converting enzyme inhibitor, ramipril, on death from cardiovascular causes, myocardial infarction, and stroke in high-risk patients. *N. Engl. J. Med.*, **342**: 145–153.

The INDANA (Individual Data Analysis of Antihypertensive intervention trials) Project Collaborators (1997) Effect of antihypertensive treatment in patients having already suffered from stroke. Gathering the evidence. *Stroke*, **28**: 2557–2562.

Lancaster T, Stead L, Silagy C, *et al.* (2000) Effectiveness of interventions to help people stop smoking: findings from the Cochrane Library. *BMJ*, **321**: 355–358.

PROGRESS Collaborative Group (2001) Randomised trial of a perindopril-based blood pressure-lowering regimen among 6105 individuals with previous stroke or transient ischaemic attack. *Lancet*, **358**: 1033–1041.

Prospective Studies Collaboration (1995) Cholesterol, diastolic blood pressure and stroke: 13000 strokes in 450 000 people in 45 prospective cohorts. *Lancet*, **346**: 1647–1653.

Rodgers A, Neal B, MacMahon S (1997) The effects of blood pressure lowering in cerebrovascular disease. *Neurology Reviews International*, 2(1): 12–15.

Sacco RL, Wolf PA, Gorelick PB (1999) Risk factors and their management for stroke prevention: Outlook for 1999 and beyond. *Neurology*, **53** (Suppl 4): S15–S24.

Sandercock P (2001) Statins for stroke prevention? *Lancet*, **357**: 1548–1549.

Viscoli CM, Brass LM, Kernan WN, *et al.* (2001) A clinical trial of estrogen-replacement therapy after ischemic stroke. *N. Engl. J. Med.*, **345**: 1243–1249.

White HD, Simes RJ, Anderson NE, *et al.* (2000) Pravastatin therapy and the risk of stroke. *N. Engl. J. Med.*, **343**: 317–326.

See TIA (above) for further reading about antiplatelet therapy and carotid revascularization, and Cardioembolic stroke (below) for further reading about anticoagulation.

Miscellaneous
Yonehawa Y, Taub E (1999) Moyamoya disease: status 1998. *The Neurologist*, **5**: 13–23.

ATHEROSCLEROTIC ISCHEMIC STROKE
The French Study of Aortic Plaques in Stroke Group (1996) Atherosclerotic disease of the aortic arch as a risk factor for recurrent ischemic stroke. *N. Engl. J. Med.*, **334**: 1216–1221.

Hassan A, Markus HS (2000) Genetics and ischaemic stroke. *Brain*, 123: 1784–1812.

Atherosclerotic plaque
Davies MJ (1996) Stability and instability: two faces of coronary atherosclerosis. *Circulation*, **94**: 2013–2020.

Davies MJ (1997) The composition of coronary artery plaques. *N. Engl. J. Med.*, **336**: 1312–1314.

Fuster V, Fallon JT, Badimon JJ, Nemerson Y (1997) The unstable atherosclerotic plaque: clinical significance and therapeutic intervention. *Thromb. Haemost.*, 78(1): 247–255.

Kullo IJ, Edwards WD, Schwartz RS (1998) Vulnerable plaque: pathobiology and clinical implications. *Ann. Intern. Med.*, **129**: 1050–1060.

Rauch V, Osende JI, Fuster V, *et al.* (2001) Thrombus formation on atherosclerotic plaques: pathogenesis and clinical consequences. *Ann. Intern. Med.*, **134**: 224–238.

Inflammation
Bittner V (1998) Atherosclerosis and the immune system. *Arch. Intern. Med.*, **158**: 1395–1396.

Cook PJ, Honeybourne D, Lip GYH, Beevers G, Wise R, Davies P (1998) *Chlamydia pneumoniae* antibody titers are significantly associated with acute stroke and transientcerebral ischemia. The West Birmingham Stroke Project. *Stroke*, **29**: 404–410.

Danesh J, Collins R, Peto R (1997) Chronic infections and coronary heart disease: is there a link? *Lancet*, **350**: 430–436.

Danesh J, Whincup P, Walker M, *et al.* (2000) Low grade inflammation and coronary heart disease: prospective study and updated meta-analysis. *BMJ*, **321**: 199–204.

Danesh J, Whincup P, Walker M, *et al.* (2000) *Chlamydia pneumoniae* IgG titres and coronary heart disease: prospective study and meta-analysis. *BMJ*, **321**: 208–213.

DeGraba TJ (1997) Expression of inflammatory mediators and adhesions molecules in human atherosclerotic plaque. *Neurology*, **49** (Suppl 4): S15–S19.

Grau AJ, Buggle F, Becher H, *et al.* (1998) Recent bacterial and viral infection is a risk factor for cerebreovascular ischemia: Clinical can biochemical studies. *Neurology*, **50**: 196–203.

Gurfinkel E, Bozovich G, Daroco A, Beck E, Mautner B, for the ROXIS Study Group (1997) Randomised trial of roxithromycin in non-Q-wave coronary syndromes: ROXIS Pilot Study. *Lancet*, **350**: 404–407.

Koenig W (2000) Heart disease and the inflammatory response. *BMJ*, **321**: 187–188.

Markus HS, Mendall MA (1998) *Helicobacter pylori* infection: a risk factor for ischaemic cerebrovascular disease and carotid atheroma. *J. Neurol. Neurosurg. Psychiatry*, **64**: 104–107.

Ridker PM, Cushman M, Stampfer MJ, Tracy RP, Hennekens CH (1997) Inflammation, aspirin, and the risk of cardiovascular disease in apparently healthy men. *N. Engl. J. Med.*, **336**: 973–979.

Ross R (1999) Atherosclerosis – an inflammatory disease. *N. Engl. J. Med.*, **340**: 115–126.

Rothwell PM, Villagra R, Gibson R, Donders RCJM, Warlow CP (2000) Evidence of a chronic systemic cause of instability of atherosclerotic plaques. *Lancet*, **355**: 19–24.

Wald NJ, Law MR, Morris JK, Zhou X, Wong Y, Ward ME (2000) *Chlamydia pneumoniae* infection and mortality from ischaemic heart disease: large prospective study. *BMJ*, **321**: 204–207.

Thrombosis
Broze GJ Jnr (1992) The role of tissue factor pathway inhibitor in a revised coagulation cascade. *Semin. Haematol.*, 29(3): 159–69.

Coller BS (1997) Platelet GPIIb/IIIa antagonists: the first anti-integrin receptor therapeutics. *J. Clin. Invest.*, **99**: 1467–1471.

George JN (2000) Platelets. *Lancet*, **355**: 1531–1539.

Furie B, Furie BC (1992) Molecular and cellular biology of blood coagulation. *N. Engl. J. Med.*, **326**: 800–806.

Hirsh J, Weitz JI (1999) New antithrombotic agents. *Lancet*, **353**: 1431–1436.

Rosenberg RD, Rosenberg JS (1984) Natural anticoagulant mechanisms. *J. Clin. Invest.*, 74(1): 1–6.

Topol EJ, Byzova TV, Plow EF (1999) Platelet GPIIb-IIIa blockers. *Lancet*, **353**: 223–227.

van Kooten F, Ciabattoni G, Patrono C, Dippel DW, Koudstaal PJ (1997) Platelet activation and lipid peroxidation in patients with acute ischemic stroke. *Stroke*, **28**: 1557–1563.

Clinical
Min WK, Park KK, Kim YS, *et al.* (2000) Atherothrombotic middle cerebral artery territory infarction. Topographic diversity with common occurrence of concomitant small cortical and subcortical infarcts. *Stroke*, 31: 2055–2061.

CARDIOEMBOLIC STROKE
General
Oppenheimer SM, Lima J (1998) Neurology and the heart. *J. Neurol. Neurosurg. Psychiatry*, **64**: 289–97.

Atrial fibrillation
Yamanouchi H, Nagura H, Mizutani T, *et al.* (1997) Embolic infarction in nonrheumatic atrial fibrillation: A clinicopathologic study in the elderly. *Neurology*, **48**: 1593–1597.

Other embolic sources
De Castro S, Cartoni D, Fiorelli M, *et al.* (2000) Morphological and functional characteristics of patent foramen ovale and their embolic implications. *Stroke*, **31**: 2407–2413.

Freed LA, Levy D, Levine RA, *et al.* (1999) Prevalence and clinical outcome of mitral-valve prolapse. *N. Engl. J. Med.*, **341**: 1–7.

Gilon D, Buonanno FS, Joffe MM, *et al.* (1999) Lack of evidence of an association between mitral-valve prolapse and stroke in young patients. *N. Engl. J. Med.*, **341**: 8–13.

Libman R, Wein T (1999) 'Newer' cardiac sources of embolic stroke. *The Neurologist*, **5**: 231–246.

Mas J-L, Arquizan C, Lamy C, *et al.* (2001) Recurrent cerebrovascular events associated with patent foramen ovale, atrial septal aneurysm, or both. *N. Engl. J. Med.*, **345**: 1740–1746.

Imaging
Blackshear JL, Brott TG (1999) Transesophageal echocardiography in source-of-embolism evaluation: the search for a better therapeutic rationale. *Mayo Clin. Proc.*, **74**: 941–945.

Channon KM, Banning AP (1999) Echocardiography in stroke and thromboembolism: transoesophageal imaging for all? *Q. J. Med.*, **92**: 619–621.

Acute treatment
Berge E, Abdelnoor M, Nakstad PH, *et al.* (2000) Low molecular-weight heparin versus aspirin in patients with acute ischaemic stroke and atrial fibrillation: a double-blind randomised study. *Lancet*, **355**: 1205–1210.

Secondary prevention
Cromheecke ME, Levi M, Colly LP (2000) Oral anticoagulation self-management and management by a specialist anticoagulation clinic: a randomised cross-over comparison. *Lancet*, **356**: 97–102.

EAFT (European Atrial Fibrillation Trial) Study Group (1993) Secondary prevention in non-Rheumatic atrial fibrillation after transient ischaemic attack or minor stroke. *Lancet*, **342**: 1255–1262.

Hart RG, Halperin JL (1999) Atrial fibrillation and thromboembolism: a decade of progress in stroke prevention. *Ann. Intern. Med.*, **131**: 688–695.

Lip GYH (1999) Thromboprophylaxis for atrial fibrillation. *Lancet*, **353**: 4–6.

Thomson R, Parkin D, Eccles M, *et al.* (2000) Decision analysis and guidelines for anticoagulant therapy to prevent stroke in patients with atrial fibrillation. *Lancet*, **355**: 956–962.

INFECTIVE ENDOCARDITIS
Dajani AS, Bisno AL, Chung KJ, *et al.* (1990) Prevention of bacterial endocarditis: recommendations of the American Heart Association. *JAMA*, **264**: 2919–2922.

Heiro M, Nikoskelainen J, Engblom E, *et al.* (2000) Neurologic manifestations of infective endocarditis. A 17-year experience in a teaching hospital in Finland. *Arch. Intern. Med.*, **160**: 2781–2787.

Heiro M, Nikoskelainen J, Hartiala JJ, *et al.* (1998) Diagnosis of infective endocarditis. Sensitivity of the Duke vs Reyn Criteria. *Arch. Intern. Med.*, **158**: 18–24.

Ling R, James B (1998) White-centred retinal haemorrhages (Roth spots). *Postgrad. Med. J.*, **74**: 581–582.

Mylonakis E, Calderwood SB (2001) Infective endocarditis in adults. *N. Engl. J. Med.*, **345**: 1318–1330.

ANTIPHOSPHOLIPID SYNDROME AND OTHER PROTHROMBOTIC STATES
Bushnell CD, Goldstein LB (2000) Diagnostic testing for coagulopathies in patients with ischemic stroke. *Stroke*, **31**: 3067–3078.

Greaves M (1999) Antiphospholipid antibodies and thrombosis. *Lancet*, **353**: 1348–1353.

Haviv YS (2000) Association of anticardiolipin antibodies with vascular injury: possible mechanisms. *Postgrad. Med. J.*, **76**: 625–628.

Markus HS, Hambley H (1998) Neurology and the blood: haematological abnormalities in ischaemic stroke. *J. Neurol. Neurosurg. Psychiatry*, **64**: 150–159.

Stewart AJ, Penman ID, Cook MK, Ludlam CA (1999) Warfarin-induced skin necrosis. *Postgrad. Med. J.*, **75**: 233–235.

DISSECTION OF THE CAROTID AND VERTEBRAL ARTERIES
Crum B, Mokri B, Fulgham J (2000) Spinal manifestations of vertebral artery dissection. *Neurology*, **55**: 304–306.

Guillon B, Levy C, Bousser MG (1998) Internal carotid artery dissection: an update. *J. Neurol. Sci.*, **153**: 146–158.

Guillon B, Tzourio C, Biousse V, *et al.* (2000) Arterial wall properties in carotid artery dissection. An ultrasound study. *Neurology*, **55**: 663–666.

Hill MD, Hwa G, Perry JR (2000) Extracranial cervical artery dissection. *Stroke*, **31**: 799.

Leys D, Moulin Th, Stojkovic, Begey S, Chavot D, DONALD investigators (1995) Follow-up of patients with history of cervical artery dissection. *Cerebrovasc. Dis.*, **5**: 43–49.

Schievink WI, Mokri B, O'Fallon WM (1994) Recurrent spontaneous cervical-artery dissection. *N. Engl. J. Med.*, **330**: 393–397.

Schievink WI, Wijdicks EF, Michels VV, *et al.* (1998) Heritable connective tissue disorders in cervical artery dissections. A prospective study. *Neurology*, **50**: 1166–1169.

Schievink WI (2001) Spontaneous dissection of the carotid and vertebral arteries. *N. Engl. J. Med.*, **344**: 898–906.

Silbert PL, Mokri B, Schievink WI (1995) Headache and neck pain in spontaneous internal carotid and vertebral artery dissections. *Neurology*, **45**: 1517–1522.

CENTRAL NERVOUS SYSTEM VASCULITIS
Demiroglu H, Özcebe OI, Barista I, *et al.* (2000) Interferon alfa-2b, colchicine, and benzathine penicillin versus colchicine and benzathine penicillin in Behçet's disease: a randomised trial. *Lancet*, **355**: 605–609.

Hankey GJ (1991) Isolated angiitis/angiopathy of the central nervous system. *Cerebrovasc. Dis.*, **1**: 2–15.

Kontogiannis V, Powell RJ (2000) Behçet's disease. *Postgrad. Med. J.*, **76**: 629–637.

Lanthier S, Lortie A, Michaud J, *et al.* (2001) Isolated angiitis of the CNS in children *Neurology*, **56**: 837–842.

Moore PM (1998) Central nervous system vasculitis. *Curr. Opin. Neurol.*, **11**: 241–246.

Moore PM, Richardson B (1998) Neurology of the vasculitides and connective tissue diseases. *J. Neurol. Neurosurg. Psychiatry,* **65**: 10–22.

Numano F, Okawara M, Inomata H, Kobayashi Y (2000) Takayasu's arteritis. *Lancet,* **356**: 1023–1025.

Sakane T, Takeno M, Suzuki N, Inaba G (1999) Behçet's disease. *N. Engl. J. Med.,* **341**: 1284–1291.

GIANT CELL ARTERITIS

Hayreh SS (2000) Steroid therapy for visual loss in patients with giant-cell arteritis. *Lancet,* **355**: 1572–1574.

Jover JA, Hernández-García C, Morado IC, *et al.* (2001). Combined treatment of giant-cell arteritis with methotrexate and prednisone. A randomised, double-blind, placebo-controlled trial. *Ann. Intern. Med.,* **134**: 106–114.

Swannell AJ (1997) Polymyalgia rheumatica and temporal arteritis: diagnosis and management. *BMJ,* **314**: 1329–1332.

Zeidler M, Hughes T, Zeman A (2000) Confused by arteritis. *Lancet,* **355**: 374.

PRIMARY INTRACEREBRAL HEMORRHAGE

Broderick JP, Adams HP Jr, Barsan W, *et al.* (1999) Guidelines for the management of spontaneous intracerebral haemorrhage. A statement for healthcare professionals from a special writing group of the Stroke Council, American Heart Association. *Stroke,* **30**: 905–915.

Fernandes HM, Gregson B, Siddique S, Mendelow AD (2000) Surgery in intracerebral hemorrhage. The uncertainty continues. *Stroke,* **31**: 2511–2516.

Knudsen KA, Rosand J, Karluk D, Greenberg SM (2001) Clinical diagnosis of cerebral amyloid angiopathy: Validation of the Boston criteria. *Neurology* **56**: 537–539.

Querishi AI, Tuhrim S, Broderick JP, *et al.* (2001) Spontaneous intracerebral hemorrhage. *N. Engl. J. Med.,* **344**: 1450–1460.

Sacco RL (2000) Lobar intracerebral haemorrhage. *N. Engl. J. Med.,* **342**: 276–279.

ARTERIOVENOUS MALFORMATION

Al-Shahi R, Warlow C (2001) A systematic review of the frequency and prognosis of arteriovenous malformations of the brain in adults. *Brain,* **124**: 1900–1926.

The Arteriovenous Malformation Study Group (1999) Arteriovenous malformations of the brain in adults. *N. Engl. J. Med.,* **340**: 1812–1818.

SUBARACHNOID HEMORRHAGE

Epidemiology

The ACROSS Group (2000) Epidemiology of aneurysmal subarachnoid haemorrhage in Australia and New Zealand. Incidence and case fatality from the Australasian Cooperative Research on Subarachnoid Haemorrhage Study (ACROSS). *Stroke,* **31**: 1843–1850.

Ingall T, Asplund K, Mähönen M, *et al.* (2000) A multinational comparison of subarachnoid haemorrhage epidemiology in the WHO Monica Stroke Study. *Stroke,* **31**: 1054–1061.

Etiology

Schievink WI, Wijdicks EFM (2000) Origin of pretruncal nonaneurysmal subarachnoid haemorrhage: Ruptured vein perforating artery, or intramural haematoma? *Mayo Clin. Proc.,* **75**: 1169–1173.

Diagnosis

Edlow JA, Caplan LR (2000) Avoiding pitfalls in the diagnosis of subarachnoid haemorrhage. *N. Engl. J. Med.,* **342**: 29–36.

Ruigrok YM, Rinkel GJE, Buskens E, *et al.* (2000) Perimesencephalic haemorrhage and CT angiography. A decision analysis. *Stroke,* **31**: 2976–2983.

van Gijn J (1997) Slip-ups in the diagnosis of subarachnoid haemorrhage. *Lancet,* **349**: 1492–1493.

van Gijn J, Rinkel GJE (2001) Subarachnoid haemorrhage: diagnosis, causes and management. *Brain,* **124**: 249–278.

Treatment

Brilstra EH, Rinkel GJE, Algra A, van Gijn J (2000). Rebleeding, secondary ischaemia, and timing of operation in patients with subarachnoid haemorrhage. *Neurology,* **55**: 1656–1660.

Feigin VL, Rinkel GJE, Algra A, Vermeulen M, van Gijn J (2001) Calcium antagonists for aneurysmal subarachnoid haemorrhage (Cochrane Review). In: *The Cochrane Library,* Issue 4. Oxford: Update Software.

Koivisto T, Vanninen R, Hurskainen H, *et al.* (2000) Outcomes of early endovascular versus surgical treatment of ruptured cerebral aneurysms. A prospective randomised study. *Stroke,* **31**: 2369–2377.

Roos YBWEM, Rinkel GJE, Vermeulen M, Algra A, van Gijn J (2001) Antifibrinolytic therapy for aneurysmal subarachnoid haemorrhage (Cochrane Review). In: *The Cochrane Library,* Issue 4. Oxford: Update Software.

Prognosis

Hop JW, Rinkel GJE, Algra A, van Gijn J (1997) Case-fatality rates and functional outcome after subarachnoid haemorrhage – a systematic review. *Stroke,* **28**: 660–664.

UNRUPTURED ANEURYSMS

Broderick JP (2000) Coiling, clipping, or medical management of unruptured intracranial aneurysms: time to randomise? *Ann. Neurol.,* **48**: 5–6.

International Study of Unruptured Intracranial Aneurysms Investigators (1998) Unruptured intracranial aneurysms – risk of rupture and risks of surgical intervention. *N. Engl. J. Med.,* **339**: 1725–1733.

Wardlaw JM, White PM (2000) The detection and management of unruptured intracranial aneurysms. *Brain,* **123**: 205–221.

CEREBRAL VENOUS THROMBOSIS

Allroggen H, Abbott RJ (2000) Cerebral venous sinus thrombosis. *Postgrad. Med. J.* **76**: 12–15.

Benamer HTS, Bone I (2000) Cerebral venous thrombosis. *J. Neurol. Neurosurg. Psychiatry,* **69**: 427–430.

Biousse V, Ameri A, Bousser M-G (1999) Isolated intracranial hypertension as the only sign of cerebral venous thrombosis. *Neurology,* **53**: 1537–1542.

de Bruijn SFTM, Stam J, for the CVST Study Group (1999) Randomized, placebo-controlled trial of anticoagulant treatment with low-molecular-weight heparin for cerebral sinus thrombosis. *Stroke,* **30**: 484–488.

de Bruijn SFTM, Budde M, Teunisse S, *et al.* (2000) Long-term outcome of cognition and functional health after cerebral venous sinus thrombosis. *Neurology,* **54**: 1687–1689.

de Bruijn SFTM, de Haan RJ, Stam J, for the Cerebral Venous Sinus Thrombosis Study Group (2001) Clinical features and prognostic factors of cerebral venous sinus thrombosis in a prospective series of 59 patients. *J. Neurol. Neurosurg. Psychiatry,* **70**: 105–108.

VASCULAR DEMENTIA

General

Amar K, Wilcock G (1996) Vascular dementia. *BMJ,* **312**: 227–231.

Epidemiology

Bousser MG, Tournier-Lasserve E. (2001) Cerebral autosomal dominant arteriopathy with subcortical infarcts and leukoencephalopathy: from stroke to vessel wall physiology. *J. Neurol. Neurosurg. Psychiatry,* **70**: 285–287.

Hebert R, Lindsay J, Verreault R, *et al.* (2000) Vascular dementia. Incidence and risk factors in the Canadian Study of Health and Aging. *Stroke,* **31**: 1487–1493.

Pathogenesis

de Groot JC, de Leeuw F-E, Oudkerk M, *et al.* (2000) Cerebral white matter lesions and cognitive function: The Rotterdam scan study. *Ann. Neurol.,* **47**: 145–1451.

Garde E, Mortensen EL, Krabbe K, *et al.* (2000) Relation between age-related decline in intelligence and cerebral white-matter hyperintensities in healthy octogenarians: a longitudinal study. *Lancet,* **356**: 628–634.

Merino JG, Hachinski V (2000) Leukoaraiosis. Reifying rarefaction. *Arch. Neurol.,* **57**: 925–926.

Reed BR, Eberling JL, Mungas D, *et al.* (2000) Memory failure has different mechanisms in subcortical stroke and Alzheimer's disease. *Ann. Neurol.,* **48**: 275–284.

van Gijn J (1998) Leukoaraiosis and vascular dementia. *Neurology,* **51** (Suppl 3): S3–S8.

van Gijn J (2000) White matters: small vessels and slow thinking in old age. *Lancet,* **356**: 612–613.

Clinical features

Dichgans M, Mayer M, Uttner I, *et al.* (1998) The phenotypic spectrum of CADASIL: clinical findings in 102 cases. *Ann. Neurol.,* **44**: 731–739.

Diagnosis

Chui HC, Mack W, Jackson JE, *et al.* (2000) Clinical criteria for the diagnosis of vascular dementia. A multicenter study of comparability and interrater reliability. *Arch. Neurol.,* **57**: 191–196.

Pohjasvaara T, Mäntylä R, Ylikoski R, *et al.* (2000) Comparison of different clinical criteria (DSM-III, ADDTC, ICD-10, NINDS-AIREN, DSM-IV) for the diagnosis of vascular dementia. *Stroke,* **31**: 2952–2957.

Wetterling T, Kanitz R-D, Borgis K-J (1996) Comparison of different diagnostic criteria for vascular dementia (ADDTC, DSM-IV, ICD-10, NINDS-AIREN). *Stroke,* **27**: 30–36.

HYPERTENSIVE ENCEPHALOPATHY

Vaughan CJ, Delanty N (2000) Hypertensive emergencies. *Lancet,* **356**: 411–417.

PITUITARY APOPLEXY

Anderson JR, Antoun N, Burnet N, Chatterjee K, Edwards O, Pickard JD, Sarkies N (1999) Neurology of the pituitary gland. *J. Neurol. Neurosurg. Psychiatry,* **66**: 703–721.

Biousse V, Newman NJ, Oyesiku NM (2001) Precipitating factors in pituitary apoplexy. *J. Neurol. Neurosurg. Psychiatry,* **71**: 542–545.

Infections of the Nervous System

BACTERIAL INFECTIONS

ACUTE PYOGENIC (BACTERIAL) MENINGITIS

DEFINITION
Inflammation of the leptomeninges (pia and arachnoid membranes) caused by bacterial infection.

EPIDEMIOLOGY
* Annual incidence: 1.9 per 100 000 for *Neisseria meningitidis*; 1.6 per 100 000 for *Haemophilus influenzae*; 1.0 per 100 000 for *Streptococcus pneumoniae*.
* Incidence rates are influenced by country, ethnic group, social class and deprivation, and immunization programmes.
* Lifetime prevalence: 1(95% CI: 0.8–2) per 1000.
* Age: any age (see *Table 33*); most common in the first month of life.

Table 33 Empirical therapy for suspected bacterial meningitis*

Age	Likely bacterial pathogens	Empirical therapy**
0–4 weeks	*Escherichia coli* (50%) Group B Streptococci(30%) *Listeria monocytogenes* (10%) *Klebsiella pneumoniae*	Amoxycillin + cefotaxime, or amoxycillin + aminoglycoside
4–12 weeks	*Escherichia coli* Group B Streptococci (*S. agalactiae*) *Listeria monocytogenes* *Haemophilus influenzae* *Streptococcus pneumoniae* *Neisseria meningitidis*	Amoxycillin + a third generation cephalosporin (cefotaxime or ceftriaxone)
3 months–18 years	*Haemophilus influenzae* *Neisseria meningitidis* *Streptococcus pneumoniae*	Third generation cephalosporin (cefotaxime or ceftriaxone) ± amoxycillin***, or amoxycillin + chloramphenicol
18–50 years	*Streptococcus pneumoniae* (40%) *Neisseria meningitidis* (30%)	Third generation cephalosporin (cefotaxime or ceftriaxone) ± amoxycillin**
>50 years	*Streptococcus pneumoniae* *Neisseria meningitidis* Aerobic Gram-negative bacilli *Listeria monocytogenes*	Amoxycillin + a third generation cephalosporin (cefotaxime or ceftriaxone)

*Applies only to the immunocompetent patient
**Add vancomycin to empirical regime when pneumococcal meningitis highly resistant to penicillin or cephalosporin is suspected
***Add if *L. monocytogenes* meningitis suspected (i.e. deficiencies in cell-mediated immunity)

PATHOLOGY

The fundamental process is inflammation of the lepto-meninges (**325, 326**). Complications include vasculitis, cerebral infarction, hydrocephalus (**327**), brain abscesses, and cerebral edema.

ETIOLOGY

The most common organisms causing meningitis are:
- *Haemophilus influenzae*: 45% of cases.
- *Streptococcus pneumoniae* (pneumococcus): 18%.
- *Neisseria meningitidis* (meningococcus): 14%.

However, there are important differences in the patterns of organisms encountered in different age groups (see *Table 33*). *Listeria monocytogenes*, although uncommon, occurs especially during pregnancy and the neonatal period. Among neonates (<1 month of age), group B streptococci (*S. agalactiae*) and coliforms (particularly *Escherichia coli*, but also *Proteus* and *Pseudomonas*) predominate.

In the 1980s, *H. influenzae* was the most common cause of meningitis in children 1 month–4 years of age, *N.*

meningitidis predominated in older children and young adults (5–29 years old) and *S. pneumoniae* in older adults.

During the 1990s widespread use of conjugate *H. influenzae* type b (Hib) vaccines, consisting of protein combined with the Hib polysaccharide capsule, has virtually eliminated Hib disease from several developed countries (and is now being introduced in developing countries). This reduction means that *S. pneumoniae* and *N. meningitidis* have become the predominant causes of meningitis in children. There are at least 13 known groups of meningococcal disease, but the most important are group B (which is the most common, accounting for about 60% of cases) and group C (which accounts for about 40% of cases and causes most deaths). Meningitis due to meningococcus group C is most common in babies, and next most common in adolescents (15–17 years old). A second epidemiologic trend is the worldwide increase in infection with strains of *S. pneumoniae* that are resistant to penicillin and other β-lactam antibiotics, mediated by alterations in the penicillin-binding proteins involved in the synthesis of bacterial cell walls.

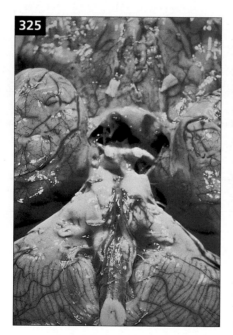

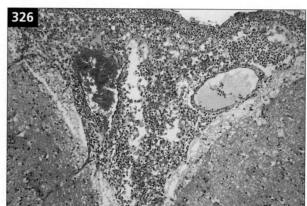

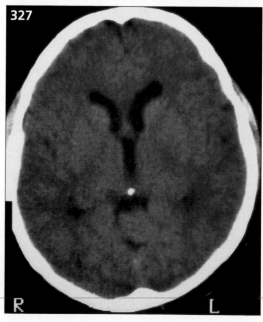

325 Base of the brain of a patient who died from acute pyogenic meningitis showing purulent meningeal exudate. (Courtesy of Professor BA Kakulas, Royal Perth Hospital, Western Australia.)

326 Histologic section of the meninges and cerebral cortex of a patient who died of acute pyogenic meningitis showing neutrophilic infiltration of the subarachnoid space, pia, arachnoid and Virchow–Robin spaces of the outer part of the brain. Bacteria are numerous, lying free in the subarachnoid space and inside neutrophilic leukocytes (phagocytosis).

327 CT brain scan showing early hydrocephalus in a patient with pneumococcal meningitis. Their symptoms had started 18 hours previously.

Risk factors
CSF leak due to:
- Recent craniotomy: risk of staphylococcal meningitis.
- Recent open skull fracture: risk of pneumococcal meningitis, and Gram-negative bacillary (coliform) pathogens, such as *Klebsiella* spp., *E. coli* and *Pseudomonas* spp.

PATHOGENESIS
Organisms may reach the meninges by direct spread from adjacent structures in the skull and spine (middle ear, paranasal sinuses, skull fractures) and via the blood stream.

Bacterial cell wall materials and bacterial products such as endotoxin stimulate the local release of proinflammatory cytokines such as tumor necrosis factor alpha, interleukin 1 and interleukin 6 from host cells and thereby initiate the inflammatory response. Hyperemia of the meninges is followed by migration of neutrophils into the walls of blood vessels and into the subarachnoid space where the inflammatory infiltrate extends along cranial and spinal nerves. Foci of necrosis develop in vessel walls, sometimes with thrombosis sufficient to cause cerebral infarction and seizures. Fibrino-purulent exudate accumulates in the subarachnoid space and may block the flow of CSF at the base of the brain or in the arachnoid granulations causing hydrocephalus. Infection may become loculated to form abscesses. Cerebral edema may develop also and raise intracranial pressure.

CLINICAL FEATURES
Meningeal inflammation
Fever, headache, meningismus (neck stiffness), and signs of cerebral dysfunction (confusion, delirium, vomiting or declining consciousness) are found in about 85% of patients at presentation. Meningismus is accompanied by Kernig's and/or Brudzinski signs in about half of adults.

Complications
- Cranial nerve palsies, particularly nerves III, IV, VI and VII (30% of cases).
- Deafness due to cochlear damage either by a direct effect of bacterial toxins or by an indirect cytokine-mediated effect.
- Epileptic seizures (30%) or focal neurologic signs (10–20% of cases), due to inflammation and thrombosis of cortical arteries and veins and venous sinuses (causing cerebral infarction), or subdural effusion.
- Signs of increased intracranial pressure (coma, cranial nerve III palsy, hypertension, bradycardia) due to hydrocephalus or cerebral edema, or subdural effusion. Papilledema is unusual at presentation (<1% of cases), and should suggest an alternative diagnosis at that time, but is more common among acutely ill patients who are deteriorating.

ETIOLOGIC CLUES
- Sources of infection: evidence of suppuration may be present in the ears (otitis media), paranasal sinuses, skin, lungs, and heart (infective endocarditis).
- Skin rash: primarily on the limbs, that is typically erythematous and macular early in the infection, but may quickly evolve into a petechial phase with further coalescence into a purpuric form, is present in about 50% of patients with meningococcemia, with or without meningitis (**328, 329**).
- Features of *a rhombencephalitis*, such as ataxia, cranial nerve palsies, and nystagmus early in the clinical course may indicate *Listeria monocytogenes* meningitis.

Atypical presentations
Neonates and infants
Change in affect or state of alertness, irritability, lethargy, listlessness, feeding difficulties, weak suck, high-pitched crying, fretfulness, vomiting, diarrhea, respiratory distress, temperature instability (fever or hypothermia), or jaundice. Neck stiffness may be absent. A bulging fontanelle is found in one-third of cases and usually occurs late in the course of the illness.

Elderly patients (particularly with diabetes or cardiopulmonary disease)
May present insidiously with lethargy or obtundation, no fever, and variable signs of meningeal inflammation.

Neutropenic patients
Symptoms and signs may be subtle because of the impaired ability to mount an inflammatory response in the subarachnoid space.

328, 329
Purpuric skin rash. Rash in an unconscious child (**328**) and adult (**329**) with meningococcal meningitis and septicemia. (Courtesy of Dr AM Chancellor, Tauranga, New Zealand.)

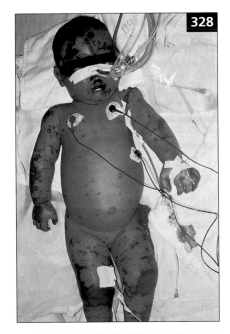

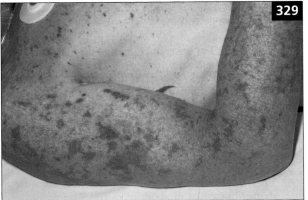

may occur and be painful, frightening and cause difficulty opening the jaw (trismus), a grimacing facial appearance 'risus sardonicus' due to contraction of the facial muscles (**341**), and difficulty swallowing, sometimes prompting the patient to complain of a 'sore throat'. The patient is usually afebrile unless there is concurrent local infection.

With severe tetanus, all muscles contract, with the stronger overpowering the weaker. There is opisthotonos, flexion of the arms, extension of the legs, periods of apnea due to spasm of the intercostal muscles and diaphragm, and rigidity of the abdominal wall. Spasms are precipitated by startle, cough, touch, and a full bladder. Laryngeal spasm can be precipitated by swallow or the passage of a nasogastric tube. Late in the disease autonomic dysfunction develops with tachycardia and hypertension alternating with bradycardia and hypotension, cardiac arrhythmias, sweating, fever, salivation and gastric stasis. Ophthalmoplegia and facial weakness are rare.

DIFFERENTIAL DIAGNOSIS
- Dystonic reactions to neuroleptic drugs (which typically involve lateral turning of the head, often with protrusion of the tongue [symptoms that are rarely, if ever, seen in tetanus]).
- Strychnine poisoning.
- Local infection in the pterygomandibular space (e.g. dental or in the masseter muscle) with trismus.
- Dislocation of the mandible leading to 'lockjaw'.
- Facial or jaw trauma.
- Rabies.
- Hysteria.

INVESTIGATIONS
- Laboratory tests are of virtually no value except to exclude strychnine poisoning.
- Blood counts and blood biochemistry findings are unremarkable.
- Imaging studies of the head and spine reveal no abnormalities.
- A LP is not necessary; the CSF is normal except for a raised opening pressure, particularly during spasms.

DIAGNOSIS
Clinical.

TREATMENT
- Nurse in quiet surroundings.
- Excise and debride any wound.
- Control muscle spasms: benzodiazepines are the mainstay of treatment; intravenous diazepam 10–40 mg every 1–8 hours may be required to prevent spasms that last more than 5–10 seconds. At high doses, lactic acidosis can occur, possibly as a result of the solvent vehicle, propylene glycol. There are γ-aminobutyric acid agonists that indirectly antagonize the toxin, but they do not restore glycinergic function.
- Maintain ventilation and oxygenation and prevent pulmonary aspiration of gastric contents:
- Control the muscle spasms.
- Tracheostomy is indicated if rigidity and spasms cannot be controlled and interfere with swallowing or breathing.

- Paralysis and ventilation are required if spasms become severe.
- Maintain nutrition and fluid balance with oral feeds if mild, or i.v. line or nasogastric tube if spasms are moderate but not severe. If severe, the patient must be intubated and ventilated.
- Human antitetanus immunoglobulin (500 units) is recommended, although its efficacy is controversial.
- Antitetanus toxin.
- Antimicrobial chemotherapy: metronidazole (0.5 g every 6 hours or 1.0 g every 12 hours intravenously) is as good as, or better than, penicillin G which is no longer the drug of choice. Also, penicillin is an antagonist of γ–aminobutyric acid, just as is tetanus toxin.
- Prevent gastric stress ulcers: H2 receptor antagonists.
- Prevent deep vein thrombosis: low dose heparin 5000 units subcutaneously twice daily.
- Control autonomic dysfunction: beta-blockade or combined alpha and beta-blockade as necessary for labile blood pressure and heart rate.

PROGNOSIS
- The disease progresses over about a week, stabilizes for another week, and then recovers over several weeks.
- The severity is very variable.
- Case fatality ranges from 10 to >50% worldwide. At least half of deaths from tetanus worldwide occur in neonates. These deaths are preventable through antepartum maternal immunization.
- In the USA, 75% of deaths occur in people who are 60 years of age or older (who make up 59% of all cases of tetanus).

PREVENTION
Tetanus is a serious preventable disease that remains a threat even in developed countries, particularly in older people. A case of tetanus reflects the failure of our health care delivery system to provide immunization. Routine boosters every 10 years should be emphasized in older people.

About 70% of a random sample of Americans aged 6 or more years had protective levels of tetanus antibodies. The prevalence of protective antibodies is less than 50% in people aged 60–69 years, and about 30% in people aged 70 years and older.

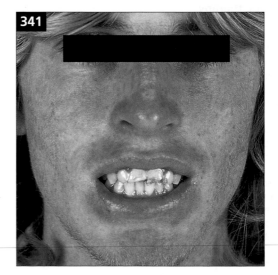

341 Facial photograph of a patient with facial muscle stiffness and grimacing (risus sardonicus) and difficulty opening the jaw (trismus) due to tetanus.

WHIPPLE'S DISEASE

DEFINITION
A rare, chronic, relapsing, multisystem granulomatous disorder that is caused by infection by *Tropheryma whippelii*, a Gram-positive bacillus; it primarily involves the intestine causing chronic diarrhea, together with fever and migratory polyarthralgias. About 5% of patients present with neurologic manifestations and 6–43% eventually develop symptomatic CNS involvement.

HISTORY
Described in 1907 by George Whipple. The patient was a missionary who had weight loss, diarrhea, and abdominal pain associated with polyarthralgia and lymphadenopathy. At autopsy, numerous argyrophilic rod-shaped organisms were present in mesenteric lymph nodes. In 1949 Black-Schaffer showed that the bacilli gave a strongly positive result when stained with periodic acid Schiff reagent. In 1991 and 1992 specific DNA sequences were amplified from affected tissue. The nucleotide sequence had phylogenetic similarities to the actinomyces group, and the organism was named *T. whippelii*.

EPIDEMIOLOGY
- Incidence: rare; fewer than 800 cases have been reported (<10 cases per year).
- Age and gender: usually presents in middle-aged men.

PATHOLOGY
- Symptomatic neurologic involvement occurs in at least 10% (6–43%) of patients at some stage in their illness. Autopsy more frequently reveals brain involvement, even in the absence of neurologic symptoms.
- Sites of predilection are the basal ganglia, insular cortex, midbrain, pons and cerebellum.
- Microscopic examination of the brain reveals widespread inflammation (encephalitis) throughout the cerebral hemispheres and brainstem (particularly the striatum, other basal nuclei and pons) characterized by mononuclear cell perivascular cuffing and infiltration of white and gray matter, marked astrocytosis, proliferation of microglia, and focal necrosis of many nerve cells.
- With hematoxylin and eosin (H&E) stain some nerve cells appear swollen and the cytoplasm has a very fine, granular, bluish-purple staining appearance.
- Fat stains demonstrate nerve cells containing numerous, rather coarse, varying-sized pale granules and globules of fat.
- PAS stain shows that the cytoplasm of neurons, astrocytes and perivascular inflammatory cells contain abundant foamy macrophages filled with masses of coalescent PAS-staining granules.
- Electron microscopy shows numerous bacilli in the distended macrophages and in the intercellular spaces. The bacilli measure 1.5–3.0 μm in length and 200 nm in diameter. The bacilli are lined by a thin surface membrane and a thick (20 nm) cell wall. Whipple's bacteria are most frequently found in microglial and ependymal cells in the brain but they are also found within astrocytes, pericytes, and choroid plexus cells. The internal layers of the retina also show many large, pale, granule-containing cells.

ETIOLOGY AND PATHOPHYSIOLOGY
Infection by *T. whippelii*, a Gram-positive bacillus.

CLINICAL FEATURES
The most common clinical presentation is the insidious onset of a malabsorption syndrome (e.g. diarrhea), sometimes preceded by migratory polyarthralgia and fever. Cardiac (pericarditis, myocarditis, marantic endocarditis) and CNS involvement is also common, and a few present with primarily neurologic manifestations.

Neurologic triad
- Dementia, apathy and personality change: progressive.
- Myoclonus (facial) and tonic-clonic seizures; oculomasticatory myorhythmia (facial myoclonus) is pathognomonic: the eyes converge synchronously (convergent nystagmus) with involuntary jaw, palatal and tongue movements. Rhythmic spinal myoclonus has also been described.
- Supranuclear ophthalmoplegia (voluntary vertical and, less so, horizontal gaze palsy; not caused by cranial nerve involvement but by lesions in the brainstem).

Other features
- Ataxic gait.
- Hypothalamic dysfunction (sleep [hypersomnolence], drinking [polydipsia], and eating [hyperphagia] disorders).
- Coma.
- Chronic meningitis.
- Blurred vision or visual loss due to vitritis, uveitis, retinitis, retinal hemorrhage, choroiditis, papilledema, optic atrophy or keratitis.
- Progressive peripheral neuropathy and myopathy are rare.

DIFFERENTIAL DIAGNOSIS
Depends on the clinical features:
- Progressive supranuclear palsy.
- Pituitary tumor.
- Alzheimer's disease.
- Vascular dementia.
- Cerebral tumor: primary or metastatic.
- Sarcoidosis.
- Syphilis.

INVESTIGATIONS
Full blood count, ESR and other blood tests
Minimal neutrophil pleocytosis; ESR and serum ACE may be raised.

Molecular DNA analysis
Amplification of sequences of bacterial 16S ribosomal RNA (rRNA) specific for Whipple bacillus (*T. whippelii*) from peripheral blood mononuclear cells using PCR.

Cranial CT scan
May be normal, show cortical atrophy, areas of low attenuation with or without contrast enhancement, areas of mixed density with multifocal enhancement and regions of vasogenic edema.

MRI brain
May be normal in the early stages or show diffuse abnormalities on T2W images. Areas of increased T2W signal intensity on MRI scans are a sensitive indicator of disease activity and the lesions may enhance intensely with contrast medium.

The lesions may be seen in the hypothalamus, midbrain and basal ganglia and may have slight mass effect (**342, 343**).

CSF
CSF is normal or more commonly contains excess white cells and protein, oligoclonal banding and increased IgG. It may reveal sickle-particle-containing cells. Staining of the CSF with periodic acid Schiff reagent may give a positive result. PCR can be used to amplify sequences of bacterial 16S rRNA specific for Whipple bacillus (*T. whippelii*) in the CSF.

Other
- EEG: non-specific.
- Biopsy of jejunal mucosa, lymph nodes, vitreous or brain.

DIAGNOSIS
Definite CNS Whipple's disease
Must have any one of the following three criteria:
- Oculomasticatory myorhythmia (OMM: pendular vergence oscillations of the eyes that are synchronous with masticatory myorhythmia) and oculo-facial-skeletal myorhythmia (OFSM: similar to OMM, also involves myorhythmia of non-facial skeletal muscle).
- Positive tissue biopsy: ultrastructural findings of distinctive periodic acid Schiff-positive bacillary rods and sickle-shaped inclusion bodies in macrophages in the CSF, vitreous or in a jejunal or brain biopsy.
- Positive PCR amplification of sequences of bacterial 16S rRNA gene corresponding to the Whipple's disease bacillus (*T. whippelii*) in infected tissues.
- If histologic or PCR analysis is not performed on CNS tissue, then the patient must also demonstrate neurologic signs. If histologic or PCR analysis is performed on CNS tissue, then the patient need not demonstrate neurologic signs (i.e. asymptomatic CNS infection).

Possible CNS Whipple's disease
Must have any one of four systemic symptoms, not due to another known etiology:
- Fever of unknown etiology.
- Gastrointestinal symptoms (steatorrhea, chronic diarrhea, abdominal distension, or pain).

- Chronic migratory arthralgias or polyarthralgias.
- Unexplained lymphadenopathy, night sweats, or malaise.
- Also must have any one of four neurologic signs, not due to another etiology:
  - Supranuclear vertical gaze palsy.
  - Rhythmic myoclonus.
  - Dementia with psychiatric symptoms.
  - Hypothalamic manifestations.
- A favorable response to trimethoprim-sulfamethoxazole or chloramphenicol therapy helps to confirm the diagnosis.

TREATMENT
Antimicrobial treatment
- Oral trimethoprim (160 mg) and sulfamethoxazole (800 mg) twice daily for 1 year plus folate (folic acid) supplementation.
- If allergic: intravenous penicillin G (2 million units, 4 hourly) and oral doxycycline (100 mg bd).

The choice of antimicrobial treatment is based mainly on taxonomy, which has been known for only the past few years. The organism has not been cultured, and therefore *in vitro* susceptibilities are not available. There are no data on comparison of antibiotics. However, empirical clinical experience suggests that patients initially treated with drugs that do not penetrate the blood–brain barrier are at risk of neurologic relapse.

Myoclonus (see p.124)
- Valproate 500 mg bd.
- Clonazepam 0.5 mg nocte, increasing up to 8 mg per day (or tolerance).

PROGNOSIS
- The clinical course is usually one of progression to death within 6–12 months but can be fulminant, leading to death within weeks, in spite of treatment with appropriate antibiotics.
- Involvement of the neuraxis carries a poor prognosis, even when the intestinal disease has been eradicated.
- Relapses are most common with CNS Whipple's disease and are often resistant to antibiotics.

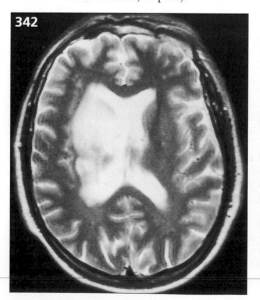

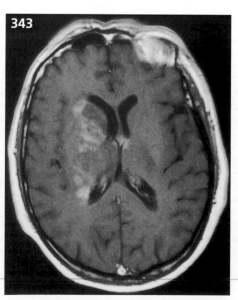

342, 343 T2W axial (**342**) and T1W axial (**343**) post contrast MRI in a patient with biopsy-proven Whipple's disease. Note the areas of increased signal with mass effect and some enhancement in the basal ganglia. The lesion was initially mistaken for an infarct but, because it involves the carotid and basilar territory, this would be distinctly unusual.

VIRAL INFECTIONS

ACUTE ASEPTIC MENINGITIS

DEFINITION
Acute meningeal irritation, benign and self-limiting, with sterile pleocytic CSF and complete recovery.

EPIDEMIOLOGY
- Incidence: 2–27 cases per 100 000 per year are reported. The incidence is probably higher by several multiples because of under-reporting.
- Lifetime prevalence: 0.9 (95% CI: 0.6–1.0) per 1000.
- Infections occur throughout the year, with a preponderance in summer and autumn in temperate climates.
- Age: mostly in children and young adults.

ETIOLOGY AND PATHOPHYSIOLOGY
Virus infection: at least 70% of cases
- Enteroviruses (over half cases of viral meningitis):
- – Coxsackie-B.
- – Echovirus.
- Herpes simplex virus (HSV) type 1 and type 2.
- Varicella-zoster.
- Mumps.
- Lymphocytic choriomeningitis.
- HIV.

Other causes
- Chemical and physical agents:
- – Myelography with oil-based contrast media.
- – Intrathecal drug administration.
- – Craniopharyngiomas.
- – Cholesterol crystals discharged from cholesteatoma.
- – Pituitary apoplexy.
- Parasites.
- Granulomatous inflammation: sarcoidosis.
- Connective tissue disease.
- Malignant infiltration.
- Drugs:
- – Cytotoxic drugs.
- – Non-steroidal anti-inflammatory drugs such as ibuprofen.
- – Immunoglobulins.
- – Antibiotics such as penicillin, isoniazid, ciprofloxacin, trimethoprim-sulfamethoxazole.

PATHOPHYSIOLOGY
Viral infections of the CNS are complications of systemic viral infections. The virus gains access to the brain by the bloodstream or, less commonly, by travelling along peripheral nerves. In order for viruses to enter the CNS from the blood they must cross the endothelial cell junctions of the blood–brain barrier (the ability to do this is dependent on surface adhesion molecules on the cells, and surface charges and cellular receptor of the virus).

Certain viruses preferentially infect the meninges, choroid plexus, and ependyma rather than cerebral parenchyma, causing meningitis; others infect neurons and glia to cause encephalitis. There is, however, considerable overlap, and some viruses may cause meningo-encephalitis. Drug-induced meningitis is either a direct chemical irritation or a hypersensitivity reaction.

CLINICAL FEATURES
Usually a rapid onset over hours of fever, headache, malaise, neck stiffness, photophobia, lethargy, myalgia and irritability. The patient usually remains coherent and can be roused easily. The occurrence of depressed consciousness, focal neurologic signs, or epileptic seizures usually implies encephalitis. The physical signs are not so marked and the illness is not as severe and prolonged as bacterial meningitis. The pathogen is seldom identified clinically:
- Myalgia and myocarditis point to coxsackie.
- Skin rash to enteroviruses, or herpes zoster virus (**344**).
- Parotitis and orchitis to mumps.
- Arthralgia and lymphadenopathy to HIV.

SPECIAL FORMS
Mollaret's meningitis
A benign recurrent 'non-infectious' meningitis of hitherto unknown cause characterized by fever, malaise and CSF pleocytosis (lymphocytes, neutrophils and endothelial cells), which may respond to corticosteroids, colchicine or phenylbutazone. New diagnostic techniques, such as the PCR for detecting viral DNA in CSF have shown HSV, predominantly type 2, to be a major cause of benign recurrent lymphocytic meningitis.

DIFFERENTIAL DIAGNOSIS
- Meningitis:
- – Early bacterial meningitis (see p.273).
- – Partially treated bacterial meningitis.
- – Meningitis caused by fastidious bacteria.
- – Fungal and parasitic meningitis (fungi and parasites do not grow readily in routine culture).
- – Parameningeal inflammation, infection or neoplasia.
- Subarachnoid hemorrhage (see p.249).

INVESTIGATIONS
Blood
Serologic studies of acute and convalescent serum samples (e.g. coxsackie, echovirus, HSV, varicella-zoster, mumps, HIV, measles, adenovirus, Epstein–Barr virus [EBV], cytomegalovirus [CMV]).

CT or MRI brain scan
Typically neither scan will show any abnormality. The main reason for imaging is to exclude other causes of headache, such as a space-occupying lesion or raised intracranial pressure, and ensure that it is safe to do an LP.

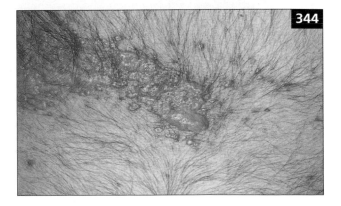

344 Herpes zoster skin rash in a patient with aseptic meningitis.

CSF

- May be normal in about 5% of cases.
- Pressure: increased.
- Microscopy: cell count raised; 5–1000 (typically 5–100) white cells per mm^3.
- Cell type: lymphocytes; polymorphs may predominate early, red cells may be present.
- Organisms: not seen.
- Protein: normal or raised up to 2 g/l.
- Glucose: normal.
- IgG index and oligoclonal bands: raised IgG; oligoclonal bands may be present.
- HSV antibody titers: an increased CSF:serum quotient for the HSV antibody titer, adjusted for CSF-blood barrier integrity, indicates a specific intrathecal antibody response.
- HSV antigen: virus isolated in less than 5% of cases.
- PCR for detection of HSV DNA in CSF: sensitive but not 100% reliable. If positive, it remains positive for at least 5 days after initiation of acyclovir therapy; the method of choice for diagnosis of HSE.
- Viral culture: low sensitivity in detecting HSV in adults but HSV can be retrieved from CSF in about half of babies with encephalitis or disseminated disease.

Blood viral serology

Acute and convalescent serum samples to demonstrate seroconversion or seroboosting.

Brain biopsy

The definitive diagnostic technique (characteristic histologic changes, immunofluorescence for HSV antigens, culture of HSV, and detection of viral DNA by *in situ* hybridization), but has little role because it is neither sensitive or specific (or safe), and in many cases it is appropriate to treat on the basis of clinical, EEG and radiologic findings and observe the clinical response to acyclovir. It does have a role in clarifying the differential diagnosis of a mass lesion that could be an abscess, granuloma, tumor or inflammatory mass, particularly if no response to acyclovir.

DIAGNOSIS

The diagnosis is suggested by neurologic, electrophysiologic and neuroimaging signs of fronto-temporal lobe necrosis with serologic evidence of seroconversion or seroboosting in paired acute and convalescent serum. However, a specific diagnosis can only be achieved by virologic studies of the CSF, PCR of the CSF, or by examination of brain tissue obtained by biopsy or at post mortem. Nested PCR amplification is a rapid, sensitive, inexpensive, and relatively non-invasive method for establishing the initial diagnosis of HSE and for monitoring the response to therapy. Although nested PCR is more susceptible to contamination artefact (false positive) than traditional methods such as virus isolation or serology, diagnostic PCR has been successfully incorporated into many laboratories and is likely to become the gold standard. HSV sequences can be detected for up to 5 days after commencing acyclovir and can differentiate between HSE due to HSV-1 and HSV-2.

TREATMENT

Prompt antiviral chemotherapy

Acyclovir must be commenced immediately in any patient with suspected HSE. The dose is 10 mg/kg given by intravenous infusion over 1 hour, every 8 hours for 10–14 days. Acyclovir is extremely well tolerated with few adverse effects in patients with normal renal function, and so it is often appropriate to treat patients with suspected HSE presumptively pending the results of further investigations. New anti-HSV agents with enhanced bioavailability, such as famciclovir are also available.

Symptomatic

Adequate oxygenation with assisted ventilation if necessary, optimal fluid and electrolyte balance and hydration, nutrition and analgesia.

Complications

- Cerebral edema and raised intracranial pressure: dexamethasone (4 mg 6 hourly i.v. or orally), mannitol (1 g/kg i.v. as a 20% solution over 1 hour), glycerol (glycerin) and intubation and hyperventilation may be required but remain controversial. Dexamethasone is often used despite the theoretical disadvantage that interferon synthesis may be inhibited. There is no consensus on the correct treatment.
- Epileptic seizures: anti-epileptic drugs such as sodium valproate or carbamazepine, if seizures occur.
- Secondary infections: treat as necessary.

CLINICAL COURSE AND PROGNOSIS

Untreated, HSE is rapidly progressive, typically leading to brain edema and death after 7–14 days; the 1 month mortality rate exceeds 70%, and only about 2.5% regain normal function.

Early aggressive antiviral therapy with acyclovir reduces mortality to 28% at 18 months, and is superior to that of vidarabine which reduces mortality to 28% at 1 month and 44% at 6 months. At 2 years after treatment with acyclovir about 38% are normal or have mild impairment, 9% have moderate sequelae, and 53% have died or are severely impaired. Among vidarabine recipients, only 15–20% are judged to be normal on long term follow-up.

Outcome is influenced by:

- Age.
- Level of consciousness (if Glasgow coma score is ≤6, outcome is uniformly poor).
- Duration of untreated disease (if treatment is commenced within 4 days of onset of symptoms, the chance of survival increases from 72% to 92% at 1 month).
- Infants with HSV-1 encephalitis have a significantly better neurologic outcome than those with HSV-2 infection of the CNS.

Relapse

Relapse of HSE after acyclovir or vidarabine therapy can occur in up to 5% of cases. In the few cases in which HSV isolates were tested for resistance to acyclovir, they remained sensitive. Re-institution of treatment with a higher dose of acyclovir (15 mg/kg every 8 hours) for a longer course (21 days) or in combination with vidarabine has been tried in a few patients but the results are inconclusive.

VARICELLA-ZOSTER VIRUS ENCEPHALOMYELITIS

DEFINITION
Inflammation of the brain or spinal cord caused by infection with the varicella-zoster virus (VZV), an α-herpes virus.

EPIDEMIOLOGY
- Incidence: rare, about 1 case per million population per year.
- Prevalence: about 0.1% of VZV infections involve the nervous system and 90% of these are in the form of encephalitis. VZV encephalitis has become more prevalent in the era of acquired immunodeficiency syndrome and other immunosuppressive diseases.
- Age: in immunocompetent individuals, herpes zoster is predominantly a disease of the elderly.
- Gender: M=F.

PATHOLOGY
A combination of ischemic and demyelinative features.

Multifocal demyelinating leukoencephalomyelitis
Infection of oligodendrocytes causes demyelinative lesions in the deep white matter which are smaller and less coalescent than those seen in PML. Target-like lesions with central necrosis and surrounding myelin pallor, and Cowdry type A intranuclear inclusions in surrounding glia and neurons are the pathologic hallmarks of varicella-zoster multifocal leukoencephalitis. Cowdry type A inclusions are virtually specific for herpes viruses but their absence does not rule out subtle infections.

Angiopathy causing cerebral infarction and hemorrhage
- Non-inflammatory angiopathy: involves mainly large cerebral arteries with non-inflammatory hyperplasia of intima and media, sometimes resulting in thrombosis and multifocal large ischemic and hemorrhagic infarcts in the cerebral cortex and subcortical white matter.

- Arteritis: involves small vessels with fibrinoid necrosis and granulomatous inflammatory infiltrates causing thrombosis and multifocal deep white matter lesions (demyelination or infarction). In purely ischemic lesions, characteristic Cowdry A inclusions may be scant or absent. Rarely, mycotic aneurysms may form and rupture, causing hemorrhage.

Brain infarction does not usually occur until weeks to months after trigeminal nerve distribution herpes zoster rash (shingles).

ETIOLOGY AND PATHOPHYSIOLOGY
Chickenpox
Primary VZV infection causes the typical rash of chickenpox. During chickenpox, VZV establishes latency in multiple dorsal root ganglia.

Shingles
After a variable, but usually long period, the VZV reactivates to cause shingles (herpes zoster), which is a disease of the peripheral nervous system causing severe radicular pain, herpetic vesicles on the skin usually in the distribution of one to three dermatomes (353–355), and pain after the vesicles have healed (post herpetic neuralgia). Focal muscle weakness

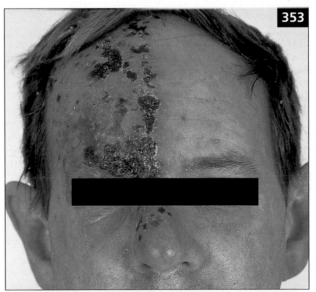

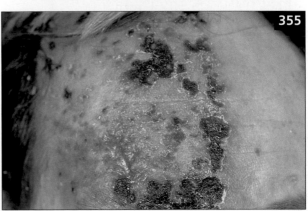

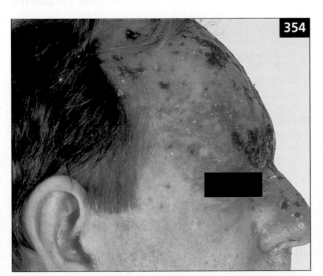

353–355 Herpes zoster infection (shingles) in the distribution of the ophthalmic division of the trigeminal nerve.

(zoster paresis) occurs in about 5% of cases, of whom about 60% recover completely, 25% incompletely, and 15% do not improve. Encephalitis may rarely follow shingles.

Post herpetic pain probably occurs because reactivation of VZV in the dorsal root ganglia appears to cause structural damage which results in chronic stimulation of the CNS. This re-sets the homeostatic mechanisms controlling pain, so that the patient perceives chronic pain, severe pain from minor stimuli, and allodynia (abnormal sensations).

Encephalomyelitis

Caused by reactivation of the VZV, latent in sensory ganglia after primary infection. Several mechanisms have been proposed, including hematogenous, transaxonal (transneural) and/or vascular spread to the CNS, and an immune-mediated effect. VZV may enter the CNS via transaxonal spread from ocular or dermatomal zoster and directly invade and infect small blood vessels, ultimately leading to ischemic infarction and necrosis of brain or spinal cord, or directly infect oligodendrocytes, leading to demyelination. The finding of an active 'centrifuge wave' of infection at the periphery of lesions and their random distribution in the brain however, suggests hematogenous spread during viremia.

Risk factors

Immunocompromised: elderly, acquired immunodeficiency syndrome (AIDS), immunosuppressive therapy.

CLINICAL FEATURES

In about half of cases, usually young people with chicken pox, the encephalitis predominantly affects the cerebellum, causing cerebellar ataxia, dysarthria, headache and drowsiness. The skin rash often precedes the neurologic symptoms by about a week but occasionally the rash of chicken pox may follow.

In immunocompromised and older individuals zoster encephalomyelitis and granulomatous arteritis (the latter after zoster ophthalmicus) usually develops concurrent with rash or weeks to months after acute herpes zoster rash (**353–355**) and is characterized by fever, seizures, mental status changes and multifocal or isolated focal neurologic deficits.

DIFFERENTIAL DIAGNOSIS

- Other forms of viral encephalitis (see p.292): CMV, HIV-1 related encephalitis, HSE (see p.295).
- Hemorrhagic multifocal leukoencephalopathy secondary to angiopathy caused by toxoplasmosis, aspergillus, CMV, HSV, ameba, HIV-1 (see p.301).
- Isolated angiitis of the CNS (see p.227).
- Stroke: ischemic (see p.202) or hemorrhagic (see p.238).
- Progressive multifocal leukoencephalopathy: typically causes hemiparesis, aphasia, visual-field defects and confusional states; MRI reveals larger and more coalescent zones of demyelination than VZV encephalitis; and CSF PCR detects JC virus DNA.

INVESTIGATIONS

Blood viral serology

Acute and convalescent serum samples to demonstrate seroconversion or seroboosting.

Cranial CT scan

CT shows focal or multifocal areas of low attenuation and swelling, and sometimes petechial or frank hemorrhage. Intracranial calcification may occur as a sequelae to zoster encephalitis.

MRI brain

MR may reveal a spectrum of lesions from multifocal ischemic and hemorrhagic infarction of varying size, depending on the caliber of the vessel involved, to a leukoencephalopathy characterized by multifocal small ovoid lesions involving white matter more than gray matter, and often more concentrated at gray-white matter junctions, due to both demyelination and necrosis caused by a small vessel vasculopathy. There are no specific distinguishing features however.

CSF

Findings are similar to viral encephalitis (see p.292). Enzyme immunoassay for antibody to VZV and PCR for detection of VZV DNA.

EEG

Abnormal, most often non-specific focal or diffuse slow wave activity, occasionally with epileptiform activity.

Cerebral angiography

May reveal segmental narrowing of large and medium-sized arteries in cases of angiopathy.

Brain biopsy

Necrosis and gliosis consistent with infarction; immunohistochemical localization of viral antigens and *in situ* hybridization or PCR detection of VZV DNA.

DIAGNOSIS

- The finding of brain infarction (ischemic or hemorrhagic) and/or demyelination lesions in an immunocompromised patient with or without a history of zoster rash, and with a fever and encephalopathy, should suggest the diagnosis of VZV encephalitis.
- Serologic evidence of seroconversion or seroboosting in paired acute and convalescent serum or the detection of antiviral antibody and VZV DNA in CSF can confirm the diagnosis.
- Brain biopsy or autopsy evidence of immunohistochemical localization of viral antigens and *in situ* hybridization or PCR detection of VZV DNA are required for the unequivocal demonstration of virus-specific antigens or nucleic acids.

TREATMENT

Encephalomyelitis

- General management is as for viral encephalitis (see p.292).
- Specific antiviral therapy with intravenous acyclovir 10 mg/kg every 8 hours for 10–14 days, or alternatively famciclovir.

PROGNOSIS

Patients with the cerebellar form usually recover completely but at least 10% of those with the general form die.

HUMAN IMMUNODEFICIENCY VIRUS (HIV)-ASSOCIATED COGNITIVE/MOTOR COMPLEX (HIV-CMC)

DEFINITION

A distinct neurologic syndrome of subcortical dementia characterized by slowness and imprecision of cognition and motor control, and called the AIDS dementia complex or HIV-1-associated cognitive/motor complex. It is the most important 'primary' neurologic complication of HIV infection.

EPIDEMIOLOGY

HIV dementia usually occurs late in the course of HIV disease, when CD4 lymphocyte counts are less than 200 cells/mm^3, but in 3–10% of patients it is the first manifestation of AIDS.
- Incidence:
  - 2 (95% CI: 0.8–5) per 100 000 per year.
  - 7% annual incidence during the first 2 years after AIDS diagnosis.
  - 7.3 cases per 100 person years for people with CD4 counts of ≤100.
  - 3.0 cases per 100 person years if CD4 count 101–200.
  - 1.3 to 1.7 cases per 100 person years if CD4 count 201–500.
  - 0.5 cases per 100 person years if CD4 count >500.
- Prevalence: 0.4% during the asymptomatic phase, 7.5–27% during the late stages of HIV disease; at least 15% of AIDS patients develop moderate to severe dementia, and up to another 20–25% have less severe cognitive dysfunction.

PATHOLOGY
Key features
- Multiple foci of microglia, macrophages, and multinucleate giant cells or the presence of HIV-infected cells in the CNS (**356**).
- Other abnormalities: inflammatory cell infiltrate, multinucleate giant cells (HIV encephalitis), reactive gliosis and diffuse white matter pallor (HIV leukoencephalopathy).

The pathologic changes are often less prominent than the clinical symptoms.

PATHOGENESIS
Complex and obscure but determined by :
- The effectiveness of the immune defences and their capacity to suppress viral replication within the brain.
- The genetic variance of the virus and its macrophage tropism (i.e. capacity to replicate well in macrophages and related cells but not well in lymphocyte-derived chronic cell lines).
- The genetic predisposition of the individual.

Probably due to indirect effects of HIV infection on the CNS. Infected and activated macrophages and microglia produce increased intracerebral cytokines and neurotoxins leading to secondary neuronal damage, principally in the subcortical and basal ganglia regions, but also in neocortical areas. White matter pallor may be due to demyelination or changes in the blood–brain barrier that are mediated by cytokines and contribute to extravasation of serum proteins

into the brain and viral entry into the brain. Certain strains of HIV-1, characterized by specific sequences in the envelope region, may have a predilection for infecting the brain and causing dementia.

CLINICAL FEATURES
Subtle early in the course, and may only be identified by formal neuropsychologic evaluation.
Three main categories:
- Cognitive: initially a predominantly subcortical dementia characterized by forgetfulness and slowed mental and motor abilities.
- Motor: loss of balance and occurrence of spastic leg weakness.
- Behavioral: apathy and social withdrawal (often mistaken as depression); sometimes organic psychosis, such as acute mania.

The disease stages have been classified from normal (stage 0) to profoundly impaired (stage 4).

Examination findings
- Cognitive: psychomotor slowing, and abnormalities of reaction time, memory, executive function and complex attention.
- Eye movements: abnormal: saccadic pursuit and hypometric saccades.
- Limbs: bradykinesia; impairment of rapid alternating and repetitive movements and tandem (heel-to-toe) gait.
- Reflexes: brisk and symmetric; primitive reflexes may manifest in later stage disease.

Concurrent illness
Subclinical HIV-associated dementia may be 'unmasked' by intercurrent illnesses, such as depression, metabolic derangements, systemic and cerebral opportunistic infections (e.g. toxoplasmosis, PML, cryptococcal meningitis), and lymphoma, which are important to look for (and treat).

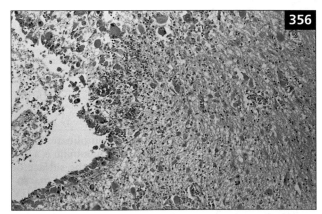

356 Histologic section of the brain of a patient who died with the HIV-associated cognitive/motor complex showing an inflammatory cell infiltrate with multiple foci of macrophages and multinucleate giant cells. (H&E stain, magnification ×16.) (Courtesy of Professor BA Kakulas, Royal Perth Hospital, Western Australia.)

SUBACUTE SCLEROSING PANENCEPHALITIS (SSPE)

DEFINITION
A rare slowly progressive disease of the CNS in children and young adults that is probably caused by chronic infection by defective measles virus not expressing its M protein.

EPIDEMIOLOGY
- Incidence: extremely rare, about 1 case per million children per year; measles vaccination has greatly reduced the incidence. Many ethnic groups are affected.
- Age: affects children and adolescents; mean age of onset of 7–8 years; rarely beyond 18 years.

PATHOLOGY
- Cerebral cortex and white matter of the cerebral hemispheres and brainstem (**360**):
- Nerve cell destruction, neuronophagia, and perivenous cuffing by lymphocytes (**361**) reflect the viral nature of the infection.
- Degeneration of medullated fibers (myelin and axis cylinders) of the white matter, accompanied by perivascular cuffing with mononuclear cells and fibrous gliosis (sclerosing encephalitis).
- Eosinophilic inclusions in the cytoplasm and nuclei of neurons and glial cells are the hallmark of the disease (**362–364**).
- Virions, thought to be measles nucleocapsids, may be seen with electron microscopy in inclusion-bearing cells.
- Immunohistochemical studies reveal measles virus antigen (**365**).
- Paired helical filament-tau immunohistochemistry and electron microscopy reveal early stages of neurofibrillary tangle formation in hippocampal neurons.

ETIOLOGY AND PATHOPHYSIOLOGY
- Measles virus infection acquired pre-natally or in infancy or early childhood: measles virus infection below 1 year of age is a risk factor.
- Persistent measles virus infection of the brain.

- Mutations of the measles virus, resulting in a lack of production of an M (matrix) protein in the measles virus, which allows the virus to remain relatively protected in an intracellular form and environment, away from the extracellular host defence mechanisms, and spread by cell-to-cell contact.

CLINICAL FEATURES
- History of primary measles infection at a very early age; often before 2 years.
- Latent interval of 6–8 years after measles infection, or in rare cases live measles vaccination.
- First stage:
- Cognitive decline: less proficient at school, language difficulties.
- Behavioral changes: temper outbursts, loss of interest in usual activities, and other changes in personality.
- Second stage:
- Intellectual deterioration: severe and progressive.
- Myoclonic jerks; widespread.
- Seizures: focal or generalized.
- Visual disturbance sometimes: due to progressive chorioretinitis.
- Third stage: neuromotor retardation with spasticity, rigidity, autonomic dysfunction and unresponsiveness.
- Final stage: insensate, virtually 'decorticated'.

DIFFERENTIAL DIAGNOSIS
- Lipid storage diseases.
- Schilder disease.
- HIV infection.
- Neurosyphilis.
- Creutzfeldt–Jakob disease (CJD).

INVESTIGATIONS
Serum
High titers of measles virus specific IgG antibody; negative syphilis and HIV serology.

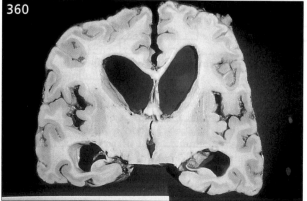

360 Section of the brain at autopsy, coronal plane, showing severe generalized atrophy of the brain due to subacute sclerosing panencephalitis.

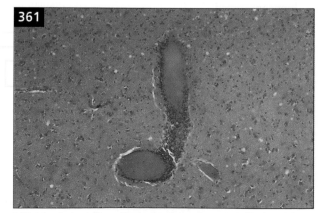

361 Histologic section of brain showing perivenous cuffing by lymphocytes and destruction of neurons.

EEG

Characteristic periodic bursts (every 3–10 seconds) of symmetrically bisynchronous slow and sharp wave complexes (Rodermacker complexes), with an amplitude around 500 µV, and often associated with myoclonic jerks, appear early in the clinical disease process and may be diagnostic (**366**). The periodic discharges are more complicated in outline and separated by longer intervals than in CJD. Unlike other types of periodic phenomena, they may occur on a fairly normal background in SSPE.

CSF

- Cell count: normal.
- Protein: normal or raised.
- Immunoglobulin levels: high.
- Oligoclonal bands of IgG: present (measles virus-specific antibody).
- Measles virus antibody titer: extremely high titers of measles specific IgG.

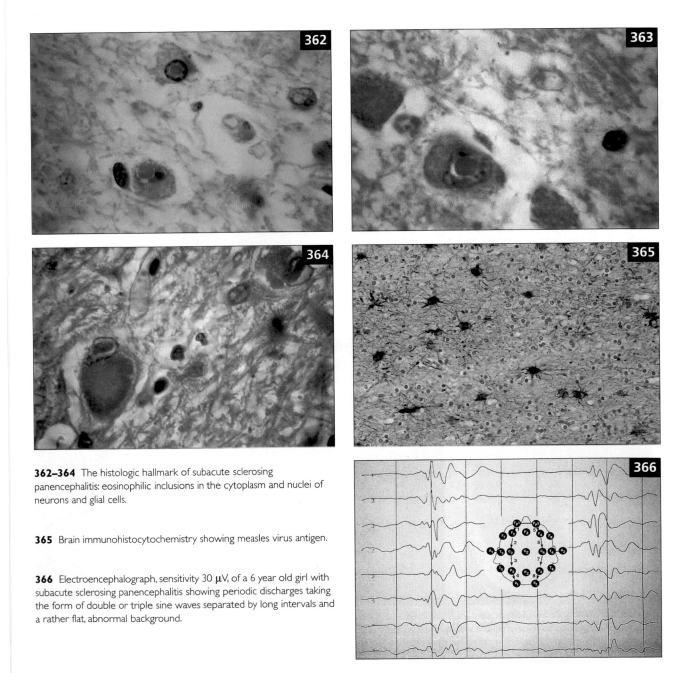

362–364 The histologic hallmark of subacute sclerosing panencephalitis: eosinophilic inclusions in the cytoplasm and nuclei of neurons and glial cells.

365 Brain immunohistocytochemistry showing measles virus antigen.

366 Electroencephalograph, sensitivity 30 µV, of a 6 year old girl with subacute sclerosing panencephalitis showing periodic discharges taking the form of double or triple sine waves separated by long intervals and a rather flat, abnormal background.

OTHER INFECTIONS: SPIROCHETAL, FUNGAL, PROTOZOAN, WORM AND PRION

NEUROSYPHILIS

DEFINITION
Syphilis is an infectious disease caused by *Treponema pallidum*, which is a natural pathogen only in humans. Four stages can be distinguished in the natural history of syphilis: primary, secondary or disseminated, latent and tertiary syphilis. Neurosyphilis is one of the tertiary forms of syphilis.

EPIDEMIOLOGY
- Incidence: the incidence of syphilis is rising in the United States, mainly due to an increase in the number of cases of cocaine/crack addiction.
- Prevalence: in Florida, USA, the prevalence of syphilis in 1987 was 66 per 100 000 persons, particularly among homosexual men. Neurosyphilis occurs in less than 3% of all syphilis cases due to administration of antibiotics in the first stages of the disease.
- Age: adults of any age.
- Gender: M>F.

PATHOLOGY
Meningovascular syphilis
- Diffuse thickening and lymphocytic infiltration of the leptomeninges and perivascular spaces.
- Vasculitis (endarteritis obliterans) of terminal arterioles, which show concentric proliferative thickening of the endothelium as well as appearance of fibroblasts (**377**). The most commonly involved artery is the MCA.

Tabes dorsalis
Degeneration with neuronal loss in the dorsal root entry zones of the spinal cord and fibers in the dorsal columns (**378**).

ETIOLOGY AND PATHOPHYSIOLOGY
- Acquired infection, mainly by sexual intercourse with an infected individual but also by vertical transmission at delivery, by laboratory accidents or blood transfusions.
- If the CNS is to be invaded, this usually occurs within 2 years after primary infection.

Stages of neurosyphilis
- Acute syphilitic meningitis usually occurs within the first 2 years of the primary infection. May involve the brain or the spinal cord.
- Meningovascular syphilis may occur any time from the onset of the secondary syphilis rash to 10 years after the primary infection but generally does not occur until 4–7 years after the primary infection. It is due to granulomatous syphilitic infiltration and vasculitis around the brainstem, spinal cord and spinal roots.
- Tabes dorsalis develops 20 years or so after the primary infection. Degeneration of dorsal roots and fibers in dorsal columns interrupt the stretch reflex arc to cause hypotonia and loss of reflexes, and lightning (stabbing) pains mainly in the legs.

- General paralysis of the insane develops about 15–20 years after the primary infection. It is due to widespread spirochetal invasion of the brain and chronic meningovascular syphilis.

CLINICAL FEATURES
Clinically, neurosyphilis can be classified into well defined syndromes, representing different clinical expressions of the same disease.

Asymptomatic neurosyphilis
- The manifestations of primary or secondary syphilis (e.g. skin rash [**379–382**]) have resolved, and there are no neurologic gray signs.
- The CSF is abnormal, such as positive serology, an increased cell count and, occasionally, an increased protein content.

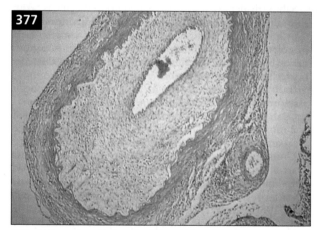

377 Cross section of a branch of the middle cerebral artery showing intimal hyperplasia due to meningovascular syphilis.

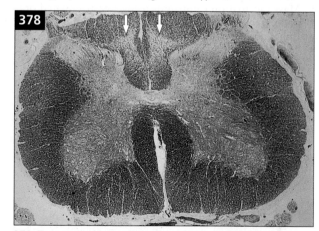

378 Transverse section of the spinal cord in a patient with tabes dorsalis showing degeneration of the posterior columns (arrows) secondary to *Treponema pallidum* infection and inflammation along the dorsal roots. (Courtesy of Professor BA Kakulas, Royal Perth Hospital, Western Australia.)

Acute syphilitic meningitis

- Symptoms include headache, nausea and vomiting, neck stiffness, seizures and changes in mental status; patients are often afebrile.
- Ocular or cranial nerve abnormalities, especially VII and VIII, may occur due to involvement at the base of the brain.
- Some patients can develop leptomeningeal granulomas, hydrocephalus or neuritis.

Meningovascular syphilis

Generally presents with a prodromic phase, weeks or months before the onset of identifiable vascular syndromes. Specific clinical features include:

- TIA or stroke-like syndrome (if focal inflammation of intracranial arteries).
- Slowly progressive cognitive decline and personality changes (if multifocal involvement of small intracranial arteries).
- Epileptic seizures.
- Argyll Robertson pupils.

(Continued overleaf)

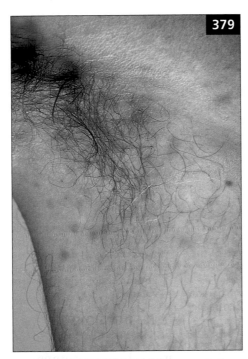

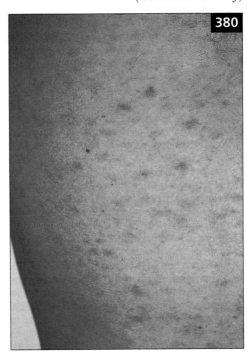

379, 380 Skin rash on the axilla and trunk of a patient in the initial stages of secondary syphilis. The lesions are bilaterally symmetric, pale red/pink, non-pruritic, discrete, round macules, about 5–10 mm (0.2–0.4 in) in diameter, distributed on the trunk and proximal extremities. After 1–2 months, red, papular lesions 3–10 mm (0.1–0.4 in) in diameter also appear on the palms, soles, face and scalp.

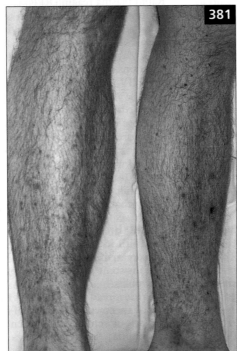

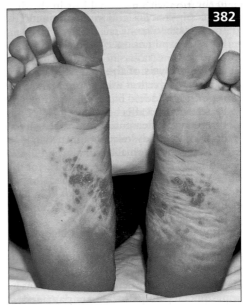

381, 382 Skin rash on the legs and foot soles of a patient in the later stages of secondary syphilis. The lesions are red/copper-colored, papular and papulosquamous, about 3–10 mm (0.1–0.4 in) in diameter and were also present on the palms, face and scalp.

CSF

- Gram stain: spherical cells, 5–15 μm in diameter, which retain the Gram stain and are surrounded by a thick refractile capsule.
- India ink stain for cryptococcal antigen. The carbon particles fail to penetrate the capsule, producing a white halo around the double refractile wall of the yeast.
- Latex agglutination test or ELISA for the cryptococcal polysaccharide antigen.
- Cryptococcal antigen titer (more than 1 : 8 is diagnostic).
- Culture: positive in 4–12 days. Isolation of yeast confirms the diagnosis and allows for sensitivity tests *in vitro*.
- Opening pressure should be measured because elevated intracranial pressure may have important prognostic implications, particularly for visual impairment.
- White cell count: may be normal or only mildly elevated.
- Protein: normal or elevated.
- Glucose: normal or decreased.

N.B. It is essential to test the CSF for cryptococcal organisms and antigen in patients with suspected cryptococcal meningitis because the CSF cell count, protein and glucose can all be normal, particularly in AIDS patients. Large volumes of CSF (20–40 ml) may be needed to find the organism.

Other

- Serum cryptococcal antigen: positive. AIDS patients have higher antigen titers in blood than in CSF.
- Blood and urine cultures are often positive.

DIAGNOSIS

Serum cryptococcal antigen is almost always positive in cryptococcosis, but meningitis should be confirmed by CSF examination. Positive India ink staining or CSF cryptococcal antigen titer will provide rapid diagnosis, which is confirmed subsequently by CSF culture.

TREATMENT

Treatment is determined by the severity of the illness.

Primary therapy (treatment of acute infection)

Severe case

Altered consciousness, CSF white blood cell count >20/mm^3, CSF antigen titer >1 : 1024 and a positive blood culture:

- Amphotericin B 0.5–0.7 mg/kg body weight per day by intravenous injection. Amphotericin is limited by frequent adverse effects, such as fever, renal dysfunction with renal tubular acidosis and, rarely, leukoencephalopathy. A liposomal form of amphotericin B may have less adverse effects.
- ±5-flucytosine (100–150 mg/kg/day by mouth or intravenously) for 2–3 weeks (the value of adding flucytosine remains undetermined). Flucytosine adverse effects include myelosuppression and gastrointestinal toxicity.
- Followed by fluconazole (an oral triazole antifungal agent) 400 mg/day by mouth, for an additional 8–10 weeks; fluconazole is as effective as amphotericin B but fluconazole causes delayed clearance of cryptococcus from the CSF.

Mild case

- Fluconazole 800 mg loading dose by mouth, then 400 mg daily by mouth.
- Itraconazole may be used instead of fluconazole but experience with itraconazole is limited.

Most patients respond clinically within 1–2 weeks, with an early mortality of 5–10%. Continue therapy for 4–6 weeks or until the CSF is sterile.

Management of raised intracranial pressure

- Mechanical drainage (repeated LPs, intraventricular shunt).
- Acetazolamide treatment.
- Corticosteroids are being studied in a controlled trial.

Maintenance therapy to prevent relapses

Triazole antifungal agents (fluconazole 200–400 mg daily by mouth, and itraconazole) have a more favorable toxicity profile and may be preferable for long term suppressive treatment necessary to avoid the high incidence of relapse (more than 50%) in patients with AIDS. With maintenance therapy, relapses are uncommon and usually related to non-compliance with treatment, but may also occur because of development of drug resistance and drug interactions which lower fluconazole levels. Monitoring serum cryptococcal antigen titers is not useful in predicting relapse.

CLINICAL COURSE/PROGNOSIS

A steadily progressive course occurs over several weeks or months. In a few patients, the course may be remarkably indolent with periods of clinical improvement and normalization of the CSF. In others, it may be fatal within a few weeks if untreated.

Unfavorable prognostic factors are:
- Altered mental status.
- High CSF cryptococcal antigen titer.
- Low CSF leukocyte count.
- Positive extrameningeal culture for cryptococcus, hyponatremia, and raised intracranial pressure (for vision).

MUCORMYCOSIS OF THE NERVOUS SYSTEM

DEFINITION
An opportunistic, malignant infection of the brain vessels caused by zygomycete fungi, including those of the genera *Absidia*, *Rhizomucor* and *Rhizopus*.

EPIDEMIOLOGY
- Incidence: rare.
- Age: often adolescents and young adults.
- Gender: M=F.

PATHOLOGY
Several forms
- Orbital.
- Rhino-orbital.
- Rhino-orbito-cerebral.
- Cutaneous.
- Pulmonary.
- Gastrointestinal.
- Disseminated.

Rhino-orbito-cerebral form
- Mucosal thickening of the paranasal sinuses on one or both sides.
- Soft tissue retro-orbital mass.
- Numerous broad, irregular non-septate fungal hyphae with non-parallel margins, within the arterial wall and often extending into the surrounding brain parenchyma.
- Secondary intraluminal arterial thrombosis.
- Secondary hemorrhagic infarction of the brain.
- Intracranial granuloma from hematogenous spread are unusual.
- Cavernous sinus thrombosis following invasion of orbital apex.
- Brain abscess following direct intracranial extension.

ETIOLOGY AND PATHOPHYSIOLOGY
The fungi are acquired from the environment and infect the lungs, paranasal sinuses and, less commonly, the skin.

The brain infection begins in the nasal turbinates and paranasal sinuses and spreads along infected vessels through the orbital apex to the retro-orbital tissues and through the cribriform plate to the brain, where it may cause a cerebral vasculitis with secondary arterial and venous thrombosis and hemorrhagic infarction.

RISK FACTORS/PREDISPOSING CONDITIONS
- Diabetes mellitus:
- Present in about three-quarters of cases.
- A risk factor for cutaneous and localized paranasal infection.
- The fungus thrives in an environment rich in glucose and acid pH.
- Poor glycemic control and ketoacidosis impair phagocytic activity of neutrophils.
- Diabetic ketoacidosis is associated with increased serum free-iron levels, which facilitates growth of rhizopus, an iron-requiring organism.
- Burns (for skin invasion).
- Neutropenia (for widespread mucor infection).
- Leukemia.
- Lymphoma.
- Cytotoxic drug treatment.
- Corticosteroid treatment.
- Post organ transplant.
- Renal failure.
- AIDS.
- Amebiasis.
- Malnutrition.
- Kwashiorkor.
- Intravenous drug abuse.

CLINICAL FEATURES
Retro-orbital mucormycosis
History
- Headache (75%).
- Eye pain.
- Facial swelling.
- Dark, blood-stained nasal discharge (45%).

Examination
- Sick (i.e. looks unwell).
- Altered sensorium (30%)
- Fever (55%)
- Orbito-fascio- cellulitis (35%): swelling, mucopurulent discharge from the eye.
- Proptosis.
- Edema of the eyelids.
- Reduced visual acuity and direct light reflex.
- Relative afferent pupillary defect.
- Retinal edema.
- Rapid reduction in visual acuity, resulting in blindness in one eye.
- Ophthalmoplegia (35%).
- Hemiparesis (30%).

Cerebral mucormycosis
Carotid territory hemorrhagic infarction of the brain (e.g. hemiparesis, dysphasia).

DIFFERENTIAL DIAGNOSIS
- Cavernous sinus syndrome such as cavernous sinus thrombophlebitis (see p.258).
- Retro-orbital tumor.

CT (400, 401)

CT shows single or multiple hypodense cysts that are localized or generalized and contain a small, asymmetrically located 'off-center', internal, hyperdense nodule (with or without calcification) corresponding to the dead and hyalinized larval scolex (calcification occurs where cysts have died). The cyst fluid is of CSF density. The cysts or nodules enhance with intravenous contrast as the cysticerci degenerate. This occurs early on, together with edema and mass effect, but the enhancement wears off as the lesion ages and the edema disappears. CT may reveal complications, which include hydrocephalus and basal meningitis.

MRI (402, 403)

MRI shows similar features to CT, with the cysts of CSF signal. MRI is more sensitive than CT for detecting edema (which indicates lesion activity; edema occurs as the parasite dies) and non-calcified cysticercosis lesions in the ventricles and subarachnoid space, such as in the basal cisterns.

Blood

- Full blood count and film: leukocytosis due to peripheral eosinophilia
- ESR: elevated.
- Serum immunochemistry: ELISA for IgM antibodies against the cysticercus antigen, and the enzyme-linked immunoelectrotransfer blot (EITB), which has a sensitivity of greater than 93% and a specificity of 100%.

CSF

- CSF is negative in 49–63% of cases of the intraparenchymal form; pleocytosis, eosinophilia, elevated protein, and occasionally hypoglycorrhachia occur in the encephalitic, racemose and basilar meningitic forms.
- Immunochemistry: ELISA for IgM antibodies against the cysticercus antigen shows a sensitivity of 87% and specificity of 95% in active disease. False positives can occur in neurosyphilis and meningeal tuberculosis. The EITB has a sensitivity of about 80% and a specificity of 100%.

Other

Anal scrapings and fecal examination for ova and parasites: frequently negative.

DIAGNOSIS

- A definitive diagnosis requires identification of the proglottids or eggs of the larval form of *T. solium* in stool. The gravid segments of the eggs must be examined for their characteristic morphologic features.
- As this can be difficult to identify positively, a positive diagnosis can be made by detecting antibodies to *T. solium* by Western blot analysis. Biopsy can also be used to make a positive identification.

TREATMENT

Treatment depends on the presenting syndrome, nature of the neurologic impairment, location and activity of cysticerci and host immune response.

Calcified neurocysticerci represent inactive cysts, and neither require nor respond to anticysticercal drug treatment.

Anticysticercal drugs

- Praziquantel, an isoquinolone antihelminthic agent, 50 mg/kg of body weight, given daily for 15–30 days, depending on the number and size of the cysts.
- Albendazole, an imidazole antihelminthic agent, 15 mg/kg body weight per day for 21 days, is the preferred drug as its plasma levels increase by 50% when used concurrently with dexamethasone, in contrast to praziquantel whose bioavailability is decreased by 50%. Albendazole produces an 80% reduction in total number of cysts after a single course of therapy, compared to a 65% reduction after praziquantel.

Anti-inflammatory drugs

A host inflammatory reaction to the death of cysticerci as a result of anticysticercal drug treatment may lead to cerebral edema and increased intracranial pressure. Concurrent treatment with:
- Prednisolone (1–2 mg/kg/day oral for 7 days), or
- Dexamethasone.

Surgery

- A CSF shunting procedure may be required for hydrocephalus due to cisternal cysticercosis and chronic arachnoiditis.
- Excision/decompression of large subarachnoid or intraventricular cysts that obstruct CSF flow.

Anti-epileptic drug therapy

If required (i.e. symptomatic epileptic seizures).

Prevention

- Disposal of human feces in a sanitary manner.
- Cook or freeze all meat or fish thoroughly before it is eaten.
- Mass treatment with albendazole or praziquantel could eliminate cestodes from the world, but this would be a formidable task, given the widespread distribution of the pork tapeworm.

PROGNOSIS

Initially treatment may seem to exacerbate neurologic symptoms, with an increase in cells and protein in the CSF, but then the patients improve and many become asymptomatic, with a striking decrease in the size and number of cysts on CT scanning.

Cisternal and racemose cysticercosis are less responsive to anticysticercal drugs than parenchymal cysticercosis.

The outcome of patients with epilepsy due to neurocysticercosis is better after anticysticercal drug therapy than when the primary disease is left to follow its natural course. This is true for both those in whom the cysticerci remain unchanged for long periods and for those in whom there is an intense inflammatory reaction that eventually destroys the cysticerci. Also, there are fewer seizures after medical treatment than after surgical removal of the cystic lesion.

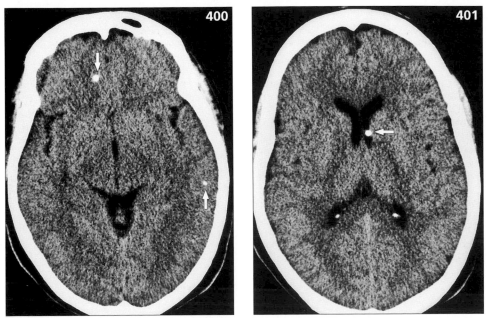

400, 401 Plain cranial CT scan showing multiple small hyperdense areas of calcification (arrows – dead cysts) in a patient with inactive cysticercosis.

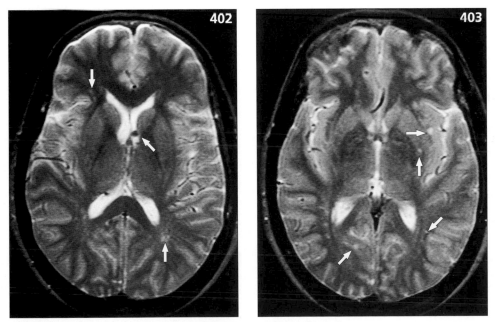

402, 403 MRI brain scan showing subtle inactive cysticercosis lesions (arrows).

CREUTZFELDT–JAKOB DISEASE (CJD)

DEFINITION
A neurodegenerative condition that is the most common clinicopathologic subtype of the transmissible spongiform encephalopathies or prion diseases.

The transmissible spongiform encephalopathies are all characterized by the deposition in brain of an abnormal, protease resistant, isoform of a membrane-bound glycoprotein, the prion protein. Since the spongiform change can be variable, the term prion disease is more accurate.

EPIDEMIOLOGY
- Incidence: 1 per million per year.
- Age: median age of onset: 61 years; rare (but increasingly reported [nvCJD]) younger than 30, and older than 80 years.
- Gender: M=F.

PATHOLOGY
Macroscopic
Normal or slightly atrophic brain.

Microscopic (404)
A triad of:
- Neuronal loss.
- Reactive astrocytic proliferation and gliosis.
- Spongiform degeneration (status spongiosus and spongiform change: vacuolation of the neuropil [405, 406]): particularly in deeper laminae of the gray matter of the frontal and temporal lobes, but also the gray matter of the striatum, thalamus, tegmentum of the upper brain stem, and cerebellar cortex.

Kuru plaques are also present: eosinophilic, round, compact extracellular depositions of prion protein (PrP); pathognomonic of a prion disease but found in only a few sporadic cases.

Ultrastructural
Intraneuronal, complex, clear vacuoles whose membranous septa look curled in profile.

ETIOLOGY
Inherited mutation in the *PrP* gene
Familial CJD (10–15% of cases)
Autosomal dominant pattern of inheritance; point mutations or insertions in the prion protein gene located on the short arm of chromosome 20. The codon 200^{Lys} and 178^{Asp} mutations (in association with codon 129$^{Val/Met}$ polymorphism) are associated with neuropathologic changes essentially indistinguishable from sporadic CJD.

Acquired
Iatrogenic transmission of CJD (<5% of cases)
- Human cadaveric pituitary-derived growth hormone (hGH): >100 cases worldwide.
- The estimated risk of developing cadaveric hGH-induced CJD for patients treated with cadaveric-derived hGH is 1 in 200–300.
- Foreign dura mater grafts: 69 cases.

- Inadequately sterilized neurosurgic instruments and depth electrodes: 6 cases.
- Human gonadotrophin: 4 cases.
- Corneal transplant: 2 cases.

Sporadic, randomly distributed illness of unknown cause (85% of cases)

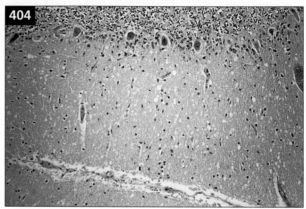

404 Microscopic section of the gray matter of cerebellum of a patient with CJD showing neuronal loss, reactive astrocytic proliferation and gliosis, and spongiform degeneration (vacuolation of the neuropil).

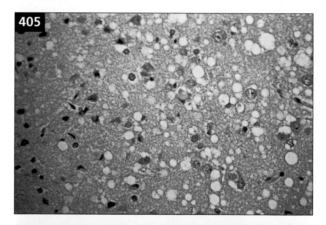

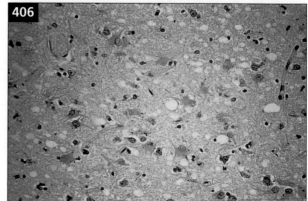

405, 406 Neuronal vacuolation and spongiform change in the brain of a patient with CJD.

PATHOGENESIS
- Transmissible to experimental animals following inoculation or dietary exposure.
- Long incubation period, hence the initial concept of a slow virus infection, but no infective agent has been found.

Prion hypothesis
- The transmissible agent is a proteinaceous infectious particle, or prion.
- The prion appears to consist principally or entirely of a modified abnormal, partially protease-resistant isoform of a normal host-encoded cellular glycoprotein, the prion protein (PrP).
- Normal prion protein, described as PrP^C, is a constituent of the surface of the neuronal cell.
- In the presence of mutations, now discovered in CJD and other transmissible spongiform encephalopathies (kuru, Gerstmann Straussler Scheinker syndrome [GSS], fatal familial insomnia [FFI], and atypical prion disease), PrP^C may change into a disease-related isoform, PrP^{Sc}, which differs from the normal cellular isoform by a post-translational modification that appears to involve a conformational change.
- The post-translational change in protein structure from PrP^C to the abnormal PrP^{Sc} is probably a critical pathologic event, causing either loss of function of PrP^C or, less likely, toxicity due to gain of function of PrP^{Sc}.
- The structural change of PrP^C to PrP^{Sc} occurs as an inevitable event (predisposed by the change in primary structure due to mutations in the PrP gene) in familial disease, as an induced event by exogenous PrP^{Sc} in transmitted cases (exogenous PrP^{Sc} interacts with endogenous PrP^C and induces the structural change), and as a rare spontaneous event in sporadic disease. Sporadic cases may also arise from a somatic mutation of the PrP gene (in addition to spontaneous conversion of the cellular isoform PrP^C to PrP^{Sc} as a rare stochastic event).
- The prion hypothesis may explain the paradoxic observation that the disease can be genetically inherited, transmitted, and sporadic.
- The clinical heterogeneity (see below) may reflect differences in host genotype (e.g. polymorphism at codon 129 of the PrP gene) and different isoforms of PrP^{Sc} (e.g. types 1 and 2).

Genetic susceptibility to acquired iatrogenic and sporadic CJD
- The general population has a common silent protein polymorphism at position (codon) 129 of the human PrP gene, where either a methionine (Met) or valine may be encoded (present). About 40% of whites are homozygous for the more frequent Met alleles, 50% are heterozygous for Met, and 10% are homozygous for the valine allele.
- Homozygosity at PrP 129 (present in about 50% of the general population) appears to confer susceptibility to iatrogenic and sporadic disease.
- Most patients with sporadic CJD are homozygous for either allele. The new variant cases of CJD (see below) are Met 129 homozygous, suggesting that about 40% of the general population are susceptible.

- Most patients with iatrogenic CJD (treatment with cadaveric pituitary-derived hGH) are also homozygous, mostly for the valine allele at this codon.
- Heterozygosity for the PrP gene appears to be protective.

Risk factors
- Iatrogenic routes of exposure.
- Growth hormone deficiency.
- Family history.
- Homozygosity for the valine or Met allele at codon 129 of the PrP gene.
- Mutations in the PrP gene.
- Occupational exposure to bovine prions.

CLINICAL FEATURES
- Variable (particularly with familial cases, and even within single pedigrees).
- Insidious onset.
- Early behavioral abnormalities (initial symptom in about 10% of cases):
  - Personality change, withdrawal, apathy, depression, sleep disturbance.
  - Agitation, fear and paranoia may prompt a psychiatric referral.
- Rapidly progressive and profound dementia: forgetful, confused, visual distortion and hallucinations.
- Myoclonus, usually stimulus-sensitive (>80% of patients).
- Motor abnormalities:
  - Cerebellar ataxia.
  - Extrapyramidal signs: tremor, rigidity, bradykinesia, dystonic posturing; choreoathetosis.
  - Pyramidal signs: weakness, spasticity, hyper-reflexia, and Babinski signs.
- Generalized seizures may occur.
- Positive family history of CJD in 6–15% of cases.

Syndromes of iatrogenic CJD
- Psychiatric disturbance (e.g. anxiety and depression) and progressive ataxia and clumsiness before the appearance of dementia and myoclonus: iatrogenic CJD associated with peripheral inoculation of prions (i.e. cadaveric hGH cases).
- Progressive dementia: iatrogenic CJD associated with central inoculation of prions (i.e. foreign dura mater or neurosurgic instruments).

Clinical variants (the spectrum)
Heidenhain variant
Early pathologic involvement of the occipital cortex leading to cortical blindness.

Brownell–Oppenheimer variant
Early and prominent ataxia (cerebellar ataxia is also prominent in iatrogenic CJD due to pituitary-derived hormones).

Thalamic variant
Insomnia and dysautonomia.

Spastic paralysis with dementia (Worster–Drought)

Amyotrophic form
Loss of anterior horn cells causing significant wasting, weakness and areflexia due to lower motor neuron changes.

More chronic and indolent form
Progresses over more than 2 years.

New variant CJD
- Linked causally to bovine spongiform encephalopathy (BSE), nvCJD is believed to be caused by the oral transmission of the BSE agent through consumption of bovine tissues containing significant infectivity (e.g. beef products containing bovine spinal cord).
- Young age of onset (below 42 years of age).
- Early behavioral/psychiatric disturbance (anxiety, depression), cerebellar ataxia and dysesthesiae.
- Absence of typical EEG changes, although the EEG is abnormal.
- High signal changes in the pulvinar of the thalamus on T2W MRI imaging of the brain.
- Clinical course is more prolonged and protracted, with average duration of 13 months compared with a mean of 6 months in other types.
- Specific neuropathologic profile with extensive formation of cerebellar prion plaques resembling those seen in kuru: they have a dense eosinophilic center and pale periphery surrounded by a zone of spongiform change.
- Homozygous for Met at codon 129 of the *PrP* gene.
- Associated with a specific pattern of protease-resistant PrP on Western blot analysis. The biochemical signature of the prions is distinct from other types of CJD and matches that of animals experimentally infected with BSE.

DIFFERENTIAL DIAGNOSIS
- Alzheimer's disease with myoclonus, but the course is usually more prolonged.
- Non-convulsive status epilepticus.
- Metabolic/toxic encephalopathy (e.g. drugs).
- Bilateral subdural hematomata.
- CNS vasculitis.
- Subacute sclerosing panencephalitis (SSPE).
- Infiltrating corpus callosum glioma.
- Huntington's disease.
- Motor neuron disease, but normal cognition.

- GSS disease: autosomal dominant inheritance, prominent cerebellar ataxia, dementia.
- Psychiatric illness (anxiety, depression).

INVESTIGATIONS (see Table 36)
CT or MRI brain
- Scans are normal (45%) or show cerebral atrophy (30%).
- T2W and PDWI MRI may reveal high-signal changes in the basal ganglia (**407**) and thalamus (5%) (e.g. the 'pulvinar sign' in variant CJD) or in scattered areas such as the cortex (7%). The sensitivity and specificity of these findings are uncertain.
- Diffusion-weighted MRI, which rapidly detects tiny changes in water mobility, such as shifts from the extracellular to the intracellular space when cellular homeostasis is disturbed, has been reported to not only show basal ganglia abnormalities but also gross abnormalities involving most of the cerebral hemispheres.
- MRI is probably the imaging modality of choice, though both MRI and CT are insensitive. Their main role is to exclude other differential diagnoses.

EEG
- Early: non-specific disorganization and generalized slow wave activity.
- Later (within 12 weeks of onset of symptoms):
- Slow background rhythm.
- Periodic sharp wave complexes (**408–411**): bisynchronous, and most commonly anterior and central (but may be lateralized and localized: occipital preponderance in Heidenhain's variant); duration: 100–600 ms; amplitude: up to 300 mV; may be monophasic, biphasic, triphasic or multiphasic; repetitive, occurring every 0.5–2.0 seconds; may be associated with myoclonic jerks; may be activated by startle; present in >60% of cases, particularly sporadic CJD, rarely in 'peripheral' iatrogenic CJD; non-specific: also occur in several encephalopathies, epilepsy and post ictal states, or during barbiturate overdose and deep anesthesia.
- 20–40% of patients do not exhibit a typical EEG (cf. nvCJD).

Table 36 Investigation findings in Creutzfeldt–Jakob disease

Disease	'Typical EEG'	14-3-3 +ve CSF	High signal on MRI brain	Other
Sporadic CJD	+ (65%)	+ (90%)	+ (>70%) (caudate and putamen)	
Familial CJD	±	±	±	PRNP analysis
Iatrogenic CJD				
CNS route	±	?	?	
Peripheral route	–	± (50%)	±	
New variant	– (100%)	± (50%)	+ (>70%) (posterior thalamus)	Tonsil biopsy

% of cases with a positive investigation, where known, are in parentheses
PRNP = prion protein

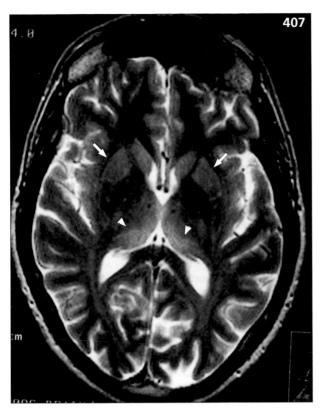

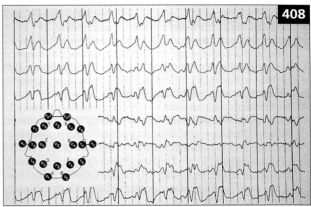

408 Electroencephalograph showing periodic triphasic wave complexes that are rather simple in contour and recurring every 0.7–0.8 seconds, against a slow polymorphous background, in a patient with rapidly progressive dementia and myoclonus due to CJD. Occasionally, the periodic discharges begin unilaterally and may resemble periodic lateralized epileptiform discharges.

407 T2W MRI from a patient with pathologically proven CJD. Note increased signal (whiteness) of the basal ganglia (arrows). Normally the basal ganglia become darker due to iron deposition with age. There is also a minor degree of atrophy. Also note the increased signal in the pulvinar (arrowheads). This was variant CJD.

409–411 Serial electroencephalographs, every 3 days, from a patient with CJD showing the progressive evolution of periodic triphasic wave complexes and the background rhythm.

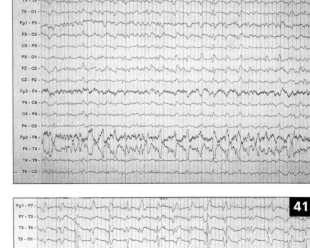

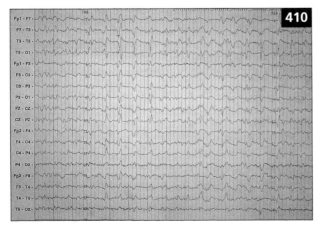

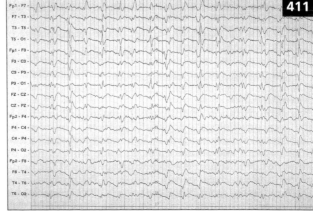

MULTIPLE SCLEROSIS (MS)

DEFINITION
A chronic autoimmune inflammatory demyelinating disease of the CNS in which the lesions are disseminated in time and space (different sites in the CNS are affected at different points in time).

EPIDEMIOLOGY
- Prevalence: higher in temperate climates further from the equator (e.g. Hobart, Tasmania, Australia, 76/100 000); lower in tropical and subtropical climates close to the equator (e.g. tropical Queensland, Australia, 12/100 000).
- Age: rare before puberty and beyond 60 years of age.
- Age of onset: <20 years: 20% of cases; 20–50 years: 50–60% of cases; >50 years: 20–30% of cases.
- Gender: F>M (2 : 1).
- Race: Northern European ancestry most common; uncommon in Australian aboriginals, Maori, Chinese, Japanese, black African.

PATHOLOGY
Multiple plaques of demyelination in the white matter of the CNS.

Acute lesion
- Demyelination of nerve fibers in the white matter of the CNS.
- Loss of oligodendrocytes.
- Perivenular infiltration of T and B lymphocytes, macrophages (filled with myelin debris) and plasma cells.
- Secondary axonal degeneration.

Chronic lesion
- Some axonal loss and remyelination.
- Glial cell proliferation resulting in discrete gray colored areas of gliosis (or sclerosis) that are called plaques.

Sites of demyelination
Any part of the CNS, particularly:
- Periventricular white matter of the cerebral hemispheres (414–416).
- Optic nerves (417).
- Cerebellum.
- Brainstem.
- Spinal cord (particularly subpial regions of the spinal cord) (418, 419).

The peripheral nervous system is not affected.

ETIOLOGY
- Unknown, but likely to be a misdirected autoimmune disease (because of the predilection of women, the human leukocyte antigen (HLA) association, the relapsing and remitting course, and the finding of immunologically active cells in the brain, spinal cord and CSF). This, and other evidence, suggests that MS is an autoimmune disease resulting from an immune attack on the myelin sheaths and axons in the CNS by autoreactive T lymphocytes and autoantibodies.
- Environmental factors, such as a virus infection (e.g. herpes virus-6), may trigger immune-mediated demyelination in genetically predisposed individuals.

Epidemiologic evidence points to environmental factors at a young age:
- Prevalence of MS increases with increasing latitude.
- Risk of MS for an individual corresponds to the risk of their area of residence before the age of about 15 years.

Genetic factors
Also likely to be relevant:
- A family history of MS is present in about 10% of people with MS.
- The concordance rate for MS in monozygotic twins is 25%, 2.5% in dizygotic twins and 1.9% in non-twin siblings.
- HLA associations with MS:
  - HLA-A3, HLA-D7, and HLA-DR2 common in Caucasians with MS (HLA-DR2: present in >60% of people with MS and 15–20% of controls).
  - HLA-DR4 common in Arabs with MS.

PATHOPHYSIOLOGY
Exposure to an unidentified non-self antigen that 'mimics' constitutive peptides of myelin evokes an antigen-specific, T cell mediated immune response. Lymphocytes, macrophages and humoral factors enter the CNS and the blood–brain barrier breaks down. B-lymphocytes produce oligoclonal immunoglobulin G (IgG) in the CSF. Sensitized T cells produce cytokines which may damage oligodendrocytes and myelin. Nerve conduction is blocked in demyelinated axons and can be restored by remyelination. In contrast, axonal loss leads to a permanent loss of neurologic function, as the CNS axonal regenerative capacity is severely limited.

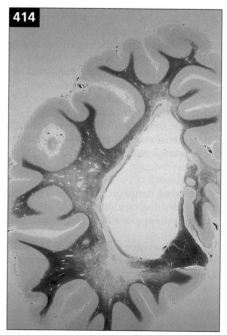

414

414 Section of one cerebral hemisphere (parietal lobe) showing a lack of staining due to periventricular demyelination in the white matter. (Courtesy of Professor BA Kakulas, Royal Perth Hospital, Western Australia.)

CLINICAL FEATURES
Onset
- Subacute onset of neurologic symptoms over several hours to days. Infrequently the symptoms evolve quickly over minutes or slowly over weeks or months.
- The onset is monosymptomatic in about 50% of cases. The remainder have initial symptoms of multiple lesions within the CNS.

Nature
The symptoms usually reflect dysfunction of the optic nerves, brainstem or spinal cord.

Reduced visual acuity
Reduced visual acuity, which varies from a slight dulling of color vision to complete monocular blindness, together with

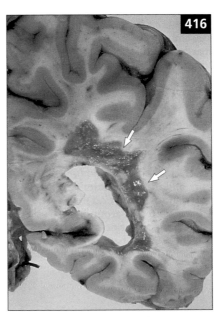

415, 416 Autopsy specimens of brain, coronal sections, showing periventricular demyelination (arrows).

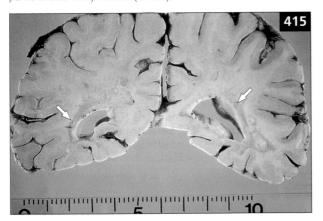

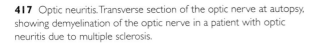

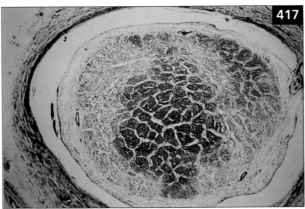

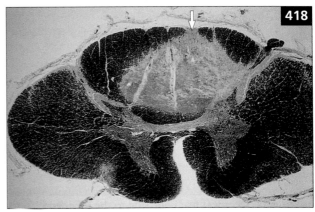

417 Optic neuritis. Transverse section of the optic nerve at autopsy, showing demyelination of the optic nerve in a patient with optic neuritis due to multiple sclerosis.

418 Transverse section of the thoracic spinal cord showing a large plaque of demyelination in the dorsal columns (arrow) in a multiple sclerosis patient who had a high stepping gait due to sensory ataxia in the lower limbs. (Courtesy of Professor BA Kakulas, Royal Perth Hospital, Western Australia.)

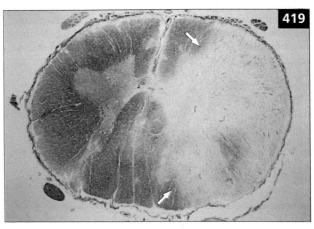

419 Transverse section of the spinal cord showing a large plaque of demyelination (arrows) in almost one-half of the spinal cord in a multiple sclerosis patient with a Brown–Sequard syndrome. (Courtesy of Professor BA Kakulas, Royal Perth Hospital, Western Australia.)

Optic neuropathy
- Leber's hereditary optic neuropathy: a maternally inherited disease, usually leading to severe bilateral visual loss, and associated with several mitochondrial DNA point mutations; the major ones at nucleotide positions 11 778, 3460, and 14 484 (see p.491).
- Other hereditary optic neuropathies.
- Ischemic optic neuropathy.
- Neurosyphilis.

Acute non-compressive spinal cord syndrome
Vascular
- Anterior spinal artery infarction: paraparesis with loss of pain and temperature sensation, develops over minutes to hours, and usually persists if infarction occurs.
- Intramedullary hemorrhage.

Inflammation of the spinal cord
- MS: usually a partial cord syndrome (e.g. unilateral loss of pain and temperature, deafferentation of one limb, or an asymmetric incomplete paraparesis) develops over hours to days with partial or complete recovery over several weeks.
- Transverse myelitis: complete loss of sensory and motor function below the level of the lesion, resulting in a flaccid, areflexic paraplegia; develops over hours to days, commonly after an infection (e.g. upper respiratory tract).
- Acute necrotizing myelitis: tuberculosis, lymphoma, carcinoma.
- Connective tissue disease: systemic lupus erythematosus.
- Sarcoidosis.

Infection of the spinal cord
- Herpes zoster.
- Herpes simplex types I and II.
- HIV.
- Tuberculosis.
- Syphilis.

Chronic non-compressive spinal cord syndrome
Inherited
Hereditary spastic paraparesis: usually a family history of autosomal dominant inheritance.

Vascular
Dural arteriovenous malformation: the most common type of spinal angioma. Usually affects the thoracolumbar segments and tends to present in middle-aged men as a chronic progressive myelopathy with symptoms that may fluctuate or be aggravated by exercise. A combination of upper and lower motor neuron signs may be present.

Inflammation of the spinal cord
- MS.
- Sarcoidosis.

Infection of the spinal cord
- Herpetic necrotizing myelitis.
- Cytomegalovirus.
- Varicella-zoster granulomatous myelitis.
- Human T lymphocyte virus-1 (HTLV-1) associated myelopathy ('tropical spastic paraparesis') in adults from endemic regions or with other risk factors (e.g. Afro-Caribbeans). A progressive spastic paraplegia develops over a number of years. However, sphincter disturbance is the rule and considerable neuropathic lower limb pain is common.
- Tuberculosis.
- Syphilis.
- Toxoplasmosis.
- Schistosomiasis.

Intramedullary tumor of the spinal cord
- Astrocytoma.
- Ependymoma.
- Lymphoma.
- Lipoma.
- Hemangioma.
- Metastases.

Metabolic
- Vitamin B_{12} deficiency: presents over weeks or months as a subacute spinal cord syndrome with intense paresthesia and a combination of pyramidal and dorsal column signs.
- Adrenomyeloneuropathy: an X-linked inherited disorder that affects males and some heterozygous females with a progressive myelopathy. A peripheral neuropathy and adrenal insufficiency may be present.

Toxic/iatrogenic
- Radiation myelopathy (see p.565): steadily progressive spastic paraplegia, months to years after radiotherapy. Pathologically there is necrosis of the irradiated cord segments with obliterative changes in blood vessels in the same region.
- Lathyrism: endemic in parts of India and presents as a subacute or chronic spastic paraparesis in people who regularly ingest chickling pea vetch over several months. It is thought to be caused by a toxin in the chickling pea.

Degenerative
- Syringomyelia (see p.541).
- Motor neuron disease (see p.534): purely motor; usually a combination of lower and upper motor neuron signs.

INVESTIGATIONS
MRI of the brain
MRI is the imaging investigation of choice. T2W images show:
- Areas of increased signal (brightness) in the white matter which can be anywhere in the brain but are typically seen in the immediate periventricular white matter and corpus callosum (**423–428**).
- The areas of brightness can be of varying size, may show some swelling, and may be multiple or only a few.
- A small proportion of patients with definite MS will have a normal MR.
- It is important to differentiate other causes of bright spots which are non-pathologic from MS plaques, for example enlarged perivascular spaces which are usually small. Normal young persons are allowed to have up to three white spots (if small).

T1W images show:
- Low signal areas (dark spots), but the T1W image is not so sensitive and demonstrates fewer lesions than T2W.

423, 424 MRI of brain in the sagittal plane, proton density image (**423**), and axial plane T2W image (**424**), showing multifocal areas of high signal intensity adjacent to the corpus callosum (**423**) and lateral ventricles (**424**) due to demyelination (arrows).

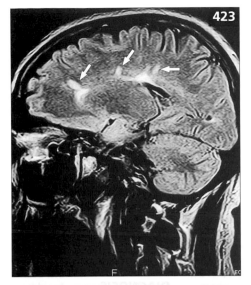

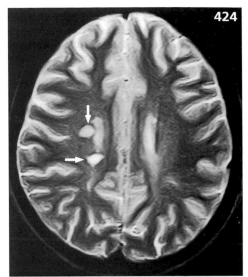

425 T2W MRI showing multiple areas of increased signal in the periventricular white matter. The involvement of the corpus callosum (lesions right down at the top of the lateral ventricles) is said to be characteristic of MS.

426 T1W MRI following contrast (same patient) shows that some of the lesions enhance (arrows) and some do not, indicating that they are of different ages and confirming the most likely diagnosis to be MS.

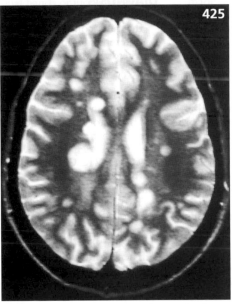

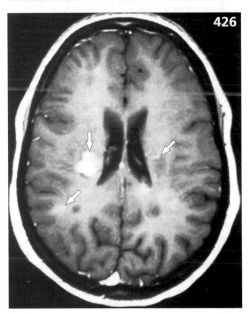

427, 428 MRI cervical spine, T2W image, in the axial plane (**427**) and sagittal plane (**428**), showing a focal area of high signal intensity in the high left cervical spinal cord posteriorly (arrows) due to demyelination, in a patient who presented with symptoms and signs of left dorsal column dysfunction (ascending tight feeling in left leg like a stocking around it).

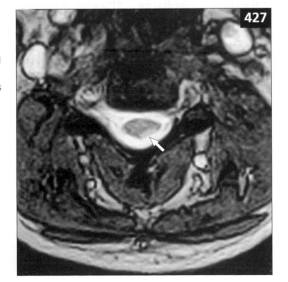

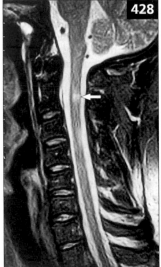

Imaging

- Chest x-ray: may show bilateral hilar adenopathy (**433**) but occasionally a similar pattern is seen in lymphoma, tuberculosis, brucellosis and bronchogenic carcinoma.
- Gallium scan: more sensitive than chest x-ray and the appearance of diffuse uptake in the lungs (or parotid, salivary and lacrimal glands), even in the absence of clinical involvement, is relatively specific but not diagnostic.
- CT brain scan without and with contrast: hydrocephalus, leptomeningeal thickening and enhancement, intra-axial mass lesions, extra-axial mass lesions.

MRI brain/spinal cord scan

Several patterns may be visible on cranial MRI (**434**) (CT is much less sensitive):

- Chronic basal leptomeningitis with thickened enhancing meninges involving the hypothalamus, pituitary stalk, optic nerve (**435**) and chiasm.
- Communicating hydrocephalus.
- Involvement of the lenticulostriate arteries by spreading up the Virchow–Robin spaces causing thrombosis and granulomatous angiitis.
- Parenchymal nodules (granulomas) which may be iso- or hyperdense, may calcify and appear as a mass lesion and may or may not enhance. These may cause obstruction to the ventricles. They occur particularly around the skull base, pituitary, pons, hypothalamus and periventricular region.
- Diffuse high signal areas in the white matter on T2W images indistinguishable from MS may also occur.
- Extra-axial sarcoid may mimic a meningioma by causing a dural enhancing mass with hyperostosis.
- Spinal sarcoid may mimic leptomeningeal metastases.

Cerebral angiography

Changes suggestive of cerebral angiitis may occur.

CSF

- Mild pleocytosis (mostly lymphocytes).
- Mild increased protein.
- Increased T4 : T8 lymphocyte ratio.
- Low CSF glucose in 20–39% of cases.
- Elevated CSF ACE, oligoclonal banding and increased IgG index in nearly one-third of patients may occur.

EMG

- Compound muscle action potentials and sensory nerve action potentials: normal or mild to moderately decreased.
- Motor and sensory nerve conduction velocities: mild to moderately decreased.
- EMG features of chronic partial denervation may be present.

Kveim test

A suspension of sarcoid tissue is injected intradermally and produces a sarcoid granuloma in about 75% of patients with subacute active sarcoidosis and in about two-thirds of those with chronic sarcoidosis of >2 years duration. False-positives occur in <5% of cases.

Tissue

- Bronchoalveolar lavage: abnormally increased T4 : T8 lymphocyte ratio: relatively specific but not diagnostic.
- Bone marrow: non-caseating granuloma.
- Biopsy of muscle (even in the absence of myopathic symptoms), lymph node, conjunctiva, skin, lung, liver or brain may reveal the diagnosis.
- Nerve biopsy:
- An axonopathy sparing unmyelinated fibers.
- Marked loss of myelinated fibers.
- Demyelination is not prominent nor is it in the usual central predominant pattern seen in vasculitic neuropathies.
- Epineural and perineural granuloma with or without periangiitis and panangiitis.
- Brain biopsy: in most cases involving intracranial mass lesions which are difficult to access safely with stereotactic brain biopsy, biopsy can be deferred until a trial of steroids is given if sarcoidosis can be inferred clinically.

Other

- Skin: skin-test unreactivity (anergy).
- Urine: 24 hour urinary calcium level: typically elevated. but not diagnostic, of sarcoidosis.

DIFFERENTIAL DIAGNOSIS
Meningo-encephalitis

- Granulomatous inflammation:
- Infection by bacteria (brucellosis, chlamydia, tularemia), mycobacteria (tuberculosis, atypical mycobacteria), fungi (histoplasmosis, coccidioidomycosis, cryptococcosus), spirochetes (treponemal infections such as syphilis), and parasites (toxoplasmosis, leishmaniasis).
- Occupational and environmental exposure to organic or inorganic agents (e.g. methotrexate, talc, metals).
- Neoplasia (lymphoma).
- Autoimmune disorders (Wegener's granulomatosis, Churg–Strauss syndrome).
- Histiocytosis X:
- Viral encephalitis (see p.292): HIV infection (see p.301).
- Carcinomatous meningitis
- Granulomatous angiitis of the CNS (see CNS vasculitis, p.227). The meningeal inflammatory reaction is consistently localized to blood vessel walls and typically produces extensive disruption of the vascular wall.
- Meningiomatosis
- Limbic encephalitis associated with occult neoplasm (see p.401).

Multifocal white matter disease

Multiple sclerosis.

Mass lesions

- Primary brain tumor (see p.357): glioma (including optic nerve glioma), meningioma, germ cell tumor, leukemia, primary CNS lymphoma.
- Metastatic brain tumor (see p.396).
- Granulomatous inflammation: syphilitic gumma, tuberculoma, cryptococcoma, toxoplasmosis, histiocytosis X.
- Spinal cord glioma, ependymoma, myelitis.

Non-caseating granulomas

Non-specific: found in infections and malignancy.

Increased level of serum ACE

- Youth.
- Hyperthyroidism.

- Diabetes.
- HIV infection.
- Leprosy.
- Tuberculosis.
- Coccidioidomycosis.
- Histoplasmosis.
- Amyloidosis.
- Multiple myeloma.
- Hodgkin's disease.
- Lymphoma (including intravascular lymphoma).
- Malignant histiocytosis.
- Primary biliary cirrhosis.
- Whipple's disease.
- Gaucher's disease.
- Silicosis.
- Asbestosis.

DIAGNOSIS

A positive biopsy finding of non-caseating granulomas in the context of characteristic clinical features, blood test (elevations of serum gamma globulin, ESR, or serum ACE), chest x-ray evidence of enlarged hilar and mediastinal lymph nodes, gallium scan, defects in cell mediated immunity, and MRI and CSF findings, having excluded other causes of granulomatous inflammation.

TREATMENT

Inferred from experience with pulmonary sarcoidosis; no controlled studies:

- Prednisone 60 mg (1 mg/kg) oral, daily for 4–6 weeks, followed by a slow taper over 3–6 months or longer.
- If steroids fail, or cannot be tapered eventually, other immunosuppressive agents, such as cyclophosphamide, azathioprine, and cyclosporine (4–6 mg/kg/day, which inhibits interleukin-2 secretion by T cells) allow reduction of steroids to 30–50% of the original dose.
- Surgery may be indicated for hydrocephalus, expanding mass lesions, or mass lesions causing increased intracranial pressure.
- Cranial irradiation of intracranial neurosarcoidosis that is refractory to treatment with steroids may be successful.

PROGNOSIS

- Most patients respond to treatment and can have medication withdrawn over months but about one-third will relapse, often in the same location as the initial disease.
- Neurosarcoidosis limited to peripheral nerves and cranial nerves may respond spontaneously.
- Intracranial neurosarcoidosis, such as mass lesions or hydrocephalus, have a more malignant course and a higher rate of relapse.
- Patients with relapsing disease and more ominous clinical features (e.g. intracranial neurosarcoid such as mass lesions or hydrocephalus) should probably remain on low-dose steroids as a maintenance dose between exacerbations.

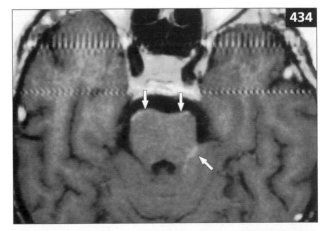

433 Chest x-ray showing bilateral hilar adenopathy due to sarcoidosis.

434 T1W MRI of the brain stem following contrast. Note the thin rim of enhancement (arrows) around the brain stem. It is unusual to see this in sarcoid, but its presence should certainly prompt the diagnosis, though is not specific for sarcoid.

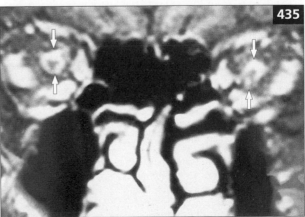

435 MRI of the orbits, coronal plane, after gadolinium injection showing brightness, due to contrast enhancement, of the dural sheath of the optic nerves (arrows) bilaterally in the patient in **431, 432**, with bilateral optic neuropathy due to sarcoidosis.

CAVERNOUS SINUS SYNDROME

DEFINITION
Involvement of two or more of the IIIrd, IVth, Vth (V^1, V^2), or VIth cranial nerves or oculosympathetic fibers on the same side.

EPIDEMIOLOGY
- Incidence: rare.
- Age: any age; mean age: 40 years.
- Gender: M=F.

PATHOPHYSIOLOGY
The cavernous sinus (really a venous plexus) lies within a dural envelope that funnels upper cranial nerves to the orbit. Consequently, small lesions, adjacent to or within the cavernous sinus, can produce dramatic localizing signs.

ETIOLOGY
Tumor: 30–70% of all cases
Malignant tumors: two-thirds
In marked contrast to the high incidence of benign tumors causing chiasmal compression:
- Nasopharyngeal cancer: 22–46% of tumors.
- Metastases: 16–33%.
- Lymphoma: 0–18%.
- Pituitary adenoma: 9–22%.

Benign tumors
One-third.
- Meningioma: 4–9% of tumors.
- Chordoma: 2–11%.
- Neuroma: 0–8%.

Aneurysm or fistula: 5–35% of all cases
- Cavernous carotid artery aneurysm.
- Carotid-cavernous fistulas.

Trauma: 5–25% of all cases

Surgery: 10% of all cases

Inflammation (idiopathic cavernous sinusitis): 0–23% of all cases
The Tolosa–Hunt syndrome eponym, with its promise of making a specific diagnosis on clinical grounds, has not proved reliable. One of the five patients who helped establish the Tolosa–Hunt syndrome later was shown to have a meningioma. A generic description, such as idiopathic cavernous sinusitis, seems preferable. Overlap with orbital inflammatory pseudotumor and idiopathic multiple cranial neuropathy syndromes suggest a similar underlying mechanism.

Infection: 0–5% of all cases
Spread of fungus or bacteria, usually from the sphenoid sinus:
- Mucormycosis.
- Meningitis.
- Bacterial sphenoid sinusitis.
- Septic cavernous sinusitis.

Diabetes: 1% of all cases

CLINICAL FEATURES
Cranial nerve palsy
- Oculomotor (IIIrd) nerve: almost all patients; pupil is involved in three-quarters of cases and generally parallels the severity of the ophthalmoplegia.
- Abducens (VIth) nerve: 95% of patients.
- Trochlear (IVth) nerve: 30% of patients; may be difficult to confirm in the presence of a partial IIIrd nerve palsy.
- Trigeminal (Vth) nerve: 40% of patients.
- Optic nerve or chiasmal dysfunction: 40% of patients.

Horner's syndrome
- 5–10% of patients.
- Difficult to diagnose in the presence of IIIrd nerve palsy without pharmacologic pupillary testing.

HISTORY
- Age of onset.
- Presence or absence of pain.
- Speed of progression.
- Past infections and tumors.

Tumor
Average age: 47 years:
- Nasopharyngeal cancer: preferentially involves the VIth nerve and mandibular division of the Vth nerve.
- Metastases: often present with rapid complete ophthalmoplegia.
- Lymphoma: other signs may be present, such as abdominal mass.
- Pituitary adenoma: lateral extension tends to involve the IIIrd nerve and ophthalmic division of the Vth nerve. Apoplectic onset usually, and involves the oculomotor nerves with a relative frequency ratio of about 4 (IIIrd nerve), 2 (VIth nerve) and 1 (IVth nerve).
- Benign tumors: a single cranial nerve is involved for long periods.

Aneurysm
- Average age: 52 years.
- Typically progressive, painful involvement of multiple cranial nerves.
- Multiple cranial nerves are affected in two-thirds, VIth nerve only in one-quarter, and IIIrd nerve only in 10%.
- Despite IIIrd nerve involvement, the pupil on the involved side is often the same size or smaller than the normal pupil, perhaps because the parasympathetic fibers are less vulnerable within the cavernous sinus.
- Painful onset in almost all patients.
- Sudden onset in about 10% of cases.

Trauma
- Average age: 30 years.
- Usually severe head trauma with basal skull fractures.

Inflammation (idiopathic cavernous sinusitis)
- Average age: 35 years.
- Painful, non-specific inflammation of the superior orbital fissure.

Infection
- Underlying diabetes common.
- Rapid, complete ophthalmoplegia.
- Life-threatening.

DIFFERENTIAL DIAGNOSIS
Unilateral ophthalmoplegia
- Orbital inflammatory pseudotumor syndrome.
- Idiopathic multiple cranial neuropathy syndrome.
- Wernicke's encephalopathy.
- Myasthenia gravis.

Rapid onset, severe ophthalmoplegia
- Trauma.
- Pituitary apoplexy.
- Carotid aneurysm.
- Mucormycosis.
- Metastatic tumor.

Bilateral cavernous sinus syndrome: <10% of all cases
- Nasopharyngeal carcinoma.
- Lymphoma.
- Leukemia.
- Craniopharyngioma.
- Pituitary apoplexy.
- Mucormycosis.

INVESTIGATIONS
- Contrast-enhanced MRI brain scan (**436**) is the key investigation: it clearly demonstrates any tumor mass or aneurysm large enough to cause a cavernous sinus syndrome, and usually shows carotid-cavernous fistulas, clues to bacterial or fungal nasal sinusitis and adjacent basilar meningeal enhancement. Idiopathic cavernous sinusitis is often not apparent on non-contrast imaging but, after contrast injection, the affected cavernous sinus usually appears mildly or moderately enlarged. Abnormal signal tissue, which may have mass effect in the cavernous sinus (similar to muscle on T1WI and to fat on T2WI), may extend into the orbital apex. The differential diagnosis includes sarcoid, meningioma, lymphoma, metastatic or local spread of tumor, infections like actinomycosis.
- MR angiography or catheter contrast carotid angiography.
- CSF, including cytology: if meningitis, lymphoma, or leukemia is suspected.
- Tensilon test: if myasthenia gravis is suspected.

DIAGNOSIS
Idiopathic cavernous sinusitis is a diagnosis of exclusion, made only after the passage of considerable time (at least 6 months) after the onset of acute painful ophthalmoplegia to confirm complete or almost complete remission and eliminate the possibility of a subacute infection or a subtle tumor in the cavernous sinus. MRI enhancement of a mildly enlarged cavernous sinus supports, but does not establish, the diagnosis; it may also be caused by infection, lymphoma, meningioma, dural arteriovenous malformation.

TREATMENT
- Specific medical (anti-microbial, anti-inflammatory) or surgical treatment, depending on the cause.
- Idiopathic cavernous sinusitis may respond to corticosteroid therapy but patients need to be carefully observed for a facilitated fungal infection.

PROGNOSIS
Tumor
- Malignant tumors: rapid deterioration.
- Benign tumors: prolonged course.

Aneurysm
- Typically progressive, prolonged course.
- One-quarter have some recovery of eye movements; residual damage often consists of elevator paresis and mild ptosis due to permanent damage to the superior division of the IIIrd nerve.

Inflammation (idiopathic cavernous sinusitis)
Remitting course, usually self-limiting.

Infection
Life-threatening and usually fatal, despite intensive antibiotic treatment.

Close clinical follow-up is essential and the MRI should be repeated if a sustained remission is not forthcoming.

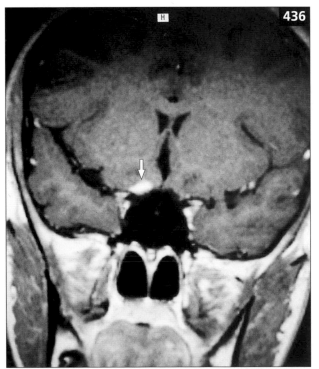

436 T1W coronal MRI with contrast of a 20 year old man with a painful right ophthalmoplegia, visual loss, sensory disturbance in the V¹ distribution. This section was taken just posterior to the orbital apex. Note the enhancement (whiteness, arrow) around the right optic nerve which extended from the orbital apex.

FURTHER READING

ACUTE DISSEMINATED ENCEPHALOMYELITIS

Davis LE (2000) Diagnosis and treatment of acute encephalitis. *The Neurologist,* **6**: 145–159.

Sahlas DJ, Miller SP, Guerin M, *et al.* (2000) Treatment of acute disseminated encephalomyelitis with intravenous immunoglobulin. *Neurology,* **54**: 1370–1372.

MULTIPLE SCLEROSIS (MS)
General

Noseworthy JH, Lucchinetti C, Rodriguez M, Weinshenker BG (2000) Multiple sclerosis. *N. Engl. J. Med.,* **343**: 938–952.

Pathogenesis

Confavreux C, Suissa S, Saddier P, *et al.* (2001) Vaccinations and the risk of relapse in multiple sclerosis. N. *Engl. J. Med.,* **344**: 319–326.

Lucchinetti C, Brück W, Parisi J, *et al.* (2000) Heterogeneity of multiple sclerosis lesions: implications for the pathogenesis of demyelination. *Ann. Neurol.,* **47**: 707–717.

Weatherby SJM, Hawkins CP (2001) Multiple sclerosis: New pathophysiological and therapeutic concepts. *Proc. R. Coll. Physicians Edinb.,* **31**: 134–148.

Clinical entities

Chan JW (2000) Optic neuritis in multiple sclerosis: an update. *The Neurologist,* **6**: 205–213.

Rudick RA (1998) A 29-year-old man with multiple sclerosis. *JAMA,* **280**: 1432–1439.

Diagnosis

McDonald WI, Compston A, Edan G, *et al.* (2001) Recommended diagnostic criteria for multiple sclerosis: guidelines from the International Panel on the diagnosis of multiple sclerosis. *Ann. Neurol.,* **50**: 121–127.

Poser CM, Brinar VV (2001) Problems with diagnostic criteria for multiple sclerosis. *Lancet,* **358**: 1746–1747.

Thompson AJ, Montalban X, Barkhof F, *et al.* (2000) Diagnostic criteria for primary progressive multiple sclerosis: a position paper. *Ann. Neurol.,* **47**: 831–835.

Poser CM, Paty D, Scheinberg LS, *et al.* (1983) New diagnositic criteria for multiple sclerosis. *Ann. Neurol.,* **13**: 227–231.

Drug treatment

Bryant J, Clegg A, Milne R (2001) Systematic review of immunomodulatory drugs for the treatment of people with multiple sclerosis: is there good quality evidence on effectiveness and cost? *J. Neurol. Neurosurg. Psychiatry,* **70**: 574–579.

Campbell SK, Almeida GL, Penn RD, *et al.* (1995) The effects of intrathecally administered baclofen on function in patients with spasticity. *Physical Therapy,* **75**: 352–362.

Comi G, Filippi M, Barkhof F, *et al.* (2001) Effect of early interferon treatment on conversion to definite multiple sclerosis. A randomised study. *Lancet,* **357**: 1576–1582.

Ebers GC (2001) Preventing multiple sclerosis? *Lancet,* **357**: 1547.

Edan G, Miller D, Clanet M, *et al.* (1997) Therapeutic effect of mitoxantrone combined with methylprednisolone in multiple sclerosis: a randomised multicentre study of active disease using MRI and clinical criteria. *J. Neurol. Neurosurg. Psychiatry,* **62**: 112–118.

Fischer JS, Priore RL, Jacobs LD, *et al.* (2000) Neuropsychological effects of interferon ß–1a in relapsing multiple sclerosis. *Ann. Neurol.,* **48**: 885–892.

Hartung HP, Gonsette RE, the MIMS Study Group (1998) Mitoxantrone in progressive multiple sclerosis: a placebo controlled randomised, observer-blind European Phase III multicentre study. Clinical data. *Multiple Sclerosis* (Abstract), **4**: 380.

INFß Multiple Sclerosis Study Group (1993) Interferon Beta–1b is effective in relapsing–remitting multiple sclerosis. I. clinical results of a multicentre, randomised, double-blind, placebo-controlled trial. *Neurology,* **43**: 662–667.

Jacobs LD, Beck RW, Simon JH, *et al.* (2000) Intramuscular interferon beta-1a therapy initiated during a first demyelinating event in multiple sclerosis. *N. Engl. J. Med.,* **343**: 898–904.

Polman CH, Uitdehaag BMJ (2000) Drug treatment of multiple sclerosis. *BMJ,* **321**: 490–494.

Prisms Study Group (1998) Randomised double-blind placebo-controlled study of interferon Beta-1a in relapsing/remitting multiple sclerosis. *Lancet,* **352**: 1498–1504

Rehabilitation

Freeman JA, Langdon DW, Hobart JC, Thompson AJ (1999) Inpatient rehabilitation in multiple sclerosis. Do the benefits carry over into the community? *Neurology,* **52**: 50–56.

Freeman JA, Thompson AJ (2001) Building an evidence base for multiple sclerosis management: support for physiotherapy. *J. Neurol. Neurosurg. Psychiatry,* **70**: 147–148.

Kraft GH (1999) Rehabilitation still the only way to improve function in multiple sclerosis. *Lancet,* **354**: 2016–2017.

Solari A, Filippini G, Gasco P, *et al.* (1999) Physical rehabilitation has a positive effect on disability in multiple sclerosis patients. *Neurology,* **52**: 57–62.

Wiles CM, Newcombe RG, Fuller KJ, *et al.* (2001) Controlled randomized cross-over trial of the effects of physiotherapy on mobility in chronic multiple sclerosis. *J. Neurol. Neurosurg. Psychiatry,* **70**: 174–179.

Prognosis

Bjartmar C, Kidd G, Mörk S, *et al.* (2000) Neurological disability correlates with spinal cord axonal loss and reduced *N*-acetyl aspartate in chronic multiple sclerosis patients. *Ann. Neurol.,* **48**: 893–901.

Weinshenker BG (2000) Progressive forms of MS: classification streamlined or consensus overturned? *Lancet,* **355**: 162–163.

NEUROSARCOIDOSIS

James DG (2001) Sarcoidosis 2001. *Postgrad. Med. J.,* **77**: 177–180

Newman LS, Rose CS, Maier LA (1997) Sarcoidosis. *N. Engl. J. Med.,* **336**: 1224–1234.

Nikhar NK, Shah JR, Tselis AC, Lewis RA (2000) Primary neurosarcoidosis: a diagnostic and therapeutic challenge. *The Neurologist,* **6**: 126–133.

Scott TF (1993) Neurosarcoidosis: Progress and clinical aspects. *Neurology,* **43**: 8–12.

Vinas FC, Rengachary S (2001) Diagnosis and management of neurosarcoidosis. *J. Clinical Neuroscience,* **8**(6): 505–513.

Zajicek JP, Scolding NJ, Foster O, *et al.* (1999) Central nervous system sarcoidosis – diagnosis and management. *Q. J. Med.,* **92**: 103–117.

CAVERNOUS SINUS SYNDROME

Keane JR (1996) Cavernous sinus syndrome. Analysis of 151 cases. *Arch. Neurol.,* **53**: 967–971.

Tumors of the Central Nervous System

BRAIN TUMORS

DEFINITION
Neoplastic lesions of the brain which may be benign or malignant, and primary or secondary (metastatic).

EPIDEMIOLOGY
- Incidence:
- Primary brain tumors (benign and malignant): 12–15/100 000/year (adults); 2–5/100 000/year (children).
- Primary benign CNS tumor: 7 (95% CI: 3–13) per 100 000 per year.
- Primary malignant CNS tumor: 3 (95% CI: 0.7–7) per 100 000 per year.
- Secondary brain tumors (metastases): 4 (95% CI: 1–9) per 100 000 per year.
- Age:
- Adults: supratentorial tumors predominate (e.g. glioma, meningioma, pituitary adenoma, metastases).
- Children: infratentorial tumors predominate (e.g. medulloblastoma, ependymoma, astrocytoma, pinealoma). After 10 years of age, the incidence of neuroepithelial tumors increases steadily with increasing age to a peak incidence of 20/100 00/year at age 70 years.
- Gender: M=F overall.
- Men: gliomas more common; women: meningiomas and nerve sheath tumors are more common.

PATHOLOGY
A. Histologic classification of brain tumors. (A more recent World Health Organization classification also exists [Kleihues and Cavenee, 2000; De Angelis, 2001].)

Neuro-epithelial (50%): cellular derivatives of the neural tube
- Glial cells (Gliomas, see p.364)
- Neurons:
- Embryonal tumors: medulloblastoma (20% of all childhood tumors, <5% of adult brain tumors) and primitive neuroectodermal tumors.
- Gangliocytoma/ganglioglioma.
- Dysembryoblastic neuroepithelial tumor (DNET).
- Neuroblastoma.
- Pineal cells: pineal cell tumors (pineocytoma, pineoblastoma).

Cellular derivatives of the neural crest
- Arachnoid cells:
- Meningioma (15%) (see p.374).
- Meningeal sarcoma.
- Schwann cells:
- Schwannoma (7–8%) (see p.383).
- Neurofibroma.

Other cells
- Adenohypophyseal cells (see p.379): pituitary adenoma (10%), pituitary carcinoma.
- Reticuloendothelial cells: primary cerebral lymphoma (see p.385).
- Vascular cells: hemangioblastoma (see p.392).
- Glomus jugulare cells: glomus jugulare tumors.
- Connective tissue cells: sarcomas.

Embryonal remnants
- Ectodermal derivatives: craniopharyngioma (2–3%) (see p.377).
- Notochord: chordoma.
- Germ cells (see p.388): germinoma (0.5%).
- Derived from the three germ layers: teratoma.

GLIOMAS

DEFINITION
A glioma is any neuroepithelial tumor of the brain and arises from glial cells such as astrocytes (astrocytoma and other astroglial neoplasms), oligodendrocytes (oligodendroglioma) and ependymal cells (ependymomas). The term does not imply any degree of differentiation.

CLASSIFICATION OF GLIOMAS ACCORDING TO NEUROEPITHELIAL CELLS OF ORIGIN
- Astrocytes.
- Astrocytoma (25–30% of brain gliomas):
  Pilocytic astrocytoma.
  Low grade astrocytoma.
  Anaplastic astrocytoma.
  Pleomorphic xanthoastrocytoma.
  Subependymal giant cell astrocytoma.
- Glioblastoma multiforme (50% of gliomas).
- Oligodendrocytes:
- Oligodendroglioma (10–20% of gliomas).
- Anaplastic oligodendroglioma.
- Ependymal cells:
- Ependymomas (5% of all brain gliomas, 8% of gliomas in childhood).
- Anaplastic ependymoma.
- Myxopapillary ependymoma.
- Subependymoma.
- Choroid plexus tumors (papilloma, carcinoma).
- Colloid cysts.
- Mixed gliomas (oligoastrocytoma, anaplastic oligoastrocytoma).

EPIDEMIOLOGY
The most common primary brain tumors in adults.
- Incidence: 6 (range 2–10) per 100 000 per year.
- Gender-specific incidence (per 100 000 per year):

	Males	Females
Glioblastoma	2.8	1.8
Astrocytoma	1.7	1.3
Oligodendroglioma	0.15	0.10
Ependymoma	0.15	0.15

- Age: any age:
- Glioblastoma: peak incidence in middle adult life: mean age 56 years.
- Anaplastic astrocytoma: mean age 46 years.
- Oligodendroglioma: any age: most often 20–40 years; early peak at 6–12 years.
- Ependymoma: peak incidence at 5 years of age:
  Supratentorial: any age.
  Infratentorial: 40% occur in the first decade of life; make up 5–10% of childhood tumors.
- Gender: M>F (2:1).

PATHOLOGY
- Malignant tumors of glial cells.
- Tumors are graded in various ways. A simple and reproducible method is based on four histologic features: pleomorphism of cells and presence or absence of nuclear atypia, mitosis, endothelial/microvascular proliferation and necrosis. Any two features classify a tumor as grade 3, and three or four features constitute a grade 4 tumor.

About 80% of gliomas are 'high grade' (malignant, anaplastic), and 20% 'low grade'.

Glioblastoma multiforme
Macroscopic
- Sites: about half occupy more than one lobe or are bilateral, and 5% show multicentric foci of growth.
- Appearance: variegated: mottled gray, red, brown or orange, depending on the degree of necrosis and the presence, degree and age of hemorrhage (**441**).
- Highly vascular.
- Mass effect.

Microscopic
- Very cellular with pleomorphism of cells and hyperchromatism of nuclei.
- Astrocytes with fibrils and astroblasts, tumor giant cells, mitotic cells.
- Vascular proliferation with hyperplasia of endothelial cells of small vessels.
- Necrosis, hemorrhage and thrombosis of vessels.

Growth
- Arises from anaplasia of mature astrocytes.
- Highly malignant.
- May extend to the meningeal surface or the ventricular wall. Malignant cells, carried in the CSF may form distant foci on spinal roots or cause widespread meningeal gliomatosis.
- Extraneural metastases are rare, and usually involve bone and lymph nodes after craniotomy.

Anaplastic astrocytoma
- Moderate hypercellularity and pleomorphism.
- Vascular proliferation.

Astrocytoma (grades 1 and 2)
Macroscopic
- Sites: anywhere in the CNS, particularly the cerebral hemispheres (usually in adults, aged 20–40 years) and the cerebellum (**442**), hypothalamus, optic nerve and chiasm and pons (the latter of which are more common in children and adolescents).
- Appearance: solid, grayish white, firm, relatively avascular tumor, almost indistinguishable from normal white matter. Calcium deposits may be present.
- Often forms large cavities or pseudocysts.

Microscopic
- Well differentiated astrocytes of fibrillary type and less frequently plump gemistocytic (gemistos-filled) type.
- Mildly hypercellular, with pleomorphism (**443**).
- No vascular proliferation or necrosis.
- Glial fibrillary acidic protein.
- Many cerebral astrocytomas are mixed astrocytomas and glioblastomas.

Growth
- A slowly growing, infiltrative tumor.
- May transform to a higher grade tumor.

Oligodendroglioma
Many oligodendrogliomas have deletions of chromosomes 1p and 19q, and molecular changes such as these may prove to be the defining criteria for this kind of tumor.

Macroscopic
- Sites: commonly frontal lobe (40–70%), deep in white matter; sometimes lateral ventricle; and rarely in other parts of the CNS.
- Appearance: multi-lobular, pink-gray, moderately firm, and relatively avascular.
- Tends to encapsulate and form calcium and small cysts.
- Little or no surrounding edema.

Microscopic
- Oligodendrocytes: small, round nucleus and a halo of unsustained cytoplasm. Cell processes are few and stubby, seen only with silver carbonate stains.
- Calcification is common, mainly in relation to zones of necrosis.
- Myelin basic protein.
- Many oligodendrogliomas are mixed oligodendroglioma-astrocytomas.

Growth
- Slow.

- May extend to the pial surface or ependymal wall, and metastasize distally in the ventriculosubarachnoid spaces (accounts for about 10% of gliomas with meningeal dissemination; less frequent than medulloblastoma and glioblastoma).
- Malignant degeneration (greater cellularity and numerous and abnormal mitoses) in about a third of cases.

Ependymoma
Macroscopic
- Sites: most commonly the wall of the fourth ventricle (70%) (**444**); other sites include the lateral ventricles of the brain and the conus or filum terminale of the spinal canal.
- Appearance: gray-pink, cauliflower-like, firm tumors in the fourth ventricle; large (up to several centimetres in diameter), gray-red, softer tumors in the lateral ventricles.
- May be cystic.
- Not encapsulated but well defined and homogeneous.
- More clearly demarcated from surrounding brain than astrocytomas.

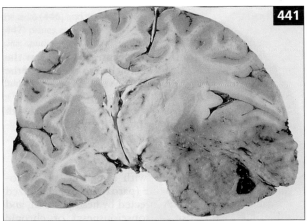

441 Coronal section of the brain at autopsy showing a large hemorrhagic and necrotic glioblastoma multiforme in the temporal lobe causing mass effect with compression of the lateral ventricle and shift of the midline.

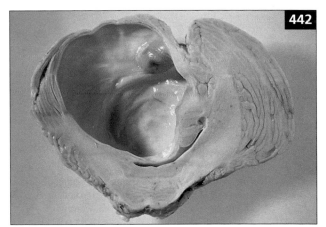

442 Autopsy specimen, section in the axial plane through the cerebellum and pons, showing a cystic cerebellar astrocytoma in an adult. On CT scan (see **452**), the mass is partly enhancing, partly cystic and has some calcification.

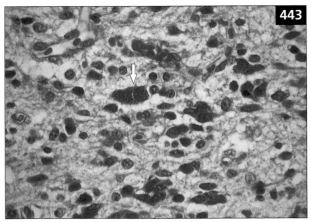

443 Histologic section of astrocytoma of the brain showing hypercellularity, pleomorphism of cells and mitoses (arrow).

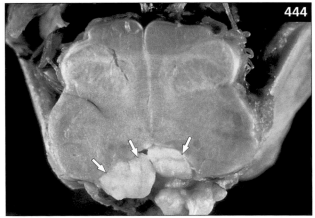

444 Section through the medulla and floor of the fourth ventricle at autopsy showing an ependymoma in the floor of the fourth ventricle (arrows).

OPTIC NERVE GLIOMA

DEFINITION
Glial tumor (usually pilocytic astrocyoma) of the optic pathway.

EPIDEMIOLOGY
- Incidence: uncommon: about 1% of primary intracranial tumors; about 2–5% of all brain tumors in childhood, about 5% (1.5–7.5%) of children with neurofibromatosis-1 (NF1).
- Age: 50% present before the age of 5 years, 90% before age 20. Chiasmal lesions are more frequent in adolescents than in children.
- Gender: F>M (2:1).

PATHOLOGY
- The vast majority are pilocytic astrocytomas (histologically identical to pilocytic astrocytomas elsewhere in the CNS), WHO grade 1 (**459, 460**); anaplastic astrocytoma occurs rarely.
- Two architectural forms:
- Diffuse expansion and obstruction of the optic nerve without extensive subarachnoid spread.
- Predominant infiltration of the subarachnoid space leaving the mildly involved nerve surrounded by a rim of tumor tissue.
- Most are slowly growing and grow along optic pathways (causing enlargement of the optic nerve [50%], optic chiasm [45%], or optic tract [5%]) and invade the subarachnoid space, causing hyperplasia of the overlying arachnoid mater, known as arachnoid gliomatosis. Optic nerve gliomas may also invade the anterior hypothalamus and cause obstruction of the foramen of Monro and obstructive hydrocephalus. Tumor growth is generally limited by dura.

ETIOLOGY AND PATHOPHYSIOLOGY
15–20% of optic gliomas occur in patients with neurofibromatosis; 50–70% of optic gliomas in children are associated with neurofibromatosis; 15–25% (50–70% of children) are associated with neurofibromatosis (see p.147).

CLINICAL FEATURES
- Slowly progressive visual deterioration: dimness of vision with decreased visual acuity and color vision; abnormal pupillary function; constricted fields, followed by variable visual field defects, depending on the location of the tumor, that can be monocular, binocular, eccentric, centrocecal homonymous, heteronymous, and bitemporal, and progressing to blindness; and optic atrophy with or without papilledema. Papilledema with or without a field cut implies involvement of the hypothalamus and obstructive hydrocephalus whereas papillitis and central visual field loss suggests an orbital lesion.
- Ocular proptosis due to the orbital mass.
- Nystagmus, if chiasmatic involvement.
- Hypothalamic and pituitary dysfunction occur occasionally in gliomas involving the optic chiasm (e.g. accelerated linear growth due to precocious puberty; adiposity, polyuria, somnolence).
- Secondary hydrocephalus.

DIFFERENTIAL DIAGNOSIS
- Optic neuritis (see p.489): sarcoidosis, multiple sclerosis.
- Optic nerve hamartoma (NF1, see p.147).
- Meningioma (see p.374): medial sphenoid, olfactory groove, intraorbital.
- Pituitary adenoma (see p.379).
- Diencephalic glioma: gliomas arising in the hypothalamus or thalamus.
- Hand–Schuller–Christian disease.
- Craniopharyngioma (suprasellar epidermoid cyst) (see p.377).

INVESTIGATIONS
CT brain scan
Coronal, sagittal and axial studies:
- The optic nerve appears enlarged (fusiform or nodular) and tortuous.
- Calcification is rare.
- Enhancement is variable.
- There may be cystic components.
- The optic canal may be enlarged (also visible on plain films of the orbit) if the tumor extends that far back.
- The tumor may be bilateral and extend back into the chiasm.

MRI scan
- The appearance is similar to that on CT but the detail is more clearly seen.
- The lesion appears isointense on T1WI (**461**) and iso- to hyperintense on T2WI (**462**).
- It is impossible to separate the tumor from the nerve radiologically (as opposed to meningiomas where it is often possible to distinguish the tumor from the nerve).
- MRI also defines the intracranial portion of the tumor better than CT.
- Magnetic resonance spectroscopy enables assessment of the biochemical composition of focal areas within the tumor and other regions of the brain.

Visual evoked potentials
Help establish and localize the lesion and establish the functional integrity of the visual system.

Blood for DNA analysis
Mutation of the *NF1* gene located on chromosome 17q11.2.

Chiasmal biopsy
Contraindicated since it is the main cause of visual deterioration and is associated with significant but unexplained mortality.

DIAGNOSIS
The clinical diagnosis of an optic pathway tumor is confirmed by CT or MRI scan, and the pathology by tissue biopsy.

TREATMENT
- Depends on the nature of the symptoms, and the location and rate of growth of the tumor; there is no universal approach to treatment
- Children with symptomatic optic pathway glioma, particularly if it involves the chiasm and either the optic nerves or the posterior regions of the visual pathway, should be closely followed, particularly for the development of precocious puberty (e.g. signs of premature secondary sexual characteristics, or accelerated linear growth rate, detected by yearly measurements of height and weight plotted on standard pediatric growth charts) and evidence of reduced visual acuity, color vision or visual fields or changes on slit lamp examination and fundoscopy.

- Treatment is indicated for progressive proptosis or loss of vision, or neuroradiographic progression.
- Therapeutic options include surgery, radiation, chemotherapy, or a combination of these modalities.
- A blind eye due to intraorbital glioma can be removed surgically for cosmetic reasons or to prevent potentially further extension of the tumor into the chiasm (which must be very rare). Surgery has a limited role in the treatment of chiasmatic gliomas that may or may not also involve the optic nerve or the posterior portion of the visual pathway. Otherwise, surgical excision is generally inappropriate because the short term risks outweigh the longer term benign course.
- Radiotherapy should be reserved primarily for patients with isolated intraorbital gliomas and residual useful vision, progressive (either visual or radiographic) isolated optic nerve gliomas (because tumor progression may be halted, at least temporarily) or extraorbital (e.g. optic chiasm) optic pathway glioma, but the long term efficacy for disease control is questionable. As many patients are children, and as these tumors may be quite extensive, large volumes of normal young brain may be included in the radiation portal; there are significant potential neurocognitive and endocrinologic sequelae of radiotherapy to consider before embarking on this treatment, let alone the theoretical possibility of radiotherapy inducing more malignant transformation of the tumor.
- There are few data to support the efficacy of chemotherapy in intraorbital glioma. The combination of carboplatinum and vincristine appears promising for extraorbital optic pathway glioma but this therapy still remains experimental.

PROGNOSIS

- May vary from extreme indolence to rapid progression but most are very slow-growing.
- Optic pathway gliomas in children with NF1 infrequently progress once the tumors have come to medical attention: in one study, demonstrable tumor growth or progression of visual disturbances occurred in only 3 of 26 children over a mean follow-up period of 4.2 years.
- 20-year survival rate: 40–50%.

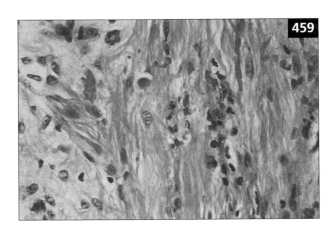

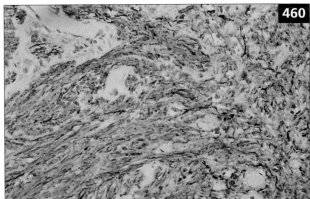

459, 460 Histology of optic nerve glioma showing infiltration of the optic nerve by glioblasts and astrocytes.

462 T2W axial MRI of the brain in NF1 showing areas of increased signal in the basal ganglia bilaterally, worse on the right, also visible in the periventricular white matter (arrows). The precise nature of these is the subject of debate.

461 T1W MRI of the orbits showing an optic nerve glioma in NF1. Note the thickened optic nerves bilaterally (arrows).

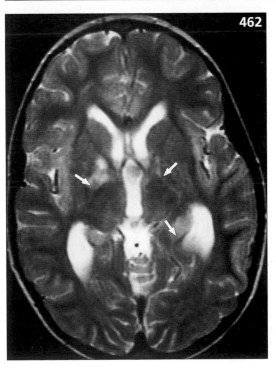

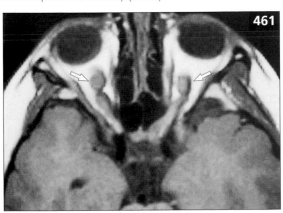

DIFFERENTIAL DIAGNOSIS
Tuberculum sellae meningioma
- Pituitary adenoma.
- Aneurysm of the terminal carotid artery.

Sphenoid ridge meningioma
- Sarcoma arising from skull bone.
- Orbitoethmoidal osteoma.
- Benign giant cell bone cyst.
- Optic nerve tumors.
- Orbital angioma.
- Metastatic carcinoma.

INVESTIGATIONS
CT brain scan (467, 468)
- Meningiomas arise from any dural surface and push the brain away.
- They are usually rounded or lobulated, iso- or slightly hypodense lesions that have well-defined, sharply demarcated contours and enhance strongly with i.v. contrast.
- There may be an enhancing dural 'tail' extending from the tumor margin.
- White matter edema varies from none (usually) to extensive (occasionally).
- Thickening of the adjacent bone (hyperostosis) may be visible.
- Calcification is occasional though can be dense.
- Large dilated venous sinuses around the tumor may be visible.
- The mass effect is usually less than for a similar sized intrinsic tumor as the slow growth allows time for the normal brain to shift and adapt to the presence of the meningioma.

MRI brain scan
- Meningiomas are often isointense to gray matter on T1WI and T2WI, so if small may be overlooked.
- They enhance strongly with i.v. contrast (gadolinium).
- Their other features are as described for CT.

Cerebral angiography
- There is usually enlargement of the meningeal arteries (branches of the external carotid) which supply the meningioma.
- Some arterial supply may come from the internal carotid arteries also.
- The venous drainage is usually to the intracranial dural venous sinuses.
- Some centres offer particulate embolization of meningiomas prior to surgery to reduce the vascularity and blood loss during tumor removal.

CSF
Increased protein; may be very high (2.0–4.0 g/l [200–400 mg/dl]) with olfactory groove meningioma.

DIAGNOSIS
- Some meningiomas reach an enormous size before the diagnosis is established.
- Diagnosis is suggested by contrast-enhanced CT and MRI, and angiography, but is confirmed histologically.

TREATMENT
Conservative
Incidentally discovered meningiomas can be followed safely with CT or MRI.

Surgical excision
- The mainstay of therapy.
- Effective for accessible surface tumors that can be totally resected, such as meningiomas of the convexity dura, falx, lateral sphenoid wing, frontal base and posterior-fossa dura. A cuff of normal dura should be removed to reduce the chance of marginal recurrence.
- Tumors that lie beneath the hypothalamus, along the medial part of the sphenoid bone and parasellar region and anterior to the brainstem are the most difficult to remove surgically. They are inoperable if they invade adjacent bone.

Stereotaxic radiosurgery
Appropriate for some well localized (i.e. not adjacent to the optic nerve or other critical structures) and small (<3 cm [<1.2 in] in diameter) meningiomas, particularly in the skull base.

Radiotherapy
Fractionated, external beam, radiation therapy can delay regrowth or recurrence and is indicated if the tumor is inoperable, incompletely resected or histologically aggressive.

Interstitial brachytherapy
- Used for recurrent benign and malignant meningiomas that have failed to respond to standard therapies, are amenable to repeat operation, and have a residual tumor thickness that does not exceed a few millimetres.
- Both stereotactic and open craniotomy techniques have been used for placement of the radiation sources (e.g. iodine-125).

Cytotoxic chemotherapy
Little success to date. Hydroxyurea appeared promising in preliminary reports. But shown recently to be ineffective.

Biologic therapies
Experimental (e.g. hormone receptor antagonists).

PROGNOSIS
- Slow rate of growth.
- Not always curable; the rate of recurrence depends on the site of the tumor, its biologic aggressiveness, and the completeness of the resection.
- Complete excision is associated with permanent cure in many cases; invasive growth leads to recurrence in about 2% of patients per year (i.e. 20% at 10 years).
- Subtotal resection and malignancy are associated with a higher rate of recurrence: for benign meningiomas, the 5 year rate of survival free of progression is about 90% and at 10 years about 75%; whereas for malignant meningiomas, 5 year survival free of progression is only about 50%. More than 80% recur after partial resection.
- Histology alone may be inadequate to characterize accurately the biologic behavior of meningiomas. Age is an important independent prognostic factor for survival.

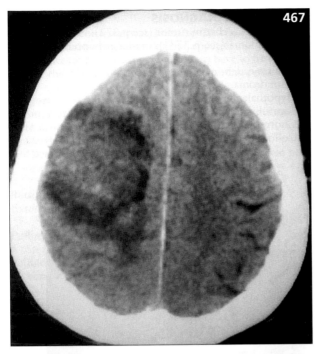

467

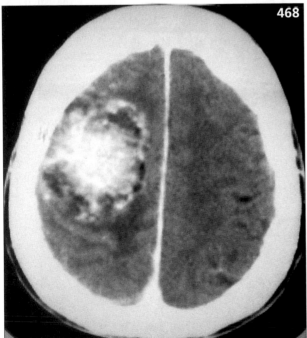

468

467, 468 CT brain scan pre- (**467**) and post (**468**) i.v. contrast. Pre-contrast the meningioma appears similar to adjacent brain and is causing relatively little displacement of the normal brain for its size. Post i.v. contrast there is intense enhancement (whiteness) making the tumor very obvious. Note the rounded shape, the flat surface against the inner skull table where it arises from the dura, the small granular calcifications (white spots), and the relative lack of white matter edema and mass effect. Also see **715** and **716** for spinal meningioma.

CRANIOPHARYNGIOMA

DEFINITION
A rare, congenital cystic tumor which arises from cell rests (embryologic remnants of pharyngeal epithelium in Rathke's pouch) above the pituitary fossa and gives rise to a suprasellar mass that compresses and infiltrates adjacent local structures, causing endocrine or visual symptoms in children and young adults.

EPIDEMIOLOGY
- Incidence: rare, 2–3% of all brain tumors.
- Age: children predominantly, but may present in adults of all ages.
- Gender: M=F.

ETIOLOGY AND PATHOGENESIS
- Congenital.
- The tumor arises from cell rests (embryologic remnants of Rathke's pouch) above the pituitary fossa at the junction of the infundibular stem and pituitary gland.

PATHOLOGY
- Usually the tumor lies above the sella turcica, depressing the optic chiasm and extending up into the third ventricle.
- Less often it is subdiaphragmatic, within the sella, where it compresses the pituitary body and erodes one part of the wall of the sella or a clinoid process, but seldom does it balloon the sella like a pituitary adenoma.
- A cystic tumor, containing dark albuminous fluid, cholesterol crystals, and calcium deposits; it is partly calcified by the time it is 3–4 cm (1.2–1.5 in) in diameter.
- Infiltrates locally.
- The sella beneath the tumor becomes flattened and enlarged.

CLINICAL FEATURES
Presents in children and young adults with any one or a combination of the following syndromes:
- Hypothalamic dysfunction: hypopituitarism (growth failure in children: delayed physical and mental development, diabetes insipidus, adiposity, amenorrhea, disturbed temperature regulation, sexual dysfunction).
- Progressive or intermittent optic nerve or chiasm compression (visual loss).
- Obstructive hydrocephalus (raised intracranial pressure: headaches, vomiting).
- Frontal lobe symptoms (mental dullness, confusion, spastic leg weakness).

Cerebellopontine angle origin
Compression of nearby structures
- Atypical trigeminal neuralgia (V).
- Tic douloureux (V).
- Loss or reduction of corneal reflex.
- Facial numbness (V).
- Hemifacial spasm.
- Progressive painless lower motor neuron facial weakness (VII).
- Hoarse weak voice (X).
- Dysphagia (IX, X).

Compression of brainstem and raised intracranial pressure (hydrocephalus)
- Headache.
- Unsteadiness, clumsiness, poor balance.
- Vertigo.
- Spontaneous nystagmus*.
- Vomiting.
- Hearing loss and/or tinnitus in the other ear.
- Altered mental state.
- Visual changes.

*Nystagmus:

	Peripheral nystagmus	Central nystagmus
Direction	Fast phase in same direction, irrespective of direction of gaze	Usually changes direction
	Horizontal or rotary/torsional Never vertical	May be bizarre Often vertical
Prognosis over 2 weeks	Decreasing severity	Does not improve significantly

DIFFERENTIAL DIAGNOSIS
- Trigeminal neuralgia (that fails to respond or responds erratically to standard treatment with carbamazepine).
- Eustachian tube obstruction.
- Cerebellopontine angle tumor:
- Acoustic neuroma: (75% of cases).
- Meningioma: (6% of cases).
- Cholesteatoma: (6% of cases):
  Epidermoid cyst.
  Arising from temporal bone.
- Glioma: (3% of cases).
- Other types: (10% of cases):
  Metastatic tumors.
  Osteomas.
  Osteogenic sarcomas.
  Neuromas of trigeminal, facial or glossopharyngeal nerve.
  Angiomas.
  Papillomas of choroid plexus.
  Teratomas.
  Lipomas.

INVESTIGATIONS
CT or MRI brain
- MRI is the method of choice, though thin section CT with i.v. contrast or air meatography are alternatives in patients who cannot have or tolerate MRI.
- The standard MRI sequence is a T1W thin section sequence through the petrous bones with i.v. contrast.
- Acoustic neuromas show up as an enhancing mass, within the VIIIth nerve canal if very small (**483**), and extending into the cerebellopontine angle if larger (**484**).

- They are rounded, may be very large and cause brainstem displacement.
- The main differential diagnosis is meningioma, which does not usually extend into the acoustic canal.

Pure tone audiometry
Sensorineural hearing loss.

Brainstem auditory evoked potentials
Not usually necessary, but if so may reveal prolongation of waves I–III.

DIAGNOSIS
The definitive investigation is gadolinium-enhanced MRI in a patient with a suggestive clinical history.

TREATMENT
- Treatment depends on a complex interplay of the needs and expectations of the patient, the size of the tumor and the local expertise.
- Treatments include expectant care with repeat scanning to assess tumor growth in elderly people and surgery with or without radiotherapy.
- Surgical approaches and techniques vary but generally involve micro-surgical techniques, an ultrasonic surgical aspirator, intraoperative monitoring of brainstem auditory evoked potentials and facial nerve function (by electromyography), and access to intensive care facilities for immediate post operative care.

Mortality varies from 2–4% depending on the size of the tumor. Other risks include deafness, facial palsy, vertigo, lower cranial nerve palsy, brainstem damage, brainstem and cerebellar infarction.

The risks increase with the size of the tumor and decrease with the experience of the operating team. The chances of surgery preserving useful hearing are slight unless the tumor is small or medium sized; surgical resection of tumors <2.5 cm (<1 in) in diameter carries a one in four to one in three chance of preserving hearing. Surgical resection of an acoustic neuroma measuring <2 cm (<0.8 in) in diameter should however provide an 80% chance of immediate preservation of facial nerve function and a 95% chance of long term facial nerve function.

- Stereotactic radiotherapy can deliver highly localized levels of radiation with minimal damage to surrounding structures. Because of the morbidity of surgery, especially to the facial nerve and hearing, there is a move toward stereotactic radiotherapy for tumors with a maximum diameter of <3 cm (<1.2 in), particularly in the elderly and for those with bilateral acoustic neuromas.
- Combined surgery and radiotherapy. Surgery to debulk a large tumor has a lower operative morbidity compared with attempted total removal. Post operative stereotactic radiotherapy in such cases may be a useful combination but the long term effects remain to be evaluated.

PROGNOSIS
Acoustic neuromas grow but the rate of growth seems to be slower in older people and they may not cause serious symptoms; 0.8–2.7% of post mortem studies find an acoustic neuroma that had not contributed to the death of the person.

PRIMARY CNS LYMPHOMA

DEFINITION
A tumor of lymphocytes or lymphoblasts, usually B cells, confined to the CNS.

EPIDEMIOLOGY
- 1–2% of cases of non-Hodgkin's lymphoma.
- 3% of all intracranial neoplasms.
- Marked increase in incidence in the last decade as part of the AIDS epidemic but also within the immunocompetent population (for unknown reasons).
- Age: median: 57 years (non-AIDS); young adults (AIDS).
- Gender: M>F (1.5:1).

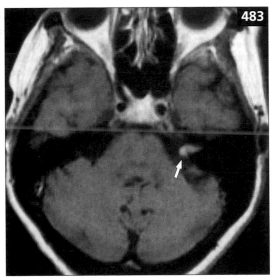

483 MRI brain, T1W image with i.v. contrast showing a small left intracanalicular acoustic neuroma (arrow).

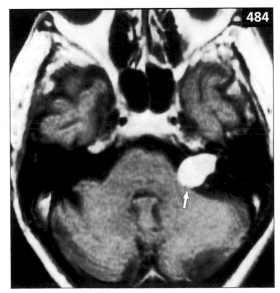

484 MRI brain, T1W image of a large acoustic neuroma projecting into the cerebellopontine angle (arrow).

PATHOLOGY
Macroscopic
- Multifocal mass deposits in the brain in two-thirds of cases.
- Solitary mass within the subcortical white matter in one-third.
- Sites:
- Brain:
  Supratentorial (75% of cases with brain lymphoma):
    Periventricular lesions are frequent.
    Corpus callosum (41%).
    Deep central nuclei (33%).
  Infratentorial (20% of cases with brain lymphoma).
  Diffuse leptomeningeal (5% of cases with brain lymphoma).
  Diffuse neuropil involvement: rare.
- Eye: posterior segment (retina and vitreous): present in 25% of cases with intracranial lymphoma.
- At autopsy, parenchymal lesions are always in contact with either the leptomeninges or the ependymal surface.

Microscopic
- The tumor cell of origin is the lymphocyte or lymphoblast (B cell, usually diffuse, large cell subtype: >2/3, T cell: <1/3; this ratio is different to systemic lymphoma).
- The fine reticulum and microgliacytes are interstitial and derived from fibroblasts and microglia (histiocytes).
- The tumor is highly cellular, with little tendency to necrosis. Mitotic figures are numerous. The nuclei are oval or bean-shaped with scant cytoplasm. The stainability of reticulum and microglial cells, the latter by silver carbonate, serves to distinguish this tumor microscopically. B cell markers identify the tumor cell type.
- Most tumors are high-grade immunoblastic or diffuse large cell type but many are arrested at relatively mature stages of differentiation.
- Although B cell immunophenotype predominates in immunocompromised (e.g. AIDS) and immunocompetent (e.g. non-AIDS) cases, the tumor cells that arise in immunocompromised patients are usually polyclonal, tending to have high-grade histologic characteristics (immunoblastic and small, non-cleaved cells) and contain Epstein–Barr virus (EBV) genomic material in about 80% of cases; whereas immunocompetent patients usually have monoclonal, large-cell lymphomas of B cell origin with a low-grade histologic appearance and no evidence of EBV infection.
- The lymphocytes express either kappa or lambda light-chain immunoglobulin. Molecular studies have also demonstrated consistent profiles of light-chain and heavy-chain immunoglobulin gene rearrangements in primary, recurrent, and metastatic CNS lymphomas.
- Regardless of cell type, a perivascular pattern predominates, with malignant cells surrounding blood vessels in concentric layers (resembling the inflammatory response of encephalitis).

N.B. Systemic non-Hodgkin's lymphoma, arising in lymph nodes and other somatic organs, spreads to the CNS in about 25–30% of cases, and tends to infiltrate the leptomeninges (sparing the parenchyma), particularly in the spinal region (and causing spinal cord compression), in contrast to PCNS lymphoma which tends to originate in the parenchyma.

TREATMENT

Management is determined by the histologic and serologic diagnosis and extent of disease.

Pineal region tumors

- Frequently non-germinomatous germ cell tumors.
- Huge masses should be biopsied. If malignant, neoadjuvant chemotherapy should be given before the second radical surgical resection.
- Smaller tumors can be debulked safely, and if malignant, radically removed.
- Shunting procedures for hydrocephalus, such as ventriculo-peritoneal shunt, are rarely necessary and may lead to fatal peritoneal metastases.
- Histologically verified pineal germinomas can be remarkably reduced in size only through a course of low-dose radiotherapy or chemotherapy alone (see Germinomas, below).

Neurohypophyseal and hypothalamic region tumors

- Preferentially infiltrate the optic pathways.
- Biopsy or partially remove when possible.

Suprasellar tumor confined to the optic pathways:

- Usually germinomas (see below).
- May require craniotomy for biopsy.

Germinoma (solitary or multifocal)

- Highly radiosensitive and historically associated with a high surgical mortality.
- Radiotherapy to the localized field, via appropriate irradiation ports, following active chemotherapy, can be curable. A reduced dose of 24 Gy (2400 rads) in daily fractions of 2 Gy (200 rads) or less, minimizes adverse effects of radiotherapy such as cognitive retardation and neuroendocrine deficiencies (growth hormone deficiency occurs with radiation doses >24 Gy (2400 rads) to the posterior hypothalamus).
- Prophylactic craniospinal or ventricle irradiation is not indicated because of associated morbidity in the growing child.
- Adjuvant pre-radiation chemotherapy, with a combination including either cisplatin or carboplatin and etoposide, may decrease the total dose of radiation necessary for inducing tumor resolution, and enhance control in malignant germ cell tumors. Chemotherapy alone is insufficient, and is often associated with an early relapse of disease.
- Disseminated germinoma should be treated with craniospinal irradiation.
- If the initial treatment was 24 Gy (2400 rads) of local irradiation, recurrent germinoma can be treated with the same or a larger dose of radiotherapy, and the craniospinal field can be selected.

Malignant germ cell tumors

Examples include mixed germ cell tumors, with numerous combinations of diverse histology and prognosis, such as a mixed germ cell tumor composed of immature teratoma with embryonal carcinoma:

- High incidence of subarachnoid dissemination and spinal metastases.

- Craniospinal radiotherapy with a high dose local boost, and intensive combination chemotherapy (regimens including ifosfamide, cisplatin [or carboplatin] and etoposide) is used.
- High dose chemotherapy with autologous bone marrow transplant or peripheral blood stem-cell support has not been successful to date but may have a role in the salvage setting of patients with relapsed or disseminated non-germinomatous germ cell tumors in the CNS.
- Daily oral etoposide cycles may be employed in patients with extracranial germ cell tumors who have failed to respond to first-line chemotherapy but have shown a response to salvage therapy; and also as a maintenance chemotherapy in patients with poor prognosis non-germinomatous germ cell tumors.
- Malignant teratomas should be surgically removed if possible because this can be curable, but its applicability depends on the site and size of the tumor.

COMPLICATIONS OF TREATMENT AND THEIR MANAGEMENT

Lack of neurohypophyseal and pituitary hormones

- Infertility, hypogonadism, small stature.
- Caused by tumor invasion or high-dose radiotherapy.
- Pituitary hormone replacement therapy is required by most children.

Lack of regulation of essential endocrine processes (e.g. sleep cycle)

Oral melatonin may improve sleep disturbance in children with pineal tumors.

VON HIPPEL–LINDAU DISEASE (VHL)

DEFINITION

A rare autosomal dominantly inherited, and occasionally sporadic, neuroectodermal disorder that is characterized by a predisposition to tumor development in the retina, cerebellum, spinal cord, pancreas and kidneys; and usually presents in early adulthood with visual or neurologic symptoms due to a hemangiomatous malformation of the retina or an associated hemangioblastoma of the cerebellum. It is one of the phakomatoses (disseminated hereditary hamartomas), along with conditions such as Sturge–Weber syndrome and von Recklinhausen's disease. Dr Eugen von Hippel, a German ophthalmologist, first described the familial nature of retinal hemangioblastomas, and Dr Arvid Lindau, a Swedish ophthalmologist, first recognized that cerebellar and retinal hemangioblastomas are part of a larger 'angiomatous lesion of the CNS' and the condition is inherited.

EPIDEMIOLOGY

- Prevalence: 1 in 40 000.
- Age: mean age of onset 26 years; range 1–78 years:
- Retinal hemangioblastoma: mean age at diagnosis 25 years (range 1–67 years).
- Cerebellar hemangioblastoma: mean age at diagnosis 30 years (range 1–78 years).
- Renal cell carcinoma: mean age at diagnosis 37 years (range 16–67 years).
- Gender: M=F.

PATHOLOGY

Capillary hemangioblastomas

Comprising endothelial cells and pericytes of:

- Retina (45–59% of patients), bilateral in half .
- Cerebellum (44–83%), brainstem (up to 18%), spinal cord (13–44%), or adrenal glands. Cerebellar hemangioblastoma is the most common primary intrinsic tumor in the posterior fossa in adults (10% of all cerebellar tumors). Up to 20% of cerebellar hemangioblastomas secrete erythropoietin sufficient to cause symptomatic polycythemia. Spinal cord hemangioblastomas have a predilection for the conus medullaris and craniocervical junction, and are associated with a syringomyelic lesion in >70% of cases.

Additional lesions

Present in some cases, including:

- Angiomas and cysts of the liver, pancreas, and kidneys (59–63%).
- Adenomas of the liver, epididymis and adrenals.
- Renal cell carcinoma (24–45% of patients, onset beyond age 20 years): secretes erythropoietin which can cause polycythemia.
- Pheochromocytoma (7–18%): probably of neural crest origin, generally considered benign but can metastasize.
- Ectopic paraganglioma, histologically identical to pheochromocytoma, may arise in the carotid body, glomus jugulare, periaortic tissues, spleen and kidney.
- Pancreatic islet cell tumor: probably of neural crest origin, more frequent in patients with pheochromocytoma; islet cell tumors are capable of metastasizing and may become symptomatic with biliary obstruction or endocrinopathy.
- Papillary cystadenoma of the epididymis: (10–26% of men with VHL), when bilateral are virtually pathognomonic of VHL disease; histologically similar lesions are seen in the broad ligament of females with VHL disease.

ETIOLOGY AND PATHOPHYSIOLOGY

- Inherited:
- Autosomal dominant inheritance.
- High penetrance (i.e. a high proportion of people with the gene develop the disease; penetrance is in excess of 90% by 60 years of age).
- Variable expression (i.e. the severity of the disease varies substantially between affected patients, even within a family), although some families seem to have a propensity for pheochromocytoma.
- The gene responsible for VHL is located on the short arm of chromosome 3, 3p25-26, the same region that is associated with renal cell carcinoma, and close to the locus of the *RAF-1* oncogene.
- The VHL disease gene is a tumor suppressor gene, a gene whose normal function is to regulate cell growth. When both copies of the gene are inactivated by means of mutation or loss (e.g. recombination or somatic deletion), cell growth is unchecked and tumors result.
- Patients with VHL disease inherit the germ line mutation on the short arm of one allele of chromosome 3 from the affected parent, and one normal allele from the unaffected parent.
- A 'two-hit hypothesis' has been proposed to explain the development of tumors: the abnormal germ line mutation is present in all cells, but only those cells in target organs that develop a second mutation in the normal allele go on to develop tumors.

- The susceptible target organs in VHL disease can be grouped as:
- Cerebellar and retinal cells (resulting in hemangioblastomas).
- Neural crest cells (resulting in pheochromocytomas, paragangliomas, and possible islet cell tumors).
- Glandular viscera (resulting in renal, pancreatic, epididymal and endolymphatic sac tumors).

CLINICAL FEATURES

- Symptoms usually do not become evident until late adolescence or adulthood.
- Progressive visual loss:
- Presenting symptom in up to 50% of patients due to enlargement of the retinal angioma (bilateral in half of cases), exudative or tractional retinal detachment, vitreous hemorrhage, macular edema or epiretinal membrane formation causing macular distortion.
- Ophthalmologic examination may reveal a decrease in visual acuity, a visual field defect, enlargement of the 'feeder' retinal vessels leading to a peripheral retinal capillary hemangioma (**495**) and exudative changes (signs of lipid deposition) in the macula.
- Progressive ataxia of limb movements, speech (dysarthria) and swallowing (dysphagia) due to cerebellar hemangioblastoma, or symptoms of increased intracranial pressure such as headache, nausea, and vomiting: presenting symptoms in about 20% of patients.
- Spinal pain, focal sensory and motor deficits from spinal tumors.
- Polycythemia due to production of erythropoietin by cerebellar hemangioblastomas and renal cell carcinomas.
- Episodes of uncontrolled hypertension, perspiration, headaches and anxiety attacks due to massive release of catecholamines by pheochromocytoma.

A thorough search for other manifestations of the disease (see Pathology, above) is also required.

DIFFERENTIAL DIAGNOSIS

- Cerebellar tumor.
- Cerebellar degeneration.
- Multiple sclerosis.

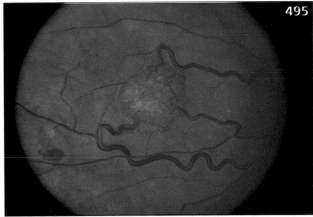

495 Ocular fundus showing a peripheral retinal capillary hemangioma with enlarged 'feeder' retinal vessels. (Courtesy of Dr AM Chancellor, Tauranga, New Zealand.)

Microscopic

Argyrophilic senile (neuritic) plaques (518–521)

- Plaques are large extracellular lesions in which the principal component of the core of the plaque is the insoluble 40–42/43 amino acid peptide called β-amyloid protein which is a minor breakdown product of amyloid precursor protein (APP).
- Plaques result from the accumulation of several proteins and an inflammatory reaction around deposits of β-amyloid.
- Degenerating nerve terminals in the plaques also contain the microtubular protein tau.
- Amyloid burden and the number of plaques do not correlate with the severity of the disease.

Neurofibrillary tangles (522–524)

- Tangles are intracellular lesions principally composed of aggregations of an abnormal form of a cytoskeletal-associated microtubular protein, tau, which is hyperphosphorylated. The aggregated neurofibrils are visualized as paired helical filaments on electron microscopy.
- They are present, together with plaques, in the projection neurons of the limbic and association areas of the cerebral cortex, particularly the parietal cortex and hippocampus, especially the CA1 zone and the entorhinal cortex, subiculum, and transitional cortex of the hippocampus.
- The number of tangles increases with the duration and severity of disease.
- Tangles are not specific for AD however, they are also found in other conditions such as dementia pugilistica, subacute sclerosing panencephalitis, and tuberous sclerosis.

Dystrophic neurites

Loss of neocortical neurons (>40%)

Loss is widespread (hippocampus, entorhinal cortex, association areas of neocortex, and nucleus basalis of Meynert [the substantia innominata] and locus ceruleus) and predominantly a loss of cholinergic, noradrenergic, and dopaminergic neurons. N.B. There is no loss of neocortical neurons in the course of normal ageing.

Loss of neuronal synapses

- Assessed using antibodies to synaptic proteins such as synaptophysin.
- The degree of synaptic loss is the best correlate with the severity of dementia.

N.B. It is not known if senile plaques or neurofibrillary tangles come first, or which is the primary factor causing AD, but as these cellular changes progress, neurons are lost.

Associated pathologic states (525)

- Concomitant Parkinson's disease changes (nigral degeneration and Lewy bodies at various sites) are present in about 20–30% of AD autopsies.
- Diffuse Lewy body disease (see p.430).
- 'Punch-drunk' syndrome, or 'dementia pugilistica': neurofibrillary changes in boxers.

Chemical pathology

- A cholinergic deficit secondary to degeneration of subcortical neurons (e.g. in the basal nucleus of Meynert) which project to the cortex and hippocampus. A family of neurotrophic factors (small proteins), of which the archetypal neurotrophin is nerve growth factor (NGF), are important (protective) for the survival of cholinergic cells.
- Diminution of monoaminergic neurons and noradrenergic, GABAergic and serotonergic functions occur in affected neocortex.
- Decreased neuropeptide transmitters: substance P, somatostatin, cholecystokinin.

ETIOLOGY

- Most cases are probably polygenic (caused by the action of several different genes), and the penetrance of disease is influenced by age and environmental factors (e.g. possibly herpes simplex virus type 1 infection in the brain).
- The concordance rate is higher (1.2–2.7) in monozygotic (MZ) and dizygotic twin pairs, suggesting the contribution of genetic factors, but MZ twins are not fully concordant, implicating non-genetic and environmental factors are involved.
- Genetic factors appear to lead to quantitatively worse disease but not to a qualitatively different pattern of brain involvement. β-amyloid deposition seems to be the neuropathologic factor most strongly influenced by genetic factors.

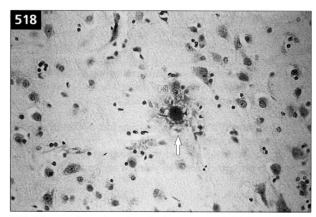

518 Microscopic section of cerebral cortex, cresyl violet stain, showing neuronal loss and an extracellular senile or 'neuritic' plaque containing a homogeneous central core of amyloid (arrow).

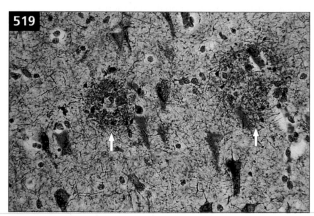

519 Microscopic section of cerebral cortex, Cajal stain, showing two senile or 'neuritic' plaques (arrows).

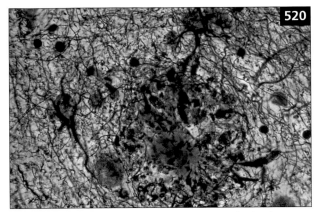

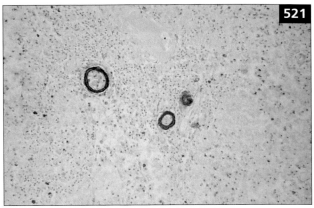

520 Microscopic section of cerebral cortex, silver stain, showing an extracellular senile or 'neuritic' plaque as a deposit of amorphous material that contains a central core of amyloid, surrounded by numerous short fibrils (resembling a bird's nest) that represent products of degenerated nerve terminals, mainly dendritic, containing lysosomes, abnormal mitochondria, and often twisted tubules.

521 Amyloid in the walls of small blood vessels near senile plaques (amyloid or congophilic angiopathy).

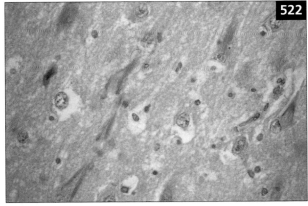

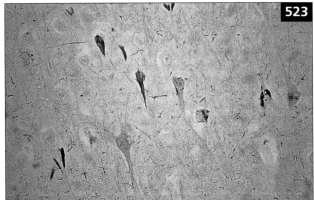

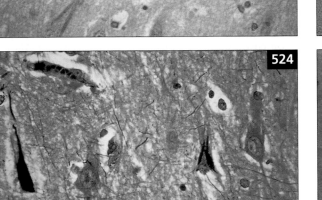

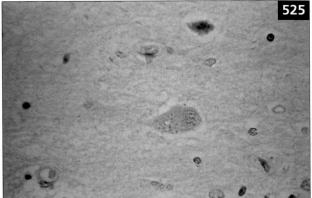

522–524 Microscopic section of brain showing neurofibrillary tangles as thick, fiber-like strands of silver-staining material, often in the form of loops, coils or tangled masses, in the nerve cell cytoplasm.

525 Microscopic section of brain showing granulovacuolar degeneration of neurons in the pyramidal layer of the hippocampus.

Frontal lobe dysfunction
- Abulia.
- Apathy.
- Behavioral change: disinhibited and inappropriate, stereotyped and perseverative behavior.
- Personality change: varying from emotionally dull, inert, lacking initiative, spontaneity and impulse, and taciturn, to emotional, social and sexual indifference or disinhibition.
- Inattention.
- Loss of judgement and insight.
- Difficulty planning.
- Variable memory loss.
- Motor perseveration.
- Speech reduction: decreased fluency followed by echolalia and mutism.
- Hyperorality.
- Prominent grasp and suck reflexes.
- Unable to perform sequences of motor tasks.
- Unable to cope with unaccustomed problems.
- Deterioration of social and work habits.
- Gait impairment.

Temporal lobe dysfunction
- Dysphasia: receptive (slow comprehension), jargon aphasia, dysnomia.
- Forgetfulness.
- Disorientation in time and place.
- Behavioral change: lighthearted, anxious or happy, physically active and on the move constantly, talkative, occupied with trivia, and attentive to all passing incidents.
- Bulimia.
- Altered sexual behavior.
- Apraxia involving articulatory, buccofacial, limb and truncal movements.

Exceptionally
- Cerebellar ataxia.
- Extrapyramidal syndrome: shuffling gait, rigidity, pseudocontractures of limbs.

DIFFERENTIAL DIAGNOSIS
- AD:
- May coexist with Pick's disease.
- Frontal lobe presentations of AD (e.g. behavioral disturbance) are unusual, particularly before 65 years.
- Atrophy is relatively mild and diffuse.
- Paired helical filaments, not straight fibrils of Pick bodies.
- More severe granulovacuolar degeneration of neurons.
- Vascular dementia: e.g. Binswanger's disease:
- May share clinical features with frontal lobe dementia syndromes, such as irritability, jocularity, hyperactivity, and mood fluctuation.
- Neurologic signs are common.
- CT scan usually reveals diffuse or multifocal white matter disease.
- Dementia with Lewy bodies (see p.430).
- Alcoholic brain damage:
- May affect the frontal lobes.
- Patients with Pick's disease may also abuse alcohol, however.
- Huntington's disease:
- Involuntary choreiform movements are usually, but not always, present.
- Positive family history.

- Creutzfeldt–Jakob disease: a rapidly progressive dementia that may be indistinguishable from that seen in Pick's disease.
- Gerstmann–Straussler–Scheinker syndrome: dementia and cerebellar ataxia or extrapyramidal dysfunction.
- Corticobasal degeneration: language disturbances and frontal lobe-type behavior may be seen but there is usually evidence of limb dystonia, ideomotor dyspraxia, myoclonus, and anasymmetric akinetic-rigid syndrome with late-onset of gait or balance disturbances.
- Depression: the profound apathy of frontal lobe dementia may be erroneously attributed to depression. However, the absence of neurovegetative symptoms and depressive ideation (e.g. guilt, worthlessness) should be clear.
- Mania: manic symptoms are reported in about one-third of cases.
- Schizophrenia: persecutory ideas and bizarre, hypochondriacal delusions may occur in some cases and suggest schizophrenia.
- Obsessive compulsive disorder: compulsive hoarding and ritualized routines occur in up to one-quarter of cases of Pick's disease, but primary obsessive compulsive disorder usually occurs in young people.
- Primary progressive aphasia:
- Linguistic disturbance varying from agrammatic, non-fluent speech to fluent aphasia with comprehension deficits, due to focal cerebral atrophy in the perisylvian region of the dominant hemisphere.
- Social conduct, judgement, insight and memory are preserved, as well as the capacity to develop strategies to circumvent any impairments.
- It is uncertain whether this disorder is a prodrome of AD, a discrete disorder without progression to global dementia, or part of a spectrum involving both. Long term follow-up studies are required.

INVESTIGATIONS
- Neuropsychologic evaluation: frontal or temporal lobe dysfunction.
- CT or MRI brain: striking atrophy of the cortex and white matter of the frontal and/or temporal lobes.
- Dynamic/functional neuroimaging, such as SPECT and PET, is often more informative than static techniques such as CT and MRI, and shows an anterior perfusion deficit, in contrast to AD which usually shows posterior perfusion deficits.
- EEG: normal.

DIAGNOSIS
- Neuropathologic.
- The best clinical predictors for the early diagnosis include 'frontal dementia', early 'cortical' dementia with severe frontal lobe disturbances, absence of apraxia, and absence of gait disturbance at onset.

TREATMENT
No specific treatment.

CLINICAL COURSE
Progressive.

PROGNOSIS
The average time from diagnosis to death is about 8 years, i.e. longer than in AD.

HUNTINGTON'S DISEASE (HD)

DEFINITION

An autosomal dominant inherited disorder characterized by progressive involuntary choreiform movements, cognitive decline, and emotional and psychiatric disturbance, due to severe neuronal loss, initially in the neostriatum and later in the cerebral cortex, as a result of an increase in the number of trinucleotide CAG repeats in the *HD* gene on chromosome 4p16.3 that encodes the protein huntingtin.

EPIDEMIOLOGY

- Prevalence: 1 per 10 000; all races.
- Age of onset: average: 35–42 years, but may start in childhood (juvenile or Westphal variant) or old age.
- Gender: M=F.

PATHOLOGY

Macroscopic

- Atrophy of the caudate nuclei and frontal lobes (**532, 533**).

- Ventricular dilatation, most marked in the frontal horns of the lateral ventricles.

Microscopic (534, 535)

- Loss of neurons occurs first in the striatum (putamen and caudate nucleus), and later to a lesser extent throughout the brain in most of the gray matter of the cerebral hemispheres and cerebellum.
- Neuronal loss is predominantly of medium sized spiny neurons which make up 80% of the neurons in the striatum; larger neurons are spared.
- Neurons in the striatum and cerebral cortex have intranuclear inclusions of huntingtin and ubiquitin.
- Reactive gliosis occurs with prominent characteristic astrocytes in the basal ganglia.
- Biochemically, GABA, acetylcholine, substance P, and dynophin are decreased in the striatum. The dopaminergic nigrostriatal pathway and dopamine concentrations are preserved.
- An imbalance between GABA, acetylcholine, and dopamine may account for the involuntary choreiform movements.

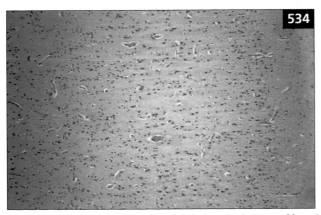

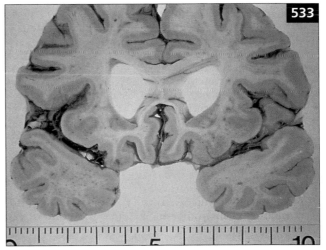

532 Coronal section through the frontal lobe of one cerebral hemisphere from a patient with advanced Huntington's disease (left) and a person with a normal brain (right) showing severe atrophy of the caudate nucleus and frontal lobe with dilatation of the frontal horn of the lateral ventricle of the brain of the patient with Huntington's disease on the left.

533 Brain at post mortem of a patient with severe Huntington's disease showing atrophy of the caudate nuclei and frontal lobes bilaterally.

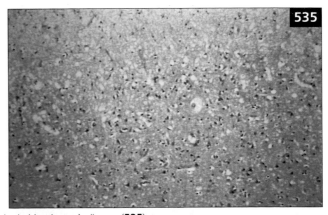

534, 535 Normal cerebral cortex (**534**) and cerebral cortex of frontal lobe in Huntington's disease (**535**).

DIFFERENTIAL DIAGNOSIS

- Structural cerebellar, brainstem or spinal cord lesion (tumor, arteriovenous malformation).
- Alcoholic cerebellar degeneration.
- Multiple sclerosis.
- Hypothyroidism.
- Neurosyphilis.
- Subacute combined degeneration of the spinal cord (sensory, not cerebellar, ataxia).
- Wilson's disease.
- Mitochondrial cytopathy.
- Paraneoplastic cerebellar degeneration: usually a subacute ataxic syndrome.
- Iatrogenic cadaveric human growth hormone-induced Creutzfeldt–Jakob disease: a drug history of hormonal therapy should be taken from all young well-muscled, or previously well-muscled, patients and top athletes with cerebellar signs.
- Idiopathic late-onset cerebellar ataxia: age of onset 25–70 years (onset after 55 years: often a relatively pure midline cerebellar syndrome with marked gait ataxia, mild appendicular ataxia).

- Other spinocerebellar degenerations (see Friedreich's ataxia, p.441).
- Progressive supranuclear palsy (dementia and supranuclear ophthalmoplegia).

INVESTIGATIONS

- Blood DNA analysis using PCR for gene mutations, commonly CAG repeat expansions, on chromosomes 3,6,11,12,14,16,19.
- Cranial CT or, preferably, MRI scan of the brain and craniocervical junction: pronounced cerebellar atrophy, particularly affecting the superior vermis (**558–560**).
- Full blood count and film.
- Urea and electrolytes, plasma cortisol, very long chain fatty acids (in males, adrenoleukodystrophy).
- Thyroid function tests.
- Liver function tests (alcoholic cerebellar degeneration).
- VDRL, TPHA.
- Vitamin B_{12} and vitamin E.
- Plasma lactate and pyruvate, mitochondrial DNA analysis (mitochondrial cytopathy).
- Plasma copper, ceruloplasmin (Wilson's disease).

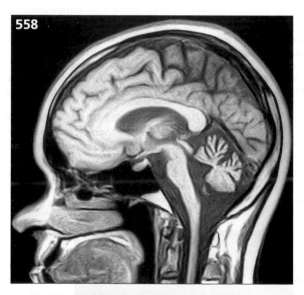

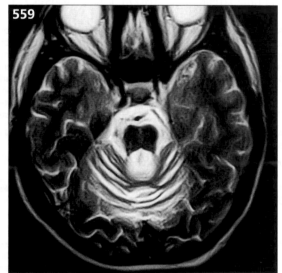

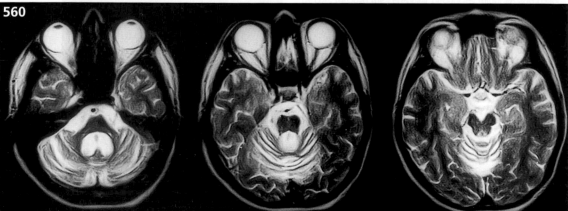

558–560 T1W midline sagittal (**558**) and T2W axial (**559, 560**) MRI of the brain in a patient with autosomal dominantly inherited cerebellar ataxia due to a mutation of the gene for spinocerebellar ataxia 1 on chromosome 6 causing expansion of the trinucleotide CAG repeat. Scans show pronounced atrophy of the medulla, pons and cerebellum, particularly affecting the superior vermis.

- Alpha fetoprotein (ataxia telangiectasia).
- Antipurkinje cell antibodies (paraneoplastic syndrome).
- EKG, and if abnormal, echocardiograph.
- Nerve conduction studies and EMG.
- Visual evoked potentials and somatosensory evoked potentials.

DIAGNOSIS
Clinical syndrome of cerebellar ataxia, positive family history, and positive DNA analysis.

TREATMENT
Symptomatic rather than curative:
- Cholinergic agents: physostigmine, lecithin, and choline chloride.
- GABAergic drugs: baclofen and sodium valproate.
- Serotonergic compounds:
- L-5-hydroxytryptophan combined with a peripheral decarboxylase inhibitor.
- Buspirone hydrochloride, a serotonin (5-hydroxy-tryptamine^{1A}) agonist, 20 mg/day in four divided doses and increased by 5–10 mg/day up to 60 mg/day. Adverse effects include transient light-headedness and nausea.

PROGNOSIS
Gradually progressive.

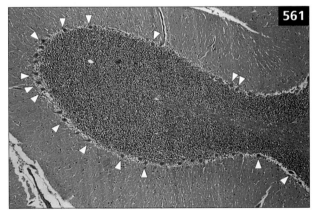

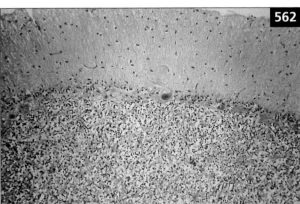

561, 562 Normal cerebellar cortex, H&E stain, with plentiful Purkinje cells (**561**, arrowheads), and higher magnification view of the cerebellar cortex of a patient with Freidreich's ataxia showing Purkinje cell loss (**562**).

FRIEDREICH'S ATAXIA

DEFINITION
An autosomal recessively inherited disease caused by a large increase in the number of trinucleotide GAA repeats within the first intron of the *FRDA* gene (X25) on the proximal long arm of chromosome 9. This results in decreased expression of the target protein frataxin, and dysfunction of the central and peripheral nervous systems and the heart. Clinically, Friedreich's ataxia is characterized by the onset before age 25 years of progressive limb and gait ataxia, cerebellar dysarthria, depressed deep tendon reflexes, pyramidal signs, distal vibration and proprioceptive sensory loss, axonal sensory neuropathy and often skeletal deformities and hypertrophic cardiomyopathy.

EPIDEMIOLOGY
- Prevalence: 2 per 100 000; the most common form of hereditary ataxia.
- Carrier frequency: 1 in 120 in European populations.
- Age: adolescence and early adult life. Onset usually occurs at 8–15 years.

PATHOLOGY
Nervous system
- Dorsal root ganglia: degeneration/loss of large sensory neurons
- Dying back of axons in:
- Large myelinated sensory nerve fibers in peripheral nerves.
- Posterior columns of the spinal cord.
- Nucleus gracilis and cuneatus, and the medial lemniscus.
- Dorsal and ventral spinocerebellar tracts.
- Corticospinal tracts: demyelination, with increasing involvement caudally.
- Cerebellum:
- Loss of Purkinje cells (**561, 562**).
- Degeneration of dentate nucleus.
- Axonal loss and demyelination of superior cerebellar peduncles.

Heart
Degeneration leading to hypertrophy and diffuse fibrosis.

Pancreas
Degeneration, giving rise to:
- Diabetes mellitus in about 10% of patients.
- Carbohydrate intolerance in an additional 20%.
- A reduced insulin response to arginine stimulation in all patients.

ETIOLOGY AND PATHOPHYSIOLOGY
Inheritance
Autosomal recessive.

Gene mutation
Friedrich's ataxia is due to a mutation in the *FRDA* gene (X25), which is located on the proximal long arm of chromosome 9 (9q13-q21.1). It has five exons spread over 40 kb that encode a novel 210-amino acid protein, named 'frataxin'. More than 95% of patients with classic Friedreich's ataxia are homozygous for the increase in GAA repeats, but a few have a combination of an increase in GAA repeats in one allele and a point mutation in the other allele,

Clinical

Korczyn AD (2001) Hallucinations in Parkinson's disease. *Lancet,* **358**: 1031–1032.

Winikates J, Jankovic J (1999) Clinical correlates of vascular parkinsonism. *Arch. Neurol.,* **56**: 98–102.

Treatment

De Bie RMA, de Haan RJ, Nijssen PCG, *et al.* (1999) Unilateral pallidotomy in Parkinson's disease: a randomized, single-blind, multicentre trial. *Lancet,* **354**: 1665–1669.

The Deep-brain Stimulation for Parkinson's Disease Study Group (2001) Deep-brain stimulation of the subthalamic nucleus or the pars interna of the globus pallidus in Parkinson's disease. *N. Engl. J. Med.,* **345**: 956–963.

Freed CR, Greene PE, Breeze RE, *et al.* (2001) Transplantation of embryonic dopamine neurons for severe Parkinson's disease. *N. Engl. J. Med.,* **344**: 710–719.

Friedman JH, Fernandez HH (2000) The non-motor problems of Parkinson's disease. *The Neurologist* **6**: 18–27.

Hely MA, Fung VSC, Morris JGL (2000) Treatment of Parkinson's disease. *J. Clin. Neurosci.,* **7**(6): 484–494.

Kieburtz K, Hubble J (2000) Benefits of comt inhibitors in levodopa-treated Parkinsonian patients. Results of clinical trials. *Neurology,* **55 (Suppl 4)**: S42–S45.

Marsh L, Dawson TM (2000) Treatment of early Parkinson's disease. *BMJ,* **321**: 1–2.

Munchau A, Bhatia KP (2000) Pharmacological treatment of Parkinson's disease. *Postgrad. Med. J.,* **76**: 602–610.

Parkinson Study Group (2000) Pramipexole vs levodopa as initial treatment for Parkinson Disease. *JAMA,* **284**: 1931–1938.

Quinn N (1999) Progress in functional neurosurgery for Parkinson's disease. *Lancet,* **354**: 1658–1659.

Schuurman PR, Bosch A, Bossuyt PMM, *et al.* (2000) A comparison of continuous thalamic stimulation and thalamotomy for suppression of severe tremor. *N. Engl. J. Med.,* **342**: 461–468.

Tanner CM (2000) Dopamine antagonists in early therapy for Parkinson Disease. Promise and Problems. *JAMA,* **284**: 1971–1973.

Complications

Agid Y, Chase T, Marsden D (1998) Adverse reactions to levodopa: drug toxicity or progression of disease? *Lancet,* **351**: 851–852.

Allain H, Schuck S, Mauduit N (2000) Depression in Parkinson's disease. *BMJ,* **320**: 1287–1288.

Chaudhuri KR, Clough C (1998) Subcutaneous apomorphine in Parkinson's disease. *BMJ,* **316**: 641.

Donnan PT, Steinke DT, Stubbings C, *et al.* (2001) Selegiline and mortality in subjects with Parkinson's disease. A longitudinal community study. *Neurology,* **55**: 1785–1789.

Fahn S (2000) The spectrum of levodopa-induced dyskinesias. *Ann. Neurol.,* **47** (Suppl 1): S2–S11.

Ferreira JJ, Rascol O (2000) Prevention and therapeutic strategies for levodopa-induced dyskinesias in Parkinson's disease. *Curr. Opin. Neurol.,* **13**: 431–436.

The Parkinson Study Group (1999) Low-dose clozapine for the treatment of drug-induced psychosis in Parkinson's disease. *N. Engl. J. Med.,* **340**: 757–763.

Rascol O (2000) Medical treatment of levodopa-induced dyskinesias. *Ann. Neurol.,* **47** (Suppl 1): S179–S188.

Rascol O, Brooks DJ, Korczyn AD, *et al.* (2000) A five-year study of the incidence of dyskinesia in patients with early Parkinson's disease who were treated with ropinirole or levodopa. *N. Engl. J. Med.,* **342**: 1484–1491.

DIFFUSE LEWY BODY DISEASE

Galasko D (1999) A clinical approach to dementia with Lewy bodies. *The Neurologist,* **5**: 247–257.

McKeith I, Del Ser T, Spano PF, *et al.* (2000) Efficacy of rivastigmine in dementia with Lewy bodies: a randomised, double-blind, placebo-controlled international study. *Lancet,* **356**: 2031–2036.

McKeith IG, Galasko D, Kosaka K, *et al.*, for the Consortium on Dementia with Lewy Bodies (1996) Consensus guidelines for the clinical and pathologic diagnosis of dementia with Lewy bodies (DLB): Report of the consortium on DLB international workshop. *Neurology,* **47**: 1113–1124.

McKeith IG, O'Brien JT, Ballard C (1999) Diagnosing dementia with Lewy bodies. *Lancet,* **354**: 1227–1228.

McKeith IG, Perry EK, Perry RH, for the Consortium on Dementia with Lewy Bodies (1999) Report of the second dementia with Lewy body international workshop. Diagnosis and treatment. *Neurology,* **53**: 902–905.

PROGRESSIVE SUPRANUCLEAR PALSY

Daniele A, Moro W, Bentivoglio AR (1999) Zolpidem in progressive supranuclear palsy. *N. Engl. J. Med.,* **341**: 543–544.

Golbe LI (2000) Progressive supranuclear palsy in the molecular age. *Lancet,* **356**: 870–871.

Morris HR, Wood NW, Lees AJ (1999) Progressive supranuclear palsy (Steele-Richardson-Olszewski disease). *Postgrad. Med. J.,* **75**: 579–584.

Schrag A, Ben-Shlomo Y, Quinn NP (1999) Prevalence of progressive supranuclear palsy and multiple system atrophy: a cross-sectional study. *Lancet,* **354**: 1771–1775.

MULTIPLE SYSTEM ATROPHY

Adams RD, Van Bogaert L, Van der Eecken H. (1964) Striato-nigral degeneration. *J. Neuropathol. Exp. Neurol.,* **23**: 584–608.

Ben-Shlomo Y, Wenning GK, Tison F, Quinn NP (1997) Survival of patients with pathologically proven multiple system atrophy: A meta-analysis. *Neurology,* **48**: 384–393.

Consensus Committee of the American Autonomic Society and the American Academy of Neurology (1996) Consensus statement on the definition of orthostatic hypotension, pure autonomic failure, and multiple system atrophy. *Neurology,* **46**: 1470.

Gilman S, Quinn NP (1996) The relationship of multiple system atrophy to sporadic olivopontocerebellar atrophy and other forms of late-onset cerebellar atrophy. *Neurology,* **46**: 1197–1199.

Graham JG, Oppenheimer DR (1969) Orthostatic hypotension and nicotine sensitivity in a case of multiple system atrophy. *J. Neurol. Neurosurg. Psychiatry,* **32**: 28–34.

Rehman HU (2001) Multiple system atrophy. *Postgrad. Med. J.,* **77**: 379–382.

Schrag A, Ben-Shlomo Y, Quinn NP (1999) Prevalence of progressive supranuclear palsy and multiple system atrophy: a cross-sectional study. *Lancet,* **354**: 1771–1775.

Shy GM, Drager GA (1960) A neurologic syndrome associated with orthostatic hypotension. *Arch. Neurol.,* **2**: 511–527.

Tu PH, Galvin JE, Baba M, *et al.* (1998) Glial cytoplasmic inclusions in white matter oligodendrocytes of multiple system atrophy brains containing insoluble alpha-synuclein. *Ann. Neurol.,* **44**: 415–422.

AUTOSOMAL DOMINANT CEREBELLAR ATAXIAS

Devos D, Schraen-Maschke S, Vuillaume I, *et al.* (2001) Clinical features and genetic analysis of a new form of spinocerebellar ataxia. *Neurology,* **56**: 234–238.

Durr A, Brice A (2000) Clinical and genetic aspects of spinocerebellar degeneration. *Curr. Opin. Neurol.,* **13**: 407–413.

Evidente VGH, Gwinn-Hardy KA, Caviness JN, Gilman S (2000) Hereditary ataxias. *Mayo Clin. Proc.,* **75**: 475–490.

Gosalakkal JA (2001) Ataxias of childhood. *The Neurologist,* **7**: 300–306.

Hurko O (1997) Recent advances in heritable ataxias. *Ann. Neurol.,* **41**: 4–6.

Jen J (2001) Atana and calcium channels. What a headache? *Arch. Neurol.,* **58**: 179–180.

Nagaoka U, Takashima M, Ishikawa K, *et al.* (2000) A gene on SCA4 locus causes dominantly inherited pure cerebellar ataxia. *Neurology,* **54**: 1971–1975

FRIEDREICH'S ATAXIA

Evidente VGH, Gwinn-Hardy KA, Caviness JN, Gilman S (2000) Hereditary ataxias. *Mayo Clin. Proc.,* **75**: 475–490.

Klockgether T (2000) Recent advances in degenerative ataxias. *Curr. Opin. Neurol.,* **13**: 451–455.

Pandolfo M (1999) Molecular pathogenesis of Friedreich's ataxia. *Arch. Neurol.,* **56**: 1201–1208.

Sherer T, Greenamyre JT (2000) A therapeutic target and biomarker in Friedreich's ataxia. *Neurology,* **55**: 1600–1601.

ATAXIA TELANGIECTASIA

Lewis RF, Lederman HM, Crawford TO (1999) Ocular motor abnormalities in ataxia telangiectasia. *Ann. Neurol.,* **46**: 287–295.

Acquired Metabolic Diseases of the Nervous System

HYPOXIC ENCEPHALOPATHY

DEFINITION
Brain dysfunction caused by a lack of oxygen to the brain as a result of failure of the circulation or respiration.

EPIDEMIOLOGY
- Incidence: uncommon.
- Age: middle-aged and elderly.
- Gender: either sex.

PATHOLOGY
Acute, global brain hypoxia (571–573)
- Laminar cortical necrosis (**571**): extensive, multifocal or diffuse, and almost invariably involving the hippocampus.
- Scattered small areas of infarction or neuronal loss may be present in the deep forebrain nuclei, hypothalamus or brainstem. Sometimes, relatively selective thalamic necrosis occurs.
- Most, if not all, of the gray matter of the cerebral, cerebellar and brainstem structures, and even the spinal cord is severely damaged if the hypoxia is severe enough and prolonged.

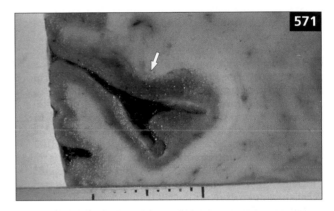

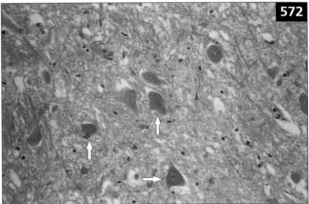

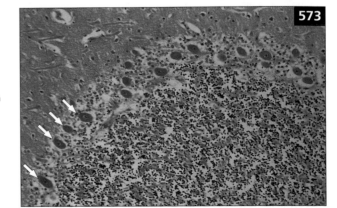

571 Section of the cerebral cortex showing laminar necrosis due to cerebral hypoxia (arrow). (Courtesy of Professor BA Kakulas, Royal Perth Hospital, Western Australia.)

572 Hypoxic neurons in the brain (arrows): swollen, more eosinophilic, indistinct outline, faint-staining nuclei, and loss of Nissl substance.

573 Hypoxic, eosinophilic purkinje cells in the cerebellum (arrows).

MRI brain
- Increased signal in the basal ganglia (particularly pallidum but midbrain may also be affected) on T1WI (**578, 579**).
- The substances which may cause an increased signal on T1WI include manganese, melanin, calcium, and blood. The differential diagnosis of increased signal in the basal ganglia on T1WI includes hyper-, hypo-, pseudohypo- and pseudopseudohypoparathyroidism (calcium), hyper-alimentation, Hallevorden–Spatz disease, carbon monoxide poisoning, hemorrhage and neurofibromatosis.

CSF
Usually normal apart from elevated levels of glutamine, the end product of cerebral ammonia metabolism.

Abdominal ultrasound
Size and echostructure of liver.

Liver biopsy (transjugular route)

DIAGNOSIS (Table 43)
There are two components to making the diagnosis:
- To determine that encephalopathy (subclinical or overt) is present.
- To establish hepatocellular insufficiency and increased portal-systemic shunting.

The diagnosis is based on the history, physical examination and laboratory findings.

TREATMENT
Treatment is determined by the underlying cause.

Hepatic encephalopathy due to the rare condition of acute liver failure is rapid in onset and progression, almost always complicated by cerebral edema in the later stages, and has a poor prognosis. Orthotopic liver transplantation should therefore be considered in these patients and meanwhile those who are grade 3 or 4 should be electively sedated with fentanyl, paralysed with atracurium, and ventilated to protect the airway and facilitate the management of cerebral edema by preventing surges in intracranial pressure related to psychomotor agitation. The cerebral edema is treated with mannitol given in repeated bolus injections of 0.5 g/kg body weight over a period of 10 minutes, and acetylcysteine can be given by continuous infusion to improve cerebral blood flow and metabolic rate for oxygen in grade 4 patients.

Hepatic encephalopathy due to the much more common chronic liver disease can be managed quite differently because it is usually due to a clinically apparent precipitating event (or combination of events), or to the spontaneous development of porto-systemic shunting, and because cerebral edema is much less frequent.

General
- Nasogastric tube.
- Central venous line.
- Indwelling urinary catheter.
- Monitor intracranial pressure (extradural monitor) if encephalopathy reaches grades 3 or 4.
- Avoid maneuvers that increase intracranial pressure (such as sensorial stimuli).
- Control restlessness.
- Hydrate carefully.
- Elevate patient's head 20–30°.
- Avoid (or use with extreme caution) drugs such as sedatives, phenytoin, phenobarbitone (phenobarbital), valproate, and dantrolene because drug metabolism and protein binding are frequently disturbed in liver disease.
- Avoid/be careful with benzodiazepines because plasma half-life of benzodiazepines is increased four- to fivefold in hepatic failure, so substantial toxicity may ensue (e.g. when used for endoscopy or nocturnal sedation).
- Avoid hypoglycemia (monitor blood glucose).

Specific
- Remove the underlying cause:
  - N-acetylcysteine for early paracetamol overdose.
  - Forced diuresis and activated charcoal for mushroom poisoning.
  - Acyclovir for herpes virus infection.
  - Surgery for acute hepatic-vein occlusion.

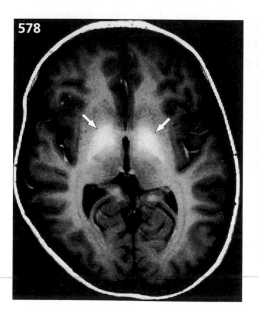

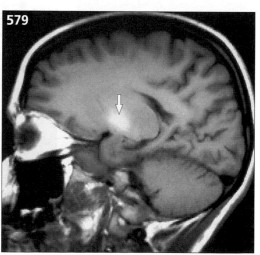

578, 579 T1W axial (**578**) and T1W sagittal (**579**) MRI of the brain in a patient with hepatic encephalopathy. Note the increased signal in the basal ganglia (arrows). (Courtesy of Dr R Gibson, Department of Neuroradiology, Western General Hospital, Edinburgh, UK.)

- Lower blood ammonia levels:
- Reduce ammonia production (restrict intake of dietary protein and inhibit urease-producing colonic bacteria). Low protein diet (20 g a day initially, increasing gradually later).
  Vegetable, rather than animal, protein diet.
  Carbohydrate enemas.
  Oral non-absorbable disaccharides: lactulose or lactisol (lactose 100 g daily in lactase deficiency): 30–60 g/day to produce 2–4 soft stools daily.
  Oral antibiotics: neomycin 6 g daily, metronidazole 800 mg daily, or rifaximin 1200 mg daily.
  Oral *Enterococcus faecium*.
- Increase ammonia metabolism: sodium benzoate 10 g daily; ornithine aspartate 9 g tds; phenylacetate.
- For patients who have previously been treated with benzodiazepines (e.g. for treatment of behavioral disturbance caused by hepatic encephalopathy), the administration of a benzodiazepine antagonist, such as flumazenil, may improve conscious level.
- Consider pharmacologic manipulation of glutaminergic and monoaminergic systems (experimental).
- If intracranial pressure exceeds 2.7–4 kPa (20–30 mmHg), apply hyperventilation (paCO$_2$ 3.3–4 kPa [25–30 mmHg]), then mannitol 0.5 g/kg in bolus; then hemodialysis or venovenous hemofiltration; then barbiturate coma.
- Orthotopic liver transplantation: acute liver failure; severe, refractory hepatic encephalopathy.

CLINICAL COURSE AND PROGNOSIS
- The encephalopathy usually evolves over a period of days to weeks and, if untreated, often terminates fatally. Sometimes the symptoms spontaneously regress completely or partially and may fluctuate in severity for several weeks or months.
- Most manifestations are reversible with medical treatment.
- Some patients have progressive debilitating neurologic syndromes such as dementia, spastic paraparesis, cerebellar degeneration, and extrapyramidal movement disorders that are associated with structural abnormalities of the CNS and were hitherto regarded as irreversible, but now may gradually improve after successful orthotopic liver transplantation.

CENTRAL PONTINE MYELINOLYSIS

DEFINITION
A disorder characterized by rapidly developing quadriparesis and a large, symmetric, demyelinating lesion of the greater part of the basis pontis. It may also affect extrapontine brain areas.

EPIDEMIOLOGY
- Prevalence: up to 0.25% of autopsies.
- Age: any age; reported in children (particularly those with severe burns) as well as adults.
- Gender: M=F.

PATHOLOGY
Demyelination occurs in the centre of the pons (**580**) and occasionally other parts of the brainstem.

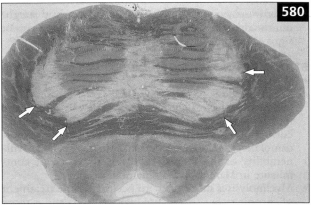

580 Transverse section of the pons showing demyelination of corticospinal tract fibers in the center of the basis pontis (arrows) with preserved neurons in the pontine nuclei and no evidence of inflammation.

Table 43 Grading system based on clinical and EEG features

Grade	Conscious level	Personality and intellect	Neurologic signs	EEG abnormalities
0	Normal	Normal	None	None
Subclinical	Normal	Normal	Only on psychometric testing	None
1	Inverted sleep pattern, restlessness	Forgetfulness, mild confusion, agitation, irritability	Tremor, apraxia, incoordination, impaired handwriting	Triphasic waves
2	Lethargy, slow responses	Disorientation in time, amnesia, disinhibited, inappropriate behavior	Asterixis, dysarthria, ataxia, hypoactive reflexes	Triphasic waves
3	Somnolent but rousable, confusion	Disorientated in place, aggressive behavior	Asterixis, rigidity, hyperactive reflexes, Babinski signs	Triphasic waves
4	Coma	None	Decerebration	Delta activity

Disorders of the CSF Circulation

HYDROCEPHALUS

DEFINITION
Hydrocephalus is defined as an increase in volume of the CSF in association with dilatation of the cerebral ventricles.

EPIDEMIOLOGY
- Incidence:
- Neonatal hydrocephalus: 1/1000 births.
- Adult hydrocephalus: depends on the incidence of precipitating causes (e.g. meningitis, subarachnoid hemorrhage); 1–2% of patients presenting to dementia clinics.
- In the UK: 3000 shunt operations annually (1500 new, 1500 recurrent).
- Prevalence (lifetime): 0.1 (95% CI: 0.01–0.3) per 1000.
- Age: any age.
- Gender: either sex.

PHYSIOLOGY OF CSF CIRCULATION
- CSF contains little protein; bicarbonate is its only buffer.
- The total volume of CSF in the cranial and spinal cavity of the adult is about 150 ml, of which about 30 ml is in the ventricular system.
- About 70% of CSF is actively secreted by the cells of the choroid plexus of the lateral, third and fourth ventricles and the remaining 30% comes from the brain's capillary bed and from metabolic water production.
- CSF is produced at a rate of 0.35 ml/min (500 ml/day), which is equivalent to a turnover of total CSF every 6 hours.
- The CSF flows slowly through the ventricular system and the foramina of Luschka and Magendie into the subarachnoid space and then up and over the cerebral convexities. Some of the fluid flows into the central canal of the spinal cord.
- Circulation of the CSF is achieved by arterial pulsation in the brain and choroid plexus, and by changes in posture, exercise and coughing, creating a pressure differential between the newly formed CSF and its site of drainage (a hydrostatic gradient).
- The CSF drains passively from the subarachnoid space into the venous system (principally the superior sagittal sinus) via the arachnoid granulations in the cranial and spinal compartments (open channels that connect the subarachnoid side to the venous side of the arachnoid villi).

- The primary function of the CSF is to provide buoyancy and allow the brain to float, protecting it from repetitive trauma whenever the head moves. Movement of CSF through the foramen magnum compensates for the changes that occur in cerebral blood volume with each heart beat.

ETIOLOGY
Overproduction of CSF
Rare, if ever (choroid plexus papilloma usually obstructs).

Obstruction to CSF outflow within the ventricles (obstructive hydrocephalus)
Congenital
- Aqueduct stenosis, with or without gliosis, 'forking' (in which the aqueduct is replaced by a number of small, inefficient channels), septum formation, or atresia. May be caused by mumps and possibly other intra-uterine infections.
- Dandy–Walker syndrome (atresia of the foramina of Luschka and Magendie associated with failure of development of the vermis of the cerebellum).
- Hind brain abnormalities, spina bifida.
- Vein of Galen aneurysm.

Space-occupying lesions
- Acquired aqueduct stenosis.
- Colloid and arachnoid cysts.
- Thalamic glioma.
- Intraventricular tumors.
- Tentorial herniation.
- Posterior fossa tumor, hemorrhage, infarct.
- Colloid cyst or tumor of the third ventricle.
- Basilar artery dolichoectasia.

Ventricular hemorrhage
- Prematurity.
- Aneurysm, arteriovenous malformation.

Defective flow in the subarachnoid space (communicating hydrocephalus)
- Meningitis:
- Pyogenic.
- Tuberculous.
- Fungal.
- Neoplastic.
- Subarachnoid hemorrhage.
- Hyperviscosity of CSF due to high CSF protein (e.g. spinal neurofibroma).

Defective absorption of CSF at the arachnoid granulations
- Congenital deficiency of arachnoid granulations (rare).
- Raised cerebral venous sinus pressure due to venous sinus thrombosis (controversial).

Idiopathic
Particularly in the elderly (see Normal pressure hydrocephalus, p.473).

Loss of brain tissue (hydrocephalus ex-vacuo)
Accumulation of CSF in the ventricular system and cerebral sulci due to loss of brain tissue as a result of atrophy, infarction and so on.

PATHOPHYSIOLOGY
Obstruction to CSF flow raises intraventricular pressure which reverses the direction of flow of CSF from the ventricles through the ependyma and into the periventricular brain parenchyma causing periventricular edema. It also reduces periventricular cerebral blood flow which, if not treated, results in periventricular demyelination and gliosis.

CLINICAL FEATURES
Infancy/early childhood
- Asymptomatic, or symptoms of irritability, poor appetite, vomiting, and poor head control.
- Rapid head enlargement (crossing percentile lines) with distortion of the normal proportions of the cranial cavity.
- Prominent scalp veins.
- Open, enlarged, tense fontanelle.
- Delayed fusion of sutures.
- 'Cracked-pot' tympanitic sound produced by percussion of the thinned skull (late).
- Brilliant transillumination of the skull (late sign).
- Delayed motor skills and milestones but alert.
- Papilledema (unusual in infants).
- Upward gaze and horizontal gaze paresis ('setting sun' eyes) occur, due to pressure of dilated third ventricle on the posterior commissure in the tectum of the midbrain.
- Paralysis or spasm of convergence.
- Spastic paraparesis with lower limb hyperreflexia and extensor plantar responses: the corticospinal tracts emanating from the parasagittal region of the motor cortex and destined for the legs have a long course around the lateral ventricles and tend to be most compressed and stretched by enlarged lateral ventricles.

N.B. Head circumference measurement should be compared with normal values on a standard head-size chart. Serial measurements which show a crossing of percentiles are important signs.

Transillumination of the skull with a torch held against the baby's head in a dark room reveals increased redness around the torch light in the presence of an excessive amount of fluid beneath the torch light.

Older children and adults (skull sutures have begun to fuse)
Raised intracranial pressure causing
- Headache, often worse in the early morning.
- Nausea and vomiting.
- Blurred vision, occasionally.
- Diplopia, due to VIth nerve palsy may occur.
- Papilledema sometimes; its absence does not exclude raised intracranial pressure.
- Optic atrophy with progressive visual loss and poor pupillary reaction to light: a late complication of chronic papilledema due to raised intracranial pressure.
- Upgaze paresis.
- Increasing unsteadiness of gait occurs, culminating in frequent falls due to a combination of ataxia, spasticity and dyspraxia of gait.
- Urgency of micturition and eventual incontinence.
- Personality change and behavioral disturbance.
- Dementia.
- Eventually, depressed consciousness.

Symptoms and signs of the primary obstructive lesion
For example, cerebellar signs of a posterior fossa tumor.

Elderly
Normal pressure hydrocephalus (NPH) syndrome
This is characterized clinically by Hakim's triad of gait apraxia, urinary incontinence and progressive dementia. Difficulty initiating movement, such as getting out of a chair, is characteristic (see p.473).

DIFFERENTIAL DIAGNOSIS
Infancy/early childhood
Enlarged head
- Achondroplasia.
- Rickets.
- Subdural hematoma.
- Megalencephaly (brain of excessive size and weight).

Transillumination of the head
Localized brain cysts.

Elderly
- Alzheimer's disease.
- Vascular (multi-infarct) dementia.
- Binswanger's disease.
- Parkinson's disease.
- Progressive supranuclear palsy.
- Multiple sclerosis.

INVESTIGATIONS
Imaging
The role of imaging is to:
- Exclude other causes of the patient's symptoms.
- Try to decide whether the hydrocephalus is obstructive (communicating or non-communicating) or non-obstructive.
- Follow-up patients being managed conservatively to check for the need for a shunt in future and in those who have been shunted to check for shunt failure.

If obstructive non-communicating hydrocephalus is diagnosed, it may be possible to identify the cause such as a third ventricular colloid cyst, posterior fossa tumor or aqueduct stenosis (**590, 591**). Communicating hydrocephalus can be identified when all the ventricles appear large but the basal cisterns are still patent (**592–597**). Non-communicating hydrocephalus is present when the lateral ± the third ventricle are much larger than the fourth ventricle. Meningitis and subarachnoid hemorrhage may cause either communicating or non-communicating hydrocephalus.

CT and MRI brain scan
In general, CT scan is satisfactory. In obstructive hydrocephalus it shows ventricular dilatation above the site of obstruction and possibly the causative lesion (e.g. tumor). If there is no obstruction to CSF flow then all ventricles will be dilated. The cortical sulci are usually compressed due to the rise in intracranial pressure. MRI is required, however, in particular circumstances such as the diagnosis of aqueduct stenosis, posterior fossa lesions, and malignant meningitis, to name but a few. For example, MRI of aqueduct stenosis shows disproportionate dilatation of the lateral and third ventricles and a small fourth ventricle. On midline sagittal MRI the aqueduct appears small. Bands or webs may be visible in the aqueduct causing obstruction. Normally the CSF flows through the aqueduct fast enough to result in a flow void on MRI, so the absence of a flow void (on carefully chosen sequences) is good corroborative evidence of aqueduct stenosis.

Usually, the temporal horns of the lateral ventricles are the first to dilate (this is a useful sign after subarachnoid hemorrhage as an early warning of possible complicating hydrocephalus). Note that the fourth ventricle is the last to dilate, so may appear small in communicating hydrocephalus simply because it has not yet had time to dilate. Therefore it can be very difficult to decide which sort of hydrocephalus is present on any imaging modality in some cases.

Periventricular white matter lucencies on CT and high signal on T2WI are common due to transependymal seepage of CSF usually sited around the angles of the lateral ventricles when due to hydrocephalus.

Other imaging methods
- Transfontanelle ultrasonography/echo-encephalography are safe, non-invasive methods of imaging and monitoring lateral ventricular size in infants and young children.
- Skull x-ray: children <10 years: large head and widened skull sutures; older children and adults (closed skull sutures): erosion of the dorsum sellae and clinoid processes (raised ICP).
- Radioactive cisternography, which is performed by injecting a radiopharmaceutic into the lumbar subarachnoid space, shows prolonged retention of the radioactive material within the ventricular system and impaired movement of radioactive material over the cerebral convexities.

CSF
CSF pressure is usually elevated, but may be normal in so-called NPH (see p.473). The appearance, cell count, protein and glucose are commonly normal, but may be abnormal in the presence of an underlying causal lesion (e.g. tumor, meningitis).

Intracranial pressure monitoring
A saline-filled catheter or catheter-tipped transducer inserted into the lateral ventricle, brain or subdural space records a pulsatile pressure of 0–1.3 kPa (0–10 mmHg) relative to the foramen of Monro when the patient is lying flat. As a mass or the ventricles enlarge within the skull, the mean intracranial pressure rises and spontaneous periodic waves become more pronounced, particularly during rapid eye movement sleep.

Non-invasive techniques include tympanic membrane displacement and transcranial doppler studies of the pulsatility index.

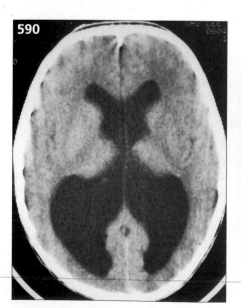

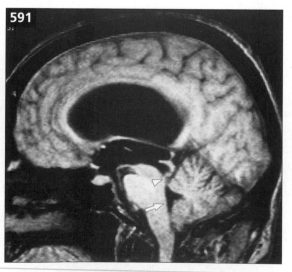

590, 591 CT brain scan at the level of the lateral ventricles (**590**) and T1W midline sagittal MR (**591**) in a patient with aqueduct stenosis. Note the large ventricles (obviously longstanding because there is no periventricular edema) with typical shape (**590**), the narrowed inferior aqueduct (**591**) (arrowhead) and the small fourth ventricle (arrow).

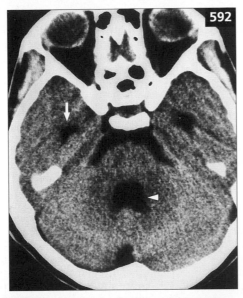

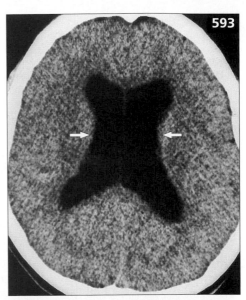

592–594 Communicating hydrocephalus. Cranial CT scans showing dilatation of the fourth ventricle (arrowhead) and temporal horns of the lateral ventricles (**592**, arrows), and lateral ventricles (**593**, arrows); and narrowing of the cortical sulci at the vertex of the brain (**594**, arrows).

595 MRI brain scan, T1W image, sagittal plane, showing dilated ventricular system without focal obstructive lesion.

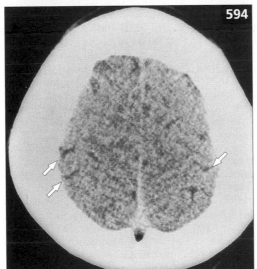

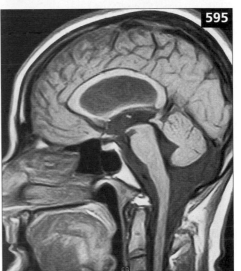

596 MRI brain scan, T2W image, axial plane, showing dilated lateral ventricles.

597 CT brain scan showing marked dilatation of the lateral ventricles in a patient with communicating hydrocephalus of unknown cause.

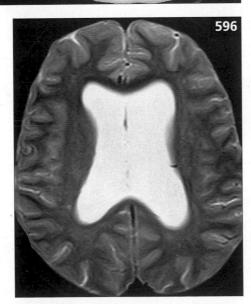

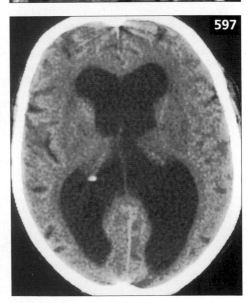

Cognitive function testing
- Mini-mental state examination and other mental screening tests are often insensitive to slight 'subcortical' cognitive impairment.
- Psychometric tests are usually needed, particularly to detect frontal lobe dysfunction.

TREATMENT
Indication
Neurologically symptomatic, progressive ventriculomegaly. The presence of ventriculomegaly in the absence of any supporting clinical features does not mean there is active hydrocephalus.

Treat underlying cause, if possible
Surgically excise the primary lesion if possible (i.e. papilloma of choroid plexus, or third ventricular or posterior fossa tumor).

Symptomatic treatment
Reduce CSF production
Carbonic anhydrase inhibitors (with or without corticosteroids or diuretics).

Facilitate CSF drainage (ventricular decompression with diversion of CSF flow)
- Transient hydrocephalus (e.g. after subarachnoid hemorrhage): ventricular or lumbar catheter for temporary CSF diversion.
- Non-communicating hydrocephalus with patent subarachnoid space: transventricular, endoscopic third ventriculostomy, with puncture of the floor of the third ventricle and drainage of CSF into the basal cisterns.
- Intraventricular or large arachnoid cysts: endoscopic communication of cyst with normal CSF pathways.
- Infantile hydrocephalus: ventriculoperitoneal or ventriculoatrial shunt (benefits about 80% of cases): CSF is drained from the frontal horn of the lateral ventricle (where there is no choroid to block the catheter) via a ventricular catheter (a pressure valve with reservoir mechanism and a distal catheter made of non-reactive tubing) into the peritoneal or atrial cavity.
- Communicating hydrocephalus (some patients): lumboperitoneal shunt: drains fluid from the lumbar subarachnoid space to the peritoneal cavity. These shunts usually work well for a few months only and, where they are successful, may be associated with symptomatic secondary descent of the cerebellar tonsils. Insertion of a separate ventricular access device at the time of shunting facilitates investigation should complications arise.
- Normal pressure hydrocephalus (see p.473):
- Removal of 50 ml of CSF may result in improvement in gait and predict a favorable response to a shunting procedure.
- Repeated lumbar punctures (LP), removing 15–20 ml CSF, may give rise to transient improvement in the early stages of the disease.
- Ventriculoperitoneal shunt may produce dramatic improvement in some cases. Improvement in post operative cognitive function is more likely if there was a known cause, and short history.

Shunt complications
- Shunt failure: 80% of shunts fail within 12 years. The highest risk of underdrainage is in the first year (30%), usually due to gradual occlusion of the ventricular catheters by choroid plexus. A CT brain scan is the best investigation for suspected underdrainage to compare with earlier scans.
- Shunt occlusion/blockage causing raised intracranial pressure.
- Overdrainage: particularly in tall patients. May produce slit ventricle syndrome, subdural hematomas, encysted fourth ventricles or post-shunt craniosynostosis.
- Infection of the valve: 70% occur within 1 month of insertion, often due to contamination at the time of insertion with *Staphylococcus epidermidis*. Commonly presents as intermittent pyrexia with malaise and signs of shunt obstruction. Occasionally there is cellulitis along the shunt tract or signs of meningitis. Diagnose by aspirating CSF from the shunt reservoir. Intrathecal vancomycin may eradicate the infection but often the entire shunt system has to be removed, followed by a period of external ventricular drainage before a new system can be re-inserted. The morbidity/mortality rate is 30–40% and survivors risk neurologic deficit.
- Subdural hematoma.
- Low pressure headache.
- Epileptic seizures.
- Shunt nephritis (an immunologically mediated disorder due to secondary *Staphylococcus albus* infection).
- Pulmonary thromboembolism with ventriculoatrial shunts.

PROGNOSIS
- Depends on the underlying condition.
- Untreated cases of infantile hydrocephalus develop necrosis of the scalp with leakage of CSF, infection, and death. A minority survive to childhood with arrested hydrocephalus characterized by enlargement of the head, some degree of intellectual handicap, limb spasticity, and impaired bladder function.
- 70% of infants with treated non-tumoral hydrocephalus maintain a normal IQ and attend a normal school. Children with infantile hydrocephalus should therefore undergo a shunting procedure (because they will benefit).

NORMAL PRESSURE HYDROCEPHALUS (NPH)

DEFINITION
A chronic hydrodynamic hydrocephalus that occurs in adults and is associated with a delay in the circulation or absorption of CSF and progressive neurologic deficit comprising Hakin's triad of gait apraxia, urinary incontinence, and progressive dementia. First described in 1965.

EPIDEMIOLOGY
- Prevalence: about 1 per 20 000 population. About 0–6% of cases of dementia.
- Age: middle-aged and elderly.
- Gender: M=F.

PATHOLOGY
- Impaired CSF flow within the ventricles or in the subarachnoid space (arachnoid villi) due to a variety of possible causes (see below).
- There is no pressure gradient between the ventricles and the cerebral convexity.

ETIOLOGY AND PATHOPHYSIOLOGY
Uncertain. The following are hypotheses:

Impairment of CSF flow within the ventricles or the subarachnoid space
- Non-communicating NPH: partial obstruction to CSF flow (e.g. aqueduct stenosis).
- Communicating NPH: impairment of CSF flow distal to the fourth ventricle, most often at the level of the basal cisterns ('cisternal block') or arachnoid villi.

Causes
- Idiopathic (at least 30%, probably about 50%).
- Subarachnoid hemorrhage.
- Meningitis.
- Head trauma.
- Intracranial surgery.
- Paget's disease of the skull.
- Mucopolysaccharidosis of the meninges.

N.B. Idiopathic cases have traditionally been attributed to defective CSF absorption through the arachnoid villi, but evidence is lacking. More recently, the theory of a vascular leukoencephalopathy has been proposed, with the concept that white matter lesions reduce periventricular tissue strength and elastic properties and thus predispose the ventricles to dilate under CSF pulse pressure. Systemic hypertension is frequently associated with NPH and is thought to lead to ventricular enlargement because of decreased CSF absorption due to increased superior sagittal sinus venous pressure and because of increased intraventricular pulse pressure from the choroid plexus. Other possibilities include congenital hydrocephalus becoming symptomatic in elderly persons and increasing age.

Episodes of slightly raised CSF pressure

CLINICAL FEATURES
Classic triad of:
- Slowly progressive gait disorder.
- Impairment of mental function.
- Urinary incontinence.

Gait disturbance
The first, and in some cases only, apparent symptom and sign:
- Difficulty in initiating walking: feet feel 'glued to the floor', also referred to as a 'magnetic gait' or gait apraxia.
- Postural instability.
- A short-stepped shuffling gait in more advances stages, often described as 'gait apraxia' but this term is perhaps inappropriate in NPH because patients with NPH may execute nearly intact walking movements when minimally supported or when lying down.
- Hyperreflexia (mainly in the lower limbs) and extensor plantar responses may be present but spasticity is not a feature (tone is usually normal) and objective motor weakness is seldom present (despite complaints of weakness and tiredness).

Causes
- Stretching or destruction of the paraventricular corticospinal fibers.
- Disconnection of basal ganglia from the frontal cortex.
- Uninhibited antigravity reflexes and co-contraction of agonists and antagonists during walking.

Progressive mental impairment
'Subcortical' dementia
- Forgetfulness.
- Inertia.
- Inattention.
- Decreased speed of processing complex information.
- Impaired ability to manipulate acquired knowledge.
- Delayed recall is severely impaired but delayed recognition is only relatively mildly affected or even normal.

Cause
- Compromise of the functional integrity of the frontal lobes and its connections.
- Unlikely to be caused by enlarged temporal horns and hippocampal dysfunction.

Urinary urgency and incontinence
- Urgency of micturition: almost always present.
- Urinary incontinence: a late sign.

Cause
Damaged periventricular pathways to the sacral bladder center, resulting in decreased inhibition of bladder contractions and hyperreflexia and instability of the bladder detrusor muscle, without concomitant defective sphincter control. Urinary incontinence is not due to a so-called 'incontinence sans gene' except in the most severe forms, when bladder hyperreflexia is associated with lack of concern for micturition, due to severe frontal lobe dysfunction.

Clinical features are probably due to hydrocephalic compression and stretching of the periventricular arterioles and venules, leading to a state of 'misery perfusion' characterized by diminished periventricular blood flow that is sufficient to result in axonal dysfunction but not enough

COMPLICATIONS
Visual loss
- 15–50% of patients.
- May occur early or late.
- May be sudden or gradually progressive.
- May be asymptomatic.
- Visual loss is probably due to a nerve conduction defect related to the status of axoplasmic flow found in papilledema. It is avoidable with appropriate monitoring and treatment.

PROGNOSIS
- Not well known.
- Often self-limiting; many people recover spontaneously in a few weeks and most people experience spontaneous resolution in 6–18 months, but it is a chronic process in some.

TREATMENT
Early detection and prevention of vision loss
Medical
- Avoid or correct predisposing factors (see above): weight reduction if obese.
- Serial LPs: if symptoms persist after initial LP perform 3–4 LPs within the first 2–4 weeks; further LPs are unlikely to help.

Pharmacologic
- Acetazolamide (Diamox), a carbonic anhydrase inhibitor which inhibits CSF production: start with oral dose of 250 mg four times a day and increase to 500 mg four times daily unless adverse effects develop (paresthesias, drowsiness, nausea, malaise, metabolic acidosis, altered taste, and renal calculi).
- Other diuretics: chlorthalidone 100 mg oral, daily; frusemide (furosemide), glycerol (but may cause weight gain).
- Corticosteroids: prednisone 40–60 mg/day for 10–14 days, and taper over the next 2 weeks.
- Anticoagulation if a secondary venous sinus thrombosis is present.

Surgical
If vision loss is severe initially or progresses in spite of medical treatment:
- Optic nerve sheath decompression by fenestration is the treatment of choice as it is reasonably safe with very few complications.
- Lumboperitoneal shunting (the insertion of a shunt from the spinal subarachnoid space to the peritoneum) has a higher risk of complications and failure.

FURTHER READING

NORMAL PRESSURE HYDROCEPHALUS (NPH)
Chen IH, Huang CI, Liu HC, Chen KK (1994) Effectiveness of shunting in patients with normal pressure hydrocephalus predicted by temporary, controlled-resistance, continuous lumbar drainage: a pilot study. *J. Neurol. Neurosurg. Psychiatry*, **57**: 1430–1432.

Evidente VH, Gwinn KA (1997) 73-year-old man with gait disturbance and imbalance. *Mayo Clin. Proc.*, **72**: 165–168.

Graff-Radford NR (1999) Normal pressure hydrocephalus. *The Neurologist*, **5**: 194–204.

Pleasure SJ (1999) Ventricular volume and transmural pressure gradient in normal pressure hydrocephalus. *Arch. Neurol.*, **56**: 1199–1200.

Vanneste JAL (1994) Three decades of normal pressure hydrocephalus: are we wiser now? *J. Neurol. Neurosurg. Psychiatry*, **57**: 1021–1025.

IDIOPATHIC INTRACRANIAL HYPERTENSION (IIH)
Bond DW, Charlton CPJ (2001) Benign intracranial hypertension secondary to nasal fluticasone propionate. *BMJ*, **322**: 897.

Brazis PW, Lee AG (1998) Elevated intracranial pressure and pseudotumor cerebri. *Curr. Opin. Ophthalmol.*, **9**: VI:27–32.

Digre KB, Corbett JJ (2001) Idiopathic intracranial hypertension (pseudotumor cerebri): a reappraisal. *The Neurologist*, **7**: 2–67.

Go KG (2000) Pseudotumour cerebri. Incidence, management and prevention. *CNS Drugs*, **14**: 33–49.

Karahalios DG, Rekate HL, Khayata MH, Apostolides PJ (1996) Elevated intracranial venous pressure as a universal mechanism in pseudotumor cerebri of varying etiologies. *Neurology*, **46**: 198–202.

King JO, Mitchell PJ, Thomson KR, Tress BM (1995) Cerebral venography and manometry in idiopathic intracranial hypertension. *Neurology*, **45**: 2224–2228.

Radhakrishnan K, Ahlskog E, Garrity JA, Kurland LT (1994) Idiopathic intracranial hypertension. *Mayo Clin. Proc.*, **69**: 169–180.

Walker RWH (2001) Idiopathic intracranial hypertension: any light on the mechanism of the raised pressure? *J. Neurol. Neurosurg. Psychiatry*, **71**: 1–7.

Cranial Neuropathies

OLFACTORY (IST CRANIAL NERVE) NEUROPATHY

DEFINITION
Disorder of the 1st cranial, or olfactory, nerve resulting in a disturbance of smell sensation (anosmia).

ANATOMY
- Nerve fibers subserving the sense of smell have their cells of origin in the mucous membrane of the upper and posterior parts of the nasal cavity.
- The olfactory mucosa contains three types of cells:
- Olfactory or receptor cells.
- Sustentacular or supporting cells.
- Basal cells, which are stem cells and the source of both olfactory (receptor) cells and sustentacular cells during regeneration.
- The olfactory or receptor cells are bipolar neurons that each have a peripheral process (the olfactory rod), from which project 10–30 fine hairs, or cilia, and several central processes (or olfactory filia) which are fine unmyelinated fibers that converge to form small fascicles enwrapped by Schwann cells and pass through openings in the cribriform plate of the ethmoid bone into the olfactory bulb. Collectively, the central processes of the olfactory receptor cells constitute the 1st cranial, or olfactory, nerve.
- In the olfactory bulb, the axons of the receptor cells synapse with mitral cells, the dendrites of which form brush-like terminals or olfactory glomeruli.
- The axons of the mitral cells enter the olfactory tract, which courses along the olfactory groove of the cribriform plate to the brain.
- The olfactory tract divides into medial and lateral olfactory striae. The medial striae contains fibers from the anterior olfactory nucleus which pass to the opposite side via the anterior commissure. Fibers in the lateral striae originate in the olfactory bulb, give off collaterals to the anterior perforated substance, and terminate in the medial and cortical nuclei of the amygdaloid complex and the prepiriform area (the lateral olfactory gyrus). The latter represents the primary olfactory cortex, which occupies a restricted area on the anterior end of the hippocampal gyrus and uncus (area 34 of Brodmann).
- Thus, olfactory impulses reach the cerebral cortex without relay through the thalamus; a unique feature among the sensory systems.
- From the prepiriform cortex, fibers project to the neighboring entorhinal cortex (area 28 of Brodmann), the medial dorsal nucleus of the thalamus, and the hypothalamus.
- Olfactory stimuli and emotional stimuli are thus strongly linked, as a result of their common roots in the limbic system. Yet, the ability to recall an odor is nowhere near as good as the ability to recall sounds and sights.

PHYSIOLOGY
- During quiet breathing, little of the air entering the nostril reaches the olfactory mucosa; sniffing carries the air into the olfactory crypt.
- To be perceived as an odor, an inhaled substance must be volatile – i.e. spread in the air as very small particles, and soluble in water or lipid.
- Intensity of olfactory sensation is determined by the frequency of firing of afferent neurons.
- Quality of odor is probably determined by 'cross fiber' activation, since the individual receptor cells are responsive to a wide range of odors and exhibit different types of responses to stimulants.

ETIOLOGY
Nasal
Odorants do not reach the olfactory receptors
Nasal obstruction or inflammation (rhinitis) is by far the most common cause.

Olfactory neuroepithelial
Destruction of receptors or their axon filaments
Congenital absence or hypoplasia of primary receptor neurons:
- Kallman syndrome (congenital anosmia and hypogonadotropic hypogonadism).
- Albino.

Disruption of the delicate filaments of the receptor cells as they pass through the cribriform plate:
- Head injury, particularly if severe enough to cause skull fracture (**608**). Less common with closed head injury. The damage may be unilateral or bilateral.
- Cranial surgery.
- Subarachnoid hemorrhage.
- Chronic meningitis.

Central
Olfactory pathway lesions
- Inferior frontal tumor compressing the olfactory tracts (e.g. olfactory groove meningioma).
- Large aneurysm of the anterior cerebral or anterior communicating artery.
- Anterior meningoencephalocele (CSF rhinorrhea may be present in certain head positions).
- Meningitis.
- Refsum's disease (hereditary ataxic neuropathy).
- Sarcoidosis.

Parkinson's disease

Multiple sclerosis

Idiopathic
Usually bilateral but can be unilateral.

CLINICAL FEATURES
- Smell should be tested with an aromatic odor, such as an orange or cordial bottle top, and not with an acrid odor, such as ammonia.
- Associated signs, such as unilateral optic atrophy and contralateral papilledema (Foster–Kennedy syndrome) may be present in conditions such as olfactory groove meningioma which extends posteriorly to involve the ipsilateral optic nerve and also causes raised intracranial pressure and papilledema.

Quantitative abnormalities of olfaction
Bilateral loss or reduction of the sense of smell (anosmia, hyposmia)
Commonly, but not always, recognized by the patient. It may present as impaired taste. Indeed, the patient with bilateral anosmia is usually convinced that the sense of taste has been lost as well (ageusia), because taste depends largely on the volatile particles in foods and beverages, which reach the olfactory receptors through the nasopharynx, and the perception of flavor is a combination of smell and taste. However, these patients are able to distinguish the elementary taste sensations (sweet, sour, bitter and salty).

Unilateral loss or reduction of the sense of smell (anosmia, hyposmia)
Seldom, if ever, recognized by the patient.

DIFFERENTIAL DIAGNOSIS
Quantitative abnormalities of olfaction
Loss or reduction of the sense of smell (anosmia, hyposmia)
- Unilateral anosmia. Hysteria: anosmia, if unilateral, may be on the same side as other symptoms such as anesthesia, blindness or deafness. Hysterical anosmics don't usually complain of loss of taste whereas true anosmics do, but actually show normal taste sensation on testing.

- Bilateral anosmia:
- Nasal obstruction or inflammation (rhinitis).
- Hysteria.

Qualitative abnormalities of olfaction
Distortions or illusions of smell (dysosmia or parosmia)
- Local nasopharyngeal conditions (e.g. empyema of the nasal sinuses).
- Depression.

Olfactory hallucinations or delusions
- Temporal lobe disease: complex partial seizures, anterior temporal lobectomy.
- Psychiatric disease: schizophrenia, depression.

Loss of olfactory discrimination
- Alcoholics with Korsakoff's psychosis (degeneration of neurons in the higher order olfactory systems of the medial temporal and thalamic regions).
- Temporal lobe disease: complex partial seizures, anterior temporal lobectomy.

Reduced odor recognition
- Alzheimer's disease.
- Huntington's disease.

INVESTIGATIONS
Determined by the clinical findings:
- CT or MRI brain scan.
- CSF examination.
- EEG.

TREATMENT
Remove the underlying cause, if possible.

PROGNOSIS
Depends on the cause. Anosmia due to head injury causing skull fracture is usually permanent. Anosmia due to closed head injury recovers in about one-quarter of patients.

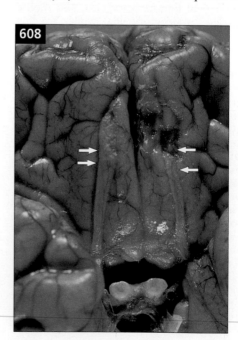

608 Ventral surface of the frontal lobes of the brain at autopsy showing disruption of the olfactory nerves bilaterally (arrows) due to traumatic brain injury.

OPTIC (IIND CRANIAL NERVE) NEUROPATHY

DEFINITION
Disorder of the optic (IInd cranial) nerve.

EPIDEMIOLOGY
Quite common.

ANATOMY
Nerve fibers from retinal nerve cells lying on the choroid at the back of the eye come straight forward and then angle sharply to run across the surface of the retina towards the optic nerve head (optic disc) where they enter the optic nerve. The macula, situated to the temporal side of the optic nerve head, is the most critical part of the retina because it is responsible for central vision. It consists of a very densely packed mass of cells. These nerve cells are particularly sensitive to a variety of toxins and, if damaged, lead to a centrocecal scotoma. Fibers from the macula form the papillomacular bundle as they shift sideways en mass and enter the temporal half of the optic disc. As they pass backwards along the optic nerve, they gradually becoming more central.

At the optic chiasm the fibers in the lateral half of the optic nerve, coming from the lateral (temporal) half of the retina, pass straight back into the optic tract on the same side. The fibers in the medial half of the optic nerve, coming from the medial (nasal) half of the retina cross (decussate) in the chiasm and pass back into the optic tract on the opposite side. However, before doing so, the fibers from the inferior nasal retina (receiving visual information from the upper temporal field), having crossed the anterior inferior optic chiasm, then loop forwards into the posterior part of the opposite optic nerve before turning back to pass in the lateral chiasm and optic tract. Consequently, pressure in the posterior optic nerve can cause not only an ipsilateral blind eye but also a small defect in the upper temporal field of the opposite eye (the anterior chiasmal syndrome). The function of the chiasm is to bring the information from the halves of each retina that look to the right and the halves of each retina that look to the left together in the same optic tract.

In the optic tract the fibers serving the identical point of each of the two retinae have to come together. The fibers in the anterior part of the optic tract rotate inwards through 90°, which brings the fibers in the lower and upper fields together in the medial and lateral halves of the tract respectively. In the posterior part of the optic tract the fibers fan out towards the six layers of the geniculate body, allowing the adjacent fibers from each retina to interdigitate. The macula fibers occupy a large central wedge of the geniculate body, with the lower fields being represented medially and the upper fields laterally.

Fibers from the lateral geniculate body sweep into the hemisphere in two fan-shaped projections, which later come together at the occipital cortex.

The lower fibers of the optic radiation (subserving the contralateral upper visual field) sweep forward into the anterior temporal lobe as Meyer's loop. The upper fibers of the optic radiation (subserving the contralateral lower visual field) follow a more direct route back into the parietal lobe. All fibers then sweep back in the deep white matter of the occipital lobe and terminate in the calcarine (visual) cortex astride the calcarine fissure.

The cells subserving the upper visual fields (i.e. lower retinae) lie in the lower half of the calcarine cortex, and those subserving the lower fields (i.e. upper retinae) are in the upper half of the cortex. The cells subserving the peripheral (temporal) visual fields are represented anteriorly (hence the finding of a temporal crescent visual field defect with an anterior striate cortex lesion), and those subserving macular vision are concentrated at the extreme tip of the occipital lobe. The longitudinal extent of the calcarine cortex is important in permitting striking localized visual field defects that may occur as a result of lesions (usually vascular) in this area.

ETIOLOGY AND PATHOPHYSIOLOGY
Optic nerve lesion
Optic nerve: unilateral
Sudden monocular visual failure:
- Ischemia: ischemic optic neuropathy (see p.487).
- Demyelination: optic neuritis (see p.488).
- Cavernous sinus thrombosis.
- Carotico-cavernous fistula.

Progressive monocular visual failure:
- Optic neuritis.
- Tumor of the orbit or optic nerve: optic nerve astrocytoma, optic sheath meningioma.
- Dysthyroid eye disease.
- Paget's disease of the skull: obstruction of foramina leading to optic atrophy.
- Anterior communicating artery aneurysm: compression of optic nerve.
- Irradiation.
- Tolosa–Hunt syndrome.
- Meningovascular syphilis.
- Subacute and chronic meningitis.

Optic nerve (bilateral) or optic chiasm
Sudden binocular visual failure:
- Bilateral ischemic optic neuropathy.
- Pituitary apoplexy.
- Raised intracranial pressure causing bilateral severe papilledema.

Sensory (tongue taste) innervation

- The sensory component of the facial nerve is small (the nervus intermedius of Wrisberg); it conveys taste sensation from the anterior two-thirds of the tongue and probably cutaneous sensation from the anterior wall of the external auditory canal.
- The taste fibers from the anterior two-thirds of the tongue first traverse the lingual nerve (a branch of the mandibular nerve) and then diverge to join the chorda tympani (a branch of the VIIth cranial nerve); thence they pass through the pars intermedia and geniculate ganglion of the VIIth nerve to the rostral part of the nucleus of the tractus solitarius in the medulla.
- Secretomotor fibers innervate the lacrimal gland through the greater superficial petrosal nerve and the sublingual and submaxillary glands through the chorda tympani.

ETIOLOGY
Brainstem
- Stroke.
- Pontine glioma.
- MS.
- Abscess.

Cerebello-pontine angle
- Acoustic neuroma.
- Meningioma.

Geniculate ganglion
Herpes zoster (Ramsay Hunt syndrome) (**638–640**).

Facial canal
Bell's palsy (see p.515).

Petrous temporal bone
- Trauma: fracture.
- Infection: *Pseudomonas aeruginosa*.
- Tumor: metastatic, invasive meningioma.

Facial nerve branches
- Parotid gland tumor or infection.
- Trauma: facial lacerations.
- Leprosy.

Facial mononeuropathy
- Ischemic: small vessel disease (e.g. vasculitis).
- Sarcoidosis.
- Behçet's syndrome.
- Sjögren's syndrome.
- Syphilis.
- Lyme disease.

CLINICAL HISTORY
Rate of onset of weakness
- Sudden or rapid onset within hours suggests trauma or a vascular etiology such as stroke or peripheral ischemic neuropathy if the weakness is unilateral, and Guillain–Barré syndrome if the weakness is bilateral.
- Subacute or gradual onset over days or weeks is most likely idiopathic (Bell's palsy) or the result of an infection or weakness.

Associated neurologic symptoms
- Ipsilateral hemiparesis, hemisensory loss, hemineglect, hemianopia suggest a supranuclear (upper motor neuron) facial palsy.
- Contralateral hemiparesis, ipsilateral limb ataxia, facial numbness and gaze palsy to the side of the facial weakness may be signs of an intra-axial low pontine lesion and indicate a nuclear/infranuclear (lower motor neuron) facial neuropathy.
- Ipsilateral sensorineural deafness indicates a lesion in the ipsilateral brainstem, cerebello-pontine angle or petrous temporal bone because of the close proximity of the vestibulocochlear nerve (see p.517).
- Ipsilateral reduced corneal reflex and ataxia are suggestive of a cerebello-pontine angle lesion. The corneal reflex can be assessed when ipsilateral paralysis of eyelid closure is present by asking the patient if a stimulus is felt, and by observing the normal consensual closure of the opposite eyelid and the upward roll of the eyeball when the cornea is touched on the paralysed side. The last sign ('Bell's phenomenon') is also apparent when the patient attempts to close the eye forcefully and is a normal event, albeit usually invisible.
- Ptosis is not found with isolated facial nerve lesions and, if present, may indicate a Horner's syndrome or an oculomotor nerve lesion.
- Vesicles in the external ear canal and on the palate are suggestive of herpes zoster infection.
- Altered taste and hyperacusis suggest a lesion of the facial nerve in the facial canal (e.g. Bell's palsy). However, Bell's palsy should not be diagnosed if deafness, reduced corneal reflex or ptosis are present.
- Otitis, trauma, and steadily worsening facial weakness suggest a lesion of the facial nerve in the petrous temporal bone.
- Parotid mass or trauma suggest a lesion of facial nerve branches.
- Peripheral nervous system signs such as sensory disturbances in the distal extremities suggest a lower motor neuron facial palsy.

Pre-existing medical conditions which could cause or predispose to facial weakness
Risk factors for ischemic stroke and ischemic neuropathy:
- Increasing age.
- Hypertension.
- Cigarette smoking.
- Hypercholesterolemia.
- Diabetes mellitus.

Ear and parotid gland infections

Head trauma with basal skull fracture

Malignancy

PHYSICAL EXAMINATION
- Drooping of one side of the face with flattening of the forehead creases, widening of the palpebral fissure, flattening of the nasolabial fold, lowering of the corner of the mouth, and impaired smiling and grinning are observed at rest.
- The eye may be red and dry as a result of impaired blinking or decreased lacrimation.

- The patient is unable to elevate the eyebrow, wrinkle the forehead, and close the eye on the affected side.
- Air escapes between the lips on the affected side when the cheeks are puffed with air.
- Emotional facial movements are also impaired.
- Corneal reflex is impaired because the lesion affects the efferent part of this reflex arc.
- Taste may be impaired if the facial nerve is lesioned proximal to the chorda tympani nerve branch, within the temporal bone, which carries taste sensation from the anterior two-thirds of the tongue.
- Speech is usually slurred (flaccid dysarthria).
- Sounds may be exaggerated (hyperacusis) if the facial nerve is lesioned proximal to the stapedius nerve branch in the temporal bone, which supplies the ipsilateral stapedius muscle to dampen loud sounds.
- Associated CNS, cranial nerve, or peripheral nervous system signs may be present such as hemisensory loss on the contralateral side or gaze palsy on the same side as the lower motor neuron facial weakness (suggesting a low pontine lesion), multiple cranial neuropathies (suggesting basilar meningitis or vasculitis) or sensory disturbances in the distal extremities or muscle wasting (which may indicate an underlying neuropathy).

- Otoscopy of the external auditory canal may reveal signs of infections and tumors in the tympanic cavity which could be relevant (e.g. vesicles of the external ear suggest herpetic facial neuropathy [Ramsay Hunt syndrome] [**639**]). Examination of the oral cavity may reveal vesicles on the palate in patients with Ramsay Hunt syndrome (**640**).

N.B. The distinction between upper and lower motor neuron facial weakness made on examination is very reliable if made during acute weakness. However, after a partial recovery has occurred, lower motor neuron facial weakness may occasionally resemble upper motor neuron weakness.

SPECIAL FORMS
Ramsay Hunt syndrome (herpes zoster facial paresis)
- Reactivation of the varicella-zoster virus.
- Otalgia.
- Hearing loss.
- Vesicles in the external ear canal and palate (**639, 640**), from which varicella-zoster virus can be easily recovered.
- Seroconversion is common, with an increase in specific antibody to VZV.
- Worse prognosis than Bell's palsy.
- Treat with oral antiviral agents: aciclovir (acyclovir), famcyclovir, valaciclovir (valacyclovir).

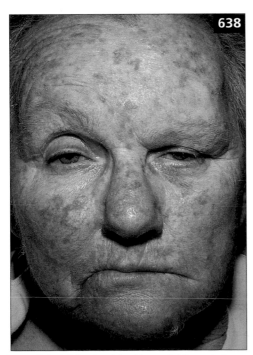

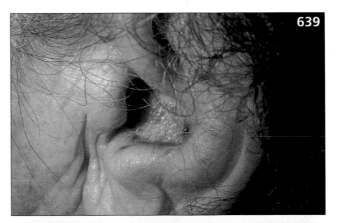

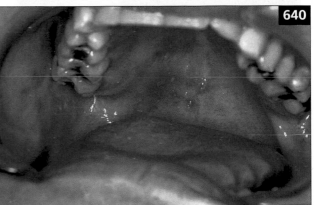

638, 639 Weakness of the left forehead (and lower facial muscles) on attempts to raise the eyebrows (**638**) and herpetic skin rash involving the external ear (**639**) due to herpes zoster infection (Ramsay Hunt syndrome) of the left facial nerve.

640 Vesicles on the right side of the palate due to varicella-zoster virus infection in a patient with a right lower motor neuron facial palsy due to varicella-zoster virus infection (Ramsay Hunt syndrome).

DIFFERENTIAL DIAGNOSIS

- Intramedullary spinal cord tumor (primary or secondary): rapid course, raised CSF protein.
- Extramedullary spinal tumor: tends to present with nerve root pain and a spastic paraparesis due to extramedullary cord compression. CSF protein is elevated.
- Hematomyelia: usually a history of trauma, sudden onset and pain in the involved area.
- Cervical spondylosis: sensory loss is usually confined to the involved nerve roots.
- Motor neuron disease: wasting of the hands but no sensory loss.
- Multiple mononeuropathy: may be associated with peculiar sensory deficits. Usually abrupt onset of loss of function of one, followed by other peripheral or cranial nerves. Sensory dissociation in the upper trunk is very uncommon.
- Diabetic neuropathy: another (but rare) cause of Charcot joints in the shoulders but other clinical features of diabetes.
- Vasculitic neuropathy (systemic: polyarteritis nodosa, rheumatoid arthritis, or non-systemic): may present with distal symmetric polyneuropathy but more commonly a mononeuropathy multiplex.
- Leprosy: tends to affect pain and temperature sensation and may cause a syringomyelia-like syndrome. However, leprosy preferentially affects the intracutaneous nerves and so the pattern of sensory loss does not follow the distribution of individual peripheral nerves or nerve roots. In lepromatous leprosy, sensory loss occurs in areas with low skin temperature, causing a superficial resemblance to a glove and stocking distribution, but other cool areas such as the nose, earlobes, breasts, abdomen and buttocks may also be affected. In addition there is usually a history of residence in an area where leprosy is endemic and there are skin lesions and enlarged nerves.
- Acute intermittent porphyria: patchy sensory loss involving the trunk or arms but usually acute onset, all four limbs are affected before the trunk, abdominal pain, psychiatric symptoms, or a deficiency of erythrocyte porphobilinogen deaminase.
- Amyloidosis: loss of sensation to pain and temperature but autonomic dysfunction is also common.
- Fabry's disease: an X-linked recessive disorder that frequently presents with severe burning pain in the hands and feet.
- Tangier disease: may cause a syringomyelia-like syndrome (spontaneous pain in the arms, wasting of the hand muscles, dissociated sensory loss in the upper trunk, and facial diplegia) due to selective loss of small myelinated and unmyelinated nerve fibers and small dorsal-root ganglion cells, but patients have large, lobulated, yellow-gray tonsils, and they may have hepatosplenomegaly, a low serum cholesterol level (unless a second lipid disorder), and nearly absent high-density lipoprotein (HDL) and apolipoprotein A-I and A-II.

DIAGNOSIS
Diagnosis is clinical and radiologic (MRI).

TREATMENT
Conservative
If a small syrinx is present associated with very slow progression/deterioration. Carbamazepine, amitriptyline or transcutaneous nerve stimulation can be used if the pain does not respond to simple analgesics.

Surgical
If increasing neurologic deficit occurs. Spinal deformity, such as kyphoscoliosis, should be first corrected. A variety of shunts, shunt materials, and shunt locations are used but there is no consensus, one reason being our lack of full understanding of the pathophysiology of syringomyelia, and lack of randomized trials of treatment strategies.

Syringomyelia associated with Chiari I malformation
The primary goal is to arrest the progression of the neurologic deficits by decompressing the Chiari I malformation with a suboccipital craniectomy and upper cervical (C1) laminectomy in combination with a duraplasty. If scarring occludes the outlet of the fourth ventricle, an opening is made in the scar to re-establish the outlet of the fourth ventricle of treatment strategies.

Syringomyelia associated with Chiari II malformation
Chiari II is a congenital malformation associated with myelomeningocele, hydrocephalus and often lower cranial nerve abnormalities. In addition to the hindbrain herniation seen in Chiari I, the posterior fossa in Chiari II is too small for the cerebellum, and there is upward herniation into the middle fossa. Consequently, decompression of the posterior fossa in Chiari II is not effective in most patients, and may result in shunt malfunction and immediate herniation into the decompression.

Post-traumatic syringomyelia
Treatment of cysts with shunts should be considered a treatment of last resort. Shunting can collapse the cyst but often complications result in re-expansion and the need for subsequent surgery and reshunting. Placing shunts in the spinal cord can also add to the neurologic deficit.

Decompression by means of a dural graft with a bypass for CSF may be helpful.

PROGNOSIS
Usually slowly progressive and ultimately severely disabling but some patients experience a stepwise deterioration, and others 'plateau' and do not progress.

CERVICAL SPONDYLOTIC MYELOPATHY AND RADICULOPATHY

DEFINITION
A condition in which the spinal cord (myelopathy) and/or nerve roots (radiculopathy) are damaged, either directly by traumatic compression and abnormal movement, or indirectly by ischemia due to arterial compression, venous stasis, or other consequences of the proliferative bony changes that characterize spondylosis.

EPIDEMIOLOGY
Most people older than 50 years have cervical spondylosis. Most have no symptoms apart from reduced mobility of the cervical spine.
- Incidence: 83 per 100 000 per year (cervical radiculopathy), 2 (95% CI: 0.5–6) per 100 000 per year (chronic spondylotic myelopathy).
- Prevalence (lifetime): 0.4 (95% CI: 0.2–0.7) per 1000 (spondylotic and compressive myelopathy).
- Age: middle-aged and elderly; peak incidence in the age group 50–54 years.
- Gender: M>F.

PATHOLOGY
Macroscopic
Spondylosis of the vertebral column
- Transverse bars occur which may extend across the posterior aspect of the vertebrae and compress the spinal cord. The lateral end of the transverse bars may encroach on an intervertebral foramen and compress the nerve root.
- Localized bosses occur centrally or laterally, which may compress the spinal cord.
- Intervertebral disc protrusions are commonly associated with the bars and bosses.
- Frequently these lesions are found at more than one vertebral level.

Spinal cord/root compression
- Indentation, flattening and distortion of the spinal cord occurs corresponding to the spondylotic protrusions (**675**).
- The C6 or C7 nerve roots are affected in two-thirds of cases of cervical radiculopathy.

Microscopic
- Demyelination of the lateral columns, ischemic change and nerve cell damage and loss in the central gray matter, and cavitation at the site of the compression are all present.
- Degeneration of the dorsal columns occurs rostral to the lesions.
- Degeneration of the lateral columns occurs caudal to the lesions.

ETIOLOGY AND PATHOPHYSIOLOGY
Predisposing factors
- Narrowing of the spinal canal in the sagittal (anteroposterior) plane: <11–12 mm (<0.4–0.5 in) results in deformation of the cord, the degree of which correlates with the clinical severity of myelopathy. The salient static measurement is however, the cross sectional area of the cord. Reduction in cross sectional area of the cord by 30% or more to a value of about 60 mm^2 or less, results in symptoms and signs.
- In patients with cervical spondylotic myelopathy caused by an ossified posterior longitudinal ligament, the dentate ligaments fix the cord against the anterior part of the canal. Sectioning of the dentate ligaments may spread the tension in the cord over a greater segment.
- Hypertrophic facet and uncovertebral joints occupy space in the root canal.
- Neck motion: predisposes to spur formation and activates symptoms and signs of cervical spondylotic myelopathy (e.g. patients with athetoid cerebral palsy).
- Deflexion (i.e. extension) of the neck.

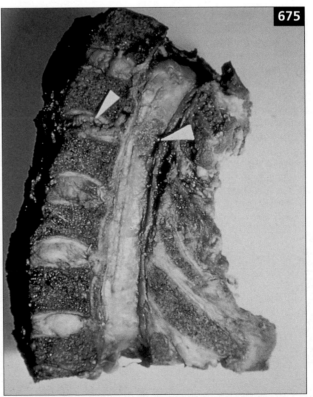

675 Autopsy specimen of the cervical spine in the sagittal plane showing a degenerate cervical intervertebral disc (oblique arrow), compressing the cervical spinal cord causing a necrosis of the cervical spinal cord at that level (horizontal arrow).

Causes

- A bulging or herniated disc (**676**).
- Degenerated yellow ligaments.
- A fixed subluxation due to disc degeneration.
- Microtrauma.

Mechanism

Direct

Traumatic compression and abnormal movement. Acute trauma is likely to exacerbate any pre-existing myelopathy in a chronically distorted, narrowly confined, cord.

Mechanical compression theory: the spinal cord is compressed by a spondylotic bar anteriorly and the ligamenta flava posteriorly, particularly during extension of the neck, when the ligamenta flava bulge into the spinal canal, decreasing its anteroposterior depth while the antero-posterior dimension of the spinal cord itself increases. People with congenitally narrow spinal canals are more vulnerable.

Dentate tension theory: the anterior spondylotic bar displaces the spinal cord posteriorly and stretches the dentate ligaments, which attach the lateral pia to the lateral dura. The attachment to the dura is fixed because the dural root sleeves are anchored in the neural foramina. Consequently, the spinal cord is pulled laterally by the dentate ligaments. The spondylotic bar may also increase dentate tension by interfering locally with dural stretch during neck flexion, the resultant increase in dural stress being transmitted to the spinal cord via the dentate ligaments.

Indirect

The role of ischemia is uncertain. There is no correlation with atherosclerosis of major vessels or with obstruction of blood flow in the anterior spinal artery. Distortion and compression of small vessels in the cord may have a pathogenetic influence. The influence of venous stasis is uncertain.

CLINICAL FEATURES

Cervical spondylosis without foraminal or spinal canal stenosis does not result in cervical spondylotic radiculopathy or myelopathy.

Cervical spondylotic myelopathy

- Neck pain in some.
- Numb, clumsy hands:
- Amyotrophic hand: localized wasting and weakness of the hand without remarkable sensory loss or gait disturbance. Correlates with a reduced cross-sectional area of the spinal cord at the C7–T1 segments. Similar to hands of patients with spinal muscular atrophy.
- Myelopathic hand: spastic dysfunction and deficient pain sensation due to reduction in spinal cord diameter at higher spinal levels.
- Spastic paraparesis: the *sine qua non* for the diagnosis.
- Loss of proprioception and vibratory sensation in the legs.
- Poorly defined cutaneous sensory loss in the legs.

Cervical radiculopathy (see Acute 'slipped disc', p.550)

- Neck and arm pain in some (**677, 678**).
- Paresthesiae, pain and cutaneous sensory loss in a radicular distribution.
- Wasting and weakness of proximal arm muscles or in the hands.
- Fasciculations in a segmental distribution in the hands and arms.

DIFFERENTIAL DIAGNOSIS

Cervical spine/spinal cord pathology

- Discogenic or degenerative cervical spine stenosis.
- Vertebral body fracture: trauma, metabolic bone disease, tumor.
- Tumor:
- Tumor of vertebral column or epidural space (or both):
  Metastases.
  Plasmacytoma or multiple myeloma.
  Primary bone tumor.
  Primary intradural tumor of spinal cord.
- Infection:
- Intervertebral discitis or osteomyelitis.
- Epidural or subdural abscess.
- Herpes zoster or other viral-based radiculopathy.
- Vascular lesion:
- Acute epidural hematoma.
- Spinal cord infarction.
- Arteriovenous malformation of the spinal cord.
- Spinal dural arteriovenous fistula.
- Amyotrophic lateral sclerosis.
- Multiple sclerosis.
- Syringomyelia.
- Diabetic radiculoneuropathy.
- Acute inflammatory demyelinating polyradiculopathy (Guillain–Barré syndrome).

Brain pathology

- Parasagittal meningioma.
- Bilateral anterior cerebral artery territory infarction.
- Bilateral corticospinal tract infarction (e.g. internal capsule and pons).
- Primary lateral sclerosis.
- Hydrocephalus.

INVESTIGATIONS

Plain films of the cervical spine

Useful because they demonstrate narrowing of the spinal canal, osteophytes arising from the posterior surfaces of degenerate discs and at the neurocentral joints, and the alignment of the vertebral bodies. Flexion and extension views may be done to look for instability with movement. They do not, however, give any information on the degree of cord or root compression or the soft tissue abnormalities around the spine.

Plain CT (679)

CT has a limited role; it images osteophytes and calcified discs, and accurately measures the dimensions of the bony spinal canal, but the cervical cord and roots cannot be assessed.

676 Illustration showing the effect of a cervical spondylitic bar, osteophyte or degenerate intervertebral disc at the C5/6 level, compressing the cervical spinal cord (causing a cervical myelopathy) and/or left C6 nerve root (causing a left C6 radiculopathy).

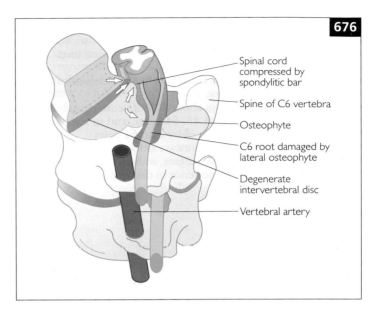

Spinal cord compressed by spondylitic bar

Spine of C6 vertebra

Osteophyte

C6 root damaged by lateral osteophyte

Degenerate intervertebral disc

Vertebral artery

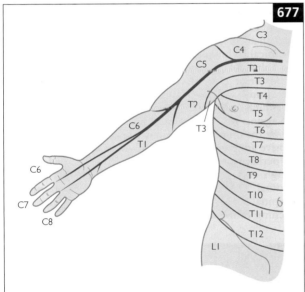

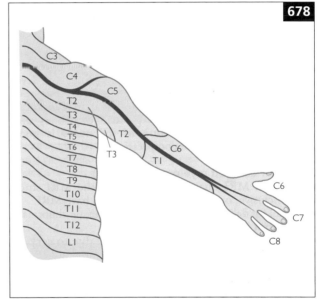

677, 678 Distribution of the cervical and thoracic dermatomes on the anterior aspect of the upper limb, chest and abdomen (**677**), and the posterior aspect of the upper limb and back (**678**).

679 CT scan of the cervical spine, axial plane at C5/6 showing very advanced spondylotic change with anterior and posterior lipping osteophytes and a large osteophyte arising from the posterior aspect of the C5 disc (circle) causing markedly severe central spinal canal stenosis.

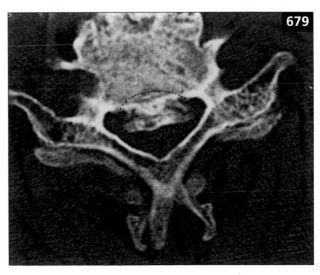

SPINAL EPIDURAL HEMATOMA

DEFINITION
Hemorrhage in the spinal epidural space.

EPIDEMIOLOGY
- Uncommon.
- Age: any age.
- Gender: M=F.

PATHOLOGY
- Blood in the spinal epidural space.
- Direct compression of the spinal cord or roots by the mass effect of the hematoma.
- Spinal cord/nerve root pressure necrosis.

ETIOLOGY AND PATHOPHYSIOLOGY
- Trauma.
- Spinal extradural arteriovenous malformation (**692**).
- Vertebral body hemangioma.
- Epidural metastases.
- Arteritis.
- Hypertension.
- Bleeding diathesis due to a coagulopathy.
- Anticoagulant therapy.
- Cocaine injection.
- Epidural anesthesia.
- Lumbar puncture in patients with a bleeding diathesis.
- Idiopathic.

CLINICAL FEATURES
Sudden and severe neck or back pain, followed in minutes to hours by progressive motor, sensory and sphincteric disturbances referable to radicular spinal cord or cauda equina origin. Other clinical features are determined by the underlying cause (e.g. vasculitis causing associated skin rash [**693–695**]).

DIFFERENTIAL DIAGNOSIS
- Hemorrhage into the spinal cord (hematomyelia) or spinal subarachnoid space (**693**).
- Intervertebral disc prolapse.
- Vertebral body collapse (spinal angulation: tuberculosis, tumor).
- Trauma.
- Spinal cord infarction.
- Epidural abscess.

INVESTIGATIONS
Blood
- Full blood count.
- ESR.
- Coagulation profile.
- Serum chemistry profile.
- VDRL/RPR and TPHA.
- Antinuclear antibody titer.
- Urine test for cocaine/amphetamine metabolites.

MRI spine
MRI is the primary method of diagnosis (**693**). The findings depend on the timing of the MR scan after the onset of the hemorrhage. At about 36 hours after onset, T1W MRI of the spine usually shows an isointense collection in the epidural space, usually anterior, with or without cord or nerve root compression. An underlying spinal vascular malformation may be seen.

CT spine
CT may also show an epidural mass, which does not tend to enhance with contrast.

Chest x-ray
Hilar lymphadenopathy, pulmonary nodules or interstitial lung disease may be seen in patients with arteritis causing spinal epidural hemorrhage.

Spinal angiography
May identify the source of the hemorrhage and even distinguish between the several types of vascular malformations and hemangioblastomas, and localize them accurately to the vertebral bodies, epidural or subdural space, or spinal cord.

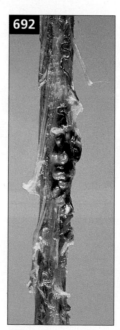
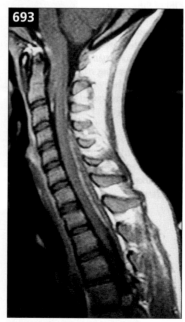

692 Autopsy specimen of spinal cord showing an epidural spinal arteriovenous malformation (a common cause of spinal epidural hematoma), containing dark clotted blood. (Courtesy of Professor BA Kakulas, Royal Perth Hospital, Western Australia.)

693 MRI cervical and upper thoracic spine, T1W image, sagittal plane, showing a linear streak of high intensity due to hemorrhage in the spinal subarachnoid space in a patient with arteritis due to Churg–Strauss syndrome (allergic angiitis and granulomatosis).

CSF

Blood and xanthochromia are present in the spinal fluid, if there has been subarachnoid hemorrhage or hemorrhage into the spinal cord (hematomyelia).

DIAGNOSIS

MRI spine or spinal angiography in a patient with appropriate clinical syndrome.

TREATMENT

- Prompt neurosurgical decompressive laminectomy, particularly if acute onset and neurologic function is deteriorating.
- Microsurgical resection or embolization of the cause (e.g. if a vascular malformation is present).

PROGNOSIS

Depends on the site, duration and degree of spinal cord and nerve root compression, and the underlying cause of the hematoma.

SPINAL EPIDURAL ABSCESS

DEFINITION

Pus or infected granulation tissue in the spinal epidural space.

EPIDEMIOLOGY

- Rare.
- Age: any age; children or adults.
- Gender: either sex.

PATHOLOGY

- An abscess containing pus or infected granulation tissue in any part of the spinal epidural space, most commonly the dorsal aspect of the thoracic spinal cord, where the loose attachment of the dura permits rapid spread of infection.
- Direct compression of the spinal cord or roots by the mass effect of the abscess.
- Spinal cord infarction secondary to pressure and thrombophlebitis of the local venous channels.

ETIOLOGY

- *Staphylococcus aureus*: most common.
- Streptococci.
- Brucella (a Gram-negative coccobacillus which may infect people in close contact with infected animals and carcasses [camels, cows, goats, sheep] or after drinking infected milk).
- Salmonella.
- Fungus.
- Tuberculosis (**696**) (complications include nerve root and/or spinal cord compression, arteritis and spinal cord infarction, spinal arachnoiditis, and spinal cord tuberculoma).
- Anaerobic organisms.

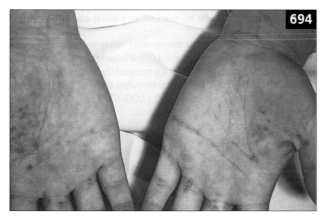

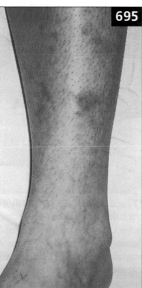

694, 695 Hands (**694**) and shin (**695**) of the patient with Churg–Strauss syndrome (**693**) showing the typical skin rash.

696 Spine of a patient with a tuberculous spinal epidural abscess due to localized spinal meningitis (Pott's disease of the spine) with vertebral body collapse and destruction of the adjacent intervertebral discs.

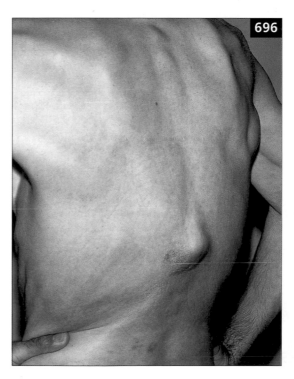

Pupillary reflexes
Light reflex
- Lesions of cranial nerve III cause ipsilateral pupil dilatation. Shining a light into either eye fails to evoke a direct or consensual response in the affected eye because of the defect in the efferent arc of the reflex. However, shining a light in the eye ipsilateral to the lesion (the affected eye) evokes a consensual reaction in the eye contralateral to the lesion (the unaffected eye).
- Bilateral occipital lobe lesions (beyond the optic nerves and tracts) which cause bilateral blindness are associated with preserved direct and consensual reflexes.

Accommodation reflex
Any lesion involving the pupilloconstrictor fibers will impair the reaction of accommodation. Selective impairment of accommodation may occur in some midbrain lesions.

Relative afferent pupillary defect
Also known as the Marcus Gunn pupil or swinging torch sign (see p.575).

Adie's pupil (tonic pupil of Adie; Holmes–Adie syndrome) (see p.497)

Horner's syndrome (see p.494)

Argyll Robertson (AR) pupil
- Described by Douglas Argyll Robertson, an Edinburgh physician.
- Small, irregular pupils that are non-reactive to light, but reactive to accommodation (AR pupils are 'accommodation retaining'.) They dilate poorly with mydriatics.
- The site of the lesion is uncertain but is probably in the pretectal region.
- Causes include syphilis and diabetes.

Clinical features of autonomic failure
Neurologic system (see Multiple systems atrophy, p.435).
- Extrapyramidal dysfunction (Parkinsonism).
- Cerebellar dysfunction.
- Pyramidal dysfunction.

Eye
- Anisocoria.
- Horner's syndrome (see p.494).
- Dry eyes, rarely excessive lacrimation.

Sudomotor system
- Sweating abnormalities (anhidrosis usually, but occasionally gustatory facial sweating in a diabetic).
- Heat intolerance.

Cardiovascular system
Postural (orthostatic hypotension): symptoms include lightheadedness, dizziness, faintness, visual disturbances or loss of consciousness (syncope) on standing upright. It is usually defined as a fall in systolic blood pressure of at least 4 kPa (30 mmHg) or to <10.7 kPa (80 mmHg) within a minute or two of standing, but such falls are neither sensitive nor specific (e.g. they can occur in the normal asymptomatic elderly, cardiac failure, Addison's disease).

Respiratory system
- Stridor.
- Inspiratory gasps.
- Apneic episodes.

Gastrointestinal system
- Constipation.
- Diarrhea (occasionally).
- Dysphagia.

Renal and urinary bladder
- Nocturia.
- Frequency.
- Urgency.
- Incontinence.
- Retention of urine.

Reproductive system
Erectile and ejaculatory failure.

ASSOCIATED FEATURES
Involvement of other neurologic systems (see Multiple systems atrophy, p.435)
- Extrapyramidal dysfunction (Parkinsonism).
- Cerebellar dysfunction.
- Pyramidal dysfunction.
- Peripheral neuropathy: peripheral autonomic fibers may be damaged in peripheral neuropathies, particularly those affecting small myelinated and unmyelinated fibers (e.g. diabetes, primary amyloidosis), or those which cause acute demyelination of the preganglionic sympathetic fibers and the vagal afferent and efferent fibers (e.g. Guillain–Barré syndrome). The usual clinical manifestations are postural hypotension, impairment of heart rate control, loss of sweating, and impotence.

SPECIAL CONDITIONS
PAF or IOH
- Degeneration of postganglionic (i.e. peripheral) sympathetic fibers.
- Age of onset: 40–60 years.
- Gender: M=F.
- Postural hypotension (dizziness and weakness on standing or walking).
- Impotence.
- Bladder disturbances.
- Loss of sweating.
- Normal neurologic examination.
- Slowly progressive course.

Autonomic failure associated with multiple system atrophy (see p.435)

DIFFERENTIAL DIAGNOSIS
Postural (orthostatic) hypotension
- Dehydration.
- Blood loss.
- Drugs.

Argyll Robertson pupils
Pseudo-Argyll Robertson pupils: pupils that do not react to light but are not small or irregular. May occur in midbrain lesions.

DIAGNOSIS

The clinical approach to the patient with clinical features of dysautonomia aims to determine:

- Whether autonomic function is affected.
- Which organ systems are affected.
- The site of the lesion (central, preganglionic and postganglionic).
- The cause of the lesion.

INVESTIGATIONS
Is autonomic function normal or abnormal?

Change of blood pressure with posture (postural hypotension)

- Normally, changing from the supine to the standing position alters the blood pressure very little.
- A fall exceeding 4/2 kPa (30/15 mmHg) is abnormal, indicating significant postural hypotension.

Change of heart rate with posture (reflex tachycardia; the 30:15 ratio)

- Normally, changing from the supine to the standing position increases the heart rate by about 11–29 beats per minute, reaching a maximum after 15 beats, after which a reflex bradycardia ensues, reaching a maximum at about the 30th beat.
- The ratio of the R–R interval (heart period) on an EKG corresponding to the 30th and 15th beats, is the 30:15 ratio. The ratio is normally considerably greater than one, but varies with age.
- Autonomic neuropathies affecting the afferent or efferent fibers of the reflex arc reduce the rise in heart rate associated with a change of posture, and reduce the 30:15 ratio.

Change of heart rate with deep breathing (sinus arrhythmia)

- Normally, inspiration is associated with an increase in heat rate and expiration with a decrease in heart rate (sinus arrhythmia). This difference is less pronounced in older individuals.
- Autonomic neuropathies involving the vagus nerve are associated with impaired variation of the heart rate with respiration (loss of sinus arrhythmia).

Valsalva maneuver

Normally, forced expiration against a closed glottis or mouthpiece (Valsalva maneuver) alters the heart rate (HR) and blood pressure (BP):

- Phase I: BP rises due to the raised intrathoracic pressure associated with the Valsalva causing mechanical compression of the aorta and increased peripheral resistance. A compensatory fall in HR, mediated by the parasympathetics in the vagus nerve, follows.
- Phase II: BP falls due to the fall in venous return (associated with continuously high intrathoracic pressure) and thus fall in stroke volume. A compensatory rise in HR (due to parasympathetic vagal withdrawal) and total peripheral resistance (due to peripheral vasoconstriction) follows.
- Phase III: forced expiration ceases and venous return increases rapidly, increasing the stroke volume and blood pressure and decreasing the heart rate.
- Phase IV: BP rises further and overshoots because the peripheral circulation is still vasoconstricted for up to 30 seconds because of the increase in peripheral sympathetic vasoconstrictor tone induced by stages II–III. Therefore, stage IV is a measure of sympathetic vascular tone.

The patient assumes the semi-recumbent posture and is asked to expire forcefully, maintaining a column of mercury at 5.3 kPa (40 mmHg) pressure for 10–15 seconds, while the EKG and BP are continuously recorded (intra-arterial catheter for BP). The ratio of the longest pulse interval to the shortest pulse interval recorded on the EKG during the maneuver (the Valsalva ratio) normally exceeds 1.45 in young adults. Increased age and parasympathetic and sympathetic neuropathies are associated with a reduced ratio.

Isometric contraction

- Normally, sustained isometric contraction (e.g. a firm handgrip) for up to 5 minutes increases the heart rate (and thus cardiac output) and total peripheral resistance (by peripheral vasoconstriction), leading to an increase in systolic and diastolic BP. Diastolic BP rises by 2 kPa (15 mmHg) or more.
- Autonomic neuropathies affecting sympathetic efferent fibers are associated with an impaired response.

Response to emotional and other stimuli

- Normally, mental arithmetic, a loud noise, or cold or painful stimuli usually evoke peripheral vasoconstriction, increase the total peripheral resistance and arterial blood pressure. In some normal people, this response may not be present.
- Autonomic neuropathies affecting sympathetic efferent fibers are associated with an impaired response.

Sweating

- Autonomic neuropathies affecting sympathetic efferent fibers are associated with impaired sweating.
- The thermoregulatory sweat test (TST) determines the distribution of sweat loss (anhidrosis). The skin is covered with a powder such as alazarine red or quinazarine that changes color when sweating occurs. The patient is warmed by radiant heat sufficient to raise the body temperature by 1°C (1.8°F).
- Local sweating may also be tested by injection or iontophoresis of acetylcholine which stimulates an axon reflex, or pilocarpine which stimulates the sweat glands directly.

Pupillary responses

- Metacholine (methacholine) 2.5%, installed into the conjunctival sac, does not affect the size of the normal pupil but it causes pupillary constriction if parasympathetic innervation is impaired. This is because of the denervation supersensitivity of the constrictor muscle of the pupil.
- Epinephrine 0.1% has no effect on the normal pupil but causes pupillary dilatation if postganglionic sympathetic innervation is impaired, also because of denervation supersensitivity.
- Cocaine 4% eye drops cause dilatation of the normal pupil because cocaine blocks the re-uptake of noradrenaline (norepinephrine), but if peripheral sympathetic innervation is impaired, pupillary dilatation does not occur.
- Tyramine 2% eye drops produce dilatation of the normal pupil because tyramine releases noradrenaline (norepinephrine) from peripheral nerve terminals, but if sympathetic innervation is impaired, noradrenaline (norepinephrine) is depleted and pupillary dilatation does not occur.

Where is the lesion (i.e. site) and what is the functional deficit?

In addition to the above tests, a number of other tests of baroreflex sensitivity, vasomotor control, and bladder control exist but are more difficult to perform.

Sudomotor function

Quantitative sudomotor axon reflex test (Q-SART): a test of postganglionic sympathetic sudomotor function. If the TST is abnormal (i.e. anhidrosis) and the Q-SART is normal, then the site of the sympathetic lesion is preganglionic.

Vasomotor function

- Skin vasomotor reflexes: measured by laser doppler flow meters (e.g. on the pulp of index finger) in response to stimuli such as standing, Valsalva, cold water. Limited if the patient is nervous and resting skin blood flow is minimal.
- Axonal flare response: measure at same time as Q-SART.
- Veno-arteriolar reflex: a test of post ganglionic adrenergic function.

Heart period (R–R interval) recordings (see above)

Responses to deep breathing, Valsalva maneuver, and standing.

What is the cause?

Underlying and associated disorders, such as diabetes mellitus and amyloidosis (see above), need to be excluded. Seropositivity for antibodies that bind to or block ganglionic acetylcholine receptors identifies patients with various forms of autoimmune autonomic neuropathy and distinguishes these disorders from other types of dysautonomia.

TREATMENT

Aims to remove the underlying cause if possible and relieve symptoms.

Postural hypotension

- General advice:
- Maintain hydration and salt intake (150 mmol/l [150 mEq] salt).
- Avoid dehydration, diuretics and other hypotensive drugs and deconditioning.
- Rise slowly from the lying and sitting positions, particularly in the morning, after hot baths and heavy meals.
- Avoid straining and extremes of temperatures.
- Wear light clothes.

- Elevate the head of the bed by 10–15 cm (4–6 in) (reduces renal arterial pressure and thus increases the secretion of renin, resulting in retention of sodium and water, and increased blood volume).
- Elastic stockings with lower abdominal constriction (reduce the volume of the venous capacitance bed).
- Drugs:
- 9-α-fluorohydrocortisone (fludrocortisone), a mineralocorticoid which increases circulating effective blood volume and probably sensitizes peripheral blood vessels to catecholamines, is the most useful drug. The dose is 0.1 mg/day and can be increased. The main adverse effects are supine hypertension, fluid retention (and heart failure), worsening of diabetes mellitus, and potassium depletion.
- Indomethacin 25–50 mg three times per day, but may cause headache.
- Alpha antagonists: ephedrine 15–50 mg three times daily; methylphenidate hydrochloride (Ritalin) 5–10 mg three times daily, and midodrine, a recently introduced α-adrenergic agonist which acts by improving arterial and venous constriction in response to standing. May be limited by supine hypertension which itself may respond to beta blockade.
- Ambulatory norepinephrine infusion via intravenous indwelling catheter and an infusion pump.
- Atrial tachypacing may help in patients who do not have a tachycardia on standing up.

Bladder dysfunction

Frequency of micturition

Anticholinergic drugs:

- Propantheline bromide 15 mg two to four times daily.
- Penthienate bromide 5 mg three to four times daily.
- Tricyclic antidepressant drugs (e.g. amitriptyline 25–100 mg/day).

Botulinum toxin injections into the detrusor muscle (2.5 MU of Botox injected per single site, up to 30 injections).

Distended bladder with incomplete emptying

Cholinergic drugs: bethanechol chloride 10 mg three to four times daily.

Gastroparesis

- Metoclopramide 10 mg before meals and at night.
- Cisapride 15–40 mg daily in two to four divided doses.

FURTHER READING

Donofrio PD, Caress JB (2001) Autonomic disorders. *The Neurologist*, 7: 220–233.

Kauffmann H (2000) Primary autonomic failure: three clinical presentations of one disease? *Ann. Intern. Med.*, **133**: 382–384.

Mathias CJ (1997) Autonomic disorders and their recognition. *N. Engl. J. Med.* **336**: 721–724.

Naumann M, Jost WH, Toyka KV (1999) Botulinum toxin in the treatment of neurological disorders of the autonomic nervous system. *Arch. Neurol.*, **56**: 914–916.

Oldenburg O, Mitchell A, Nurnberger J, et al.. (2001) Ambulatory norepinephrine treatment of severe autonomic orthostatic hypotension. *J. Am. Coll. Cardiol.*, **37**: 219–223.

Schatz IJ (2001) Treatment of severe autonomic orthostatic hypotension. *Lancet*, **357**: 1060–1061.

Vernino S, Low PA, Fealey RD, et al. (2000) Autoantibodies to ganglionic acetylcholine receptors in autoimmune autonomic neuropathies. *N. Engl. J. Med.*, **343**: 847–855.

Diseases of the Peripheral Nerve

PERIPHERAL NEUROPATHY

DEFINITION
A disorder of any or all of the peripheral nerves or nerve roots.

EPIDEMIOLOGY
- Incidence: 69 per 100 000 per year.
- Lifetime prevalence: 3 per 1000.
- Age: any age, but usually the middle-aged and elderly.
- Gender: M=F.

ANATOMY (722–725)
A peripheral nerve consists of a cell body and about six fascicles, each of which contains many myelinated and unmyelinated axons. Each fascicle has small nutrient blood vessels which are integral to its function.

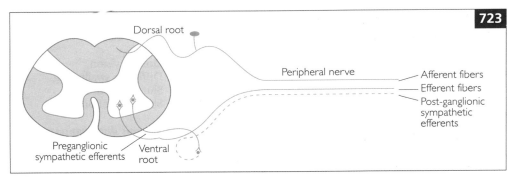

722 Diagrammatic representation of peripheral nerve trunk and its blood supply Regional arteries arranged longitudinally outside the nerve trunk give rise to nutrient arteries that penetrate the epineurium and form an anastomosis. Small arterioles penetrate the perineurium of the fascicles and form an endocapillary network.

723 Diagrammatic representation of components of the peripheral nerve trunks.

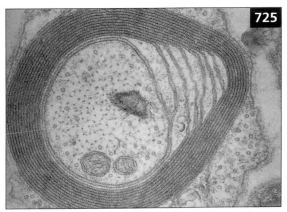

724 Transverse section of a peripheral nerve stained with toluidine blue. The circular shaped myelin is dark blue.

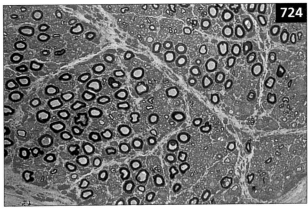

725 Electron micrograph of a transverse section through a normal myelinated nerve fiber, showing the axon in the center surrounded by several layers of myelin. The major dense lines of the myelin arise by the fusion of the inner surfaces of the Schwann cell surface membrane.

CLINICAL FEATURES
History
- Usually healthy prior to onset.
- Pain in the shoulder and neck:
- Onset quite sudden, and often in the evening or night.
- Typically severe, deep and sometimes excruciating. Rarely mild.
- May radiate to the medial part of the scapula or down the arm to involve the whole arm or part of the upper arm or forearm.
- Lasts from a few hours to a few weeks; usually several days. The pain may linger as a dull ache for some time, however.
- Mild numbness may be present over the deltoid muscle in the rough distribution of the axillary nerve; paresthesiae occur rarely.
- Severe, and often unilateral, weakness of the muscles of the shoulder, arm or both develops over a few hours, frequently overnight, during the pain or more commonly just after it has mainly subsided. The weakness is maximal soon after onset, but occasionally it progresses.

Examination
- Early wasting and flaccid weakness of one or any combination of muscles of the shoulder and arm: serratus anterior, rhomboids, supra- and infraspinatus, deltoid, latissimus dorsi, or one or more arm muscles innervated by major nerves or their branches (**734, 735**).
- Normal, depressed or absent deep tendon reflexes of the arm.
- Sensory loss is less apparent and, if present, is usually in the area of innervation of the axillary nerve.

CLINICAL VARIANTS
Involvement of single nerves or their branches rather than a large part of the brachial plexus
These nerves usually have their origin in the brachial plexus, e.g.:
- Long thoracic nerve to serratus anterior.
- Suprascapular nerve.
- Axillary nerve.
- Anterior interosseous nerve.
- Lateral antebrachial cutaneous nerve.
- Median nerve trunk.
- Median palmar cutaneous branch.

In these cases, it has been proposed that the pathology is probably within the corresponding fascicle of the brachial plexus rather than a separate trunk of the respective nerve. However, this would not explain occasional cases with involvement of nerves remote from the brachial plexus such as the lower cranial nerves (facial nerve, vagus nerve, recurrent laryngeal nerve, accessory nerve, and cranial nerves IX, X, XI and XII combined) and the phrenic nerve.

Bilateral involvement
Occurs in about 5–10%, but up to one-third, of cases.

Lumbosacral plexus involvement
Rare.

Familial neuralgic amyotrophy
- Inherited as an autosomal dominant trait.
- Associated with a mutation in distal chromosome 17q.
- Genetically distinct from hereditary neuropathy with liability to pressure palsies.

- Episodes may be precipitated by pregnancy and non-specific illness, and tend to recur.
- Congenital anomalies, such as syndactyly and hypotelorism, are common in affected members of these families.

Recurrent episodes of neuralgic amyotrophy
Rare.

DIFFERENTIAL DIAGNOSIS
- Guillain–Barré syndrome: usually involves the legs first, and pain is not commonly severe and prominent.
- Poliomyelitis: the CSF is usually abnormal (unlike neuralgic amyotrophy).
- Rucksack paralysis: direct mechanical injury to the brachial plexus from wearing a heavy back pack.
- Compression of the brachial plexus during sleep: unlikely to cause severe pain.
- Isolated lesions of the long thoracic nerve to serratus anterior: need to exclude a local cause.
- Radiation therapy: may cause painful lesions of the brachial plexus but usually a relevant history and scarring, and slower onset.
- Multifocal motor neuropathy: bilateral, but asymmetric, painless, and slower in onset.
- Lead poisoning: may cause bilateral brachial neuropathy but usually painless.

INVESTIGATIONS
Nerve conduction studies
- Motor conduction velocity to proximal muscles may be slow.
- Sensory nerve action potentials may be reduced.

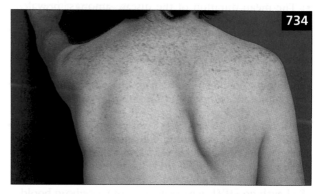

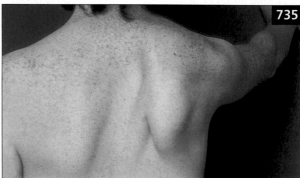

734, 735 Winging of the right scapula due to neuralgic amyotrophy of the brachial plexus causing weakness of the serratus anterior (supplied by the long thoracic nerve). (Courtesy of Dr AM Chancellor, Neurologist, Tauranga, New Zealand.)

Needle EMG

Usually reveals normal paraspinal muscles and multifocal axonal lesions within the brachial plexus or its branches, but can be consistent with an isolated lesion of a peripheral nerve.

MRI brachial plexus

If a local compressive or infiltrative cause is suspected (e.g. neuroma).

DIAGNOSIS

Typical clinical picture of rather sudden onset of neuropathic shoulder pain and weakness, supported by EMG studies, and followed by spontaneous resolution of pain and gradual, but often incomplete, resolution of weakness.

TREATMENT

- Physiotherapy, particularly passive (and later active) exercises of the shoulder joint for patients with impaired shoulder elevation, to prevent a 'frozen shoulder' syndrome.
- No effective medical treatment; no convincing evidence for corticosteroids.
- Therapeutic interventions should perhaps be directed to patients with persistent conduction block with the aim of eradicating the block and possibly minimizing subsequent axon loss. Intravenous immunoglobulin is worthy of future study.

PROGNOSIS

Pain usually resolves within 1–2 weeks but weakness may not recover for months or even years. In one series of 99 patients, one-third had made a functional recovery after one year, three-quarters after 2 years, and 89% at 3 years. Weakness of the shoulder muscles had recovered by the end of 1 year in 60% of cases whereas no patient with predominantly lower plexus involvement recovered normal function.

VASCULITIC NEUROPATHY

DEFINITION

Ischemia and infarction of one or more peripheral nerves due to vasculitis of the vasa nervorum.

EPIDEMIOLOGY

- Rare.
- Age: any age.
- Gender: M=F.

PATHOLOGY

- Vasculitis of the vasa nervorum (50–300 μm diameter).
- Ischemia and infarction of one or more peripheral nerves.

ETIOLOGY

Primary vasculitis

- Allergic granulomatosis and angiitis (Churg–Strauss syndrome): a granulomatous necrotizing vasculitis which predominantly affects the lungs. A prodromal phase of asthma and eosinophilia commonly precedes the onset of systemic vasculitis, which may involve one or more peripheral nerves. Other features include vasculitic rash, glomerulonephritis and positive anti-neutrophil cytoplasmic antibody in 60–70%.

- Polyarteritis nodosa: affects medium-sized arteries (e.g. cerebral, gastrointestinal, renal), and causes peripheral neuropathy in about half of patients, usually as a mononeuritis multiplex or symmetric polyneuropathy. Presents at any age and is twice as common in men than women. It is characterized commonly by malaise, fever, weight loss, and tachycardia; and may be associated with an acute abdomen, vascular event of the brain or heart, or severe or treated hypertension. Anti-neutrophic cytoplasmic antibodies are rare, and when present, may indicate coincident vasculitis of small vessels, and may be associated with a lupus anticoagulant and alpha1-antitrypsin deficiency.
- Wegener's granulomatosis: a systemic necrotizing granulomatous vasculitis of the upper and lower respiratory tract, with or without glomerulonephritis or arthralgia. Multiple mononeuropathy or polyneuropathy may occur, as may cranial neuropathies. Anti-neutrophil cytoplasmic antibody is positive in 90% of cases.
- Giant cell arteritis (see p.234): may be complicated by multiple mononeuropathy, as well as mononeuropathy and polyneuropathy.

Vasculitis associated with systemic autoimmune disease

- Rheumatoid arthritis: vasculitis may affect small arteries, arterioles, capillaries, and venules, and often causes few symptoms. When present, it is associated with long-standing disease, seropositivity, and florid subcutaneous nodule formation. Polyneuropathy, and particularly multiple mononeuropathy, are rare. More common causes are joint deformities and synovial swellings causing entrapment neuropathies, and medication-induced neuropathy.
- Sjögren's syndrome.
- Systemic lupus erythematosus: occasionally presents with a multiple mononeuropathy or chronic inflammatory demyelinating polyneuropathy.

Vasculitis associated with other conditions

- Cryoglobulinemia, particularly mixed (often hepatitis C positive).
- Behçet's disease: a small vessel vasculitis with mono-nuclear cell infiltrate in the skin, gastrointestinal ulcers and the CNS (occasionally), characterized by relapsing ocular lesions and recurrent oral and genital ulcers, meningo-encephalitis, and rarely peripheral neuropathy, usually in the form of multiple mononeuropathy.
- Human immunodeficiency virus (HIV) infection.
- CREST syndrome (calcinosis, Raynaud's phenomenon, esophageal dysmotility, sclerodactyly and telangiectasis).
- Non-systemic vasculitis of peripheral nerves.
- Angiitis associated with amphetamine use.
- Paraneoplastic vasculitis: lymphoma, small cell lung carcinoma.

CLINICAL FEATURES

- Depend on the size and extent of the nerves involved:
- – Large nerve infarction: multiple mononeuropathy.
- – Smaller nerve infarction: asymmetric sensorimotor neuropathy.
- – Nerve ischemia: distal symmetric sensorimotor neuropathy.
- Onset is typically rapid over several weeks.
- Pain is prominent: deep, aching and neuropathic.
- Symptoms and signs of the underlying disease may or may not accompany the neurologic deficits.
- Multiple mononeuropathy:
- – Several peripheral or cranial nerves become involved, one after another, within days or weeks.
- – Pain, paresthesia, loss of sensation, and muscle weakness in the dermatomes and myotomes supplied by the diseased nerve(s).
- – As more nerves become involved, the clinical picture resembles a polyneuropathy.
- Symmetric polyneuropathy: in polyarteritis nodosa and Wegener's granulomatosis this pattern is as common as multiple mononeuropathy.

DIFFERENTIAL DIAGNOSIS
Multiple mononeuropathy
Hematologic disorders

- Acute myeloid leukemia.
- Myelodysplastic syndrome.
- Plasmacytoma.
- Paraproteinemia.
- Waldenström's macroglobulinemia.
- Lymphoma.

Inflammation/infection

- Meningococcal septicemia.
- Infective endocarditis.
- Cutaneous polyarthritis, in children.
- Non-vasculitis, steroid-responsive form.
- Sarcoidosis (see p.350): a chronic multisystem disease of unknown cause. There is infiltration of affected tissues (most commonly lung) by T lymphocytes and mono-nuclear phagocytes, with formation of non-caseating epithelioid granuloma. The central and peripheral nervous system is involved in about 5% of cases, and the peripheral nervous system alone in about 3%. The most common neurologic presentation is cranial neuropathy, frequently involving the facial nerve. The course may be fluctuating, as with Wegener's granulomatosis. Peripheral nervous system involvement is usually as a mononeuropathy multiplex, which may be accompanied by lesions of the CNS and cranial nerves, but can also be as a symmetric polyneuropathy, compressive median neuropathy due to synovitis, or multifocal sensory neuropathy with large areas of sensory loss over the trunk.

Other conditions

- Diabetes mellitus.
- Neurofibromatosis.
- Jellyfish stings.

Symmetric sensorimotor neuropathy (see p.579)

Guillain–Barré syndrome (see p.588)
Fulminant forms of vasculitic neuropathy (e.g. Churg–Strauss syndrome) may present like this.

Mass lesions
Suspect if the affected nerves lies close together.

INVESTIGATIONS
Nerve conduction studies
Normal or mildly decreased nerve conduction velocities, compound muscle action potentials, and sensory nerve action potentials in the involved nerves. Conduction block in a few cases.

EMG
Typical changes of an axonal neuropathy (e.g. denervation and reinnervation) in most cases.

Blood tests
- ESR
- Antinuclear antibodies.
- Antineutrophic cytoplasmic antibodies.
- Rheumatoid factor.

Tissue biopsy (muscle or sural nerve)
A nerve biopsy (**736–738**) is essential as a basis for long term immunosuppression. It is positive in 90% of cases of vasculitis if the nerve is abnormal neurophysiologically. An additional muscle biopsy increases the diagnostic yield:

- Eosinophilic infiltrates: suggestive of Churg–Strauss syndrome.
- Epineurial and endoneurial granulomas, with secondary demyelination, are diagnostic of sarcoidosis.

DIAGNOSIS
A histologic diagnosis requiring confirmation by tissue biopsy.

TREATMENT
Corticosteroids are the mainstay of treatment despite the lack of evidence from controlled clinical trials. Steroids combined with cyclophosphamide are generally required for severe forms, or those with systemic features of vasculitis. The drawbacks of cyclophosphamide include opportunistic infection, gonadal failure and bladder carcinoma (15%). For patients with giant cell arteritis, steroids should be continued for many months, or even years; the clinical features and ESR are useful measures for titration of dosage.

PROGNOSIS
Depends on the cause:

- Polyarteritis nodosa: poor in untreated patients. Corticosteroid therapy is associated with partial or complete recovery of neurologic function in about half of patients over a few months to years.
- Rheumatoid arthritis: outcome varies, and may not be that bad.
- Systemic lupus erythematosus: tends to recover spontaneously.
- Wegener's granulomatosis: peripheral (and cranial) neuropathies may resolve spontaneously over several hours.
- Sarcoidosis: corticosteroids are the treatment of choice but the response is extremely variable.
- Non-systemic form confined to nerve or nerve and muscle: much better prognosis and an excellent response to therapy.

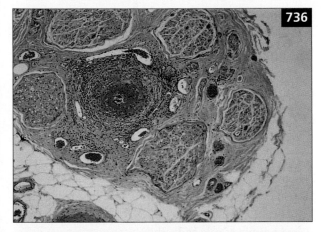

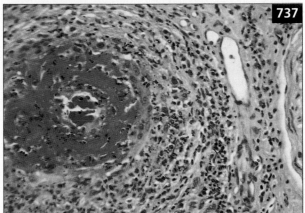

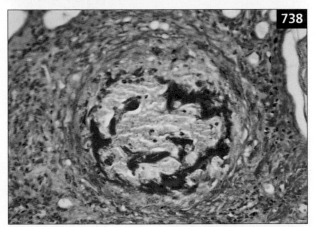

736–738 Sural nerve biopsy from a patient with ischemic neuropathy due to polyarteritis nodosa. H&E stain, ×100 magnification (**736**), and H&E, ×400 (**737**), show infiltration of the arteriolar wall by neutrophils, and fibrinoid necrosis of the vessel wall as a homogenous pink. Martius scarlet blue stain for fibrin, ×400 (**738**), shows the fibrin (of the fibrinoid necrosis) as red.

HERPES ZOSTER INFECTION

DEFINITION
A predominantly dermatologic condition caused by reactivation of the varicella-zoster virus which is latent in nerve cells.

EPIDEMIOLOGY
Varicella-zoster virus is a ubiquitous infectious agent. More than 90% of the adult population in the western world, and 50% in tropical countries, are infected with the virus.
- Incidence of shingles: 100–225 per 100 000 general population per year.
- Cumulative incidence: at least 20% of all adults suffer from zoster at some time.
- Age: any age, but the chances rise with age. 5% of cases occur in children younger than 15 years of age.
- Gender: M=F.

PATHOLOGY
- Dorsal root ganglia: inflammation (mononuclear cell infiltration) with intranuclear varicella-zoster virus inclusions in neurons and satellite cells; neuronal loss and necrosis. Destruction of ganglion cells is prominent in areas of hemorrhage. Sclerosis occurs months to years after the acute attack.
- Posterior nerve roots: inflammation, destruction of myelin and axonal swelling within 1–2 weeks after the onset of rash, followed by macrophage and fibroblastic proliferation.
- Posterior columns: myelin breakdown in severe infections.

ETIOLOGY AND PATHOPHYSIOLOGY
- Transmission is largely through inhalation of infectious aerosols. Direct contact with active varicella or zoster lesions less often leads to infection.
- Incubation period: 10–21 days.
- Primary infection in the non-immune host is chickenpox.
- Following the acute, often trivial, primary infection, the virus becomes latent in nerve cells.
- In the immune host, reactivation of the virus results in zoster, which is predominantly an infection of the skin (shingles).

Risk factors
- Increasing age.
- Immunosuppression.
- HIV infection.

CLINICAL FEATURES

- Site of involvement of nerve root dermatomes:
- – Trigeminal nerve: 12% of patients.
- – Cervical: 17%.
- – Thoracic: 50%.
- – Lumbar: 10%.
- – Sacral: 5%.
- Pain, and sometimes paresthesia, in the region of the involved dermatome may precede the skin eruption by up to 3 weeks. This may lead to misdiagnosis (e.g. of chole-cystitis) and inappropriate treatment (e.g. cholecystectomy).
- Skin lesions (vesicular eruption) and sensory loss in the affected dermatomes (**739–742**). The vesicles are initially clear, become turbid, begin to crust within 5–10 days, and occasionally leave residual scars.
- Low grade fever, general malaise, headache, neck stiffness, and regional lymphadenopathy may accompanying symptoms.
- In 3–5% of patients with cutaneous zoster, concomitant infection of the ventral roots at the same level of the spinal cord lead to weakness of the affected myotome ('segmental zoster paresis').
- Pain usually abates after the skin has healed, but at least 10–20% of patients develop post-herpetic neuralgia.

COMPLICATIONS

- Aseptic meningitis: some degree is often, although not always present, particularly in the early stages.
- Encephalitis (see p.292).
- Cerebral infarction via infiltration and arteritis of major intracranial arteries.
- Brachial plexus neuropathy.
- Myelitis.
- Acute ascending polyradiculopathy.
- Mononeuropathy (median, ulnar, long thoracic, recurrent laryngeal, or phrenic nerves).
- Post-herpetic neuralgia: point-prevalence in community studies is about 19% at 1 month, 7% at 3 months, 3% at 1 year, and 1% at 3 years. Usually mild to moderate severity. Risk factors include increased age (>60 years), prodrome of dermatomal pain before appearance of rash, and severity of pain and rash.

INVESTIGATIONS

- Swab and culture infected vesicles.
- Viral serology.
- Electromyography: may show evidence of motor denervation in paraspinal muscles adjacent to involved sensory roots, indicating concomitant involvement of ventral roots (clinically or subclinically).

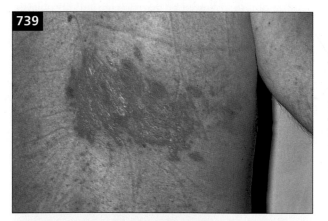

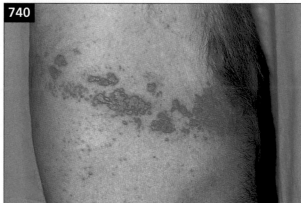

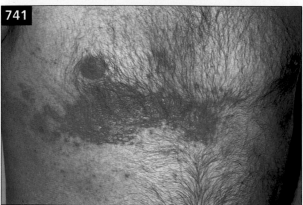

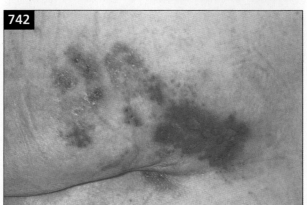

739–741 Vesicular skin rash in the distribution of the T5 dermatome, around the trunk in the mid thoracic level, due to herpes zoster infection of the right T5 dorsal root ganglia.

742 Vesicular skin rash over the left side of the sacrum in a patient with a left L5 radiculopathy due to herpes zoster infection.

TREATMENT
Herpes zoster
Acyclovir
- 800 mg five times a day, orally for 7 days (intravenously if immunocompromised).
- Speeds healing and reduces the period of pain and skin lesions.
- Reduces the incidence of post-herpetic neuralgia.
- Combining acyclovir with oral prednisolone does not prevent the occurrence of post-herpetic neuralgia.
- A related drug to acyclovir, such as valacyclovir or famciclovir, is an alternative. As they have better bioavailability, they can be given three times daily. Famciclovir oral 500 mg or 750 mg three times daily, given within 72 hours of the onset of rash for 7 days, but once- or twice-daily dosing interval in patients with renal impairment, decreases the duration and symptoms of acute herpes zoster and post-herpetic neuralgia. Adverse effects are few.

Post-herpetic neuralgia
Analgesia
- Topical:
- – Lignocaine gel 5%.
- – Capsaicin.
- – Acetylsalicylic acid (aspirin).
- Oral: tricyclic antidepressants.
- Parenteral:
- – Ketamine.
- – Narcotics.
- – Intravenous lidocaine.
- Nerve blockade/solvents:
- – Selective sympathetic or somatic nerve blockade.
- – Alcohol.
- – Chloroform.
- – Low-energy laser.
- Systemic and intralesional corticosteroids: ineffective.

Antiviral therapy
- Famciclovir (500 mg or 750 mg three times a day for 7 days) halves the duration of post-herpetic neuralgia (by about 2 months on average from 163 days [4 months] to 63 days [2 months]) in immunocompetent patients, particularly those over 50 years of age.
- Valaciclovir (valacyclovir).

PROGNOSIS
- Herpes zoster infection usually resolves spontaneously over a week or so, particularly with supplementation in the form of antiviral agent.
- Recovery from post-herpetic neuralgia occurs in most cases, but may take up to 2 years.

HUMAN IMMUNODEFICIENCY VIRUS (HIV) NEUROPATHY

DEFINITION
Peripheral neuropathy ('neuritis' in its true sense) caused by infection with the human immunodeficiency virus.

EPIDEMIOLOGY
- Prevalence: uncommon; about 1–2% of HIV positive individuals. Much more common in the late stages of the disease.
- Age: young adults.
- Gender: M≥F.

PATHOLOGY
Acute and chronic inflammatory demyelinating polyneuropathy
Segmental demyelination.

Distal, symmetric, painful, predominantly sensory axonal neuropathy
- The most common peripheral nerve syndrome associated with HIV infection, occurring clinically in about one-third of patients late in the disease course, and demonstrable pathologically in up to 100% of small series (**743**).
- A progressive axonal degeneration with endoneurial and epineurial inflammation may be found on nerve biopsy.

Sensory ataxic neuropathy
Ganglioneuronitis.

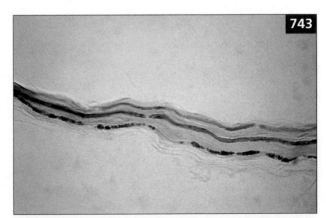

743 Sural nerve biopsy, teased osmicated preparation, three nerve fibers. In the upper and middle fibers paranodal demyelination is seen and in the lowermost fiber there are myelin ovoids indicating Wallerian degeneration.

Mononeuritis multiplex and progressive polyradiculopathy
Necrotizing arteritis of the vasa nervorum (**744, 745**).

Isolated mononeuropathy without apparent local compression (e.g. facial nerve, median nerve, lateral cutaneous nerve of thigh, common peroneal nerve)

Iatrogenic dose-related toxic neuropathy

ETIOLOGY AND PATHOPHYSIOLOGY
Acute inflammatory demyelinating polyneuropathy
- A rare event which occurs early in the course of HIV infection and may represent a reaction to seroconversion.
- Presumed to result from an immune reaction that transiently causes peripheral demyelination.
- Secondary to perivascular replication of HIV in infiltrating mononuclear cells.
- Usually recovers completely.

Chronic inflammatory demyelinating polyneuropathy
May occur at any disease stage, presumably as a result of immune mediated demyelination.

Distal, symmetric, painful, predominantly sensory axonal neuropathy
- Etiology unknown.
- Rare in the early stages of infection.
- Clear temporal relation between onset of symptoms or abrupt change in severity of symptoms and cytomegalovirus (CMV) infection.

Mononeuritis multiplex and progressive polyradiculopathy
Usually arise in AIDS patients with CD4 counts <50 and CMV infection.

Iatrogenic dose-related toxic neuropathy
Due to treatment for HIV with dideoxynucleotides, particularly ddC.

CLINICAL FEATURES
- Onset especially in the late stages of the disease, when the CNS is also commonly involved.

- Several subtypes of peripheral neuropathy: the most common patterns involve several rather than single nerves.

Acute inflammatory demyelinating polyneuropathy
- Subacute onset over days.
- Progressive motor weakness, beginning in the lower extremities and ascending.
- Areflexia.
- Variable sensory and autonomic symptoms.
- Some patients progress to respiratory insufficiency requiring mechanical ventilatory support.

Chronic inflammatory demyelinating polyneuropathy
- Progressive motor weakness, beginning in the lower extremities and ascending.
- Areflexia.
- More prominent sensory symptoms than AIDP.
- May follow a progressive or relapsing course over months

Distal, symmetric, painful, predominantly sensory axonal neuropathy
- Distal symmetric sensory involvement beginning in the feet and gradually ascending in the legs.
- Severe neuralgic pain; burning or shooting in character.
- Feet are numb, and paresthesiae in upper and lower limbs are usually present.
- Examination reveals impairment of vibration and pinprick sensation distally, loss of or diminished angle reflexes with variable depression of other reflexes and sensory ataxia.
- Motor weakness in distal muscles may be present but this is overshadowed by the sensory symptoms.

Sensory ataxic neuropathy

Progressive polyradiculopathy
Cauda equina syndrome.

Mononeuritis multiplex
Bilateral radial nerve palsy.

Isolated mononeuropathy without apparent local compression
- Facial neuropathy.
- Median neuropathy.

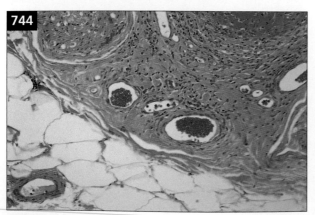

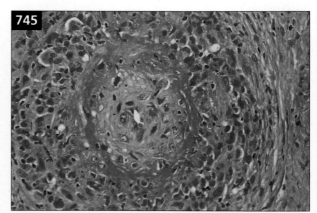

744, 745 Nerve biopsy showing mild inflammatory cell infiltrate around the veins of the vasa nervorum (**744**) and marked neutrophil infiltration (dark, nucleated cells) and fibrinoid necrosis (homogeneous pink substance) of the arteriolar wall of the vasa nervorum (**745**).

- Lateral cutaneous nerve of thigh neuropathy.
- Common peroneal neuropathy.

DIFFERENTIAL DIAGNOSIS
Acute and chronic inflammatory demyelinating polyneuropathy (see pp. 589, 593)

Distal, symmetric, painful, predominantly sensory axonal neuropathy
- Toxic effects of dideoxynucleoside antiretroviral agents, which may mimic or exacerbate this neuropathy.
- Other potentially neurotoxic agents commonly used in HIV patients such as dapsone, isoniazid, and vincristine.
- Vitamin B_{12} deficiency is common in these patients.
- Lymphoma may produce neuralgia by direct invasion or by paraneoplastic effects.
- Diabetes mellitus.
- Alcoholic neuropathy.

Sensory ataxic neuropathy due to ganglioneuronitis
- Paraneoplastic syndrome.
- Sjögren's syndrome.

Mononeuritis multiplex
- Vasculitis.
- Herpes zoster infection.

INVESTIGATIONS
CD4 lymphocyte count
Most opportunistic complications appear after significant immunosuppression has occurred, as reflected by CD4 lymphocyte counts of $200/mm^3$ or less.

Plasma HIV viral RNA load

Serology
- HIV.
- CMV.

CSF
- Acute and chronic inflammatory demyelinating polyneuropathy.
- Prominent elevation of CSF protein.
- Moderate lymphocytic pleocytosis, in contrast with the non-HIV-infected population with acute IDP.
- A polymorphonuclear pleocytosis suggests CMV infection.

Electrophysiologic studies
Acute and chronic inflammatory demyelinating polyneuropathy:
- Prominent slowing and motor nerve conduction blocks.
- Prolonged or absent F-wave responses.
- Variable degrees of axonal damage and denervation.

Distal, symmetric, painful, predominantly sensory axonal neuropathy
- Diminished amplitudes and conduction in sural nerves and variable amplitude decrements in other nerves with relatively preserved conduction.
- EMG may detect symmetric denervation and reinnervation.

Sural nerve biopsy
Performed if the differential diagnosis includes other treatable conditions that can be diagnosed by sural nerve biopsy (see Peripheral neuropathy, pp.579, 583).

TREATMENT
General principles
- Correct any metabolic deficiency and discontinue potential neurotoxic agents, particularly dideoxynucleosides, if possible.
- Physiotherapy to prevent contracture formation and improve strength and function.
- Occupational therapy.
- Subcutaneous heparin 5000 U bd and compression stockings to prevent deep vein thrombophlebitis in non-ambulatory patients.
- Disabling sensory symptoms (neuralgic pain) may respond to any of the following:
  - Amitriptyline.
  - Carbamazepine (starting with 100 mg bd and increasing by 200 mg weekly to 800–1200 mg/day if tolerated and needed).
  - Diphenylhydantoin (phenytoin) (100 mg tds).
  - Gabapentin (300–600 mg tds).
  - Mexiletene (mexiletine) (150 mg bd, increasing to 300 mg bd as required), if the above measures fail.
- Narcotic analgesia, if the above measures fail.

Acute inflammatory demyelinating polyneuropathy
- May recover spontaneously.
- If significant motor impairment:
  - Plasma exchange totalling 200–250 ml/kg divided in five exchanges over a 2-week period with 5% albumin replacement. Or:
  - Pooled human immunoglobulin 0.4 g/kg daily for 5 days given as an i.v. infusion at 0.05–4.0 ml/kg/hour as tolerated.
- Electively intubate patients with impending respiratory failure (vital capacity <1000 cm^3) until adequate ventilatory function returns.

Chronic inflammatory demyelinating polyneuropathy
- Maintenance therapy with one treatment every 2–4 weeks of pooled human immunoglobulin (or plasma exchange). Intervals can be gradually extended as response occurs.
- Corticosteroid therapy probably should not be used because of the potential for facilitating opportunistic infections.

Distal, symmetric, painful, predominantly sensory axonal neuropathy
- Direct HIV therapy has variable benefit.
- Treat disabling sensory symptoms (neuralgic pain) as above.

Iatrogenic dose-related toxic neuropathy
Discontinue potential neurotoxic agents, particularly dideoxynucleosides, if possible.

Single-lesion paucibacillary leprosy

Single dose of rifampicin (rifampin) 600 mg, ofloxacin 400 mg, and minocycline 100 mg (ROM).

Paucibacillary leprosy

Rifampicin (rifampin) 600 mg monthly, supervised, and dapsone 100 mg daily, unsupervised, for 6 months.

Multibacillary leprosy

Rifampicin (rifampin) 600 mg and clofazimine 300 mg monthly, supervised; and dapsone 100 mg and clofazimine 50 mg daily, unsupervised, for at least 12 months, if not 24 months.

Adverse effects

Uncommon

- Dapsone: mild hemolytic anemia (can be severe with glucose-6-phosphate dehydrogenase deficiency), agranulocytosis and skin eruptions. Safely taken in pregnancy.
- Clofazimine: gastrointestinal upset and skin pigmentation (which clears when the drug is discontinued). Safely taken in pregnancy.
- Rifampicin (rifampin): rarely causes side effects given as a once monthly dose of 600 mg, but experience in pregnancy is limited.

PROGNOSIS

If appropriately treated, the average relapse rate is slightly >1% for paucibacillary cases and <1% for multibacillary cases. If relapse does occur, the patient should be re-treated with the same regimen since drug resistance is very unlikely if the patient's *M. leprae* was originally fully sensitive to the drugs used.

PARAPROTEINEMIC NEUROPATHIES

DEFINITION

A group of neuropathies associated with the presence of excessive amounts of abnormal immunoglobulins, which are usually monoclonal serum proteins (termed M protein or M spike) and are the product of a single clone of plasma cells.

EPIDEMIOLOGY

- Prevalence: account for 10% of demyelinating neuropathies and 10% of neuropathies of otherwise unknown etiology.
- Age: more common in the elderly (i.e. >50 years of age).
- Gender: M>F.

ETIOLOGY

Monoclonal gammopathy of uncertain significance (MGUS) (most common):

- Comprises two-thirds of patients with paraproteinemic neuropathy.
- Among patients with MGUS and neuropathy, the paraprotein is of any immunoglobulin (Ig) class, but is usually IgM (60%) and sometimes with κ light chains, and less commonly IgG (30%) and IgA (10%).

- Some paraproteins (mostly polyclonal) react with GM1 gangliosides or disialosyl groups on gangliosides GD1b, GT1b, and GQ1b.

Systemic disorders

- Multiple myeloma.
- Osteosclerotic myeloma (solitary or multiple plasmacytomas), or the POEMS (polyneuropathy, organomegaly, endocrinopathy, monoclonal paraproteinemia, and skin hyperpigmentation) syndrome.
- Waldenström's macroglobulinemia.
- Amyloidosis.
- Cryoglobulinemia.
- Other lymphoproliferative disorders:
- Non-Hodgkin's lymphoma.
- Leukemia.
- Castleman's disease.
- Hypersensitivity lymphadenopathy.

PATHOLOGY (748)

MGUS

- The IgM polyneuropathy is usually of demyelinating type and predominantly causes large fiber sensory dysfunction.
- Immunocytochemistry may show binding of IgM to myelin with widening of the interperiod line within myelin.
- Electron microscopy may show characteristic widening of external myelin lamellae.
- The IgG polyneuropathy may be an axonal neuropathy, and there may be antibodies directed against sulfatide or chondroitin sulfate C, both of which are epitopes on the axon.

Systemic disorders

Multiple myeloma

- Usually a dying-back peripheral neuropathy with destruction of both axons and myelin; presumably primary axonal degeneration with secondary demyelination.
- Amyloid deposition is present in about one-third of cases.
- Neoplastic root infiltration occurs rarely.

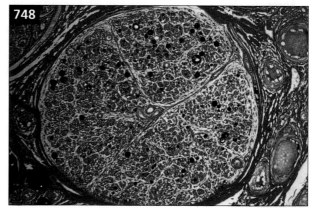

748 Transverse section though a nerve fascicle showing loss of myelinated fibers and axonal degeneration.

Osteosclerotic myeloma
- A rare plasma-cell dyscrasia characterized by single or multiple plasmacytomas that manifest as sclerotic bone lesions.
- Accounts for 3–5% of myelomas.
- 85% of patients present with a demyelinating polyneuropathy, with secondary axonal degeneration, and with or without inflammation.
- The M protein, which is usually IgG or IgA in low concentration, is present in 90% of cases, and virtually always with a λ subtype of light chain.
- Essentially the same disease as the POEMS syndrome.

Waldenström's macroglobulinemia
- Demyelination, but distal axonopathy and sensory neuropathy occur rarely.
- The IgM paraprotein is derived from lymphocytoid cells that proliferate in the marrow and lymph nodes, much the same as in IgM MGUS, from which Waldenström's macroglobulinemia may arise.

Amyloidosis
Amyloid polyneuropathies are of two types:
- Inherited amyloidosis-associated neuropathy.
- Primary (non-familial) systemic amyloidosis-associated neuropathy:
  - More common than inherited amyloidosis-associated neuropathy.
  - An M spike is present in serum or urine in 90% of patients, usually consisting of IgG with a λ light chain or the light chain alone.
  - A symmetric sensorimotor small-diameter sensory fiber axonal polyneuropathy with amyloid deposition.

Cryoglobulinemia
- Cryoglobulins are proteins (usually IgG or IgM) which precipitate when cooled, re-dissolve when warmed, and are deposited as immune complexes in blood vessels.
- The immunoglobulin may be monoclonal, both monoclonal and polyclonal (mixed essential cryoglobulinemia), or polyclonal.
- Neuropathy is quite common in patients who have mixed essential cryoglobulinemia, the type unassociated with lymphoproliferative diseases, chronic infections, or autoimmune disorders.
- The neuropathy is a confluence of complete and incomplete multiple axonal mononeuropathies caused by vasculitis in numerous nerve fascicles.

PATHOPHYSIOLOGY
- Some of the abnormal immunoglobulins have properties of antibodies which are directed against components of the myelin sheath or axolemma.
- Others have an uncertain pathophysiologic role intermediate between that of proteins associated with neuropathies and proteins associated with lymphoproliferative disorders.
- The nerves may also be damaged by deposition of the amyloid byproduct of the circulating paraprotein.
- Immunoglobulin M antibodies are more likely to be pathogenic than IgG or IgA.

- Myelin associated glycoprotein (MAG) is the most common target epitope. The carbohydrate epitope on myelin-associated glycoprotein also reacts with the HNK-1 epitope and there is shared reactivity with two other myelin proteins, P0 and PMP-22, and a sulfated glycosphingolipid sulfate-3-glucuronyl paragloboside.
- A few patients with a sensory form of axonal neuropathy have autoantibodies (usually IgG) directed against sulfatide or chondroitin sulfate C, both of which are epitopes on the axon.
- In the CANOMAD syndrome (chronic ataxic neuropathy, ophthalmoplegia, M protein, agglutination, anti-disialosyl antibodies), the antibody binds to human dorsal roots and dorsal root ganglia and to femoral and oculomotor nerves.
- In osteosclerotic myeloma, the deposition of light chains in the endoneurium suggests that the paraprotein has a proximate role in nerve damage. Greatly elevated levels of proinflammatory cytokines, such as tumor necrosis factor, have also been implicated.
- In amyloidosis, the pathogenesis of the generalized sensory neuropathy is uncertain; both a direct toxic effect of amyloid and vascular insufficiency have been proposed. Amyloid concentration in the flexor retinaculum causes carpal tunnel syndrome (see p.630).

CLINICAL FEATURES
Heterogeneous clinical picture.

Peripheral neuropathy associated with MGUS
IgM (usually κ) paraproteinemic neuropathy syndrome with antibodies to myelin-associated glycoprotein
- A relatively homogeneous subgroup clinically.
- Men, over 50 years of age are principally, but not exclusively, affected.
- Slowly progressive, predominantly sensory, sensorimotor demyelinating neuropathy characterized by foot numbness, paresthesiae, imbalance and gait ataxia progressing over a few months. Touch, joint position and vibration sensation in the legs (referable to conduction in large fibers) are most affected.
- Aching, discomfort, dysesthesiae or lancinating pains occur in half the patients.
- An upper limb postural tremor is often present.
- Weakness of the distal leg muscles with variable wasting occurs as the illness advances.
- A few patients have a pure motor disorder.

IgG and IgA paraproteinemic neuropathy syndromes
- More heterogeneous clinical picture.
- Clinical features and response to treatment commonly resemble CIDP, although a few have a sensory form of axonal neuropathy.

Neuropathic syndrome due to paraproteins (mostly polyclonal) which react with GM1 gangliosides
Purely motor syndrome.

Neuropathic syndrome due to paraproteins specific for disialosyl groups on gangliosides GD1b, GT1b and GQ1b
- Progressive sensory ataxic neuropathy due to altered position sense.
- CANOMAD syndrome develops in a subgroup of these patients.

Systemic malignant disorders (precede or accompany neuropathy)

Multiple myeloma

- Neuropathy is present neurophysiologically in about one-third of patients, and clinically in about 5–10% of patients.
- Usually mixed sensorimotor peripheral neuropathy but purely sensory or relapsing and remitting forms occur.
- Autonomic dysfunction may be present in some patients, and suggests the presence of systemic amyloidosis.
- Weakness and numbness of the distal limbs appear subacutely over several weeks, beginning occasionally in the upper limbs.

Osteosclerotic myeloma, or the POEMS syndrome

Commonly presents with a slowly progressive neuropathy which is mainly motor and demyelinating, and may be part of the POEMS syndrome (polyneuropathy associated with organomegaly, endocrinopathy, M protein, skin thickening and hyperpigmentation, and clubbing).

Waldenström's macroglobulinemia

- Sensorimotor neuropathy occurs frequently, very similar to that which occurs in IgM paraprotein associated neuropathies of benign type.
- Fatigue, weight loss, and bleeding dominate the clinical picture.
- Paresthesiae and numbness in the feet are followed by weakness and wasting of the lower legs, causing foot drop and a steppage gait, and months later, by arm weakness.

Amyloid neuropathy

- A symmetric sensorimotor small fiber polyneuropathy is the presenting feature in 15% of patients.
- Numbness in the feet is the most common presenting symptom, but the signature symptoms are burning and aching pains with lancinating electric sensations and loss of pain and temperature sensation in the distal parts of the limbs.
- Autonomic symptoms can be extreme, particularly postural hypotension, diarrhea (also from infiltration of the gut wall), impotence and bladder dysfunction.
- Carpal tunnel syndrome is common.
- Systemic symptoms include weight loss, and those referable to amyloid deposition in other organs, such as the heart and kidneys.

Cryoglobulinemia

- The most common clinical picture is that of a progressive, symmetric, distal sensorimotor neuropathy (due to a confluence of incomplete mononeuropathies) combined with one or two clearly recognizable mononeuropathies (e.g. wrist or foot drop).
- The other typical presentation is that of a multiple mononeuropathy.
- Onset is acute in about one-third of patients who have multiple mononeuritis.
- Pain is almost always present at onset.
- Paresthesiae and Raynaud's phenomenon are precipitated by cold in some patients.
- Weakness may be multifocal or generalized.

DIFFERENTIAL DIAGNOSIS

Chronic inflammatory demyelinating polyneuropathy (see p.593)

- About one-quarter of patients with CIDP also have a paraproteinemia (which is of uncertain relevance).
- The cardinal EMG feature of CIDP (a focal block of electric conduction in motor nerves) sometimes also occurs in MGUS.
- The CSF protein level is usually elevated in both CIDP and MGUS.
- Both CIDP and MGUS respond to immunomodulating treatment.

Multifocal motor neuropathy (see CIDP, p.594):

- A purely motor disorder of middle-aged men, characterized by slowly progressive, painless weakness that is asymmetric and confined to one limb.
- Linked to high titers of IgM antibodies directed at GM1 ganglioside on myelin membranes. The circulating paraprotein is often polyclonal, but monoclonal in 20% of cases.
- Electric conduction block in the proximal or middle segments of motor nerves, with normal sensory conduction in the same nerves.
- 90% of patients respond to immune globulin, but require repeated infusions.

Motor neuron disease (see p.534)

Multiple myeloma

- Absence of systemic features of myeloma (bone pain, fatigue, anemia, hypercalcemia, renal insufficiency).
- Smaller amount of paraprotein (<3 g/dl serum, and usually 0.75–1.5 g/dl).
- Amyloidosis (cf. sensory form of axonal neuropathy that may occur with IgG MGUS).

INVESTIGATIONS

Nerve conduction studies

IgM paraproteinemic demyelinating neuropathy with anti-myelin-associated glycoprotein antibodies

- Slowing of motor nerve conduction velocity which is more distal than proximal.
- Distal motor latencies prolonged representing a marked distal accentuation of conduction slowing.
- Absence of conduction block.

Multiple myeloma

Neurophysiologic evidence of axonal damage, which may be severe.

Waldenström's macroglobulinemia

Neurophysiologic evidence of demyelination, but occasionally a distal axonopathy or sensory neuropathy.

Amyloid neuropathy

Features of a symmetric sensorimotor small fiber axonal neuropathy.

Cryoglobulinemia

Neurophysiologic evidence of axonal damage in multiple nerves.

Immunoglobulins and serum protein electrophoresis
- Immunoglobulins can be detected by immunoelectrophoresis or the more sensitive immunofixation tests.
- The detection of cryoglobulins requires that the blood specimen is transported to the laboratory in a warm-water bath.

CSF
CSF protein is often raised, and in osteosclerotic myeloma the CSF protein is almost invariably elevated to >1 g/l (>100 mg/dl).

Bone marrow examination or radiologic skeletal survey
Performed if suspected plasmacytoma or myeloma (e.g. patients with IgG and IgA paraproteins, particularly if resistant to treatment).

Nerve biopsy
MGUS: most common
- Immunocytochemistry may show binding of IgM to myelin with widening of the interperiod line within myelin.
- To rule out amyloid deposition in patients with sensory axonal neuropathy due to suspected IgG MGUS.

Amyloid neuropathy
Confirms the diagnosis in 90% of cases.

Biopsy of other tissues
Amyloid neuropathy
Amyloid is detected in biopsies of bone marrow and rectal mucosa in 70% and 80% of cases, respectively.

TREATMENT
Treatment of the underlying cause may improve the neuropathy.

MGUS
IgG or IgA MGUS
- Plasma exchange (a total of 220 ml/kg, given in four or five treatments) has been shown in a controlled trial to sometimes afford at least short-term benefit within days or weeks of administration in about one-third of patients.
- Intravenous immunoglobulin in high dose (0.4 g/kg body weight daily for 5 days) appears to benefit some patients.
- Corticosteroids, sometimes in combination with immunosuppressants, may be effective but is more often ineffective.
- Cyclophosphamide, melphalan, azathioprine, chlorambucil, fludarabine and interferon-alpha have been used.
- Immunoadsorption (in which IgG and immune complexes are removed by passing the patient's blood through a plastic column containing covalently bound staphylococcal protein) generally produces only transient amelioration, and needs to be repeated every few months.

IgM MGUS
- Generally more refractory to treatment than IgG or IgA MGUS.
- May respond to same regimens as IgG or IgA MGUS, particularly if chlorambucil or cyclophosphamide is added in a dose sufficient to reduce the amount of M protein.
- Patients with anti-MAG antibodies generally require prolonged therapy with monthly plasma exchange and continuous oral or pulsed intravenous cyclophosphamide.
- Interferon-alpha was beneficial in one trial.

Systemic disorders
Multiple myeloma
Removing the paraprotein by plasma exchange has no consistent effect on the neuropathy.

Osteosclerotic myeloma
- Treatment of solitary bone lesions (e.g. resection, focused radiotherapy, or chemotherapy) may stabilize or improve the neuropathy in about half of patients but the response may not be forthcoming for several months.
- Plasma exchange is generally ineffective, as in neuropathy associated with myeloma.

Waldenström's macroglobulinemia
- Plasma exchange may slow the progression of the neuropathy.
- Prednisone, melphalan, and chlorambucil may be helpful.

Amyloid neuropathy
- Prednisone and melphalan prolongs survival in a small proportion of patients for several years but has little effect on the neuropathy.
- Autologous stem-cell transplantation may stabilize or improve the condition in a few patients in the short term at least.

Cryoglobulinemia
- Corticosteroids, cyclophosphamide, and plasma exchange are variably successful in stabilizing the neuropathy.
- Interferon alpha is promising in cases associated with hepatitis C.

PROGNOSIS
MGUS
- Usually benign, mild and stable, but about 20% of patients will in time acquire a malignant plasma-cell disorder, usually myeloma.
- The syndrome of predominantly sensory neuropathy due to IgM κ paraprotein with antibodies to myelin-associated glycoprotein is associated with a benign clinical course.
- Neuropathies associated with benign paraproteins of the IgG and IgA class respond better to treatment than those associated with an IgM paraprotein. However, patients with IgM paraprotein neuropathies may improve after plasma exchange or intravenous immunoglobulin, particularly when used in association with cyclophosphamide or chlorambucil.
- In patients with polyneuropathy associated with IgM monoclonal gammopathy, antibody tests to MAG (myelin-associated glycoprotein) SGPG (sulfoglucuronyl paragloboside), and sulfatide do not have prognostic value.

DIABETIC NEUROPATHY

DEFINITION
Neuropathic complications of diabetes mellitus.

EPIDEMIOLOGY
- Incidence: 54 (95% CI: 33–83) per 100 000 per year.
- Lifetime prevalence: 2 (95% CI: 1–3) per 1000 population. One of the most common causes of peripheral neuropathy:
  - At the time of diagnosis, 8% of non-insulin dependent diabetics have definite or probable neuropathy, compared with 2% of an age-and sex matched control population.
  - After 10 years of follow-up, the prevalence of neuropathy increases to 42% among diabetic patients and to 6% in controls.
  - At any one time, about 34% of insulin dependent diabetics and 26% of non-insulin dependent diabetics have distal symmetric polyneuropathy; and 58% of insulin dependent diabetic patients aged 30 years or more have distal symmetric polyneuropathy
  - At any one time, about 17% of diabetics have at least one abnormal test of autonomic function but, besides erectile dysfunction, only 2.4% report symptoms attributable to autonomic dysfunction.
- Age: adults, increases with duration of diabetes.
- Gender: M=F.

PATHOLOGY
Axonal degeneration of nerve fibers of all sizes, both myelinated and unmyelinated.

ETIOLOGY AND PATHOPHYSIOLOGY
- Diabetes renders nerves vulnerable to injury and may also involve the vasa nervorum.
- Hyperglycemia play a central role in the pathogenesis of diabetic peripheral neuropathy.

Risk factors for neuropathy
- Poor glycemic control.
- Duration of diabetes.
- Age.
- Height.
- Male gender.
- Alcohol consumption.

Risk factors for neuropathy in insulin- (but not non-insulin) dependent diabetics
- Systemic hypertension.
- Cigarette smoking.
- Hyperlipidemia.

CLINICAL SYNDROMES
Onset
May be acute, but more commonly insidious.

Rapidly reversible phenomena
Hyperglycemic neuropathy
- Presumably related directly to hyperglycemia or to a metabolic abnormality correlated with it (e.g. hypoxia, a switch to anaerobic glycolysis in the diabetic nerve).
- Patients with severe uncontrolled hyperglycemia.
- Uncomfortable sensory symptoms, mainly in the legs.

- Nerve conduction velocity is reduced.
- Rapidly corrected by establishing diabetic control.

Generalized polyneuropathies
Distal symmetric predominantly sensory (and motor) axonal polyneuropathy
- The most common type of diabetic neuropathy.
- Very common in diabetes, particularly with poorly controlled disease of long duration.

Pathology: a distal axonal degeneration of dying back type with relative preservation of dorsal root ganglion cells (**749**). This may well be a central-peripheral distal axonopathy in which there is also a rostral degeneration of nerve fibers in the dorsal columns of the spinal cord. An important aspect is a failure of axonal regeneration, which probably contributes to the lack of reversibility of the neuropathy once it is established, even with good glycemic control.

Pathophysiology: it remains to be established whether the mechanism is a direct metabolic effect or whether it is secondary to hypoxia from microvascular disease. A major metabolic abnormality in nerve is the accumulation of sorbitol because of increased flux in the polyol pathway secondary to hyperglycemia. The sorbitol in diabetic nerve is not sufficient in quantity to produce osmotic damage but it is possible that it may have deleterious effects on neural metabolism. However, trials with aldose reductase inhibitors that reduce the production of sorbitol have failed so far to show any substantial effects on diabetic polyneuropathy. Other possible metabolic disturbances of relevance include alterations in the metabolism of essential fatty acid and non-enzymatic glycation of proteins.

Clinical: distal symmetric predominantly sensory (and motor) loss characterized by sensory impairment in a glove and stocking distribution and distal motor weakness. The sequelae of longstanding severe distal sensory loss, such as neuropathic joints, may be present (**750**).

Treatment: strict control of blood glucose concentrations by an insulin pump or multiple daily insulin injections can prevent or greatly diminish the risk of developing neuropathy. This treatment however, is only applicable to patients with type I insulin-dependent diabetes and only a small proportion of them. Good glycemic control can only be achieved in practice in about 25% of patients. Once DSSP is established, it fails to improve significantly even with satisfactory glycemic control. Treatment is therefore required that will prevent the occurrence of neuropathy or halt its deterioration if present.

Prognosis: after 25 years of diabetes, about half will have developed neuropathy. Further research is required to help identify, perhaps by genetic markers, those patients who are more susceptible to developing neuropathy.

Autonomic neuropathy
- Symptoms include nocturnal diarrhea, postural hypotension and syncope.
- Mild degrees are common in both type I and type II diabetes, but severe forms are virtually only encountered in type I diabetic patients.

Acute painful sensory neuropathy
- Uncommon.
- Mechanism: uncertain.
- Severe burning or aching pain, mainly in the legs but sometimes more widespread.
- Precipitants include treatment with insulin.
- Examination reveals intense cutaneous contact hyperesthesia but only mild sensory loss.
- May be associated with uncontrolled hyperglycemia and precipitous weight loss.
- Nerve biopsy shows acute axonal degeneration.
- Prognosis: resolves over several months with adequate glycemic control.

Focal and multifocal neuropathies
More common in diabetics than in the general population.

Pathogenesis
The abrupt onset of a diabetic IIIrd cranial nerve palsy is consistent with an ischemic basis and this has been supported by sound pathologic studies. The pathology is a focal demyelination, accounting for the usually satisfactory recovery that occurs, presumably by remyelination. Although nerve ischemia usually gives risk to axonal loss rather than segmental demyelination, it is possible that demyelination in focal diabetic lesions is the result of reperfusion injury (which is known to produce demyelination).

Other focal peripheral nerve lesions are likely to result from an abnormal susceptibility of diabetic nerve to compression. The reasons for this is uncertain, but in non-diabetic individuals entrapment neuropathies are related to longitudinal axoplasmic displacement away from the site of compression and the consequent distortion and breakdown of the myelin sheath of larger myelinated fibers. The basal lamina surrounding nerve fibers is known to be abnormally rigid in patients with diabetic neuropathy, possibly due to increased cross linking of collagen because of abnormal glycation related to advanced glycation end product (AGE) formation.

In some patients with proximal lower limb diabetic neuropathy, inflammatory lesions, including vasculitis, affecting small epineurial vessels, are present in peripheral nerves, raising the possibility of a superimposed auto-immune process.

Cranial neuropathies
The IIIrd and VIIth cranial nerves are affected particularly.

Thoracoabdominal radiculoneuropathy

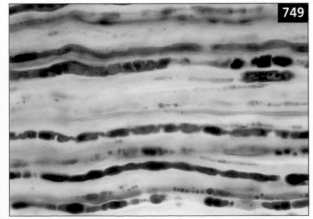

749 Teased nerve fiber (osmium tetroxide) showing segmental demyelination(yellow axons [myelin normally appears black]) and active Wallerian degeneration due to focal interruption of axons (numerous myelin ovoids which appear as black blobs).

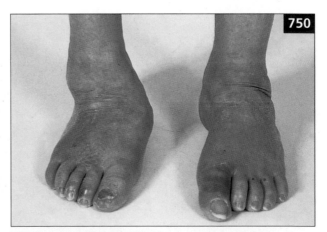

750 Deformed (Charcot) ankle joints in a patient with distal symmetric sensory neuropathy due to diabetes.

Focal limb mononeuropathies (including entrapment and compression neuropathies)

- Located at the well-known sites of entrapment or external compression, and commonly involve the median nerve at the wrist (**751**) and ulnar nerve at the elbow. Other common sites are the radial and peroneal nerves (as in patients without diabetes), as well as the superficial branch of the radial nerve (cheiralgia paresthetica).
- Symptomatic carpal tunnel syndrome is found in about 11% of patients with diabetes mellitus (**751**).
- Not uncommonly superimposed on a polyneuropathy, which may be symptomatic or asymptomatic and only evidenced from nerve conduction studies. A coexistent polyneuropathy is found in about 80% of diabetics with an ulnar nerve palsy, and about 20% of diabetics with carpal tunnel syndrome.
- Frequently it is difficult to determine whether the cause is external pressure or intrinsic focal nerve ischemia or infarction secondary to occlusion of small blood vessels supplying the nerve.
- Femoral neuropathy is not caused by entrapment.
- Acute painless peroneal neuropathy: usually caused by compression to at least some degree in diabetics.
- Brachial plexus neuropathy:
  - Unilateral or bilateral.
  - May be associated with a typical radiculo-plexopathy of the legs (symmetric or asymmetric) and a background generalized sensorimotor polyneuropathy.
  - Onset: subacute or gradual.

Proximal diabetic neuropathy (diabetic amyotrophy, 'diabetic radiculo-plexopathy', 'lower limb asymmetric motor neuropathy')

- Acute, painful, unilateral or asymmetric proximal leg weakness with particular involvement of the sensorimotor territory of the L2–L4 nerve roots (weakness of hip flexion and knee extension, absent knee jerk, and numbness of the anterior thigh and leg).
- Onset in middle-aged or elderly diabetics.
- May be the first manifestation of diabetes.
- May arise in patients with diabetes that is mild and well controlled.

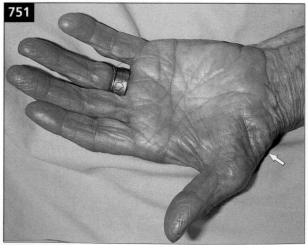

751 Wasting of the left abductor pollicis brevis muscle (arrow) in a patient with a median neuropathy at the wrist due to diabetes.

- May occur against a background of a chronic, symmetric polyneuropathy.
- Severe pain in the anterior thigh may be present at onset.
- Weakness of the quadriceps and iliopsoas is most marked, but the adductor muscles (obturator nerve) may also be weak.
- Absent knee jerk.
- Sensory deficits are rare.
- Weight loss is usual.
- Differential diagnosis includes autoimmune vasculitis: MRI scan showing enhancement of the lumbar nerve roots suggests autoimmune vasculitis rather than diabetes as the cause.
- Nerve conduction studies and EMG usually show features consistent with axonal degeneration of the lumbar spinal nerve roots.
- Pathologic studies show inflammatory change or small infarcts in the lumbosacral plexus and trunks of the femoral and other (e.g. obturator) nerves.
- Treatment is symptomatic although steroids have been used in severe cases despite the diabetes.
- At least some degree of recovery begins within weeks of onset and continues over 12–18 months; if no improvement at all has occurred after several months the diagnosis is in doubt.
- Recovery is incomplete in nearly half of patients.

Superimposed chronic inflammatory demyelinating polyneuropathy

- CIDP is more frequent in diabetics.
- A secondary autoimmune process may be responsible.

DIFFERENTIAL DIAGNOSIS
Predominantly sensory neuropathies
- Diabetes.
- Thiamine deficiency.
- Malignancy.
- Leprosy.
- Hereditary sensory neuropathies.
- Amyloid.
- Uremia.

Predominantly motor neuropathies
- Guillain–Barré syndrome.
- Porphyria.
- Diphtheria.
- Botulism.
- Lead.
- Charcot–Marie–Tooth disease.
- Disorders of the neuromuscular junction or muscle.

INVESTIGATIONS
- Nerve conduction studies: a more pronounced decrease in sensory and motor compound action potential amplitudes than in nerve conduction velocities, consistent with axonal degeneration.
- Blood glucose: fasting.
- Hemoglobin A1C.
- Nerve biopsy if the diagnosis remains uncertain.

DIAGNOSIS
A typical clinical and neurophysiologic profile in a diabetic patient, after excluding differential diagnoses.

TREATMENT

- Good diabetic control probably prevents the development of neuropathy.
- Pancreatic transplantation may relieve the progression.
- Aldose reductase inhibitors do not appear to be effective.
- Recombinant human nerve growth factor 0.1μg/kg was not effective in a recently published randomized controlled trial involving 1019 patients with diabetic polyneuropathy.
- Intravenous immunoglobulin may be helpful for diabetic amyotrophy, but controlled trials are needed.
- Painful neuropathy may respond to tricyclic antidepressants; gabapentin 900 mg/day is probably ineffective or only minimally effective.

PROGNOSIS

- Depends on the intensity of glycemic control.
- Poor glycemic control and low plasma concentrations of insulin independent of concentrations of glucose are associated with increased risk of development and progression of neuropathy.
- Autonomic neuropathy in diabetes probably carries a poor prognosis (i.e. increased risk of death).

FURTHER READING

PERIPHERAL NEUROPATHY
Epidemiology
MacDonald BK, Cockerell OC, Sander JWAS, Shorvon SD (2000) The incidence and life-time prevalence of neurological disorders in a prospective community-based study in the UK. *Brain*, **123**: 665–676.

Martyn CN, Hughes RAC (1997) Epidemiology of peripheral neuropathy. *J. Neurol. Neurosurg. Psychiatry*, **62**: 310–318.

Etiology
Bird SJ, Rich MM (2000) Neuromuscular complications of critical illness. *The Neurologist*, **6**: 2–11.

Subtypes
Bryer MA, Chad DA (1999) Sensory neuronopathies. *The Neurologist*, **5**: 90–100.

Holland NR, Crawford TO, Hauer P, et al. (1998) Small-fibre sensory neuropathies: clinical course and neuropathology of idiopathic cases. *Ann. Neurol.*, **44**: 47–59.

Windebank AJ, Blexrud MD, Dyck PJ, Daube JR, Karnes JL (1990) The syndrome of acute sensory neuropathy: clinical features and electrophysiologic and pathologic changes. *Neurology*, **40**: 584–591.

Investigation
Gabriel CM, Howard R, Kinsella N, et al. (2000) Prospective study of the usefulness of sural nerve biopsy. *J. Neurol. Neurosurg. Psychiatry*, **69**: 442–446.

McLeod JG (1995) Investigation of peripheral neuropathy. *J. Neurol. Neurosurg. Psychiatry*, **58**: 274–283.

Said G (2001) Value of nerve biopsy? *Lancet*, **357**: 1220–1221.

Wolfe GI, Nations SP (2001) Guide to autoantibody testing in peripheral neuropathies. *The Neurologist*, **7**: 195–207.

Management
Hughes RAC (2000) Management of chronic peripheral neuropathy. *Proc. R. Coll. Physicians Edin.*, **30**: 321–327.

HEREDITARY NEUROPATHIES
De Jonghe P, Timmerman V, Nelis E, et al. (1999) A novel type of hereditary motor and sensory neuropathy characterised by a mild phenotype. *Arch. Neurol.*, **56**: 1283–1288.

Lupski JR (2000) Recessive Charcot-Marie-Tooth disease. *Ann. Neurol.*, **47**: 6–8.

HEREDITARY MOTOR AND SENSORY NEUROPATHY
Kamholz J, Menichella D, Jani A, et al. (2000) Charcot-Marie-Tooth disease type 1. Molecular pathogenesis to gene therapy. *Brain*, **123**: 222–233.

HEREDITARY NEUROPATHY WITH LIABILITY TO PRESSURE PALSIES
Duborg O, Mouton P, Brice A, et al. (2000) Guidelines for diagnosis of hereditary neuropathy with liability to pressure palsies. *Neuromuscular Disorders*, **10**: 206–208.

GUILLAIN–BARRÉ SYNDROME
Feasby TE, Hartung H-P (2001) Drain the roots. A new treatment for Guillain–Barré syndrome. *Neurology*, **57**: 753–754.

Hahn AF (1998) Guillain-Barré syndrome. *Lancet*, **352**: 635–641.

Hartung H-P (1999) Infections and the Guillain-Barré syndrome. *J. Neurol. Neurosurg. Psychiatry*, **66**: 277.

Hughes RAC, Gregson NA, Hadden RDM, Smith KJ (1999) Pathogenesis of Guillain–Barré syndrome. *J. Neuroimmunol.*, **100**: 74–97.

Hughes RAC (2001) Sensory form of Guillain–Barré syndrome. *Lancet*, **357**: 1465.

Logina I, Donaghy M (1999) Diphtheritic polyneuropathy: a clinical study and comparison with Guillain-Barré syndrome. *J. Neurol. Neurosurg. Psychiatry*, **67**: 433–438.

Oh SJ, La Ganke C, Claussen GC (2001) Sensory Guillain-Barré syndrome. *Neurology*, **56**: 82–86.

Seneviratne U (2000) Guillain-Barré syndrome. *Postgrad. Med. J.*, **76**: 774–782.

Wollinsky KH, Hülser P-J, Brinkmeier H, et al. (2001) CSF filtration is an effective treatment of Guillain–Barré syndrome. A randomized clinical trial. *Neurology*, **57**: 774–780.

CHRONIC INFLAMMATORY DEMYELINATING POLYNEUROPATHY
Duarte J, Martinez AC, Rodriguez F, et al. (1999) Hypertrophy of multiple cranial nerves and spinal roots in chronic inflammatory demyelinating neuropathy. *J. Neurol. Neurosurg. Psychiatry*, **67**: 685–687.

Dyck PJ, Dyck PJB (2000) Atypical varieties of chronic inflammatory demyelinating neuropathies. *Lancet*, **355**: 1293–1294.

Haq RU, Fries TJ, Pendlebury WW (2000) Chronic inflammatory demyelinating polyradiculoneuropathy. A study of proposed electrodiagnostic and histologic criteria. *Arch. Neurol.*, **57**: 1745–1750.

Hughes R, Bensa S, Willison H, et al. (2001) Randomized controlled trial of intravenous immunoglobulin versus oral prednisolone in chronic inflammatory demyelinating polyradiculoneuropathy. *Ann. Neurol.*, **50**: 195–201.

McLeod JG, Pollard JD, Macaskill P, et al. (1999) Prevalence of chronic inflammatory demyelinating polyneuropathy in New South Wales, Australia. *Ann. Neurol.*, **46**: 910–913.

Mendell JR, Barohn RJ, Freimer ML, et al. (2001) Randomised controlled trial of IVIg in untreated chronic inflammatory demyelinating polyradiculoneuropathy. *Neurology*, **56**: 445–449.

Pestronk A (1998) Multifocal motor neuropathy: Diagnosis and treatment. *Neurology*, **51** (Suppl 5): S22–S24.

Van den Berg-Vos RM, Franssen H, Wokke JHJ, et al. (2000) Multifocal motor neuropathy: Diagnostic criteria that predict the response to immunoglobulin treatment. *Ann. Neurol.*, **48**: 919–926.

VASCULITIC NEUROPATHY
Moore PM (2000) Vasculitic neuropathies. *J. Neurol. Neurosurg. Psychiatry*, **68**: 271–276.

HERPES ZOSTER INFECTION
Choo PW, Galil K, Donahue JG, et al. (1997) Risk factors for post herpetic neuralgia. *Arch. Intern. Med.*, **157**: 1217–1224.

Cunningham AL, Dworkin RH (2000) The management of post-herpetic neuralgia. *BMJ*, **321**: 778–779.

Upper arm lesions
- Trauma: supracondylar fracture of the humerus.
- External compression against the spiral groove:
- Intoxicated sleep (e.g. with the arm folded over the back of a chair or resting on a hard ridge ['Saturday night palsy', 'Parkbanklähmung', paralysie des ivrognes']).
- Improper positioning during general anesthesia.
- Prolonged (e.g. 3 hours) shooting practice in a kneeling position with the upper arm resting on the ipsilateral knee.
- Akinetic rigid syndromes (e.g. Parkinson's disease) causing severe immobility.
- Hereditary liability to pressure palsies (see p.587): palsy after normal sleep.
- Lipoma adjacent to the nerve.
- Traumatic aneurysm of the radial artery.
- Callus bone formation following fracture of the shaft of the humerus.
- Myositis ossificans of the shaft of the humerus.
- Prolonged labor or forceps extraction in the neonate, or repeated blood pressure measurement in the premature infant.
- Athletic activities (compression by lateral head of triceps or a fibrous arch at the lower part of the humeral groove):
- Involving extension at the elbow against strong resistance.
- 'Windmill' pitching motion of competitive softball.
- Medical mononeuropathy:
- Diabetes mellitus.
- Arteritis.
- Nerve tumor.

Forearm (posterior interosseous nerve) lesions
- Congenital hemihypertrophy of the supinator muscle.
- Entrapment of the motor branch of the radial nerve, the deep radial nerve or the posterior interosseous nerve, between 'normal' anatomic structures, at the level of the supinator muscle.
- Accessory brachioradialis muscle.
- Dislocation of the elbow, fracture of the ulna with dislocation of the radial head, or Monteggias's fracture.
- Arthroscopy of the elbow joint.
- Rheumatoid arthritis of the elbow joint.
- Traumatic aneurysm of the posterior interosseous artery.
- Arteriovenous fistula for hemodialysis.
- Lipoma.
- Intramuscular myxoma.
- Cysts.
- Ganglia.

Wrist lesions (superficial terminal branch of radial nerve)
- Handcuffs and other tight wrist bands (e.g. watch band).
- Direct injury:
- Accidental.
- Post-surgery:
  Stenosing tenosynovitis (de Quervain's disease).
  Open reduction of fractures of radius and ulna.
  Shunt operations for hemodialysis.
- Transposition of a flexor tendon towards the thumb.
- Repeated movements of pronation and supination of forearm, or abduction and adduction of the wrist with the forearm in pronation and the wrist in flexion.
- Stenosing tenosynovitis (de Quervain's disease).

Finger lesions (dorsal digital nerves)
- Professional and daily use of scissors (thumb).
- Palmar ganglion.

HISTORY
Axillary lesions
- Short history of weakness stretching the elbow, wrist, all fingers and thumb.
- Pain is not prominent.

Upper arm lesions
- Often sudden onset of inability to extend wrist, fingers and thumb.
- Numbness or paresthesia of the lateral/radial part of the forearm.
- Pain in the elbow and forearm may be present.
- Precipitating injury or predisposing factors (e.g. alcohol or drug intoxication; see above).

Forearm (posterior interosseous nerve) lesions (supinator syndrome)
- Slowly progressive onset of symptoms.
- Initially, difficulty stretching the little finger (it gets curled up during tasks such as retrieving something from a trouser pocket).
- Later, inability to extend metacarpophalangeal joint of the little finger and then similar weakness begins in other fingers, one after the other.
- Consequently, difficulty playing the piano but writing remains normal and grip powerful if the fingers are passively placed around an object.
- Pain is uncommon.
- Bilateral symptoms may occur.

Wrist lesions
- Shooting pain in the radial side of the wrist.
- Painful paresthesia in the thumb and index finger evoked by touching or knocking the radial side of the wrist.
- Reduced sensation on the radial side of the hand (**764**).

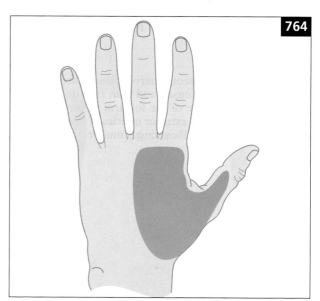

764 Areas of skin innervated by the radial nerve (superficial terminal branch of radial nerve).

EXAMINATION
Axillary lesions
- Weakness of the triceps and all muscles extending wrist, fingers and thumb.
- Mild decreased sensation on the back of the upper arm and forearm, in the web between index finger and thumb, and the radial side of dorsum of the hand.

Upper arm lesions
- Dropped hand and fingers due to weakness of extensors of wrist and metacarpophalangeal joints (**765, 766**).
- Spares triceps muscle and sensation in the upper arm, and often posterior cutaneous nerve of forearm leading to preserved sensation in the web between the index finger and thumb.
- Weakness of brachioradialis (elbow flexion with forearm pronated [not supinated cf. biceps]), supinator (supination of forearm with elbow extended [not flexed, cf. biceps]).

Forearm (posterior interosseous nerve) lesions (supinator syndrome)
- Dropped fingers without dropped hand: inability to extend the fingers and thumb at the metacarpophalangeal joints. Despite severe weakness of extensor carpi ulnaris, wrist extension remains possible because extensor carpi radialis muscles function normally (because the branch to extensor carpi radialis leaves the main stem of the radial nerve above the elbow and proximal to entry of the supinator muscle). If extensor carpi ulnaris is weak, a distinct radial deviation of the extended hand occurs when the patient is asked to make a fist.
- There may be some extension of the index finger at the interphalangeal joints (by contraction of the lumbrical muscles innervated by the median nerve) and some weakness of the supinator muscle, but brachioradialis remains powerful (unless the lesion is above the elbow).
- The interossei may appear to be weak (although they are not weak) with any radial nerve lesion above the wrist because of weakness of finger extension; in order for the fingers to be abducted they need to be extended first. If the fingers are supported on a flat surface, the action of the interossei can be assessed and, in the event of a radial nerve lesion, the fingers can spread apart (to some extent at least), whereas in an upper motor neuron lesion, a T1 root lesion, or a combined lesion of the radial and ulnar nerves, there is weakness of finger abduction.

Wrist lesions
Reduced sensation over the lateral/radial part of the dorsum of the hand, and the dorsum of the thumb (except the nail area), index finger (proximal to the middle phalanx) and first phalanx of the middle finger.

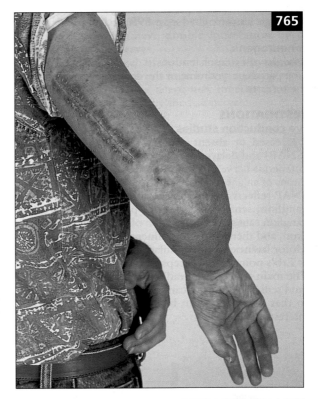

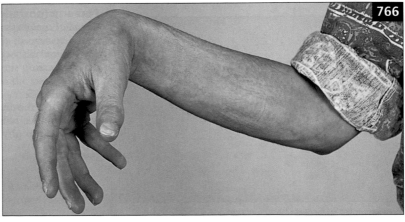

765, 766 Upper arm scar indicating the site of injury to the radial nerve (**765**), and dropped hand and fingers due to weakness of extensors of wrist and metacarpophalangeal joints following upper arm radial nerve injury (**766**).

Infections
- Leprosy.
- Tuberculosis.
- Phlegmon of the palm.

Hereditary liability to pressure palsies (see p.587)

HISTORY
Axillary and upper arm lesions
Same as elbow lesions unless evidence of concomitant median or radial neuropathy.

Elbow and forearm lesions
Sensory symptoms
- Numbness, pins and needles, and occasionally burning pain in the ring and little finger, and sometimes the hypothenar region (but not outside the sensory area of the ulnar nerve, nor causing the patient to wake at night, in contrast to the carpal tunnel syndrome).
- Leaning on the elbow (e.g. against the lower edge of a car window) or flexing the elbow (e.g. reading in bed) may precipitate or exacerbate the symptoms.
- The elbow or the nerve in the ulnar groove may be painful or tender to touch.

Motor symptoms
Weakness and clumsiness of fine finger movements (e.g. zipping trousers, releasing a belt, buttoning and unbuttoning clothing, sewing, guitar playing) may be the presenting symptoms, depending on the fascicles involved, but usually follow the sensory symptoms.

EXAMINATION
Axillary and upper arm lesions
Same as elbow lesions unless evidence of concomitant median or radial neuropathy.

Elbow and forearm lesions
Sensory signs
Altered sensation on the little finger (palmar and dorsal sides), ring finger (ulnar half), and often adjoining parts of the hand, but may be restricted to the tips of the little and ring fingers, or even absent (**774**).

Autonomic signs
- Uncommon.
- Furrowed or atrophic nails of the little and ring fingers.
- Trophic skin lesions may also be present in the cutaneous distribution of the ulnar nerve.

Motor signs
- Weakness (and wasting) of first dorsal interosseous and hypothenar eminence (adduction of the thumb and little finger respectively) may be the only initial signs (**775–778**); the flexor carpi ulnaris and flexor digitorum profundus muscles are rarely wasted (medial border of forearm) or weak in the early stages.
- A useful test of thumb adduction is to ask the patient to squeeze a sheet of paper between the base of the thumb and the index finger; weakness of the adductor pollicis is present if the interphalangeal joint of the thumb flexes, due to use of the median-innervated flexor pollicis longus (Froment's sign).

- If the patient has a radial neuropathy (in isolation or combination), it is not possible to test precisely finger abduction because the fingers need to be extended first. In this situation, finger abduction should be tested with the palm faced downwards on a hard surface, and the fingers resting in an extended position but, even then, the movements will not be quite normal even if the ulnar nerve is preserved.
- The flexor digitorum profundus III and IV are tested by testing flexion of the distal interphalangeal joint of the little and ring finger against resistance, while the middle proximal interphalangeal joint is fixed in extension.
- The flexor carpi ulnaris often escapes compression at the elbow but if not, there may only be a slight radial deviation of the hand on wrist flexion; wrist flexion remains generally unaffected because of the action of the (median-innervated) flexor carpi radialis.
- Severe ulnar neuropathy gives rise to the so-called 'ulnar claw hand' with guttering of the dorsum from atrophy of the interosseous muscles and third and fourth lumbricals, hyperextension of the fourth and fifth metacarpophalangeal joints, mild flexion of the interphalangeal joints and abduction of the little finger (**779, 780**).

Wrist and palm lesions
Deep and superficial branch: just proximal to or within Guyon's canal
- Pure weakness, and possibly wasting, of all hand muscles innervated by the ulnar nerve (adductor pollicis, interosseous muscles, hypothenar muscles [abduction of little finger], and palmaris brevis [no skin dimple on extreme abduction of the little finger]).
- Sparing of flexor carpi ulnaris and flexor digitorum profundus (as for more proximal lesions at the elbow).
- Loss of sensation on palmar aspect of the little finger and ulnar half of the ring finger, corresponding to the cutaneous innervation of the superficial terminal branch.
- Normal sensation over the proximal part of the hypothenar and the dorsal part of the ring and little fingers.
- Little pain.

Deep branch, proximal part: at the pisiform bone
- Pure weakness, and possibly wasting, of all hand muscles innervated by the ulnar nerve, excluding palmaris brevis (which contracts during strong abduction of the little finger and causes indentation of the skin overlying the hypothenar).
- Normal sensation (the lesion is beyond the branching of the superficial terminal branch within Guyon's canal).

Deep branch, distal part: at (or distal to) the hamate bone
- Weakness and wasting of the radial hand muscles innervated by the ulnar nerve (adductor pollicis, interossei), with sparing of function of the hypothenar muscles, and palmaris brevis muscle.
- Normal sensation.

Superficial branch: at or distal to Guyon's canal
- Weakness of palmaris brevis muscle (no skin dimple on extreme abduction of the little finger).
- Loss of sensation of the little and ring finger (ulnar half) on the palmar side.

774 Approximate area in which light touch and pain sensation are reduced in an ulnar nerve lesion. N.B. Nerve root, plexus and cord lesions do not 'split' the ring finger.

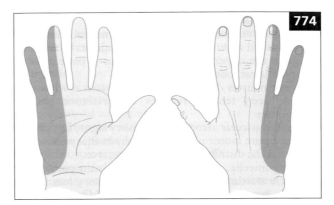

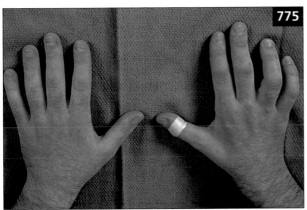

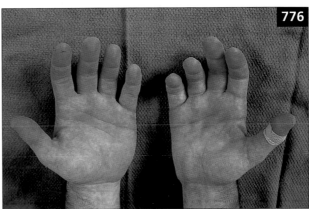

775, 776 Severe ulnar neuropathy causing wasting of the dorsal interossei (**775**) and wasting of the adductor pollicis and an 'ulnar claw hand' (**776**).

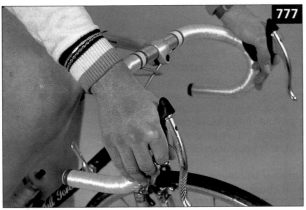

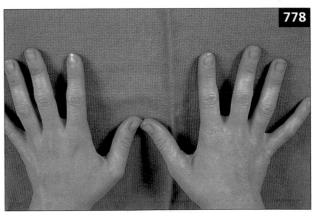

777, 778 Compressive mononeuropathy of the deep palmar branch of the ulnar nerve in a cyclist, causing wasting (and weakness) of the interossei.

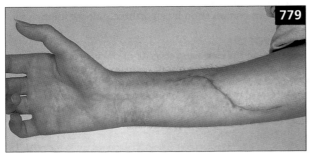

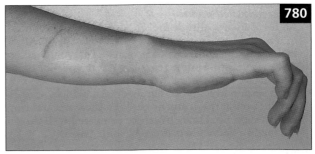

779, 780 Severe ulnar neuropathy due to forearm injury causing the so-called 'ulnar claw hand' with flexion of the interphalangeal joints and abduction of the little finger (**777**) and hyperextension of the fourth and fifth metacarpophalangeal joints (**780**).

FEMORAL NEUROPATHY

DEFINITION
Dysfunction of the femoral nerve.

EPIDEMIOLOGY
Uncommon.

ANATOMY
Course of the femoral nerve
- Arises from the L2, L3 and L4 nerve roots within the psoas muscle.
- Descends along the lateral border of the psoas muscle, within the fascia between the psoas and the iliacus muscles.
- Proximal to the inguinal ligament it gives off branches to the iliopsoas muscle.
- Descends further, beneath the inguinal ligament, lateral to the femoral artery, and gives off branches to the sartorius and the four parts of the quadriceps muscle.
- Distal to the inguinal ligament, sensory branches arise: the intermediate cutaneous nerve of the thigh, and the medial cutaneous nerve of the thigh, which innervate the skin on the anterior and medial aspects of the thigh.
- The terminal branch of the femoral nerve, the purely sensory saphenous nerve, passes within the quadriceps muscle through Hunter's canal, and about 10 cm (4 in) above the knee it leaves this canal and gives of the infrapatellar branch, which innervates the skin on the medial aspect of the knee down to the tuberosity of the tibia.
- More distally, the saphenous nerve descends along the medial side of the tibia and the anterior surface of the medial malleolus, to supply the skin at the anterior and medial surface of the knee, and the medial aspect of the lower leg, including the ankle and arch of the foot.

ETIOLOGY
Femoral nerve
Compression (in the iliac fossa most commonly, and in the inguinal region)
- Spontaneous hematoma in the psoas or iliacus muscle:
- Bleeding diathesis: anticoagulation, hemophilia (may be bilateral).
- Ruptured aortic aneurysm.
- Trauma.
- Abdominal or pelvic surgery:
- Hematoma after nerve block.
- Catheterization via the femoral artery causing retroperitoneal hematoma or pseudoaneurysm in the groin.
- Laparoscopy.
- Stapling in laparoscopic hernia repair.
- Inadvertent suturing.
- Retractor blades (self-retaining) used in abdominal surgery.
- Vaginal delivery.
- Vaginal hysterectomy in lithotomy position (extreme abduction and exorotation of the thighs may stretch the femoral nerve).
- Abdominal hysterectomy.
- Hip abscess after parturition.
- Hip arthroplasty.
- Renal transplantation, associated with pressure from retractor blades, hematoma or ischemia from 'stealing'.
- Synovial cyst of the hip.
- Prolonged pressure on the abdomen after intoxication.

Penetrating injuries
Inflammation
- Inguinal lymphadenitis.
- Rheumatoid bursitis of the iliopsoas muscle.
- Heterotopic calcification.

Irradiation
Vincristine toxicity

Saphenous nerve
Iatrogenic
- Arthroscopy or menisectomy.
- Saphenous vein graft.
- Stripping of varicose veins, endoscopic dissection of perforating veins, cryosurgery.
- Arterial reconstruction in the thigh.

Compression
- Entrapment:
- At the medial side of the knee.
- In the subsartorial canal.
- By a branch of the femoral artery.
- Neurilemmoma
- Bursitis of the pes anserinus, distal to the adductor canal.

Irradiation

HISTORY
Femoral nerve
- Sudden falls caused by buckling of the knee, particularly if walking on an uneven road surface, climbing up an incline, or descending a staircase (i.e. when the body weight has to be supported with some knee flexion).
- Deep, severe, nerve trunk pain, with or without numbness and paresthesia on the anterior aspect of the thigh or inner aspect of the lower leg, may be present, depending on the cause. Pain is common in diabetic amyotrophy and psoas hematoma, which may mimic femoral neuropathy, and is minimized by full flexion of the hip. Acute pain in the flank of the abdomen is reported particularly by patients with hematomas in the iliacus muscle that compress the femoral nerve.

Saphenous nerve
Pain, numbness and paresthesia on the inner aspect of the knee (if the infrapatellar branch is involved) and lower leg.

EXAMINATION
Femoral nerve
- Weakness of iliopsoas and the quadriceps, with iliopsoas tested in the supine position, and quadriceps tested at a mechanical disadvantage (because it is such a massive and strong muscle) with the knee in flexion and the patient sitting and trying to bring the lower leg forward against resistance. This method also avoids testing the knee in extension where a locked joint would have to be wrenched open (which is painful and mild weakness easily missed).
- The most reliable proof of normal strength of the quadriceps is the ability to rise from the floor, whilst squatting on one knee, transferring the weight to the other leg, flexed at the knee, and extending the other leg. Of course, with advanced age this is determined more and more by non-neurologic factors such as joint stability, and the test becomes less reliable.

- A decreased or absent knee jerk is consistent, but not specific.
- Wasting of the anterior aspect of the thigh invariably occurs after some time.
- Loss of sensation over the anterior and medial aspect of the thigh and the medial aspect of the lower leg is present (**784, 785**).
- With progressive weakness, the knee is locked in a hyper-extended position (genu recurvatum) during walking.

Saphenous nerve
Reduced sensation on the inner aspect of the knee (if the infrapatellar branch is involved) and lower leg.

DIFFERENTIAL DIAGNOSIS
- Lumbosacral plexopathy or lumbar radiculopathy (L2, L3, L4): it is crucial to carefully assess the strength of the adductor muscles of the hip because weakness of the hip adductors is not consistent with a femoral neuropathy and more suggestive of a lesion in the lumbosacral plexus, lumbar nerve roots L2, L3, L4; or obturator nerve.
- Diabetic lumbar radiculopathy/plexopathy: an axonal plexopathy (rather than demyelination) with EMG features of denervation in the quadriceps as well as the hip adductors and paravertebral muscles, indicating a proximal root lesion.

INVESTIGATIONS
Nerve conduction studies
The saphenous nerve can be examined using peripheral nerve conduction studies and with SSEPs.

EMG
Needle examination helps to distinguish femoral neuropathy from diabetic amyotrophy which is an axonal neuropathy (rather than demyelination) with features of denervation in the quadriceps as well as the hip adductors and paravertebral muscles.

CT scan of the pelvis
Reliably detects mass lesions in the pelvis that may cause femoral neuropathy.

DIAGNOSIS
Requires the presence of isolated weakness of the iliacus, iliopsoas, sartorius and/or quadriceps femoris and sensory loss over the anterior thigh and medial lower leg. Can be confirmed by EMG.

TREATMENT
Depends on the cause.

Conservative
Painful paresthesia may be alleviated with carbamazepine or phenytoin.

Surgical
- Only if direct penetrating trauma with severe axonal injury or complete interruption of nerve continuity.
- Retroperitoneal hematomas are usually decompressed surgically or aspirated but this is to relieve pain; there is no evidence that it improves recovery.

PROGNOSIS
Depends on the cause and severity of the neuropathy. Femoral neuropathy after operation, from stretch or compression tends to be followed by spontaneous recovery, although this may take weeks or even months.

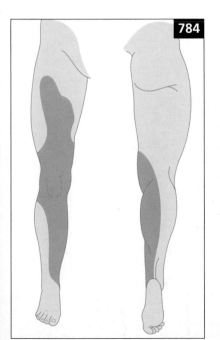

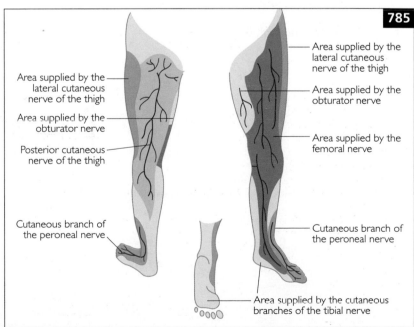

784, 785 Area of skin innervated by the femoral nerve.

OBTURATOR NEUROPATHY

DEFINITION
Dysfunction of the obturator nerve.

EPIDEMIOLOGY
Rare, in isolation.

ANATOMY
Course of the obturator nerve (786)
- Arises from the union of the ventral branches of the L2, L3 and L4 nerve roots within the belly of the psoas muscle.
- Emerges on the medial border of the psoas muscle.
- Descends over the sacroiliac joint, along the wall of the pelvis.
- Enters the obturator canal and gives off anterior branches and posterior branches, before entering the thigh.
- The posterior branches innervate the adductor muscles of the thigh (adductor brevis, adductor longus, and adductor magnus) which stabilize the hip.
- The anterior branch ends as a sensory nerve innervating an area of skin on the inner side of the thigh.

ETIOLOGY
- Obturator hernia.
- Normal labor.
- Scar formation in the thigh.
- Pelvic masses (frequently also cause a femoral neuropathy):
- Psoas muscle hematoma.
- Retroperitoneal schwannoma.
- Endometriosis
- Iatrogenic:
- Hip surgery, damaging the nerve by overstretching, retractor blades, fixation screws, and cement.
- Fixation of acetabular fracture.
- Urologic surgery with prolonged hip flexion.
- Intrapelvic surgery.
- Laparoscopic dissection of pelvic nodes.
- Gracilis flap operations.

HISTORY
- Weakness in the leg.
- Pain, numbness and paresthesia on the inner aspect of the knee (if the infrapatellar branch is involved) and lower leg.

EXAMINATION
- Weakness of hip adduction.
- Depressed adductor muscle tendon reflex.
- Normal power of quadriceps muscle and normal knee jerk.
- Reduced sensation on the inner aspect of the thigh (787).
- Broad based gait may be present.

DIFFERENTIAL DIAGNOSIS
- Lumbosacral plexopathy or lumbar radiculopathy (L2–L4).
- Femoral neuropathy: weakness of quadriceps muscle and depressed knee jerk.
- Osteitis or other disorders of the symphysis: pain in the groin and medial part of the thigh similar to the neuralgic pain of an obturator neuropathy, but usually local tenderness.

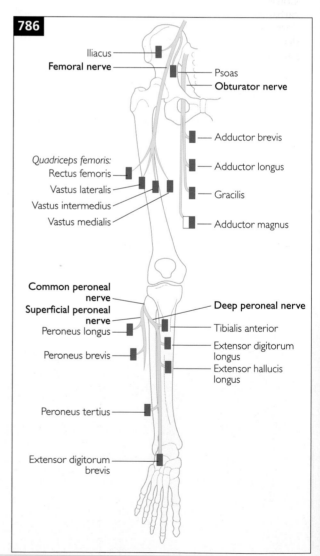

786 Diagram of the obturator, femoral and common peroneal nerves and the muscles that they supply.

INVESTIGATIONS
Nerve conduction studies
No nerve conduction technique is described.

EMG
Needle examination may indirectly confirm the diagnosis by demonstrating denervation activity confined to the hip adductors.

CT scan of the pelvis
May detect a mass lesion in the pelvis causing obturator neuropathy.

DIAGNOSIS
Requires the presence of isolated weakness of the hip adductors, with or without sensory loss over the inner thigh. Can be confirmed by EMG.

TREATMENT
Depends on the cause.
- Conservative: painful paresthesia may be alleviated with carbamazepine or phenytoin.
- Surgical: retroperitoneal hematomas are usually decompressed surgically or aspirated but this is to relieve pain; there is no evidence that it improves recovery.

PROGNOSIS
Depends on the cause and severity of the neuropathy.

GLUTEAL NEUROPATHY

DEFINITION
Dysfunction of the superior and/or inferior gluteal nerves.

EPIDEMIOLOGY
Uncommon.

ANATOMY
Course of the superior gluteal nerve (788)
- Arises from the L4, L5 and S1 nerve roots.
- Descends over the piriformis muscle, through the suprapiriform foramen, and then between the gluteus medius and minimus muscles.
- Innervates the gluteus medius and minimus and the tensor fasciae latae muscles.

Course of the inferior gluteal nerve (788)
- Arises from the L5, S1 and S2 nerve roots.
- Descends through the infrapiriform foramen, dorsolateral to the sciatic nerve.
- Innervates the gluteus maximus muscle.

ETIOLOGY
Superior gluteal nerve
Trauma
- Fall on the buttocks (acute transient entrapment of the superior gluteal nerve between the piriformis muscle and the major sciatic incisure, or more permanent damage due to secondary muscle fibrosis).
- Intramuscular injections in the buttocks:
- Incorrectly placed injections may damage the sciatic nerve and superior gluteal nerve.
- Correctly placed injections, in the upper outer quadrant of the buttock, may cause a partial lesion, with weakness of only the tensor fasciae latae muscle.
- Hip surgery via a posterior approach (the so-called 'Hardinge approach').

787

787 Area of skin innervated by the obturator nerve.

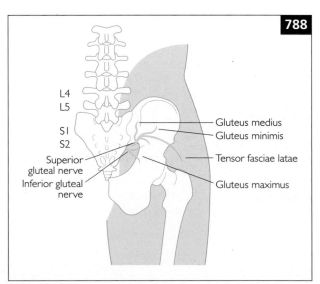

788 Diagram of the gluteal nerves and the muscles that they supply.

Compression
Coma or anesthesia injections: may damage the superior gluteal nerve and the sciatic nerve.

Inferior gluteal nerve
Compression
Colorectal tumor (often there is concurrent involvement of the posterior cutaneous nerve of the thigh, with altered sensation of the inferior lateral buttock).

Bilateral gluteal neuropathy
- Prolonged labor.
- Spondylolisthesis of L4 on L5 (perhaps by entrapment within the piriform muscle).

CLINICAL FEATURES
Superior gluteal nerve
- Pain in the buttock.
- Difficulty walking (weakness of gluteus medius and minimus leads to weakness of hip abduction, which causes defective tilting of the pelvis and difficulty swinging the contralateral leg forward).

Inferior gluteal nerve
- Pain in the buttock.
- Difficulty walking, and particularly descending stairs and arising from a chair, due to weakness of hip extension (gluteus maximus).

DIFFERENTIAL DIAGNOSIS
Proximal myopathy (all symmetric and slowly progressive)
- Dystrophinopathy.
- Limb girdle dystrophy.
- Polymyositis.
- Acid maltase deficiency.

Hip joint disorder

INVESTIGATIONS
EMG
Needle examination of the gluteii identifies denervation activity.

MRI scan pelvis

DIAGNOSIS
Requires the presence of isolated weakness of the gluteal muscles. Can be confirmed by EMG.

TREATMENT
Depends on the cause.
- Conservative.
- Surgical: if more or less total nerve damage and no evidence of recovery.

PROGNOSIS
Depends on the cause and severity of the neuropathy.

SCIATIC NEUROPATHY

DEFINITION
Dysfunction of the sciatic nerve.

EPIDEMIOLOGY
Not uncommon.

ANATOMY
Course of the sciatic nerve (789)
- Arises from the L4, L5, S1, S2 and S3 nerve roots.
- In the pelvis (or gluteal region below) the fibers that will eventually form the tibial and common peroneal nerves are arranged in two separate divisions: the medial and lateral trunk respectively. The peroneal nerve fibers within the lateral division of the sciatic nerve are more prone to compression than the tibial nerve fibers in the medial division, so that a partial lesion of the sciatic nerve at this level may be indistinguishable from that of a peroneal nerve palsy in the leg, including preservation of the ankle jerk.
- Leaves the pelvis through the sciatic foramen.
- Courses below the piriformis muscle, although the division that is destined to become the peroneal nerve (and sometimes the entire nerve) may pierce the piriformis muscle, or pass over it.
- In the gluteal region, the nerves passes laterally and then vertically downwards. Beneath the gluteus maximus it lies between the greater trochanter and the ischial tuberosity, just posterior to the hip joint.
- At the inferior part of the buttock, the nerve is situated superficially in the subgluteal space amongst collagen and fat tissue. This is a site where the nerve may be damaged by an inflammatory process or wrongly applied injection fluids that can easily spread.
- The nerve descends dorsal to the femur, between the knee flexor muscles.
- The medial division consecutively supplies the semitendinosus, biceps femoris (long head) and semimembranosus muscles, and contributes to the innervation of the adductor magnus muscle.
- The lateral division innervates the short head of the biceps femoris.
- The sciatic nerve terminates at the proximal part of the popliteal fossa, where it divides into the tibial and common peroneal nerve.
- The main sciatic trunk does not have sensory branches but the nerve is accompanied by the posterior cutaneous nerve of the thigh (S1–S3) which innervates the skin of the dorsal aspect of the thigh and the proximal part of the calf.

ETIOLOGY
Pelvis
Tumors
- Metastatic carcinoma.
- Neurofibroma, schwannoma.
- Lipoma.

Vascular abnormalities
- Arteriovenous malformation.
- False aneurysm of the abdominal aorta.
- Unruptured aneurysm of the common iliac artery or internal iliac artery.
- Ruptured aneurysm of the hypogastric artery.

Endometriosis

Childbirth
Cesarian section with epidural anesthesia.

Infection
Clostridium septicum, with immuno-incompetence.

Gluteal region
Compression
- Prolonged sitting:
- Alcoholic- or drug-induced stupor on a toilet, or hard rail.
- Anesthesia in a sitting position.
- Meditation/sleeping in a cross legged position.
- Coma (usually drug induced with rhabdomyolysis).
- 'Backpocket sciatica' from credit cards or coins.

Vascular lesions
- Hematoma (bleeding diathesis).
- Persistent sciatic artery.
- False aneurysm, loop or abnormal collateral of the inferior gluteal artery or superior gluteal artery.

Tumors
- Neurofibroma, schwannoma.
- Lipoma.
- Lymphoma.
- Hemangiopericytoma.

Iatrogenic
- Hip surgery (total hip arthroplasty):
- Ipsilateral: trochanteric wiring or extruding cement.
- Contralateral: rhabdomyolysis.
- Intramuscular injections that are not placed in the upper and outer quadrant of the buttock or, even if appropriately placed, cause muscle necrosis or fibrosis.
- Scoliosis surgery: Harrington's operation.
- Femoral fracture surgery: closed nailing.
- Heart surgery: mechanical compression or femoral artery occlusion.
- Femoral artery catheterization.

Trauma
- Hip fracture–dislocation.
- Femur fracture.

'Pyriformis syndrome'
An anatomic variation in which the piriformis muscle compresses the sciatic nerve as it emerges from the pelvis through the greater sciatic notch. There must be objective neurologic and neurophysiologic signs of sciatic nerve dysfunction (not just pain in the buttock); reproduction of pain with deep palpation via the gluteal or rectal route; negative EMG findings in the paraspinal muscles; appropriate radiologic studies excluding lumbosacral nerve root compression, and masses in the paravertebral area, lower pelvis and sciatic notch; negative CSF examination (i.e. no signs of inflammation that could reflect nerve root inflammation or infection); and ultimately confirmation by operation and subsequent relief with nerve decompression.

Thigh
Tumors
- Neurofibroma, schwannoma.
- Lipoma.

Vascular lesions
Aneurysm of persistent sciatic artery or popliteal artery.

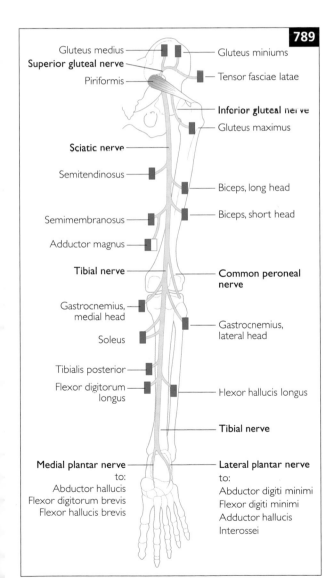

789

Gluteus medius
Superior gluteal nerve
Piriformis
Gluteus miniums
Tensor fasciae latae
Inferior gluteal nerve
Gluteus maximus
Sciatic nerve
Semitendinosus
Biceps, long head
Biceps, short head
Semimembranosus
Adductor magnus
Tibial nerve
Common peroneal nerve
Gastrocnemius, medial head
Gastrocnemius, lateral head
Soleus
Tibialis posterior
Flexor digitorum longus
Flexor hallucis longus
Tibial nerve
Medial plantar nerve to:
Abductor hallucis
Flexor digitorum brevis
Flexor hallucis brevis
Lateral plantar nerve to:
Abductor digiti minimi
Flexor digiti minimi
Adductor hallucis
Interossei

789 Diagram of the gluteal, sciatic, tibial and common peroneal nerves and the muscles that they supply.

Tumors
- Synovial cyst.
- Tibialis posterior tendon cyst.
- Malignant schwannoma.
- Plantar fibromatosis.

Lateral plantar neuropathy
Trauma to the foot
Fractures or soft tissue injuries.

Compression of its first branch between the intrinsic muscles of the sole

Entrapment
- Tight shoes.
- Prolonged standing on the rungs of a ladder with soft shoes.
- Immobilization in a bed with prolonged pressured against the footboard (usually in hospital).
- Local callus, fasciitis or arthritis.

Medial plantar proper digital neuropathy
- Ill-fitting shoes.
- Scar tissue after bunion surgery.
- Arthritis of the first metatarsophalangeal joint.

Lateral plantar proper digital neuropathy
Traumatic neuroma secondary to bunion.

Plantar interdigital neuropathy (Morton's metatarsalgia)
Compression of one of the interdigital nerves of the foot, which arise from the medial and lateral plantar nerves at the point where they course between the metatarsal heads, just before they divide into two digital nerves (**791**). The most common site of compression is between the third and fourth metatarsal bones, particularly in women. The heads of the metatarsal bones and the deep transverse ligament contribute to the compression. The swelling around the nerve consists mainly of fibrous tissue; the term 'neuroma' is a pathologic misnomer.

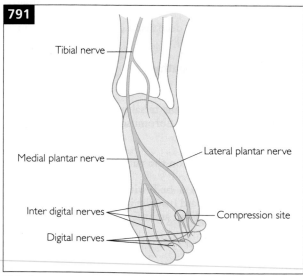

791 Compression site in Morton's metatarsalgia.

CLINICAL FEATURES
Tibial neuropathy proximal to the ankle
- Wasting and weakness of plantar flexion (gastrocnemius, soleus) and inversion (tibialis posterior), and toe flexion (flexor digitorum longus):
  - The calf muscles (gastrocnemius and soleus) are often tested together (plantar flexion) but because they are so strong, it is difficult to detect even marked weakness if plantar flexion of the foot is tested against the examiner's hand with the patient supine. If the patient can walk, it is preferable to examine the patient walking on their toes (i.e. without the heel touching the floor) and then standing on one leg, supporting the body weight on the toes, and then hopping on the forefoot, without the heel touching the floor. Of course, some people, such as the elderly, may not be able to perform this maneuver due to other impairments, despite normal power of the calf muscles.
  - The soleus muscle can be tested reasonably selectively by examining plantar flexion against resistance with hip and knee flexed and the patient supine.
- Decreased or absent ankle jerk.
- Diminished sensation of the heel (calcaneal nerve), sole of the foot (medial and lateral plantar nerves) and dorsal aspect of the toes (digital nerves) (**792**).

Tibial neuropathy at the ankle (in the tarsal tunnel)
(Posterior) tarsal tunnel syndrome
- Unilateral usually, but may be bilateral.
- Pain (often burning) in the sole of the foot.
- Paresthesia in the toes.
- Symptoms may only be present at night or while standing or exercising, such as walking, jogging, or playing tennis.
- Wasting and weakness of the intrinsic muscles at the sole of the foot (abductor hallucis and short flexor digitorum muscles, and flexor and abductor digiti minimi, abductor hallucis and the interossei) is usually asymptomatic and the muscles are difficult to see or test separately. Indeed, many normal individuals are unable to fan their toes. However, there may be a difference compared with the normal, particularly on palpating the muscle bulk of both feet.
- Sensory loss in the sole of the foot and toes in the distribution of the medial (most commonly) or lateral plantar nerve or both.
- Hoffmann–Tinel sign: local pain, paresthesia and an electric sensation radiating across the sole of the foot towards the toes, particularly the medial toes, elicited by pressure or percussion over the tarsal tunnel, beneath the medial malleolus, with the foot everted.
- An underlying cause may be apparent such as abnormal postures of the foot, hypermobility of the ankle joint, local masses and a perforating ulcer of the foot (cf. leprosy).

Calcaneal neuropathy (sensory branch of the tibial nerve at the heel)
Pain in one or both heels.

Plantar neuropathy
- Isolated paresthesia and sensory loss, usually in the medial part of the sole (the medial plantar nerve is more commonly affected).
- Weakness of the intrinsic foot muscles is usually asymptomatic (see above).

Medial plantar proper digital neuropathy
- Pain, paresthesia and sensory loss on the medial side of the great toe.
- Tenderness and thickening of the nerve.

Lateral plantar proper digital neuropathy
Pain, paresthesia and sensory loss on the lateral side of the little toe.

Plantar interdigital neuropathy (Morton's metatarsalgia)
- Severe burning pain in the sole of the foot, between the heads of the relevant metatarsal bones (usually the third and fourth), and radiating to the relevant toes (usually the third and fourth), with associated local paresthesia and numbness. The pain may also radiate proximally.
- The symptoms are initially precipitated or exacerbated by weight bearing on the feet (standing or walking), external pressure between the heads of the metatarsal bones, or passive dorsiflexion of the toes, but later become continuous, unless footwear is removed.
- A sensory deficit may be present on the adjoining sides of the toes.

DIFFERENTIAL DIAGNOSIS
Tibial neuropathy proximal to the ankle
- S1 radiculopathy (deficits of motor, reflex and sensory function in the typical distribution of the myotome (gastrocnemius/soleus and ankle jerk [S1]) and dermatome (the lateral border of the foot [S1]):
  - Disc herniation.
  - Radiculitis due to infection (e.g. borrelia).
- Lumbosacral plexopathy.

Tibial neuropathy at the ankle (tarsal tunnel syndrome)
- Musculoskeletal pain (no paresthesia, and normal conduction in the tibial nerve):
  - Plantar fasciitis.
  - Stress fractures.
  - Bursitis.
- Lumbar spinal stenosis (if pain and paresthesia in the foot and toes during exercise).
- S1 radiculopathy: may cause paresthesia in the sole of the foot, but usually other signs, such as absent ankle jerk and weakness of the calf muscles.
- Morton's neuralgia: shooting pain evoked by pressure over one of the metatarsal bones (i.e. painful trigger points over the sole of the foot).
- Medial plantar neuropathy: pain is precipitated by pressure distal to the medial malleolus (as opposed to immediately below it) and the clinical symptoms and signs do not involve the lateral sole.
- Distal polyneuropathy, especially diabetic neuropathy, causing burning feet may be quite similar to bilateral tarsal tunnel syndrome, but there are usually additional signs such as depressed ankle jerks and more extensive sensory loss on both the ventral and dorsal aspects of the feet.
- Sciatic nerve tumor may even initially mimic a tarsal tunnel syndrome.

Plantar neuropathy
S1 radiculopathy: may cause paresthesia in the sole of the foot, but usually other signs, such as absent ankle jerk and weakness of the calf muscles.

Plantar interdigital neuropathy (Morton's metatarsalgia)
- Tarsal tunnel syndrome.
- Interdigital neuroma.
- Stress fracture or avascular necrosis of a metatarsal bone.
- Soft tissue injury to the foot.

INVESTIGATIONS
Nerve conduction studies
- A tibial neuropathy proximal to the ankle may be detected by stimulating the tibial nerve in the popliteal fossa and the ankle, and measuring the conduction velocity between these points as well as the amplitude of the motor evoked potential.
- Compression of the tibial nerve at the ankle (in the tarsal tunnel) may be suspected if there is delayed motor conduction (distal latency) in the medial and lateral plantar nerves as assessed by stimulating at the ankle and recording from the abductor hallucis and abductor digiti minimi respectively. However, in order to distinguish between a lesion in the tarsal tunnel and a more distal lesion, both of which may affect one or more branches of the tibial nerve, it is necessary to stimulate the tibial nerve proximal to the tunnel and the plantar nerves distal to the tunnel. Nevertheless, motor nerve conduction velocity is not infrequently normal in tarsal tunnel syndrome and the diagnosis may depend on sensory conduction studies which are more sensitive.

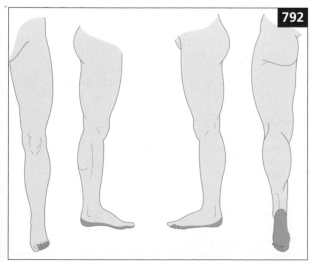

792

792 Area of skin innervated by the tibial nerve.

EMG

Needle EMG may be helpful if signs of denervation are present in the intrinsic foot muscles, particularly abnormal motor unit potentials, because fibrillation and fasciculation potentials may occur in healthy people, particularly in the abductor hallucis (and also the gastrocnemius).

Ultrasound, x-ray or MRI of the popliteal fossa, lower leg, tarsal tunnel or foot

Frequently detects any mass lesion compressing the tibial nerve (e.g. hematoma) or affecting the nerve (e.g. tumor).

DIAGNOSIS

Requires the presence of isolated weakness of plantar flexion, ankle inversion and toe flexion, a depressed or absent ankle jerk, and sensory loss over the sole of the foot. Can be confirmed by EMG.

TREATMENT

Depends on the cause.

Tibial neuropathy proximal to the ankle

Treat the cause.

Tibial neuropathy at the ankle (tarsal tunnel syndrome)

- Change footwear if it is poorly fitting.
- Antilepromatous drugs, if appropriate.
- Surgical decompression of the retinaculum: generally successful, as in the carpal tunnel syndrome.

Calcaneal neuropathy (sensory branch of the tibial nerve at the heel)

Surgical decompression.

Medial plantar proper digital neuropathy

- Change footwear or insert protective padding.
- Surgical excision of the nerve with concurrent bunionectomy, if present, often provides dramatic relief of persistent symptoms.

Plantar interdigital neuropathy (Morton's metatarsalgia)

- Review footwear and ensure appropriate fit without tight pressure on the sole. Supplement with padding if necessary.
- Injection of local anesthetic together with corticosteroid affords recovery among one-third, and is associated with later recovery after 2 years in another third.
- Carbamazepine taken orally may be helpful.
- Surgical excision of the abnormal tissue is radical but frequently successful. A dorsal approach may facilitate mobilization and prevent infection. A new 'neuroma' may form later.
- Neurolysis, by incision of the intermetacarpal ligament above resection, is an alternative.

PROGNOSIS

Depends on the cause and severity of the neuropathy.

PERONEAL NEUROPATHY

DEFINITION

Dysfunction of the peroneal nerve.

EPIDEMIOLOGY

One of the most common mononeuropathies.

ANATOMY
Course of the peroneal nerve
Proximal to the ankle

- The common peroneal nerve arises from a separate division within the sciatic nerve at a variable level above the knee, sometimes as far proximal as the upper thigh.
- It carries fibers from the L4, L5, and S1 nerve roots.
- In the popliteal fossa, the lateral cutaneous nerve of the calf arises from the common peroneal nerve to innervate the skin of the upper third of the lateral lower leg (**793**).
- Below the knee the common peroneal nerve winds around the head of the fibula, at which point it rests directly on the periosteum and is particularly prone to compression, stretch or other trauma.
- It then courses through the fibular tunnel (a fibroosseous canal between the insertion of the peroneus longus muscle and the fibula) and enters the compartment of the peroneal muscles, where it divides into a deep and a superficial branch.
- The deep peroneal nerve innervates the tibialis anterior, extensor digitorum longus and extensor hallucis longus muscles.
- The deep peroneal nerve continues to descend as the terminal branch of the deep peroneal nerve and lies superficially at the dorsum of the ankle and foot where it innervates the extensor digitorum brevis muscle and a small area of skin in the web between the first and second toes (**794**).
- The superficial peroneal nerve gives off motor branches to the peroneus longus and brevis muscles about 10 cm (4 in) proximal to the lateral malleolus and, in about one-quarter of individuals, gives rise to a terminal motor branch (the accessory deep peroneal nerve).
- The sensory branch of the superficial peroneal nerve pierces the deep fascia of the lower leg and supplies the skin of the lower half of lateral lower leg and dorsum of the foot.
- A sural communicating branch joins the medial cutaneous nerve of the calf, originating from the tibial nerve, to form the sural nerve, which supplies the skin on the lateral side of the heel, the sole and the little toe (see pp.647, 654).

ETIOLOGY (CAUSES IN ISOLATION OR COMBINATION)
Common peroneal neuropathy (or sometimes only deep or superficial branch) at the level of the fibular head

Postural change

- Prolonged squatting or kneeling (e.g. gardening, strawberry picking, farming, delivering a baby).
- Sitting with legs crossed habitually.
- Bed rest, particularly with a bed rail.

Running

Weight loss
- Starvation (e.g. voluntary, prisoners of war).
- Gastrointestinal or malignant disease.
- Anorexia nervosa.

Iatrogenic
- Plaster casts.
- Tight bandages.
- Arthroscopy of the knee.
- Arthrodesis (intramedullary) of the knee.
- High tibial osteotomy.
- Malpositioning during anesthesia.

Congenital abnormalities
- Constriction band.
- Hereditary liability to pressure palsies.

Trauma
- Fracture of the femur or fibula.
- Inversion trauma of the foot.

Vascular
Hematoma in the popliteal fossa.

Tumors
- Exostosis of the fibular head or intraosseous cyst.
- Osteochondroma.
- Cysts of the lateral meniscus or tibio-fibular joint.
- Neurofibroma.
- Intraneural cysts.
- Hemangioma.
- Lipomatosis of the popliteal fossa due to steroids.

Pretibial myxoedema

Herniation of the gastrocnemius muscle

Peroneal neuropathy between the fibular head and the ankle
Anterior compartment syndrome (deep peroneal nerve compression)
- Swelling of necrotic muscle.
- Aneurysm of the tibial artery.

Lateral compartment syndrome (superficial peroneal nerve compression)
- Compression as the superficial peroneal nerve as it courses through the deep fascia of the lower leg after giving off motor branches to the peroneal muscles. Causes include athletic exercise (most commonly) and callus formation after midshaft fracture of the fibula.
- Swelling of necrotic muscle.
- Idiopathic (may be bilateral).

Peroneal neuropathy at the ankle
Compression of the terminal branch of the deep peroneal nerve at the anterior aspect of the ankle ('anterior tarsal tunnel syndrome')
- Tight footwear (shoelaces, ski boots).
- Local contusion.
- Ganglion.
- Talotibial exostoses.

Compression of terminal branches of the superficial peroneal nerve
- Entrapment during sleep or sitting.
- Epidermoid cysts.
- Fascial bands.
- Cannulation of foot veins.
- Arthroscopic knee surgery.
- Intermittent pneumatic compression as prophylaxis for deep vein thrombosis.

Lateral cutaneous nerve of calf lesions
Isolated compression.

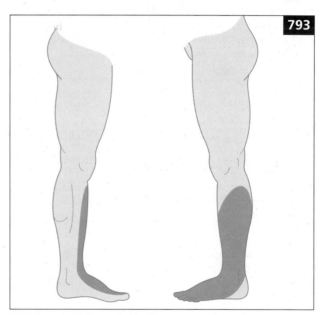

793 Area of skin innervated by the common peroneal nerve.

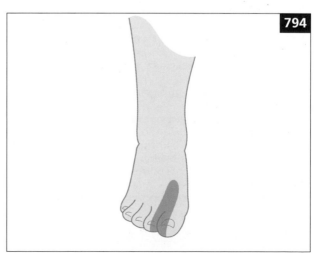

794 Area of skin innervated by the deep peroneal nerve.

CLINICAL FEATURES
Common peroneal neuropathy at the level of the fibular head

- The extent of the deficits depends on whether the lesion involves the fascicles of the deep or the superficial peroneal nerve or both, as well as the duration and severity of the compression. Isolated deficits in the distribution of the deep or superficial peroneal nerve are most commonly due to a lesion of a separate fascicle at the level of the head of the fibula than a more distal lesion involving a single one of the two branches.
- Foot drop due to weakness of dorsiflexion of the ankle (tibialis anterior; deep peroneal nerve), leading to a typical stepping gait, in which there is compensatory overaction of the hip and knee flexors to clear the sagging foot during the swing phase. With mild weakness, the gait may be normal but the foot swings with less clearance from the floor than the normal side and the patient may not be able to walk on the heel of the affected side. With moderate weakness of tibialis anterior, the foot may still land on the heel, but immediately afterwards the ankle dorsiflexors give way giving rise to a characteristic, flat-footed sound.
- Weakness of ankle eversion (peroneal muscles; superficial peroneal nerve) and extension of the toes (extensor digitorum longus and brevis and extensor hallucis longus; deep peroneal nerve).
- Normal ankle jerk.
- Altered sensation (numbness or paresthesia) of the lateral part of the lower leg and dorsum of the foot (superficial peroneal nerve) and/or web between the first two toes (deep peroneal nerve). The sensory deficit is often less extensive, however, than might be expected from the anatomic distribution of the innervation by the nerve(s). Pain is uncommon, particularly when the neuropathy is due to external compression.

N.B. Confusingly, dorsiflexors of the ankle and toes are flexor muscles in the physiologic sense because they shorten the leg, but have been called extensor muscles by anatomists.

Peroneal neuropathy between the fibular head and the ankle
Compartment syndromes (see below)
- Severe pain and red discoloration of the skin in the affected part of the lower limb. The pain may arise rapidly over hours and may also remit.
- Precipitated or exacerbated by strenuous physical exercise (e.g. running).
- Dorsalis pedis arterial pulse may be absent.

Anterior compartment syndrome (deep peroneal nerve compression)
- Weakness of dorsiflexion of the ankle (tibialis anterior) and toes (extensor hallucis longus and extensor digitorum longus), if it is possible to test in the presence of severe pain.
- Sensory loss in the web between the first and second toes.

Lateral compartment syndrome (superficial peroneal nerve compression)
- Weakness of eversion of the ankle (short and long peroneal muscles), if possible to test and if the cause involves the superficial nerve before it gives off motor branches to the peroneal muscles about 10 cm (4 in) proximal to the lateral malleolus. Otherwise the only neurologic deficits may be pain and sensory loss on the dorsum of the foot.
- Sensory loss over the lower half of the lateral calf and dorsum of the foot.

Peroneal neuropathy at the ankle
Compression of the terminal branch of the deep peroneal nerve ('anterior tarsal tunnel syndrome')
- Painful paresthesia in the web space between the first and second toes.
- Wasting of the extensor digitorum brevis on inspection.

Compression of terminal branches of the superficial peroneal nerve
Pain and numbness in part of the dorsum of the foot.

Lateral cutaneous nerve of calf lesions
Pain and/or sensory loss in the popliteal fossa and lateral part of the calf.

DIFFERENTIAL DIAGNOSIS
Common peroneal neuropathy at the level of the fibular head

- Pyramidal tract lesions (e.g. stroke): cause weakness of the flexor muscles of the leg, particularly dorsiflexion of the ankle, and so may be confused with a peroneal neuropathy, but because other flexor muscles of the leg are affected, the gait pattern is different: there is circumduction of the hip and the foot tends to be dragged, rather than causing a stepping gait. Furthermore, the muscle tone and deep tendon reflexes are increased and the plantar response extensor.
- Anterior horn cell lesions (e.g. motor neuron disease, spinal muscular atrophy): may present with wasting and weakness of the muscles innervated by the common peroneal nerve, but usually there is clinical or electrophysiologic evidence of denervation in at least three of the four regions formed by the head, arms, trunk and legs, and no sensory loss.
- L5 radiculopathy (e.g. L4/5 intervertebral disc herniation or, less commonly, an extremely lateral prolapse of the L5/S1 disc): also causes some weakness of the extensors of the ankle and toes, nerve and sensory loss in the lateral lower leg, but weakness of the extensor hallucis longus is most pronounced and there is also weakness of ankle inversion due to denervation of the tibialis posterior muscle.
- Sciatic neuropathy: may present with a foot drop because the lateral division of the sciatic nerve largely corresponds with the peroneal nerve, and is more prone to compression than the portion corresponding to the tibial nerve.
- Compartment syndrome (anterior or lateral): often involve the deep or superficial peroneal nerves.
- Distal myopathy: usually bilateral and involves muscles outside those innervated by the peroneal nerves.

INVESTIGATIONS
Common peroneal neuropathy at the level of the fibular head
Nerve conduction studies
- May be detected by stimulating the peroneal nerve at the ankle, and below and above the fibular head while recording from the extensor digitorum brevis muscle, and identifying local slowing and/or conduction block. Recording from tibialis anterior increases the chance of detecting conduction block.
- Nerve conduction studies may also give a clue to the prognosis. A reduced or absent SNAP of the superficial peroneal nerve examined in a distal segment is consistent with axonal loss in the peroneal nerve and indicates a worse prognosis than conduction block.

EMG
Needle EMG may be particularly helpful if no conduction abnormalities are found in the nerve segment across the fibular head to differentiate a suspected common peroneal neuropathy from an L4/5 radiculopathy, plexopathy or sciatic neuropathy. Important muscles to study are the short head of biceps femoris (innervated by the lateral division of the sciatic nerve), and the tibialis posterior (supplied by L5 but not the peroneal nerve).

CT or MRI scan of the brain, spinal cord, lumbosacral spine or leg
Frequently detects any lesion of the pyramidal tract or disc protrusion.

DIAGNOSIS
Requires the presence of foot drop due to weakness of dorsiflexion of the ankle (tibialis anterior), eversion of the ankle (peroneal muscles) and extension of the toes (extensor digitorum longus and brevis and extensor hallucis longus); a normal ankle jerk; and/or altered sensation of the lateral part of the lower leg and dorsum of the foot (superficial peroneal nerve) and/or web between the first two toes (deep peroneal nerve). Can be confirmed by EMG.

TREATMENT
Depends on the cause.

Conservative
- Most cases are due to external compression or stretch and recover spontaneously through remyelination within weeks or months with a conservative approach of observation and avoidance of further compression. A lightweight plastic orthosis which does not further compress the peroneal nerve at the head of the fibular should be used to facilitate a safer and more comfortable gait.
- Prolonged and severe compression during a long anesthetic or deep coma may result in a persistent deficit due to severe axonal damage (identified by EMG examination). Surgical decompression is ineffective.

Surgical decompression
- Clinical features compatible with entrapment of the distal part of the superficial peroneal nerve where the nerve pierces the fascia, 10 cm (4 in)above the lateral malleolus.
- Penetrating trauma, including immediate or delayed peroneal palsy after surgery in the region of the knee, which may have disrupted the continuity of the nerve and which necessitates immediate exploration.
- Local mass lesion causing slowly progressive deficit such as a nerve tumor, lipoma, cyst, or ganglion.
- Compartment syndrome, in which case immediate fasciotomy is indicated.

PREVENTION
High risk patients
- Coma.
- Bedridden with leg paralysis: Guillain–Barré syndrome.
- Leg in plaster that reaches as high as the head of the fibula.

Strategies of prevention
- Protect the common peroneal nerves at the head of the fibular by soft padding around the head of the fibula.
- Make an appropriate window in plaster casts near the head of the fibula.
- Instruct patients with a leg plaster to check the strength of the toe extensors each day and if weak, to open the plaster.
- Use care with removing a lower leg plaster by sawing or cutting.

SURAL NEUROPATHY

DEFINITION
Dysfunction of the sural nerve.

EPIDEMIOLOGY
Uncommon.

ANATOMY
Course of the sural nerve (795)
- Arises from the confluence of the medial cutaneous nerve of the calf (from the tibial nerve) and the lateral cutaneous nerve of the calf (from the common peroneal nerve).
- The medial cutaneous nerve of the calf arises from the tibial nerve in the popliteal fossa and descends in the middle of the calf between the two heads of gastrocnemius. After it has pierced the fascia it is joined beneath the skin by the branch from the lateral cutaneous nerve of the calf, which originates from the common peroneal nerve.

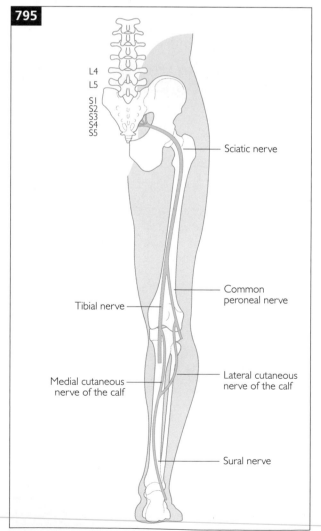

795 Origin and course of the sural nerve.

- The sural nerve descends the calf more laterally, between the Achilles tendon and the lateral malleolus.
- It curves around the lateral malleolus and ends at the lateral border of the foot.
- It innervates the skin of the lateral side of the ankle, and lateral border of the sole, up to the base of the fifth toe (796).

ETIOLOGY
Sural neuropathy in the popliteal fossa
- Baker's cyst.
- Arthroscopy, or other operations in the popliteal fossa (e.g. for varicose veins).

Sural neuropathy in the calf
- Tight chains, lacing or elastic socks around the calf.
- High-topped footwear.
- Pressure against a hard ridge.
- Calf muscle biopsy.

Sural neuropathy at the ankle:
- Sitting with, or on, crossed ankles.
- Adhesions after soft tissue injury.
- Avulsion fracture of the base of the fifth metatarsal bone.
- Fractured sesamoid bone in the peroneus longus tendon.
- Osteochondroma.
- Neuroma.
- Ganglion.
- Sural nerve biopsy (complicated by persistent pain in about 5% of cases and infections or delayed wound healing at the site of biopsy in about 20% of patients).

CLINICAL FEATURES
- Pain, paresthesia or numbness of the lateral ankle or sole.
- Local pressure may aggravate the sensory symptoms (Hoffmann–Tinel sign) and indicate the site of the lesion.

DIFFERENTIAL DIAGNOSIS
S1 radiculopathy.

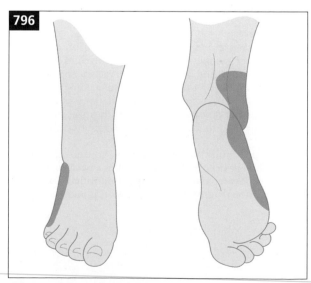

796 Area of skin innervated by the sural nerve.

INVESTIGATIONS
Nerve conduction studies
The amplitude of the SNAP is normally large and easy to elicit with lesions proximal to the sensory ganglion (e.g. S1 radiculopathy) but are decreased or absent with lesions causing axonal degeneration distal to the sensory ganglion (e.g. of the sural nerve).

DIAGNOSIS
Requires the presence of isolated sensory loss the skin of the lateral side of the ankle, and lateral border of the sole, up to the base of the fifth toe. Can be confirmed by EMG.

TREATMENT
Depends on the cause:
- Advice how to avoid external compression, if causal (e.g. special postures with crossed ankles, calves against hard ridges, high-topped boots or tight chains).
- Surgery (neurolysis or nerve section) for compression by post-traumatic fibrosis or tumors.

PUDENDAL NEUROPATHY

DEFINITION
Dysfunction of the pudendal nerve.

EPIDEMIOLOGY
Not uncommon.

ANATOMY
Course of the pudendal nerve (797)
- Arises from the S2, S3 and S4 nerve roots and innervates most of the perineum.
- Descends from the pelvis below the piriformis muscle, crosses the sacrospinous ligament, and enters the perineum through the lesser sciatic notch.
- Courses anteriorly, with its associated blood vessels, along the intrapelvic wall within a tunnel in the dense obturator fascia (the obturator canal or Alcock's canal) and terminates by dividing into three branches:
  - The inferior rectal (hemorrhoidal) nerve, which may also arise from S3 and S4, supplies the external anal sphincter, the perianal skin and the mucosa of the lower anal canal.
  - The perineal nerve innervates the muscles of the perineum (e.g. bulbocavernosus), the erectile tissue of the penis, the external urethral sphincter, the distal part of the mucous membrane of the urethra and the skin of the perineum and labia/scrotum.
  - The dorsal nerve of the clitoris/penis courses forward in Alcock's canal, pierces the urogenital diaphragm, and sends a branch to the corpus cavernosum before running forward on the dorsum of the clitoris/penis to innervate the skin, prepuce and glans.

ETIOLOGY
External compression
- Prolonged bicycle ride.
- Colposcopy with suture through the sacrospinal ligament and subsequent nerve entrapment.
- Operation on hip fracture using perineal post.

797 The pudendal nerve and its branches.

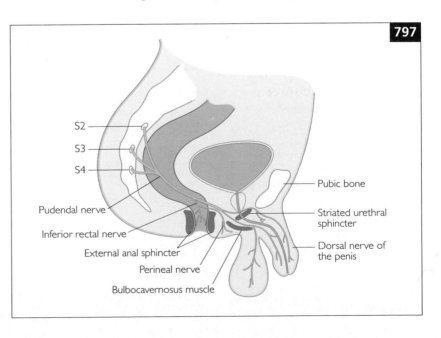

797

S2
S3
S4
Pubic bone
Pudendal nerve
Striated urethral sphincter
Inferior rectal nerve
External anal sphincter
Dorsal nerve of the penis
Perineal nerve
Bulbocavernosus muscle

Stretch injury
- Childbirth: may cause anal sphincter muscle division, and additional damage to the pudendal nerve. Vaginal delivery also causes compression of the pudendal nerves.
- Straining during defecation.
- Pelvic fracture or surgery.

Polyneuropathy
- Diabetic.
- Alcoholic.

CLINICAL FEATURES
History
- Incontinence of urine or feces (pudendal neuropathy is a common cause of fecal incontinence, mainly lesions in the distal segment of the pudendal nerve or in the inferior rectal nerve).
- Impotence.
- Altered sensation in one-half or all of the labia majora/penis and perineum.

Examination
- Absent anal reflex (S3 and S4 nerve roots and pudendal nerve): normally, pricking the perianal skin elicits a reflex contraction of the external anal sphincter which can be seen as a dimpling of the perianal skin.
- Absent bulbocavernosus reflex (S3 and S4 nerve roots and pudendal nerve): normally, compression of the glans penis evokes a contraction of the bulbocavernosus muscle, which is best assessed clinically by palpation.

DIFFERENTIAL DIAGNOSIS
- Conus medullaris or cauda equina lesion.
- Polyneuropathy.
- Disturbance of vascular supply or autonomic innervation (e.g. diabetes).
- Structural abnormalities of the pelvic floor and relevant viscera.

INVESTIGATIONS
Anorectal manometry
May assess the function of the pudendal nerve to some degree.

Urodynamics
May assess the function of the pudendal nerve to some degree.

Nerve conduction studies
Infrarectal stimulation of the terminal parts of the pudendal nerves by mounting disposable surface electrodes on the index finger of a disposable glove and recording the evoked muscle potential from the external anal sphincter (inferior rectal nerve) and urethral sphincter (perineal nerve), the latter via electrodes mounted on a Foley catheter, is possible.

EMG
Needle EMG of the external anal sphincter, external urethral sphincter (difficult and unpleasant for the patient), bulbocavernosus and puborectalis muscles may be helpful.

Reflex responses
Stimulation of the clitoris/penis and recording from the anal sphincter and bulbocavernosus.

Motor and somatosensory evoked potentials
Can be used to study central as well as peripheral nerve conduction to and from the perineal region respectively.

CT or MRI scan of the sacral spine or pelvis

DIAGNOSIS
Requires the presence of incontinence of urine or feces, impotence, and altered sensation in half or all of the labia majora/penis and perineum.

TREATMENT
Depends on the cause.

FURTHER READING

SUPRASCAPULAR NEUROPATHY
Antoniadis G, Richter HP, Rath S, et al (1996). Suprascapular nerve entrapment: experience with 28 cases. J. Neurosurg., 85: 1020–1025.
Van Zandijcke M, Casselman J (1999) Suprascapular nerve entrapment at the spinoglenoid notch due to a ganglion cyst. J. Neurol. Neurosurg. Psychiatry, 66: 245.

CARPAL TUNNEL SYNDROME
Epidemiology
Atroshi I, Gummesson C, Ornstein E, Ranstam J, Rosen I (1999) Prevalence of carpal tunnel syndrome in a general population. JAMA, 282: 153–158.
MacFarlane GJ (2001) Identification and prevention of work-related carpal-tunnel syndrome. Lancet, 357: 1146–1147.

Etiology
Stevens JC, Beard CM, O'Fallon WM, Kurland LT (1992) Conditions associated with carpal tunnel syndrome. Mayo Clin. Proc., 67: 541–548.

Pathology
Jenkins PJ, Sohaib A, Akker A, et al. (2000) The pathology of median neuropathy in acromegaly. Ann. Intern. Med., 133: 197–201.

Diagnosis
D'Arcy CA, McGee S (2000) Does this patient have carpal tunnel syndrome? JAMA, 283: 3110–3117.
Franzblau A, Werner RA (1999) What is carpal tunnel syndrome? JAMA, 282: 186–187.
Witt JC, Stevens JC (2000) Neurological disorders masquerading as carpal tunnel syndrome: 12 cases of failed carpal tunnel release. Mayo Clin. Proc., 75: 409–413.

Treatments
Dammers JWHH, Veering MM, Vermeulen M (1999) Injection with methylprednisolone proximal to the carpal tunnel: randomized double blind trial. BMJ, 319: 884–886.
Ebenbichler GR, Resch KL, Wiesinger GF, Uhl F, Ghanem A-H, Fialka V (1998) Ultrasound treatment for treating the carpal tunnel syndrome: randomized 'sham' controlled trial. BMJ, 316: 731–735.
Garfinkel MS, Singhal A, Katz WA, et al. (1998) Yoga-based intervention for carpal tunnel syndrome. A randomized trial. JAMA, 280: 1601–1603.

SCIATIC NEUROPATHY
Vroomen PCAJ, de Krom MCTFM, Slofstra PD, Knottnerus JA (2000) Conservative treatment of sciatica: A systematic review. Journal of Spinal Disorders, 13: 463–469.

Neuromuscular Junction Disorders

MYASTHENIA GRAVIS (MG)

DEFINITION

Myasthenia gravis is an acquired autoimmune neuromuscular disorder in which serum IgG antibodies (anti-AChRAb) to acetylcholine receptors (AChR) in the post-synaptic membrane of the neuromuscular junction lead to receptor loss, and skeletal muscle fatigue and weakness. Myasthenic crisis is when weakness of the muscles of respiration is severe enough for the patient to require mechanical ventilation.

EPIDEMIOLOGY

- Prevalence: 5–18 cases per 100 000 population.
- Lifetime prevalence: 0.4 (95% CI: 0.2–0.7) per 1000.
- Incidence: 3(95% CI: 0.8–7) per 100 000 per year. Incidence is age- and sex-related, with one peak in the second and third decades affecting mostly women and a peak in the sixth and seventh decades affecting mostly men.
- Age: any age, from early childhood to old age.
- Thymoma-associated myasthenia gravis has a peak incidence at 40–50 years of age.
- Non-thymoma-associated MG has a peak incidence at 10–30 and 60–70 years of age.
- Gender: M=F.

PATHOLOGY
End-plate abnormalities

A decrease in number (by about two-thirds) of nicotinic acetylcholine receptors in the post-synaptic membrane at neuromuscular junctions of skeletal muscle, with simplification of postsynaptic folds and widening of the synaptic cleft. The degree of reduction of AChRs generally correlates with the severity of MG.

Thymus
- Thymoma occurs in 10% of patients, which may be locally invasive.
- Medullary hyperplasia, characterized by lymphoid follicles with germinal centers, occurs in about 60% of patients, usually those presenting before 40 years of age.

ETIOLOGY
Autoimmune
- Anti-AChRAb reduce the number of AChRs by accelerated endocytosis and degradation of the receptors, functional blockade of acetylcholine (ACh) binding sites and complement-mediated damage to the AChRs.
- B lymphocytes produce the anti-AChRAb but T lymphocytes have a key role in the autoimmune response.
- The origin of the autoimmune response is unsolved. The thymus has been implicated because about 75% of patients have thymic abnormalities (85% thymic hyperplasia [germinal-center formation] and 10–15% thymoma) and thymectomy improves most patients.
- Genetic factors and abnormalities of immune regulation may increase the likelihood of MG: there is a moderate association with the HLA antigens B8 and DRw3; a stronger association with HLADQw2 is still controversial.
- A wide variety of other autoimmune diseases are associated with MG (see below).

Disorders or factors that may exacerbate MG
- Thyroid disease: hyperthyroidism, hypothyroidism.
- Infection.
- Drugs: aminoglycoside antibiotics (streptomycin, gentamicin, kanamycin, neomycin), polymyxin, colistin, curare, quinidine, quinine and antiarrhythmic agents such as procainamide.

PATHOPHYSIOLOGY

- Muscle contraction depends on effective neuromuscular transmission.
- Effective neuromuscular transmission depends on the number of interactions between ACh molecules released from the nerve terminal, and AChRs on the post-synaptic membrane of the neuromuscular junction (**798**).
- The nicotinic ACh receptor is a glycoprotein that projects through the muscle membrane and is composed of five subunits (two *a*, one *b*, one *d*, and one *g* or *e* subunit), arranged like barrel staves around a central channel. Each of the two *a* subunits has an ACh-binding site that is located extracellularly.
- In the resting state the ion channel of the AChR is closed.
- When ACh binds to the binding sites of both *a* subunits of the AChR, the receptor's cation channel opens transiently, allowing the rapid passage of cations and producing a localized electric end-plate potential.
- If the amplitude of this potential is sufficient, it generates an action potential that spreads along the length of the muscle fiber, triggering the release of calcium from internal stores and leading to muscle contraction.
- At the normal neuromuscular junction, the end-plate potentials are more than sufficient to generate muscle action potentials consistently, without failures.
- At the myasthenic neuromuscular junction, the decreased number of AChRs results in end-plate potentials of diminished amplitude, which fail to trigger action potentials in some fibers. When transmission fails at many junctions, the power of the whole muscle is reduced, causing muscle weakness. When contractions are repeated, due to repeated nerve stimulation, the amount of ACh released per nerve impulse normally declines (runs down) after the first few impulses because the nerve terminal is not able to sustain its initial rate of release. If there is a reduced number of AChRs, as is the case in MG, this ACh 'rundown' results in progressive failure of transmission at more and more junctions and muscle power progressively declines, causing fatiguability.
- AChRs normally undergo continuous turnover at the neuromuscular junction, depending on regulating influences of the motor nerves and neuromuscular

transmission. Impairment of transmission induces increased transcription of AChR genes. Consequently, virtual complete recovery can occur in patients with MG if the autoimmune attack can be controlled.

CLINICAL FEATURES

- The clinical hallmarks are muscular weakness and fatiguability.
- The weakness tends to increase with repeated activity and improves with rest.
- Weakness usually occurs in a characteristic distribution.

Ocular muscles

- The eyelid and extraocular muscles are the first muscles to be involved in about 65% of patients, and are affected at some stage of the disorder in >90% of patients, causing ptosis (**799**) and diplopia, which are typically asymmetric.
- Weakness remains confined to the eyelid and extraocular muscles in about 15% of patients (ocular myasthenia).
- At the bedside, fatiguable ptosis can be demonstrated by asking the patient to maintain upward gaze without blinking for 30–60 seconds.

Facial and bulbar muscle weakness

- Leads to loss of facial expression (a characteristic 'flattened' or 'snarling' smile), inability to whistle, and difficulty with speech ('mushy' or nasal speech), chewing and swallowing.
- Weakness of the neck extensors and muscles of mastication may necessitate the patient to use one of their hands to prop up their jaw.

Limb weakness

- Generalized weakness develops in about 85% of patients and may affect the proximal and distal limb muscles, neck extensors (and diaphragm).
- Initially, it may be episodic (e.g. sudden weakness of the legs) and precipitated by emotional stress or infection.
- Characteristically, the weakness is increased by exercise, tone is normal and deep tendon reflexes are generally brisk.
- At the bedside, fatiguable limb weakness can be demonstrated by asking the patient to elevate the outstretched arm against resistance for 30–60 seconds, and comparing the strength with the opposite rested limb.

798 Diagrammatic representation of the neuromuscular junction, showing the site of acetylcholine receptors of the post synaptic membrane. (ACh = acetylcholine; AChE = acetylcholinesterase.)

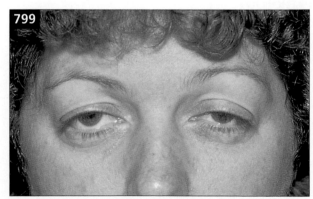

799 Bilateral ptosis in a patient with myasthenia gravis.

Respiratory muscle weakness
May lead to shortness of breath and, in severe cases, ventilatory failure.

Associated other immune conditions
Susceptibility is determined through immune response genes (e.g. HLA):
- Neuromyotonia (continuous muscle fiber activity caused by peripheral nerve hyperexcitability).
- Thyroid disease: hyperthyroidism occurs in about 5% (3–8%) of patients with MG, and hyper- and hypothyroidism may aggravate myasthenic weakness.
- Polymyositis.
- Rheumatoid arthritis.
- Systemic lupus erythematosus.

SPECIAL FORMS
Neonatal myasthenia
- A transient illness, lasting <1 month.
- It occurs in 1/8 babies of myasthenic mothers.
- It is due to placental transfer of maternal anti-AchRAb to the baby.
- Arthrogryposis (severe joint contractures occurring *in utero*) is occasionally present.

Juvenile myasthenia
Myasthenia in patients younger than 18 years of age is termed juvenile myasthenia. The illness is similar to MG in young adults.

Penicillamine-induced myasthenia
- This is similar to adult MG, including the presence of anti-AchRAb.
- It usually resolves over several months after withdrawal of the drug.

DIFFERENTIAL DIAGNOSIS
Generalized myasthenia
Congenital myasthenic syndromes
- Rare.
- Inherited, usually as recessive disorders.
- Early-onset.
- Not autoimmune disorders; anti-AchRAb is undetectable.
- Sophisticated electrophysiologic and immunocyto-chemical tests required for diagnosis.
- Most forms are non-progressive.

Drug-induced myasthenia
- Penicillamine:
  - Triggers autoimmune myasthenia.
  - Recovery within weeks after drug withdrawal.
- Curare, procainamide, quinines, aminoglycosides:
  - Weakness in normal people.
  - Exacerbation of MG.
  - Recovery after drug withdrawal.

Lambert–Eaton syndrome
- Weakness, fatigue, areflexia.
- 60% have associate small cell lung cancer.
- Nerve conduction studies: incremental response on repetitive nerve stimulation.
- Antibodies to calcium channels are present.

Venoms (snakes, scorpions, spiders)

Botulism
- Generalized weakness.
- Dilated pupils.
- Ophthalmoplegia.
- Nerve conduction studies: incremental response in repetitive nerve stimulation.

Inflammatory demyelinating polyradiculoneuropathies
- Acute (Guillain–Barré) motor type.
- Miller–Fisher syndrome.
- Chronic.

Hyperthyroidism
- Exacerbates MG.
- Generalized weakness.
- Thyroid function tests are abnormal.

'Functional' disorder
MG is sometimes misdiagnosed as a 'functional' disorder, perhaps because of the fatiguing characteristics of the muscle weakness, its worsening with stress, and the lack of other neurologic signs.

Ocular myasthenia
Progressive external ophthalmoplegia (mitochondrial cytopathy)
- Ptosis, diplopia.
- Generalized weakness in some cases.
- Mitochondrial DNA: abnormal.

Oculopharyngeal muscular dystrophy

Grave's disease
- Diplopia.
- Exophthalmos.
- Thyroid-stimulating immunoglobulin is present.

Intracranial mass compressing cranial nerves
- Ophthalmoplegia.
- Cranial nerve weakness.
- CT or MRI brain abnormality.

Bulbar myasthenia
Brainstem stroke

Motor neuron disease (pseudobulbar palsy)

INVESTIGATIONS
Anti-AChRAb assay
- 85–90% of patients with generalized MG and 60% of patients with ocular disease have elevated titers of serum antibodies to AChR that are detectable by an immuno-precipitation assay.
- Anti-AchRAb is specific to MG and is therefore useful in diagnosis.
- In an individual patient, the antibody titer generally correlates with the severity of the disease, as shown by the response to plasma exchange and, in the longer term, to immunosuppressive drugs. Correlation of titer and disease severity across patients, however, is poor (i.e. a patient with mild disease can have a high titer and a patient with severe disease can have a low titer) probably because of antibody heterogeneity.

Continued overleaf

Anti-AChRAb assay (*continued*)
- The antibody remains detectable in many patients in clinical remission.
- Among the 10–20% of patients with MG who do not have detectable anti-AChRAb, antibodies to another neuromuscular junction protein muscle specific kinase (MuSK) are present.

Antibodies to muscle specific kinase (MuSK)
- Inhibit the function of MuSK
- MuSK is a receptor tyrosine kinase that is an essential component of the developing neuromuscular function.

Anti-striated muscle antibody assay
Detectable in >90% of patients with thymoma and in about 30% of other patients with MG.

Anticholinesterase (edrophonium chloride) test (800, 801)
Edrophonium (Tensilon) is an anticholinesterase with a rapid onset (30 seconds) and short duration (5 minutes) of action.

Indications
- The diagnosis has to be made immediately because of disease severity.
- The patient is sero-negative for anti-AchRAb.

Procedure
- The test is undertaken in hospital where full resuscitative equipment must be readily available.
- Pre-treat with atropine, 0.6 mg i.v. to counteract parasympathetic overstimulation and avoid occasional adverse effects.
- Assess the strength of an objectively weak muscle or group of muscles (e.g. degree of ptosis or diplopia; vital capacity).
- Inject a test dose of edrophonium (Tensilon) 1–2 mg i.v.
- If no adverse effects develop, inject a further 5–6 mg.
- A positive response is indicated by an obvious improvement in strength within 1 minute (e.g. abolition of ptosis, an increase in the length of time that the arm can be kept outstretched, and increase in vital capacity) which disappears within 5 minutes.
- This test can be combined with EMG measurements of neuromuscular transmission.

An alternative, less commonly used, procedure
- Administer atropine intramuscularly into one leg and wait for a placebo response.
- If negative, administer neostigmine 1.5 mg i.m. into the other leg.

The atropine counteracts parasympathetic overstimulation and also serves as a placebo control for motor effects. Neostigmine i.m. provides more time for tests and is less risky than i.v. edrophonium (i.e. from anaphylaxis).

EMG
Results can be misleading in patients who are already receiving anticholinesterase medication; in such patients the drug should, if possible, be withdrawn for 1 week before the study.

Repetitive nerve stimulation
- A useful supplement to the clinical diagnosis when antibody testing is negative.

- The nerve to a clinically weak or proximal muscle is stimulated supramaximally at a rate of 3 per second and the muscle action potentials are recorded from surface electrodes over the muscle. A progressive decrement in the amplitude of the evoked action potential of 15% or more is considered abnormal (802). The test is generally unpleasant for the patient, and false positives and negatives may occur.

Single fiber EMG
- This test detects delayed or failed neuromuscular transmission in pairs of muscle fibers supplied by branches of a single nerve fiber (803, 804).
- A sensitive but not highly specific test. Positive in about 90% (88–92%) of cases, its specificity is limited because of positive findings in other disorders of nerves, neuromuscular junction, and muscle.

Chest x-ray and CT or MRI of the mediastinum (thymoma, thymic hyperplasia)
- CT and MRI reliably reveal enlargement of the thymus gland.
- The thymus is normally detectable until mid-adulthood but persistence of the thymus in a patient with MG who is over 40 years of age, or an increase in its size in any patient on repeated scanning, raises the possibility of a thymoma.
- If negative initially, it should be repeated after 2–3 years in those who are positive for anti-AchR and antistriated muscle antibody.

Screen for other disorders
- Antinuclear antibody.
- Antithyroid antibodies.
- Rheumatoid factor.
- Fasting blood glucose.
- Thyroid function tests.
- Pulmonary function tests.
- Tuberculin test.
- Bone densitometry in older patients.
- Mitochondrial DNA analysis (if ocular myasthenia).

Screen for disorders that may interfere with immunosuppressive therapy
- Hypertension.
- Unsuspected infections such as tuberculosis.
- Peptic ulcer.
- Occult gastrointestinal bleeding.
- Renal disease.
- Diabetes.
- Osteoporosis.

Tests
- Blood pressure, fundoscopy, EKG, serum creatinine.
- Occult blood.
- Fasting blood glucose.
- Chest x-ray.
- Pulmonary function tests.
- Tuberculin test.
- Bone densitometry in older patients.

DIAGNOSIS
- As a diagnosis of MG almost commits the patient to long term medical or surgical treatment that carries substantial risks, every effort should be made to establish the diagnosis before initiating treatment.

- Anti-AchRAb testing is reliable, and a positive result is virtually definitive in the majority of patients, although a negative assay result does not exclude MG. The other tests listed above may be useful in patients with doubtful anti-AchRAb results.
- Other conditions that mimic MG should be excluded, and associated conditions that may influence the choice of treatment should be searched for.

CLASSIFICATION

Four main groups of acquired myasthenia gravis can be distinguished which have implications for treatment:

Group I
- Onset: early (<40 years).
- Gender: F>M.
- Weakness: generalized usually.
- Thymus: hyperplasia.
- Anti-AChRAb titers: high.

Group II
- Gender: M=F.
- Weakness: generalized weakness usually.
- Thymus: thymoma (which may be benign or locally invasive).
- Anti-AChRAb titers: intermediate.

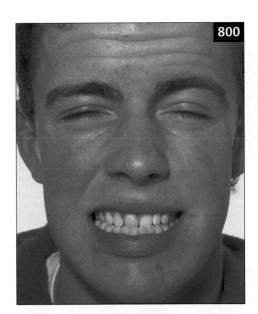
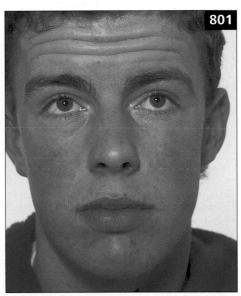

800, 801 Myasthenic 'snarl' (**800**) as the patient tries to open his eyes, due to facial weakness, before an edrophonium test. Restored muscle power (**801**) within minutes of injection of edrophonium 5 mg i.v. (Courtesy of Dr AM Chancellor, Neurologist, Tauranga, New Zealand.)

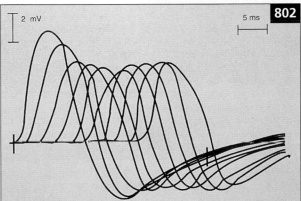

802 Supramaximal repetitive ulnar nerve stimulation at 5 Hz showing ten successive muscle action potentials recorded over abductor digiti minimi and a decrement in amplitude of more than 15% between the first and fourth response.

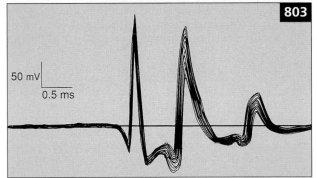

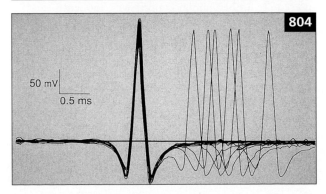

803, 804 Single fiber EMG. **803** Normal 'jitter' of the second, compared with the first muscle fiber, supplied by a single nerve fiber. The responses of the second muscle fiber, relative to the first, are virtually superimposed upon one another due to the absence of any delay in neuromuscular transmission. **804** Myasthenia gravis patient in whom 'jitter' is substantially increased due to variable delay in neuromuscular transmission.

Group III
- Onset: late (>40 years).
- Gender: M>F.
- Weakness: generalized or ocular.
- Thymus: atrophy/involution.
- Anti-AChRAb titers: low.

Group IV
- Weakness: ocular only or generalized.
- Thymus: atrophy/involution.
- Anti-AChRAb titers: absent, but autoantibodies to other muscle cell targets are implicated.

MODES OF THERAPY
In general, four methods of treatment are used:
- Anticholinesterase agents.
- Thymectomy.
- Immunosuppression.
- Short term immunotherapies.

Anticholinesterase medication
- Most useful in mild cases.
- Pyridostigmine (Mestinon) 30–120 mg p.o., or neostigmine bromide 15–30 mg p.o.; both given every 3–4 hours except at night.
- Neostigmine can also be given subcutaneously or intramuscularly (15 mg p.o. is equivalent to 1 mg subcutaneously or intramuscularly), preceded by atropine 0.5–1 mg.
- Pyridostigmine usually produces a smoother response.
- Adverse effects are caused by parasympathetic stimulation: pupillary constriction; colic; diarrhea; increased salivation, sweating, lacrimation, and bronchial secretions.
- Gastrointestinal adverse effects can be controlled with propantheline bromide, atropine or loperamide.

Thymectomy
Thymectomy has two purposes: to prevent the spread of thymoma and to induce remission, or at least improvement, permitting a reduction in immunosuppressive medication.

Indications
Thymic tumors must be removed surgically since they may spread locally and become invasive, though they rarely metastasize. The tumor and remaining thymus gland should be removed as completely as possible. If not, or if it is invasive, marker clips should be placed at the tumor site during surgery and focused radiation treatment carried out postoperatively. After removal of a thymoma, some patients become weaker, presumably as a loss of a suppressive effect of the thymoma, and require further immunosuppressive treatment.

Thymectomy is indicated for generalized MG in patients who are between adolescence and about 60 years of age. The only reason for delaying thymectomy in pre-pubertal children, if possible, is because of the role of the thymus in development of the immune system. It is uncertain whether thymic tissue persists in patients with MG who are older than 60 years.

Thymectomy has also been undertaken in purely ocular MG with good results. Thymectomy should never be performed as an emergency procedure. The patient's strength and respiratory function in particular should be optimized preoperatively, but not with immunosuppressive agents if they can possibly be avoided because they increase the risk of perioperative infection. If the vital capacity is below 2 l, plasmapheresis should be carried out preoperatively.

Technique
Thymectomy should remove as much of the thymus as possible. Although a cervical incision with mediastinoscopy is associated with a smaller scar and less postoperative pain, it has not been confirmed that this method consistently enables the thymus to be removed completely. A sternal-splitting approach with exploration extending into the neck optimizes removal of all thymic tissue and related fat. Epidural morphine minimizes postoperative pain and thereby enhances respiratory effort. For a few days after thymectomy, the requirement for anticholinesterase medication may be decreased and so only about three-quarters of the preoperative dose needs to be given intravenously postoperatively.

Outcome
The benefits of thymectomy are usually delayed until months to years after surgery. Clinical remission occurs in about one-third of patients and remission in another half, which is substantially better than if not treated surgically.
Mechanism of effect
The mechanism by which thymectomy produces benefit in MG is still uncertain. Possible reasons include removal of a source of continued antigenic stimulation, removal of a reservoir of B cells secreting AChR antibodies, and correcting a disturbance of immune regulation. Whatever, generally, anti-AChRAb levels fall after thymectomy.

Immunosuppressive treatment
Indications
Immunosuppressive treatment should be considered when weakness is not adequately controlled by anticholinesterase drugs and is sufficiently distressing to outweigh the risks of possible adverse effects of immunosuppressive drugs.

Duration
Treatment must be continued for a prolonged period, often permanently.

Corticosteroids
The most consistently effective immunosuppressive drugs but they have the largest array of adverse effects. When initiating steroid therapy in patients with moderate to severe generalized weakness, the patient should be hospitalized because of the risk of transient steroid-induced exacerbation in the first few weeks in up to one-half of patients. This risk is minimized by beginning with a daily dose of 10–20 mg of prednisone and increasing it gradually by about 5 mg every 2–3 days, according to the patient's clinical condition and response, until a satisfactory response is achieved or the dose reaches 50–60 mg a day. However, the favorable effect of steroids may take 2–4 weeks to become apparent and maximal benefit may not be realized until after 6–12 months or more.

After about 3 months of daily high-dose treatment, a switch to an alternate day regime may help to minimize adverse effects but a small dose of prednisone may be required on the 'off' day if muscle strength fluctuates significantly. Over the next few months to years, the total dose should be tapered slowly (e.g. 5 mg/month) to the minimum effective dose. Few patients are able to be weaned off prednisone completely.

The mechanisms by which corticosteroids work in MG may include a reduction in anti-AChRAb levels, diminished anti-AChRAb reactivity of peripheral blood lymphocytes, and increased synthesis of AChRs.

Azathioprine

Azathioprine is metabolized to the cytotoxic derivative 6-mercaptopurine and acts predominantly on T cells. It is most useful for patients in whom steroids are contraindicated, in whom steroids evoked an insufficient response, or as an adjunct to permit a reduction in steroid dose. The drug is well tolerated but up to 10% of patients have an idiosyncratic influenza-like reaction (fever, myalgia and malaise) and it takes many months to 1 year to show its therapeutic effect.

Treatment begins with a test dose of 50 mg daily for 1 week and, if tolerated, the dose is gradually increased to the target dose of 2–3 mg/kg total body weight (not lean body mass) per day. If patients are also taking allopurinol, the dose of azathioprine must be reduced by as much as 75% and the white blood cell count and mean corpuscular volume monitored closely. Complete blood count and liver function tests should be undertaken weekly for the first 8 weeks and every 3 months thereafter. Treatment is usually lifelong.

Combined prednisolone and azathioprine

Among patients with moderate or severe symptoms, a randomized controlled trial showed that the combination results in lower doses of prednisolone, fewer relapses, longer periods of remission, and fewer adverse effects than prednisolone alone.

Methotrexate

Weekly methotrexate, 5–10 mg, is an alternative to the few patients who are unable to tolerate, and need, azathioprine.

Mycophenolate mofetil

A novel and potent immunosuppressive agent, which blocks purine synthesis in activated T and B lymphocytes. In an open-label study, the addition of mycophenolate mofetil 1 g twice daily for 6 months to corticosteroids improved function within 2 weeks to 2 months in 8 out of 12 patients. No major adverse effects were observed. Randomized controlled trials are required.

Short term immunotherapies

Plasma exchange

Three to five daily exchanges of 50 ml/kg body weight may produce striking short term clinical improvement. The therapy is useful when combined with immunosuppressive drug treatment, if patients have severe disease and can enable patients who might normally require hospital admission to remain at home.

Intravenous immunoglobulin (IVIG)

IVIG 0.4 g/kg body weight for 5 days may be as effective as a 5-day course of plasma exchange.

TREATMENT

Treat or avoid disorders and drugs that interfere with neuromuscular transmission

- Thyroid disease: hyperthyroidism, hypothyroidism.
- Infection.
- Drugs: aminoglycoside antibiotics (streptomycin, gentamicin, kanamycin, neomycin), polymyxin, colistin, curare, quinidine, quinine and antiarrhythmic agents such as procainamide.

Anticholinesterase medication to enhance neuromuscular transmission

- First line treatment for all patients.
- Pyridostigmine (Mestinon) 30–60 mg every 4 hours has an effect within 30 minutes that peaks at 2 hours and gradually declines thereafter. The timing of administration should be tailored to the patient's needs, i.e. to avoid peaks and valleys of strength, and before meals or physical activity. The maximum daily dose rarely exceeds 120 mg every 3 hours. Higher doses may increase weakness (receptor desensitization or rarely cholinergic block). A sustained-release preparation of Mestinon (Timespan) should only be used at bedtime, and only if the patient experiences significant weakness during the night or in the early morning.
- Provides symptomatic relief in most patients, particularly when weakness is mild, but the improvement is often incomplete and wanes after a few weeks or months.
- If weakness interfering with normal activities persists, additional measures should be considered as described below.

Ocular cases

- Anticholinesterase medication suffices for a few patients.
- Prednisolone, in relatively low dose (e.g. 30 mg on alternate days), is commonly effective for these patients who have persistent symptoms despite anticholinesterase medication.

Thymoma patients

Group II patients

- Thymectomy is indicated because the tumor can infiltrate local mediastinal structures.
- The myasthenic symptoms do not usually respond to removal to the thymus and tumor in these patients.
- Immunosuppressive drug treatment (prednisolone and/or azathioprine) is often effective in controlling myasthenic symptoms before thymectomy and afterwards.

Patients without thymoma

Group I patients

- Thymectomy is indicated for patients in group I (see above) with moderate or severe weakness; about 75% of patients will show improvement or remission.
- Immunosuppressive drug treatment should be considered in those who fail to respond to thymectomy or who are too ill to undergo surgery.

Group III and IV patients

Immunosuppressive drug treatment should be considered in these patients who have persistent symptoms despite anticholinesterase medication; about 80% of patients treated with prednisolone and/or azathioprine at optimal dose regimens show marked improvement or remission.

Pregnant patients with myasthenia

Weakness does not usually increase during pregnancy, but may do so in the postpartum period for a few months:

- Maintain existing (pre-pregnancy) treatments, including immunosuppressive drugs, during the pregnancy; there is no evidence that prednisolone or azathioprine, as used in MG, are teratogenic.
- Plasma exchange can also be used if needed.

Neonatal myasthenia

General care of the infant (intubation and assisted ventilation, nasogastric feeding, and removal of pharyngeal secretions) should be provided and anticholinesterase medications given.

Myasthenic crisis

Crisis may be precipitated by infection, initiation of corticosteroid treatment at high dosage, or inadequate treatment:

- Maintain the airway and provide assisted ventilation and anticholinesterase medication.
- Intravenous immunoglobulin (IVIG) therapy or plasma exchange can be used if needed.

Cholinergic crisis

Crisis occurs due to excess anticholinesterase medication:

- Maintain the airway and provide assisted ventilation and atropine, if not already being given.
- Withdraw anticholinesterase medication temporarily, and reintroduce later at a reduced dose.
- Immunosuppressive drug therapy and/or plasma exchange can be used if needed.

PROGNOSIS

The prognosis for patients with MG has improved dramatically in recent years. Now, with optimal care, the mortality rate is zero. Remission or substantial improvement can be expected in 80% of patients and most patients lead normal lives but take immunosuppressive medication indefinitely. Without treatment, 20–30% will die within 10 years.

LAMBERT–EATON MYASTHENIC SYNDROME (LEMS)

DEFINITION

Lambert–Eaton myasthenic syndrome is an antibody-mediated autoimmune disorder of neuromuscular transmission, characterized by muscle weakness, hyporeflexia or areflexia and autonomic dysfunction.

HISTORY

In 1953 Anderson and colleagues reported a case of a 47 year old man with a bronchial neoplasm, progressive muscle weakness and hyporeflexia who developed progressive apnea following administration of succinylcholine. They concluded that there was 'strong clinical evidence for believing that the severe muscle weakness was of the myasthenic type'.

In 1956, at a meeting of the American Physiological Society, Lambert, Eaton and Rooke presented a report of six patients with defective neuromuscular transmission associated with malignant neoplasms. They identified that some of the clinical and electrophysiologic features were different from what was expected in myasthenia gravis. Subsequently in 1957, Eaton and Lambert summarized the clinical and electrophysiologic characteristics of the myasthenic syndrome.

EPIDEMIOLOGY

- Incidence: rare.
- Age: onset >40 years in >80% of patients.
- Carcinoma-associated LEMS: mean age at presentation 58 years (rarely before 30 years of age).
- LEMS without carcinoma: mean age at presentation 48 years.
- Gender: M≥F (?dependent on smoking patterns).

ETIOLOGY AND PATHOPHYSIOLOGY

The release of neurotransmitters at presynaptic motor nerve terminals of the neuromuscular junction and autonomic neurons depends on the influx of calcium through the presynaptic voltage-gated calcium channels (VGCC).

LEMS is caused by IgG autoantibodies directed against the presynaptic VGCC, particularly the P/Q type of VGCC, leading to inhibition of calcium flux, a reduction in release of acetylcholine from the motor nerve terminal into the synaptic cleft of the neuromuscular junction, and muscular weakness.

There are two broad groups of patients with LEMS: those with an underlying malignancy and those without, but both share the same clinical and electrophysiologic characteristics.

Malignancies associated with LEMS

- Small cell carcinoma of the lung (SCLC).
- Lymphoproliferative disorders.
- Carcinoma of the breast, colon, stomach, gall bladder, kidney, ovary, and bladder.
- Adenocarcinoma of the lung, pancreas and prostate.
- Intrathoracic carcinoid.

Many patients with LEMS (60%) have an associated SCLC. The SCLC tumor cells express VGCCs of L, N, and P/Q subtypes, and appear to provide the antigenic stimulus for antibody production which cross react with VGCCs in the nervous system. The prevalence of LEMS in patients with SCLC is 3%. In patients presenting with LEMS the chance of having an underlying SCLC falls sharply after 2 years and becomes very small after 4–5 years. There is a significant association of LEMS with HLA-B8, which is stronger in the group without carcinoma.

Both LEMS groups (with and without malignancy) also show an association with immunologic disorders, as suggested by the presence of autoimmune diseases in about 25% of patients, organ-specific antibodies in about 40% of patients, and also non-organ-specific antibodies. The prevalence of autoantibodies is higher in the group with no underlying carcinoma.

Immunologic disorders associated with LEMS
- Addison's disease.
- Celiac disease.
- Diabetes mellitus of juvenile-onset.
- Pernicious anemia.
- Psoriasis.
- Rheumatoid arthritis.
- Scleroderma.
- Sjögren's syndrome.
- SLE.
- Thyroiditis.
- Vitiligo.

CLINICAL FEATURES
Onset of symptoms
Usually gradual and insidious, occasionally subacute.

Cardinal clinical features
Limbs and trunk
- Weakness and fatiguability of upper and lower limb muscles (proximal>distal) occurs, with muscle pain and stiffness. A temporary increase in strength can return after voluntary exercise (unlike myasthenia gravis [MG]), but the weakness can be exacerbated by prolonged exercise, hot bath or hot weather.
- Respiratory muscle weakness (spontaneous or induced by anesthesia).
- Depressed or absent deep tendon reflexes.
- Post-tetanic potentiation of tendon reflexes (i.e. after sustained contraction of the appropriate muscle for 10–15 seconds).
- Peripheral paresthesiae may occur.
- Poor response of weakness to edrophonium and neostigmine (unlike myasthenia gravis).
- Marked sensitivity to curare (as in MG).

Cranial nerves (70% of patients)
- Symptoms: often mild and transient, such as eyelid drooping, diplopia, slurred speech, dysphagia, difficulty chewing, weaker voice, head lolling.
- Signs: rare except for ptosis (54% of patients [805, 806]) and neck flexion weakness (34% of patients); other rare signs include jaw weakness, facial weakness, and palatal weakness.

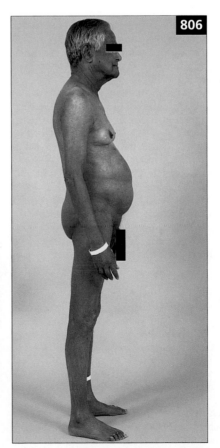

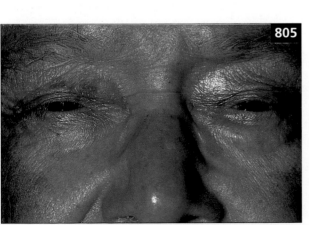

805, 806 Bilateral ptosis, proximal limb wasting and weakness, and gynecomastia in a patient with Lambert–Eaton myasthenic syndrome associated with small cell carcinoma of the lung.

Autonomic features (sympathetic and parasympathetic, 80% of patients)
- Dry mouth.
- Impotence.
- Constipation.
- Poor bladder and bowel control.
- Impaired sweating.
- Tonic pupils.
- Orthostatic hypotension/lightheadedness.
- Impaired esophageal and intestinal motility.

N.B. Severe autonomic dysfunction may be found on testing even when symptoms are minimal.

Features of underlying malignancy
SCLC, lymphoma, and other cancers listed above.

DIFFERENTIAL DIAGNOSIS
- MG.
- Myopathy.
- Chronic fatigue syndrome.

INVESTIGATIONS
Antibodies to VGCCs
- Antibodies to P/Q type VGCCs are present in >90% of patients, particularly those with carcinoma-associated LEMS.
- Antibodies to N type VGCCs are present in <50% of patients, but are more common in LEMS associated with primary lung cancer.

Electrodiagnosis
Electrophysiologic tests are useful for diagnosis as well as for monitoring the course of the illness:
- Amplitude of compound muscle action potential (CMAP) to a single supramaximal stimulus: decreased (normal or near normal in MG).
- Post activation potentiation: marked increase in CMAP amplitude by >100% immediately after maximal voluntary contraction (an increase in CMAP may be seen in MG, and when present is less marked than in LEMS).
- Post activation exhaustion: a decrease in the CMAP amplitude 2–4 min after maximal voluntary muscle contraction (as also occurs in MG).
- Repetitive nerve stimulation at slow rates (2–5 Hz): decremental pattern (MG also has a decremental pattern in which >10% decrement is considered to be abnormal).
- Repetitive nerve stimulation at fast rates (30–50 Hz): incremental pattern of over 2–20 times (MG may show an incremental pattern, but it is usually less marked than in LEMS).
- Single fiber electromyography (SFEMG): increased jitter and intermittent impulse blocking, which improve with higher firing rates (MG shows increased jitter and impulse blocking which get worse with higher firing rates).
- *In vitro* microelectrode studies:
- Miniature end-plate potential (MEPP) amplitudes: normal (small or undetectable in MG).
- End-plate potential (EPP) quantal content: low (normal in MG).
- Distribution of end-plate potential amplitudes: Poisson's distribution (normal distribution in MG).

Edrophonium test
May be positive, but the response is usually weaker than in MG.

Screen for an underlying malignancy and immunologic disorder
- Full blood count.
- ESR.
- Urea and electrolytes.
- Plasma glucose.
- Liver function tests.
- Thyroid function tests.
- Autoantibody screen.
- Vitamin B_{12}.
- Chest x-ray.
- Sputum cytology.
- Urinalysis.
- Stool occult blood.

DIAGNOSIS
Diagnosis is based on the clinical findings and results of investigations.

TREATMENT
The treatment strategy depends on the severity of the symptoms, the degree of response to symptomatic treatment, and the presence or absence of an associated malignancy.

Treatment of muscle weakness and autonomic symptoms
3,4-diaminopyridine
- Blocks voltage-gated potassium channels which leads to prolongation of the action potential at motor nerve terminals and the open time of the VGCCs, resulting in increased influx of calcium enhancing quantal neurotransmitter release.
- It improves muscle strength and autonomic disturbances without serious adverse effects.
- The optimal dose varies from 5 mg tds to 25 mg qid.
- Onset of beneficial effect occurs within 20 minutes of oral dose.
- The beneficial effect lasts about 4 hours.
- The maximum response occurs 3–4 days of treatment, due to cumulative effect of the drug.
- Adverse effects include peri-oral paresthesia and seizures (rarely).

3,4-diaminopyridine plus anticholinesterase drugs (e.g. neostigmine)
Anticholinesterases, such as neostigmine, produce mild or no improvement alone, but seem to potentiate the effects of 3,4-diaminopyridine.

Guanidine and pyridostigmine
Guanidine effectively reduces symptoms but it may have serious adverse effects which include bone marrow toxicity, nephrotoxicity, hepatotoxicity, dermatitis and atrial fibrillation.

Treatment of severe weakness

Plasma exchange
Repeated plasma exchanges may improve symptoms in both groups of LEMS, having a peak effect at 2 weeks and subsiding by 6 weeks. Protein A immunoadsorption removes IgG from plasma selectively.

Intravenous immunoglobulin (IVIG)
Given at 1 g/kg body weight/day for 2 days, IVIG significantly increases muscle strength compared with placebo, peaking at 2–4 weeks and lasting up to 8 weeks, in patients with LEMS and no carcinoma. The clinical response is associated with a significant fall in antibodies to VGCCs. There are no data on IVIG therapy in LEMS associated with carcinoma.

Treatment of any underlying malignancy

- The specific treatment of the underlying tumor usually results in improvement or remission of symptoms, and the only further treatment required may be continuation of 3,4-diaminopyridine.
- If specific treatment for the tumor fails to resolve symptoms, further treatment with prednisolone should be considered, or, if severely weak, plasma exchange or IVIG.

No response to treatment, and screening for malignancy

Steroids or steroids and immunosuppressants
- Long term prednisolone may be beneficial, and if remission is achieved, the dose can be tapered to the minimum maintenance dose.
- Prednisolone combined with azathioprine may be more effective than prednisolone alone in LEMS not associated with carcinoma (but no randomized trial evidence has been obtained).

FURTHER READING

GENERAL
Vincent A, Palace J, Hilton-Jones D (2001) Myasthenia gravis. *Lancet*, **357**: 2122–2128.

MYASTHENIA GRAVIS
Epidemiology
Robertson NP, Deans J, Compston DAS (1998) Myasthenia gravis: a population based epidemiological study in Cambridgeshire, England. *J. Neurol. Neurosurg. Psychiatry*, **65**: 492–496.

Clinical subtypes
Aarli JA (1999) Late-onset myasthenia gravis. *Arch. Neurol.*, **56**: 25–27.

Investigations
Hoch W, McConville J, Melms A, *et al.* (2001) Autoantibodies to the receptor tyrosine kinase MuSK in patients with myasthenia gravis without acetylcholine receptor antibodies. *Nat. Med.*, **7**: 365–368.

Treatment
Ciafaloni E, Massey JM, Tucker-Lipscomb B (2001) Mycophenolate mofetil for myasthenia gravis: An open-label pilot study. *Neurology*, **56**: 97–99.
Evoli A, Batocchi AP, Minisci C, *et al.* (2001) Therapeutic options in ocular myasthenia gravis. *Neuromuscular Disorders*, **11**: 208–216.

Gronseth GS, Barohn RJ (2000) Practice parameter: thymectomy for autoimmune myasthenia gravis (an evidence-base review). Report of the Quality Standards Subcommittee of the American Academy of Neurology. *Neurology*, **55**: 7–15.Kissel JT, Franklin GM, and the Quality Standards Subcommittee of the American Academy of Neurology (2000) Treatment of myasthenia gravis. A call to arms. *Neurology*, **55**: 3–4.
Pallace J, Newsom-Davis J, Lecky B, and the Myasthenia Study Group (1998) A randomised, double-blind trial of prednisolone alone or with azathioprine in myasthenia gravis. *Neurology*, **50**: 1778–1783.
Task Force of the Medical Scientific Advisory Board of the Myasthenia Gravis Foundation of America (2000) Myasthenia gravis: recommendations for clinical research standards. *Neurology*, **55**: 16–23.
Tindall RSA, Rollins JA, Phillips TJ, *et al.* (1987) Preliminary results of a double-blind, randomised, placebo-controlled tiral of cyclosporine in myasthenia gravis. *N. Engl. J. Med.*, **316**: 719–724.

Clinical research
Task Force of the Medical Scientific Advisory Board of the Myasthenia Gravis Foundation of America (2000) Myasthenia gravis: recommendations for clinical research standards. *Neurology*, **55**: 16–23.

LAMBERT–EATON MYASTHENIC SYNDROME
General
Seneviratne U, de Silva R (1999) Lambert-Eaton myasthenic syndrome. *Postgrad. Med. J.*, **75**: 516–520.

Original descriptions
Anderson HJ, Churchill-Davidson HC, Rocharson AT (1953) Bronchial neoplasm with myasthenia: prolonged apnoea after administration of succinlycholine. *Lancet*, **2**: 1291–1293.
Eaton LM, Lambert EH (1957) Electromyography and electrical stimulation of nerves in diseases of the motor unit: observations on a myasthenic syndrome associated with malignant tumours. *JAMA*, **163**: 117–124.
Lambert EH, Eaton LM, Rooke ED (1956) Defect of neuromuscular conduction associated with malignant neoplasms. *Am. J. Physiol.*, **187**: 612–613.

Treatment
Sanders DB, Massey JM, Sanders LL, Edwards LJ (2000) A randomised trial of 3,4-diaminopyridine in Lambert–Eaton myasthenic syndrome. *Neurology*, **54**: 603–607.

Muscle Disorders

X-LINKED DYSTROPHINOPATHIES

DEFINITION

Recessive disorders of muscle (Duchenne's and Becker's muscular dystrophy) caused by a mutation in the short arm, locus 21, of the X chromosome (Xp21), in the enormous gene that codes for the protein dystrophin.

Dystrophin is a filamentous protein present in striated and cardiac muscle and other tissues which is expressed at the periphery of the muscle fiber in the sarcolemmal membrane. Its function is to support the muscle membrane during muscle contraction and prevent destruction of muscle fibers in response to shearing forces.

CLASSIFICATION
Duchenne's muscular dystrophy (DMD)

The most severe dystrophinopathy, in which practically no dystrophin is detected in skeletal muscle by immuno-cytochemistry.

Becker's muscular dystrophy (BMD)

A milder allelic form in which some muscle fibers express dystrophin. First recognized by Becker in 1955 as a distinct benign form of X-linked myopathy.

EPIDEMIOLOGY (see Table 48)

- Incidence:
- DMD: 1 per 3500 male births.
- BMD: one-fifth to one-tenth that of DMD (i.e. about 1 per 35 000 births).
- Prevalence:
- DMD: 2.5 per 100 000 population (relatively low, compared with incidence, because the disease is usually fatal before the third decade).
- BMD: higher than that of DMD because of its relatively benign natural history.
- Age:
- DMD: onset in early childhood (muscle necrosis and serum enzyme elevation can be found in neonates).
- BMD: onset in teenage years or early 20s.
- Gender:
- Almost all patients are male because the inheritance is as an X-linked recessive trait.
- Girls are affected very rarely due to autosomal translocation or if there is only one X chromosome (e.g. Turner's syndrome).

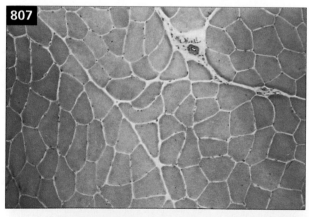

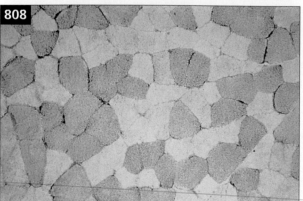

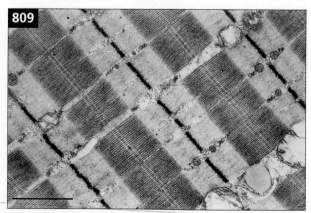

807–809 Normal muscle. H&E stain, ×30 magnification (**807**). Note the arrangement of the muscle fibers in fascicles, the close interdigitation of the muscle fibers, and the muscle fiber nuclei are nearly all subsarcolemmal. NADH-tr. ×100 (**808**): a mosaic arrangement of fibers of various staining intensities. Type 1 fibers are darkly stained and Type 2 fibers are paler, but this distinction is clearer in myosin ATPase preparation. Type 2A fibers tend to be darker than type 2B fibers. The intermyofibrillar substance has a finely granular appearance. Electron microscopy (**809**, bar = 1 μm).

Table 48 Epidemiology of X-linked dystrophinopathies

	DMD	BMD
Incidence	1/3500	1/35 000
Onset	2–7 years	3 years–adult
Creatine kinase	50x normal	10x normal
Wheelchair-bound	By 12 years of age	After 12 years of age
Respiratory failure	By 20 years of age	After 20 years of age
Dystrophin	Absent	Reduced (patchy expression)

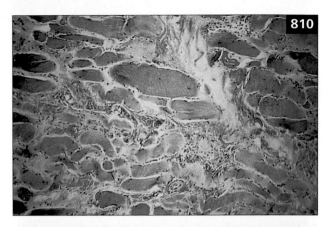

PATHOLOGY
Light microscopy (807–811)
- Abnormal variations in fiber size.
- Fiber splitting.
- Central nuclei.
- Replacement by fat and fibrous tissues.

Dystrophin immunostaining (812–814)
- DMD: <3% of fibers have dystrophin (**813**).
- BMD: severe (i.e. in a wheelchair by 15–20 years of age): 3–15% dystrophin; mild (i.e. ambulatory >20 years of age): >20% dystrophin; partial staining of circumference of muscle fibers (**814**).

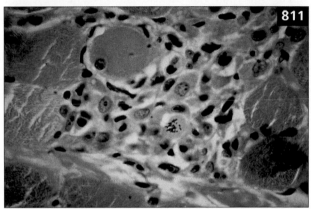

810 Duchenne muscular dystrophy. Muscle biopsy showing variability of fiber size, rounded fibers, and distortion of the muscle structure by extensive deposition of fibrous and fatty tissue between the muscle fibers.

811 Duchenne muscular dystrophy. An area of regenerative activity in muscle: regenerating fibers are usually smaller than surrounding fibers and contain central, enlarged, vesicular nuclei, with prominent nucleoli.

812–814 Cryostatic sections of human muscle biopsies stained with fluorescent labelled monoclonal antibodies to dystrophin, a cytoskeletal protein located at the periphery of muscle fibers beneath the sarcolemma from: normal muscle (**812**), showing characteristic even staining of the sarcolemma; muscle from an individual with Duchenne's muscular dystrophy (**813**) showing virtually no staining of dystrophin (<3%); muscle from an individual with Becker's muscular dystrophy (**814**), showing only dull green background staining which is reduced in intensity and varies both between and within fibers.

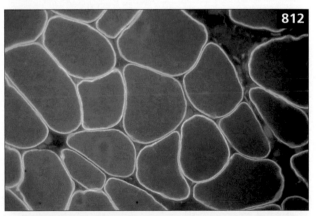

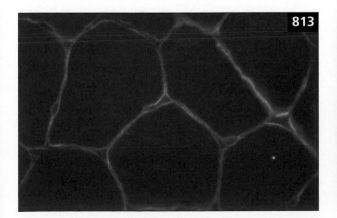

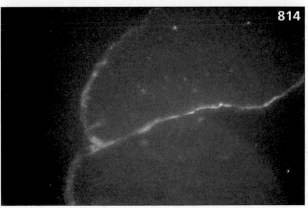

ETIOLOGY AND PATHOPHYSIOLOGY

- The dystrophinopathies involve X-linked inheritance.
- A mutation in the short arm, locus 21, of the X chromosome (Xp21), in the gene that codes for dystrophin.
- Null mutations result in no protein production and a severe progressive phenotype (DMD), whereas missense mutations result in phenotypes of intermediate severity (BMD). The dystrophin gene is the largest gene associated with a disease that has been identified (2.4 million base pairs). It consists of at least 85 exons with introns making up 98% of the gene.
- In about one-third of patients, DMD is the result of a new mutation; one-third of all patients have a family history consistent with X-linked recessive inheritance, and one-third are born to unwitting carriers.
- The mutation rate in the gene is unusually high ($7–10 \times 10^{-5}$/gene/generation), probably because of its large size.
- Dystrophin links the cytoskeleton to the sarcolemma. Absence of dystrophin results in loss of dystrophin-associated glycoprotein and disruption of the linkage between the cytoskeleton and the extracellular matrix, leading to sarcolemmal instability and muscle cell necrosis.

CLINICAL FEATURES
DMD

- Progressive symmetric proximal muscle weakness of the upper and lower limb girdles with hypertrophy of calf muscles.
- Cardiomyopathy is always present.
- Non-progressive intellectual impairment occurs in at least 10% and up to one-third of patients and is present from childhood; special schooling is required for some patients.
- Smooth muscle can be affected, causing paralytic ileus, gastric dilatation and atony of the bladder wall.

Year 2
- Motor developmental delay is noticeable after the first year.
- Onset of walking may be delayed beyond 18 months of age.

Year 5
- Difficulty running and climbing stairs, have frequent falls.
- Show tip-toe walking with a waddling gait.
- Gower's sign: in order to stand up from the floor, children employ their hands to 'climb up their legs' (**815, 816**).
- They have weakness of lower limbs, pelvic muscles and lower trunk.
- Hyperlordosis with a prominent abdomen.
- Enlarged but weak calf muscles (pseudohypertrophy), due to excess fat and connective tissue plus large but ineffective muscle fibers.

Years 6–9
- Joint contractures of the iliotibial bands, hip flexors, and heel cords are present.
- Thoracic deformity.

Year 10
Unable to walk or stand and are dependent on a wheelchair.

Mid teens
Loss of upper limb function occurs.

Late teens–early twenties
- Usually fatal.
- Death is usually related to pulmonary infections, respiratory failure, gastrointestinal complications or cardiomyopathy.

Carriers
- About 8% of female carriers have limb-girdle myopathies.
- A small number of carriers may also suffer from isolated cardiomyopathy.

BMD
- Onset is usually after 12 years of age (3–20 years of age).
- Patients show similar clinical features to DMD but milder, and myocardial and intellectual involvement is less common.
- Calf pain during exercise and myoglobinuria are common.
- Patients may live up to many decades with mild to moderate symptoms that can be indistinguishable from those of limb-girdle dystrophies.

DIFFERENTIAL DIAGNOSIS
- Congenital myopathies of the nemaline and central core types.
- Limb-girdle muscular dystrophies (see p.674).
- Spinal muscular atrophy (see p.534):
- X-linked and autosomal dominant forms of muscular dystrophy, e.g. Emery–Dreifuss muscular dystrophy:
- The defective gene for the commoner X-linked Emery–Dreifuss muscular dystrophy (EDMD), *STA* at Xq28, when normal, codes for a 34 kD nuclear membrane protein named 'emerin', which is expressed in skeletal muscle and myocardium but is still of unknown function. The gene, *LMNA* at 1q21, for the autosomal dominant form of EDMD encodes other nuclear membrane proteins, laminins A and C.
- Onset in early childhood of progressive humeroperoneal muscle weakness and wasting, and contractures of elbow flexors, Achilles tendons and paraspinal muscles. Cardiac involvement is common with conduction defects, bradycardias, and heart blocks. Appropriately timed insertion of a pacemaker may prevent a fatal conduction defect.
- The diagnosis of EDMD depends on mutation analysis rather than protein immunohistochemistry (at present).

INVESTIGATIONS
Blood
- Serum creatine kinase: markedly elevated up to the thousands or tens of thousands of units in DMD, and also elevated in BMD and female carriers.
- Molecular genetics: DNA analysis in blood leukocytes using the polymerase chain reaction (PCR) is abnormal in more than two-thirds of DMD patients.
- Electrophoresis (western blotting) biochemically demonstrates the deficiency of a particular protein, such as dystrophin.

Urine
Myoglobinuria after anesthetic exposure (DMD).

EKG
Features of a cardiomyopathy may be present (also in female carriers).

EMG
Myopathic features occur early in the course. Later, the number of motor units that are activated decreases and tissue may even become unexcitable.

Muscle biopsy
Obtain from mildly involved muscles rectus abdominus rather than from gastrocnemius or deltoid muscles because of worsening caused by immobilization.

Light microscopy (810, 811)
- Abnormal variations in fiber size.
- Fiber splitting.
- Central nuclei.
- Replacement by fat and fibrous tissues.

Dystrophin immunohistochemistry staining
- Staining uses labelled monoclonal antibodies to dystrophin, a cytoskeletal protein located at the periphery of muscle fibers and beneath the sarcolemma.
- In DMD, the majority of fibers fail to show any staining (813).
- In BMD the intensity of staining is reduced and varies both between and within fibers, as it does in the rare female carriers of DMD who manifest symptoms of the disease (814).
- Staining differentiates benign from malignant myopathies.

Role
With the advent of molecular diagnosis and in cases with documented family histories, muscle biopsy might not be required as much as in the past to establish the diagnosis. In less-documented cases, muscle biopsy can be very useful in distinguishing DMD, which is a severe disease, from other diseases that present with similar clinical features but which have a more favorable prognosis (e.g. congenital myopathies of the nemaline and central core types).

DIAGNOSIS
DMD
The diagnosis can be confirmed by muscle biopsy showing absence or near absence of dystrophin on immunostaining (813). DNA analysis in blood leukocytes using PCR is abnormal in more than two-thirds of DMD patients. Prenatal diagnosis from chorionic villi is also feasible.

PREVENTION
Prenatal diagnosis and carrier detection
Conventional strategies of detecting female carriers by pedigree analysis, clinical assessment (some mild muscle weakness), serum creatine kinase (CK) determination (elevated in about 70% of cases), EMG, and histologic study of muscle biopsy specimens, are now complemented by dystrophin analysis in muscle biopsy, PCR analysis of heterozygotes, and restriction fragment length polymorphism analysis.

Fetal abnormalities can be detected using molecular techniques in samples of chorionic villi during early pregnancy (after 8 weeks) or by amniocentesis. Muscle biopsy from fetus or dystrophin immunostaining can be obtained after 19 weeks of gestation with ultrasound guidance.

DNA analysis by molecular genetic studies is much more accurate and thus now essential for detecting female carriers of DMD and BMD, as well as for prenatal diagnostic analysis of chorion villus biopsy material.

Genetic counselling
Genetic counselling is important for all families with an affected male. A known carrier has one chance in two of giving birth to a DMD boy or to a carrier female. About one-third of patients, however, do not have family histories.

It is often necessary to know the specific gene mutation occurring in a family, which is usually accomplished by initially studying an affected male in the family. However, a major problem in genetic counselling in DMD is that some mothers transmitted a mutation to more than one offspring

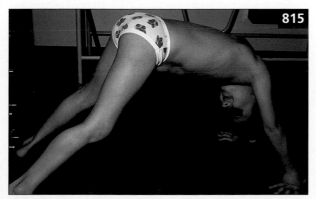

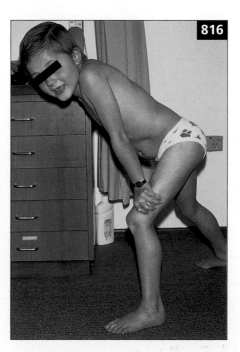

815, 816 A boy with Duchenne muscular dystrophy rising from the floor, and climbing up his legs (Gowers' sign). (Courtesy of Professor BA Kakulas, Neuropathology Department, Royal Perth Hospital, Australia.)

which they did not have in their somatic cells (in their peripheral blood leukocytes). This has been attributed to germline mosaicism. This means that prenatal testing may have to be considered in subsequent pregnancies if a mother has had an affected son, because it cannot be guaranteed that his dystrophy is the result of a new mutation and is therefore unlikely to recur.

TREATMENT

A multidisciplinary team approach to ongoing management (medical, genetic, physiotherapy, occupational therapy, nursing, social work) is required.

Family and patient education

Physical, emotional, educational and financial implications should be discussed.

Physiotherapy

- Physiotherapy aims to preserve mobility and prevent early contractures, which are common in flexor muscles of hips, knees and ankles.
- Passive range of motion exercises and appropriate orthotics may prolong ambulation.
- Exercises to maintain strength in functional muscles and prevent obesity (which further impairs ambulation and respiratory function) are also helpful.
- Patients who can no longer walk may benefit from splints (at night, kept in a neutral position), braces, crutches, and surgery (e.g. scoliosis surgery), and should try to stand at least 3 hours/day in divided periods. However, excessive exercise can be detrimental.

Respiratory therapy

- Breathing exercises or playing wind instruments may be beneficial.
- In the late stages, intermittent positive pressure ventilation is useful, particularly when CO_2 is being retained.

Medication

Prednisolone 0.75 mg/kg/day by oral administration may be appropriate in special circumstances such as acute deterioration. Neuromuscular strength may improve after 1 month of treatment and the maximum effect is reached by 3 months. In controlled studies, the benefits lasted for 3 years. Adverse effects include insomnia, difficult behavior and gastrointestinal symptoms. The mechanism by which steroids may stabilize the clinical course of DMD may be that prednisone slows muscle destruction.

Oxandrolone, an anabolic steroid, may be useful before initiating corticosteroid therapy because it is safe, accelerates linear growth, and may slow the progress of weakness.

Avoid anesthetics with halothane and succinylcholine because patients may develop episodes that resemble malignant hyperthermia. Adverse effects may be reduced by using non-depolarizing muscle relaxants.

Gene therapy

- Gene therapy is experimental.
- Myoblast transplant therapy has succeeded in the *mdx* mouse model but has failed in patients to date.
- Gene therapy administered through viral vectors or liposomes is being tested in animal models.

Other strategies for treatment (currently being researched)

- Elucidate the function of the dystrophin–glycoprotein complex.
- Restore the link between subsarcolemmal cytoskeleton and the extracellular matrix by:
- Replacing the missing protein (dystrophin): Myoblast transfer: not successful to date. Gene therapy: difficult.
- Up-regulating compensating proteins (utrophin).
- Up-regulating proteins with missense mutations (sarcoglycans).
- Gene therapy is in the experimental preclinical stage.

PROGNOSIS
DMD

Most boys start using a wheelchairs by age 12 years and die in their 20s.

BMD

The natural history is much less predictably than that of DMD but inability to walk occurs later than with DMD. Patients become confined to a wheelchair at 12–40 years or later, and many individuals marry, have children, and survive well into middle age and beyond. Death usually occurs at 30–60 years of age.

FACIO-SCAPULO-HUMERAL MUSCULAR DYSTROPHY (FSHD)

DEFINITION

An autosomal dominant inherited disorder characterized by weakness of the facial, scapulohumeral, anterior tibial and pelvic girdle muscles; sometimes associated with retinal vascular disease, sensory hearing loss and, in severe cases, even abnormalities of the CNS due to a genetic defect on chromosome 4.

EPIDEMIOLOGY

- Prevalence: 1:20 000; the third most common hereditary disease of muscle (after Duchenne and myotonic dystrophy).
- Age of onset: any age, but usually 10–50 years of age, and mostly in the second and third decades. A large proportion of gene carriers remain asymptomatic for decades.
- Gender: M=F.

PATHOLOGY
Dystrophic muscle

- Disruption of muscle architecture.
- Abnormal variation in fiber size.
- Degeneration and regeneration of muscle fibers.
- Replacement of muscle by fat and fibrous tissue.

ETIOLOGY AND PATHOPHYSIOLOGY

Autosomal dominant inheritance with high penetrance: the gene is located to the distal chromosome 4q35 where there are normally between 10 and 100 almost identical tandemly arranged repeating units each of 3.3 kb, making up an area that is greater than 35 kb in length. In patients with FSHD, a number of these repeats are deleted, due to large deletions of variable size, so that the area is <35 kb in length (as measured on an electrophoretic gel). No gene has been identified within the area of this deletion, suggesting that these deletions execute a position effect on a more centromeric located gene. In other words, the deletions do not appear to disrupt a transcribed gene but are thought to interfere with the expression of a gene or genes located proximal to the deletions.

CLINICAL FEATURES
- Weakness of the facial, scapulohumeral, anterior tibial, and pelvic girdle muscles occurs (**817, 818**).
- The spectrum of clinical severity is wide, even within families: some have only minimal facial involvement and normal life expectancy, and others are wheelchair bound in childhood with marked kyphoscoliosis and ventilatory failure.
- Although weakness is present in over 95% of affected individuals by age 20 years, up to one-third of patients have no symptoms (i.e. do not recognize the weakness), and most present to medical attention because of involvement of the shoulder rather than the facial muscles.
- However, the first sign is weakness of certain facial muscles, including the orbicularis oculi, orbicularis oris, and zygomaticus, but the actual onset of the weakness can be difficult to establish because abnormal features may be interpreted as nothing more than family traits. Bell's phenomenon and drooping of the lower lip are present, and patients may be unable to whistle. The masseter, temporalis, and extraocular muscles are not involved, and the bulbar and respiratory muscles are also spared.

- FSHD also involves the trapezii, rhomboids, and serratus anterior scapular fixators. Scapular winging is maximized with forward movement because of the serratus anterior weakness (see p.616). The pectoralis is very atrophic. Deltoid and rotator cuff musculature are better preserved.
- Later in the disease, weakness involves the lower limbs, particularly the anterolateral leg compartment (foot dorsiflexors) and finally the hip girdles. Truncal weakness may also occur.
- Side-to-side asymmetry of muscle wasting and weakness is frequent and often striking.
- Heart muscle is spared usually but a predilection for atrial tachyarrhythmias exists.
- An exudative retinopathy is present in one-third of cases.
- Retinal vascular tortuosities are usually subclinical in most cases.
- High frequency sensory hearing loss can be present but is usually asymptomatic.
- Abnormalities of the CNS are present in severe cases.

DIFFERENTIAL DIAGNOSIS
- Autosomal dominant scapuloperoneal syndromes: different pattern of involvement and progression.
- Neurogenic disorders.
- Nemaline myopathy.
- Desmin storage.
- Mitochondrial myopathy.
- Polymyositis.
- Centronuclear myopathy.

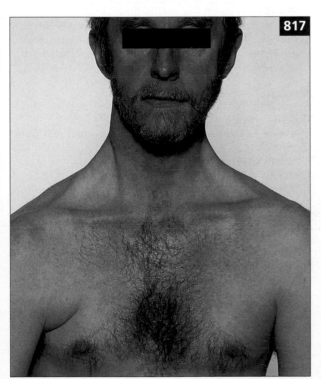
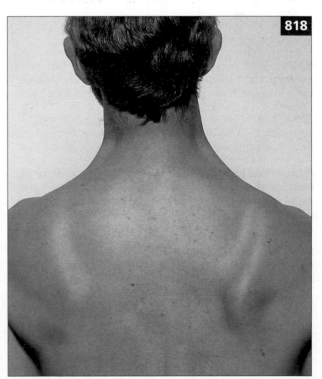

817, 818 Wasting and weakness of the muscles of the face, upper arms and shoulders with prominent weakness of the pectoral muscles and winging of the scapulae in a patient with facioscapulohumeral muscular dystrophy.

INVESTIGATIONS

- Serum CK: may be raised 2–7 times normal, but this varies by age and gender (elevated in three-quarters of affected males and two-fifths of affected females).
- EMG: myopathic.
- Muscle biopsy: may reveal minimal myopathic changes or severe dystrophic muscle, depending in part on the choice of muscle biopsied. A significant inflammatory component may be seen.
- Blood: leukocyte DNA analysis: affected individuals have small restriction fragments of 10–35 kb containing the deletion, whereas unaffected individuals have restriction fragments of 50–300 kb.

DIAGNOSIS

- Patients with characteristic facial and shoulder weakness, and an autosomal dominant family history almost always have the same molecular defect.
- The 4q35 deletion that causes FSHD can be identified in 86–95% of cases with the disease (sensitivity), and is >98% specific for the disease.
- The 5–14% of affected individuals in whom a deletion cannot be identified is attributed to: (1) technical difficulties with degraded or partially digested DNA; (2) translocation between 4q35 and homologous regions on 10q complicating the interpretation of the Southern blot data and, rarely, (3) FSHD not linked to 4q (locus heterogeneity). In such cases, if the clinical suspicion of FSHD remains high, further testing with other 4q35 and 10q probes as well as more extensive study of the kindred with linkage analysis may be required.

PRESYMPTOMATIC AND PRENATAL DIAGNOSIS

Restriction enzyme DNA fragments associated with the gene have been found to be greater than 35 kb in length in individuals who do not have muscular dystrophy; in affected individuals fragments are always less than this (as measured by electrophoretic gel).

Furthermore, there is a general tendency for shorter fragments (i.e. larger deletions) to be associated with earlier onset and more severe cases of the disease; in a sporadic case, for example, this can give an idea of the likely prognosis.

TREATMENT
Myopathy

No specific treatment for the weakness.

Physiotherapy

Posterior plastic ankle orthotics can correct foot drop. A trunk brace may help patients with prominent lumbar lordosis and abdomen. A motorized wheelchair with adjustable height control is invaluable for non-ambulatory patients.

Exudative retinopathy

Photocoagulation may be necessary to prevent retinal detachment.

PROGNOSIS

- Many patients are only mildly affected; most affected individuals remain able to work, often adapting remarkably well to profound weakness in distinct muscle groups.
- The rate of disease progression is variable but usually very slow.
- It is severely disabling for >15% who eventually become dependent on wheelchairs.

LIMB-GIRDLE MUSCULAR DYSTROPHIES (LGMD)

DEFINITION

A clinically and genetically heterogeneous group of autosomal-dominant and autosomal-recessive inherited muscle disorders.

EPIDEMIOLOGY

- Uncommon.
- Age: onset at any age but predominantly between first and fourth decades.
- Gender: M=F.

ETIOLOGY

- A small minority (<10%) of cases are inherited as an autosomal dominant trait (type 1) and are relatively mild.
- The majority are inherited as autosomal recessive traits (type 2), which is often more severe and resembles DMD.
- At least three dominant subtypes and eight recessive subtypes have been identified.
- One recessive subtype (LGMD 2A) is caused by a deficiency of a muscle-specific protease (calpain 3).
- Four other recessive subtypes (LGMD 2C, D, E and F) are caused by deficiencies of particular sarcoglycans (dystrophin associated glycoproteins) which form part of the dystrophin-associated protein complex of muscle membrane.

The dystrophin-associated complex

- A large oligomeric complex in the sarcolemmal membrane of skeletal muscle, which provides an important structural link between the actin-cytoskeleton and the extracellular matrix in skeletal muscle (**819**).
- The complex consists of several subcomplexes beneath the extracellular matrix (laminin-2, α-dystroglycan, glycoprotein complex [sarcoglycans and β-dystroglycan], dystrophin and F-actin cytoskeleton).

Laminin-2 (merosin)
- Laminin-2 is located in the extracellular matrix at the periphery of muscle fibers.
- Absent in children with congenital muscular dystrophy (onset in newborn) who have a nonsense mutation (no functioning protein produced).
- Deficient in children and even adults who have a missense mutation in the merosin gene and produce merosin but in reduced quantities.
- It is also expressed around blood vessels in the brain. Hence MRI T2W images show a leukodystrophic pattern, but the intellect is usually normal.

α-Dystroglycan

- Is a 97 kDa precursor which is encoded by a single gene, mapped to chromosome 3p21, and has a novel laminin (merosin) receptor, which connects the sarcolemma to the extracellular matrix.
- It is located outside the cell, and binds the extracellular matrix component laminin-2 with high affinity.
- It is found in muscle and also the neuromuscular junction, peripheral nerve, brain, kidney and embryo.

Sarcoglycans: α (adhalin), β, γ

- These are abnormal in some autosomal recessive forms of limb girdle muscular dystrophy (sarcoglycanopathies).
- The spectrum of disease (sarcoglycanopathies) is similar to DMD and BMD, and determined by the nature of the mutations (nonsense vs. missense).
- Girls present like DMD or BMD, with gradual onset of progressive proximal limb weakness (e.g. difficulty ascending stairs and running), lumbar lordosis, prominent calf muscles, and tight tendoachilles.
- Cardiomyopathy may occur.
- CK is high.
- Muscle biopsy dystrophic, but a normal amount of dystrophin is present. Staining for antibodies to sarcoglycans reveals a deficiency of one or more of the sarcoglycans.

Dysferlin

- Is localized in muscle membrane but its role is unknown at present.
- Dysferlinopathies have their onset in late teens or adulthood.
- Weakness begins in the lower limbs only: distal (gastrocnemius) weakness (plantar flexion: difficulty standing on toes) and painful calves.
- Weakness progresses slowly and may involve the biceps (only) in the upper limbs.
- CK is elevated (1000s).
- Muscle biopsy is dystrophic (necrotizing myopathy).
- Loss of ambulation occurs at 30–40 years of age.

β-Dystroglycan (inside the cell)

This binds to the cysteine-rich domain of dystrophin.

Dystrophin

Dystrophin links the cytoskeleton to the sarcolemma.

CLASSIFICATION (see Table 49)

Table 49 Classification of limb-girdle muscular dystrophies

Disorder	Gene location	Gene product
Autosomal dominant		
LGMD 1A	5q22-q34	(Genetic anticipation, no cardiac involvement)
1B	1q11-21	Caveolin-3 (cardiac arrhythmias may occur early)
1C	3p25	Caveolin-3 (a scaffolding protein)
1D	6q23	
1E	5q31	
Autosomal recessive		
LGMD 2A	15q15.1-q21.1	Calpain-3
2B	2p13	Dysferlin (cf. Miyoshi myopathy)
2C	13q12	γ-sarcoglycan
2D	17q12-q21.33	α-sarcoglycan (adhalin)
2E	4q12	β-sarcoglycan
2F	5q33-q34	δ-sarcoglycan
2G	17q11-q12	?
2H	9q31-q34.1	?

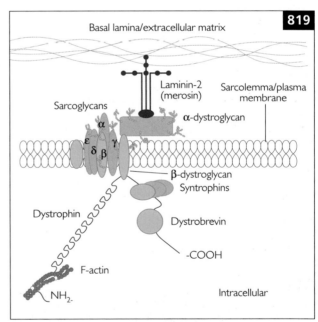

819 Diagrammatic representation of the dystrophin-associated complex in the muscle fiber membrane. Specific muscular dystrophies are caused by deficiencies of dystrophin (Duchenne and Becker muscular dystrophy), a particular sarcoglycan (limb-girdle muscular dystrophy), or laminin-2 (merosin) (congenital muscular dystrophy).

PATHOLOGY

No characteristic histologic features are present (**820, 821**).

Dystrophic muscle

- Dystrophic muscle shows disruption of muscle architecture.
- Variation in fiber size, with very hypertrophied fibers and small fibers.
- Prominent internal nuclei especially in hypertrophied fibers.
- Fiber splitting in some fibers, especially in severely involved fibers and late in disease.
- Degeneration and regeneration of muscle fibers.
- Increased fibrous tissue.

Immunohistochemistry

Deficiency of a muscle specific protease (calpain-3) or a particular sarcoglycan can be found.

PATHOPHYSIOLOGY

Disruption of the dystrophin–glycoprotein complex in skeletal muscle leads to several forms of limb-girdle (and other forms of) muscular dystrophy.

CLINICAL FEATURES

General

- Proximal muscle weakness occurs in pelvic and upper girdle muscles, sparing the face (**822, 823**).
- Cardiac involvement may occur.

Autosomal dominant LGMD

Dominant family history.

LGMD 1A

- Onset occurs in patients aged 18–35 years.
- Affected individuals may have dysarthria and Achilles tendon contractures.
- Serum CK is normal or mildly elevated.

LGMD 1B

- Onset occurs in patients aged 4–38 years.
- Cardiac conduction defects are a prominent complication.
- Serum CK is normal or mildly elevated.

LGMD 1C (caveolin deficiency)

- Onset occurs in patients aged 5 years.
- Serum CK is 4–25 times normal values.

Autosomal recessive LGMD

Sarcoglycanopathy

- Sarcoglycanopathy generally occurs as childhood-onset, but may arise in adults.
- Calf hypertrophy is common (**824, 825**).
- Early involvement of the scapular muscle, deltoid and pelvic girdle.
- Serum CK is normal or mildly elevated.

Calpainopathy

- Onset occurs in patients aged 8–15 years generally, but adult-onset is fairly common.
- Atrophic muscles, scapular winging, sparing of hip adductors, and Achilles tend contractures are present.
- Serum CK is 10 times normal values.

Dysferlinopathy

- Presentation occurs in late teens or early twenties.
- There is posterior distal lower limb involvement early on, with inability to stand on the toes.
- Serum CK is massively elevated (may be >100 times normal values).

DIFFERENTIAL DIAGNOSIS

- BMD.
- Emery–Dreifuss muscular dystrophy: contractures are a very prominent feature.
- Chronic polymyositis.
- Mitochondrial cytopathy.
- Metabolic myopathy: adult-onset acid maltase deficiency.
- Endocrine and drug-induced myopathies.
- MG.
- Spinal muscular atrophy.

INVESTIGATIONS

Blood

- Serum creatine kinase: usually elevated. If normal or mild elevation in active disease, suspect autosomal dominant LGMD. If elevated >100 times normal in the early stages, suspect dysferlinopathy.
- Molecular genetics: DNA analysis in blood leukocytes using PCR.
- Electrophoresis (western blotting): biochemically demonstrates the deficiency of a particular protein.

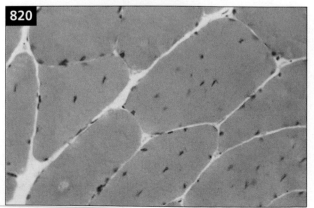 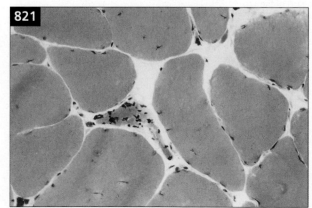

820, 821 Muscle biopsy specimens in a patient with limb-girdle muscular dystrophy showing variation in fiber size, prominent internal nuclei and degenerative and regenerative changes.

- Linkage analysis to dominant LGMD loci if dominant family history and family structure is suitable.

EKG
Features of a cardiomyopathy may be present.

EMG
Myopathic, no specific features.

Muscle biopsy
Light microscopy: dystrophic muscle (820, 821)
- Disruption of muscle architecture.
- Variation in fiber size.
- Degeneration and regeneration of muscle fibers.
- Increased fibrous tissue.

Immunocytochemistry
Use at least two sarcoglycan antibodies as well as dystrophin antibodies:
- Dystrophin: generally normal, but may be abnormal in sarcoglycanopathy.
- Sarcoglycans: a specific sarcoglycan may be absent or reduced. Sarcoglycans are normal in calpainopathy and dysferlinopathy.
- Dysferlin.

If abnormalities are detected on immunocytochemistry with dystrophin or sarcoglycan antibodies, then the full range of sarcoglycan antibodies should be used to attempt to pinpoint the primary deficiency.

Immunoblotting
Immunoblotting is necessary to examine calpain-3. Multiplex blotting may also show which sarcoglycan is primarily involved.

822, 823 The limb-girdle muscular dystrophy phenotype: note wasting of the proximal two-thirds of the deltoids (with pseudohypertrophy of the distal one-third), forearm flexors, thigh adductors, and medial heads of the gastrocnemius muscles.

DIAGNOSIS
Direct detection of the mutation is the final proof of diagnosis and allows carrier detection/prenatal diagnosis. However, given the complexity of the genes and the heterogeneity of the mutations, this is best directed by the results of protein analysis. Therefore, these dystrophies should be diagnosed using a combination of clinical studies, protein studies and genetic studies, which may only be carried out in specialized centers.

TREATMENT
A multidisciplinary team approach (medical, genetic counselling, physiotherapy, occupational therapy, speech therapy, psychology, social work) is required.

PROGNOSIS
Variably progressive.

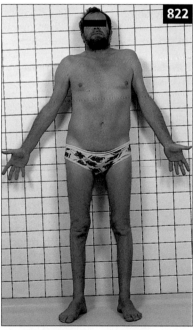

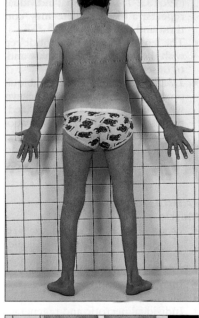

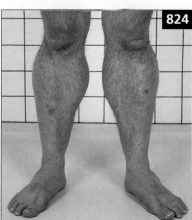

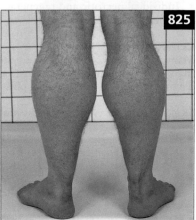

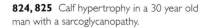

824, 825 Calf hypertrophy in a 30 year old man with a sarcoglycanopathy.

Pancreas
Diabetes mellitus.

Gonads
Tubular testicular atrophy, impotence and poor libido in men.
   N.B. These patients tend to tolerate general anesthetics poorly.

SPECIAL FORMS
Congenital myotonic dystrophy
- Present since birth.
- The abnormal gene is transmitted exclusively through maternal inheritance.
- The fetus shows hydramnios and reduced fetal movements.
- Neonates show respiratory distress, bilateral facial weakness and hypotonia.
- In children mental retardation is a major feature; 75% of patients need special education, and 75% of the remainder at mainstream schools require further assistance to achieve minimum standards in reading and counting.
- There is a high prevalence of cardiac and gastroinstestinal involvement: 20% die of cardiac dysfunction and 15% are still incontinent of feces at age 5 years.
- 25% die before 18 months of age, and 50% survive into the mid-30s.

Myotonic dystrophy type 2
- Myotonic dystrophy type 2 is linked to the long arm of chromosome 3 in a single large family.
- Clinical features are the same as those with myotonic dystrophy type 1, although the degree of facial and limb weakness and the ptosis are more like that of a mild, rather than severe, myotonic dystrophy type 1.

Proximal myotonic myopathy (PROMM)
- Proximal muscle weakness and myotonia predominates but distal weakness may also develop in some individuals with PROMM.
- The disease has a similar frequency as classic myotonic dystrophy.
- It is linked to the same region of chromosome 3 as myotonic dystrophy type 2.
- Patients show a less severe impairment than classic myotonic dystrophy .
- Congenital disease is absent.

DIFFERENTIAL DIAGNOSIS
Myotonia clinically
- Myotonic dystrophy (adults).
- Myotonia congenita (dominant and recessive forms).
- Paramyotonia congenita ± hyperkalemic periodic paralysis.
- Hypothyroid myopathy.
- Drugs: 20,25-diazacholesterol (lipid lowering agent), triparanol (lipid lowering agent), beta-blockers, and depolarizing muscle relaxants (e.g. succinylcholine) may cause or exacerbate myotonia.

Non-dystrophic myotonias
Chloride channelopathies
Myotonia congenita:
- Thompsen's disease (autosomal dominant): presents in infancy.
- Becker's disease (autosomal recessive): present in childhood.

- Generalized myotonia, worse in the cold and relieved by warmth or exercise.
- Patients show diffuse muscle hypertrophy and little if any weakness.

Sodium channelopathies
Paramyotonia congenita (autosomal dominant):
- Attacks of myotonia and flaccid weakness, usually precipitated by cold, but also by hyperkalemia and beta-blockers.
- Myotonia is relieved by hypokalemia or acetazolamide.
- There is overlap with the periodic paralyses, since in some patients the weakness is associated with hyper- or hypokalemia, and hyperkalemic periodic paralysis results from mutations in the same sodium channel gene as paramyotonia congenita. Hypokalemic periodic paralysis is a calcium channelopathy (see p.693).

Distal myopathy
Neurogenic
- HMSN 2 (Charcot–Marie–Tooth–2).
- Distal spinal muscular atrophy.
- Scapuloperoneal syndrome.

Myopathic
- Myotonic dystrophy.
- Fascioscapulohumeral dystrophy.
- Desminopathy.
- Mitochondrial myopathy.
- Congenital myopathies.
- Glycogen storage disease.
- Inclusion body myositis.

INVESTIGATIONS
Blood
- Fasting glucose.
- Thyroid function tests.
- Serum IgG reduced.
- Serum CK: normal or mildly elevated.

Slit lamp examination
Cataracts.

EKG
- Abnormalities of cardiac conduction are common, even in patients without cardiac symptoms, and progress over time.
- An annual EKG is recommended because EKG changes are often a predictor of development of cardiac symptoms.
- Ventricular late-potentials may be predictive of ventricular arrhythmias. However, potentially fatal heart block or rhythm disturbances can occur despite a normal EKG. As the perioperative period is a particularly dangerous time with respect to development of tachyarrhythmias and heart block, the anesthetist must always be made aware of the diagnosis of myotonic dystrophy.

24-hour EKG recording
This is indicated if cardiac symptoms are present or a significant change occurs on the EKG.

EMG
Multiple myotonic discharges.

Molecular DNA analysis
PCR technique: triplet repeat expansion.

DIAGNOSIS
Clinical and EMG, but confirmed by molecular DNA analysis.

TREATMENT
The main goals are prevention and treatment of systemic disease.

Myotonia
In general, patients do not complain much about myotonia:
- Phenytoin 100–200 mg bd orally can alleviate disabling and bothersome myotonia with reasonable efficacy and safety.
- Nifedipine 10–20 mg three times daily may help.
- Antimyotonic drugs such as quinine sulfate, disopyramide (100–200 mg three times daily) and procainamide (250–500 mg four times daily) prolong the PR interval and can impair cardiac conduction. Disopyramide has anticholinergic adverse effects. Procainamide may cause nausea, diarrhea, skin rash, confusion, and SLE-like syndrome and agranulocytosis.
- A short course of prednisolone may help particularly severe cases sometimes.

N.B. Any improvement in myotonia may not necessarily realize functional benefit for patients whose symptoms are more as a result of weakness than myotonia.

Excessive daytime sleepiness due to central mechanisms
- Lifestyle advice: take short naps at convenient times, such as after meals, to minimize disruption of daily activities.
- Methylphenidate may be helpful, but there have been no long term studies of risks and benefits.

Excessive daytime sleepiness due to hypercapnia
Normal assisted ventilation.

Fecal incontinence
Procainamide 300 mg bd.

PROGNOSIS
Sudden death is well recognized, and may be due to heart block or arrhythmia.

POLYMYOSITIS

DEFINITION
An acquired proximal inflammatory myopathy characterized by progressive proximal muscle weakness, elevated serum creatine kinase, and the presence of inflammatory infiltrates in muscle.

EPIDEMIOLOGY
- Prevalence: 1 in 100 000.
- Age at onset: >18 years of age.
- Gender: F≥M.

PATHOLOGY
Acute
- Predominantly endomysial (in the fascicles) inflammatory cell infiltrates (T cells), surrounding or partially invading individual muscle fibers (**832**).
- B cells are infrequent.
- T cells are of the cytotoxic type.
- Single fiber necrosis with phagocytosis.
- 'Moth-eaten' fibers.
- Atrophy of both fiber types.
- Angular atrophic fibers.
- Increased central nucleation.
- No perifascicular atrophy or microangiopathy.

Chronic
- Marked variation in fiber size (**833**).
- Hypertrophied fibers.
- Central nucleation.
- Fiber splitting.
- Regenerating and necrotic fibers.
- Endomysial and perifascicular fibrosis.
- Inflammatory cell exudates.
- Focally distributed architectural changes in individual fibers.

ETIOLOGY AND PATHOPHYSIOLOGY
Idiopathic polymyositis
T cell mediated cytotoxicity of muscle fibers.

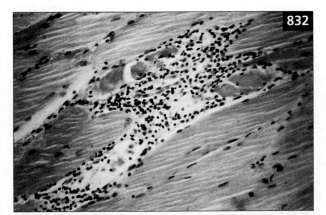

832 Polymyositis. Inflammatory infiltrate between muscle fibers within the fascicle (endomysial) and adjacent to necrotic fibers and small intrafascicular blood vessels.

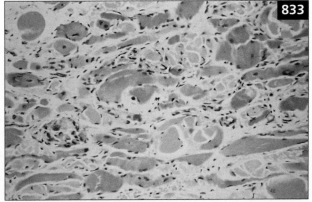

833 Chronic polymyositis, transverse section of muscle, ×140, H&E. There is marked variability in muscle fiber size, central nucleation, a marked increase in fibrous tissue, and a diffuse inflammatory cell response. Some fibers are conspicuously rounded.

Systemic autoimmune or connective tissue diseases
- Mixed connective tissue disease.
- Systemic lupus erythematosus.
- Rheumatoid arthritis.
- Scleroderma.
- Polyarteritis nodosa (**834**).
- Sjögren's syndrome.

Infection
Viral myositis
- HIV.
- Human T-cell lymphotropic virus type 1.
- Benign acute myositis:
- Influenza A and B.
- Parainfluenza.
- Adenovirus 2.
- Acute rhabdomyolysis:
- Influenza A and B.
- Echo 9.
- Adenovirus 21.
- Herpes simplex.
- Epstein–Barr virus.
- Epidemic pleurodynia: Coxsackie B5 (also B1, 3 and 4).

Bacterial myositis
Acute suppurative myositis:
- *Staphylococcus aureus.*
- Streptococcus.
- Yersinia.
- Anerobic organisms.

Fungal myositis

Parasitic myositis
- Protozoa:
- Toxoplasmosis.
- Sarcosporidiosis.
- Trypanosomiasis.
- Amebiasis.
- Cestodes:
- Cysticercosis.
- Coenurosis.
- Hydatidosis.
- Sparganosis.
- Nematodes:
- Trichinosis.
- Toxocariasis.

Drugs
- Penicillamine, zidovudine.

CLINICAL FEATURES (see Table 50)
Presentation of symptoms
- Slow onset (weeks to months).
- Usually symmetric weakness of proximal limb muscles, typically involving the pelvic more than the shoulder girdle, occasionally with pain and muscle tenderness.
- Weight loss, neck weakness, dysphagia and voice change are common.
- No skin rash, eye and facial muscle involvement, family history of neuromuscular disease, history of exposure to myotoxic drugs or toxins, endocrinopathy, neurogenic disease, or dystrophy is present.

Evolution of symptoms
Weakness usually evolves slowly over months or, frequently, several years, such that gross muscle wasting may be evident at the time of diagnosis.

Underlying carcinoma
No link.

DIFFERENTIAL DIAGNOSIS
- Myositis associated with autoimmune disorders (MCTD, SLE, RA, PSS, PAN).
- Polymyalgia rheumatica: pain with limitation of movement (which may be misinterpreted as muscle weakness), but the CK is normal and muscle biopsy shows only minimal abnormalities.
- Endocrine myopathy: thyroid disease.
- Metabolic myopathy: osteomalacic myopathy.
- Toxic myopathy: alcohol, opiates, chloroquine, D-penicillamine, zidovudine.
- Muscular dystrophy.
- Myotonic dystrophy.
- MG.
- Spinal muscular atrophy.
- Neuropathy.

INVESTIGATIONS
Blood
- Serum CK level: helpful in diagnosis and monitoring response to therapy. Levels may be normal or only moderately raised (up to five times normal).
- ESR: usually, though not invariably, elevated.
- Anti Jo-1 antibody, found in 30% of cases, is associated with lung infiltrates and greater risk of cardiomyopathy.

EKG
Occasionally shows heart block.

EMG
- Useful for confirming active or inactive myopathy and for excluding neurogenic disorders.

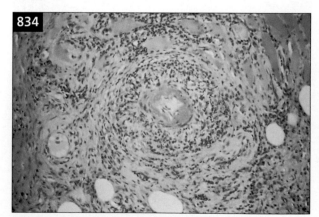

834 Polyarteritis nodosa. In this muscle biopsy there is intimal thickening and infiltration of the walls of two small arteries by macrophages and lymphocytes.

- Shows increased spontaneous activity with fibrillations, positive sharp waves, and complex repetitive discharges; and myopathic potentials characterized by short-duration, low-amplitude polyphasic motor units on voluntary activation. These findings are non-specific and occur in a variety of acute, toxic and active myopathic processes.
- Mixed myopathic and neurogenic potentials (polyphasic units of short and long duration) may also be present as a consequence of the regeneration of muscle fibers and chronicity of the disease.

Muscle biopsy

Endomysial infiltration by mononuclear inflammatory infiltrates (predominantly T8 lymphocytes), surrounding and invading muscle fibers (**832–834**).

DIAGNOSIS

A diagnosis of exclusion, based on clinical features, supported by laboratory investigations, of which the most important is muscle biopsy. Patients do not have (1) family history, (2) exposure to myotoxic drugs or toxins, (3) another acquired muscle disease caused by endocrine, metabolic, or neurogenic disease, (4) certain sporadically occurring dystrophies (dystrophinopathies, sarcoglycanopathies, dysferlinopathies), and (5) inclusion body myositis.

TREATMENT

- Empirical.
- Treatment has non-selective effects on the immune system.
- Efficacy has not been proven in randomized trials.
- No treatment is uniformly effective.
- Adverse effects can be serious.

- Encouragement of mobility (particularly in the elderly) and physiotherapy to prevent contractures are essential.
- A high protein diet is advisable.
- Attention to swallowing, adequacy of ventilation, and precautions against deep venous thrombosis must be considered.

Corticosteroids

- Oral prednisolone 1 mg/kg/day on alternate days.
- Combination therapy with methotrexate or azathioprine can be considered.
- Intravenous methylprednisolone: 0.5 g/day for 3 days (pulse therapy) if symptoms are not controlled with oral therapy.

Avoiding complications of corticosteroid treatment

- Keep initial dose of prednisolone <1 mg/kg/day, if possible, particularly if mild disease, concern about adverse effects (e.g. postmenopausal) or remission induced.
- Begin to reduce high dose prednisolone (1 mg/kg/day) within 4–6 weeks.
- Begin combination therapy at 4–6 weeks as a steroid sparing agent if the disease is slow to come under control (i.e. introduce a second line agent earlier rather than later, as opposed to continuing prednisolone for 2–3 months; too long really).
- Keep maintenance dose <10 mg/day (or 20 mg alternate days).
- Monitor muscle performance regularly (manual, myometer or isokinetic dynamometry, and functional assessment).
- Use prophylactic calcium supplements and biphosphonates, particularly in postmenopausal women.

Table 50 Major clinical features of dermatomyositis, polymyositis and inclusion body myositis (IBM)

Clinical features	Dermatomyositis	Polymyositis	IBM
Male: female	1:2	1:1	3:1
Age at onset	Any age	>18 years	>50 years
Site of weakness	Limb girdle	Limb girdle	Asymmetric
Respiratory muscle involvement	In severe cases	No	No
Dysphagia	Frequent	Rare	40% of patients
Muscle tenderness	Frequent	Infrequent	Infrequent
Skin involvement	Frequent	No	Absent
Involvement of other systems	Lung, heart	No	No
Associations			
Connective tissue diseases	PSS, MCTD	Yes	<15% of cases
Autoimmune diseases	Uncommon	Common	Uncommon
Viruses	Not proven	HIV, HTLV-1	Not proven
Parasites and bacteria	No	Yes	No
Drug-induced myotoxicity	Yes	Yes	No
Carcinoma	20%	No	No
Familial	No	No	Yes, in some cases
Course	Acute/subacute	Subacute/chronic	Chronic

Steroid resistance
Second line agents
- Methotrexate: can be given as a single weekly oral dose.
- Azathioprine 2.5 mg/kg/day.

Third line agents
- Cyclosporine.
- Cyclophosphamide.
- Plasma exchange.

Problems in management
- Late diagnosis.
- Steroid complications: cushingoid features.
- Ocular cataracts or glaucoma.
- Diabetes.
- Infection.
- Osteoporosis.
- Myopathy:
  - If prednisone >10 mg/day for a long period.
  - Detect by declining strength on myometry.
  - Normal CK.
  - Myopathic EMG with spontaneous activity.
  - Biopsy if uncertain.
- Steroid resistance.
- Relapses: it is not common to be able to withdraw treatment and avoid relapse, but using a small maintenance dose also does not seem to prevent relapses.
- Immunodeficiency.

Treatment of relapses
- Increase dose of prednisolone to 30–50 mg/day.
- Add methotrexate or azathioprine.
- Add intravenous immunoglobulin if patients do not show prompt improvement over 3 weeks.

Other 'last resort' forms of treatment
- Plasmapheresis.
- X-ray irradiation.
- Thoracic outlet drainage.
- Thymectomy.
- Stem cell transplant.

PROGNOSIS
The response is less favorable than in dermatomyositis, particularly in those with a long history at presentation. Immunosuppressive therapy usually causes improvement and prevents further progression but significant improvement may not occur in some. Antibody to signal recognition peptide, found in 5% of cases, is associated with a fulminant course and resistance to treatment. The 5-year survival rate for treated patients is nearly 80%. Up to 30% of patients may be left with residual muscle weakness.

DERMATOMYOSITIS

DEFINITION
An idiopathic inflammatory myopathy with characteristic cutaneous manifestations.

EPIDEMIOLOGY
- Prevalence: 1 in 100 000.
- Age at onset: any age, affects children and adults. Comprises 95% of childhood myositis.
- Gender: F>M (2:1).

PATHOLOGY
Inflammatory infiltration of muscle occurs by macrophages and T and B lymphocytes. B cells are frequent, and T cells are of the helper type. The inflammatory infiltrates are predominantly perivascular, or in and around the interfascicular septa, rather than within the fascicles. Therefore, they do not penetrate the muscle fiber membrane. Damage appears to occur through compression, rather than infiltration, of the fiber.

Microangiopathy: intramuscular blood vessels show endothelial hyperplasia with tubuloreticular profiles, fibrin thrombi (particularly in children) and obliteration of capillaries. Capillary numbers are reduced, there are immunoglobulin deposits on vessel walls and blood vessel endothelial cells show ultrastructural changes. The capillary loss and consequent ischemia causes microinfarcts and may be responsible for the sometimes striking perivascular atrophy seen.

The necrotic, degenerating and regenerating muscle fibers are mostly in groups involving a portion of a muscle fasciculus and are often the result of microinfarcts within the muscle.

Perifascicular atrophy, characterized by two to 10 layers of atrophic fibers at the periphery of the fascicle is found in about 90% of children and at least 50% of adults with dermatomyositis and is diagnostic of dermatomyositis, even in the absence of inflammation.

ETIOLOGY
- Unknown in most cases.
- Caused or exacerbated by drugs in a few patients:
  - Hydroxyurea.
  - Quinidine.
  - Non-steroidal anti-inflammatory drugs.
  - Penicillamine.
  - 3-hydroxy-3-methylglutaryl coenzyme A-reductase inhibitors ('statins').

PATHOPHYSIOLOGY
A humorally-mediated microangiopathy (e.g. antibodies against capillary endothelial cells with complement activation) with muscle fiber inflammation occurring secondarily to focal ischemia.

CLINICAL FEATURES
Muscle disease
- Initial symptoms include subacute onset of myalgias, fatigue and weakness, manifested as difficulty climbing stairs, raising the arms for actions such as shaving or brushing hair, rising from a squatting or sitting position, or a combination of these features.

- Weakness typically involves the proximal muscles symmetrically, and the pelvic more than the shoulder girdle.
- Pain and tenderness on palpation of the muscles is variable.
- The course is slowly progressive during a period of weeks to months.
- Difficulty swallowing (dysphagia) or symptoms of aspiration may reflect involvement of striated muscle in the pharynx or upper esophagus.
- Dysphonia.

Cutaneous manifestations
- Heliotrope rash (**835**): a violaceous to dusky erythematous rash, with or without edema, in a symmetric distribution involving the perorbital skin. The rash may be mild and only comprise a slight discoloration along the eyelid margin.
- Gottron's papules: slightly raised violaceous papules and plaques, with or without a slight scale and rarely a thick psoriasiform scale, over bony prominences, particularly the metacarpophalangeal joints, proximal interphalangeal joints, and distal interphalangeal joints. Papules may also be found overlying the elbows, knees, feet, or a combination of these. Within the lesions there is commonly telangiectasia.
- An erythematous to violaceous psoriasiform dermatitis involving the scalp.
- Malar erythema.
- Poikiloderma (which is the combination of atrophy, dyspigmentation, and telangiectasia) on sun exposed skin such as the extensor surfaces of the arms, the 'V' of the neck, and the upper back (shawl sign).
- Violaceous erythema on the extensor surfaces.
- Nailfold changes: periungual telangiectases and/or hypertrophy of the cuticle, and small hemorrhagic infarcts in the hypertrophic area.

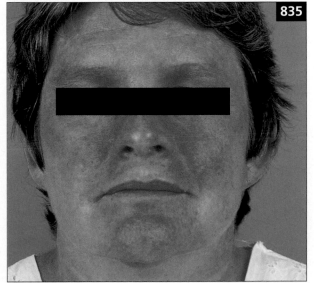

835 A blue–purple discoloration of the eyelids, cheeks and nose by a typically heliotrope and slightly edematous rash of dermatomyositis.

Systemic features
- Raynaud's phenomenon: generalized arthralgias accompanied by morning stiffness; a symmetric non-deforming arthritis involving the small joints of the hands, wrists and ankles; or both, may be present in up to 25% of patients.
- Esophageal disease, manifested by dysphagia, occurs in about 15–50% of patients. There are two main forms:
- Proximal dysphagia is caused by involvement of striated muscle of the pharynx or proximal esophagus, correlates with severity of the muscle disease, and responds to steroid treatment.
- Distal dysphagia is due to involvement of non-striated muscle and is more common in patients who have an overlap with scleroderma or another collagen-vascular disorder.
- Pulmonary disease: occurs in about 15–30% of patients, particularly those with esophageal disease, and is usually due to an interstitial pneumonitis. Less common causes include the muscle disease itself (causing hypoventilation or aspiration), and treatments for the muscle disease (causing opportunistic infections or drug-induced hypersensitivity pneumonitis). Associated with a poor prognosis.
- Cardiac disease: present in up to 50% of patients but uncommonly symptomatic. Disorders include conduction defects and primary end-rhythm disturbances, and even less commonly congestive heart failure, pericarditis, and valvular disease. Associated with a poor prognosis.
- Calcinosis of the skin (firm, yellow, or flesh-colored nodules, usually over bony prominences, and occasionally extruding through the surface of the skin) or muscle (generally asymptomatic) is unusual in adults but may occur in up to 40% of children and adolescents with dermatomyositis.

Malignancy
- About 20–25% have associated malignancy, before the onset of myositis, concurrently with myositis, or after the onset of dermatomyositis.
- Malignancy is more common in older patients (>50 years) but may even occur in children.
- The site of malignancy can be predicted by the patient's age (e.g. testicular cancer in young men, colon and prostate cancer in elderly men).
- Gynecologic malignancy, particularly ovarian carcinoma, is common. Nasopharyngeal carcinoma is common among Asians with dermatomyositis.

Evolution of symptoms
- Symptoms are usually subacute over several weeks.
- Evolution may be rapid with severe weakness, dysphagia and respiratory muscle involvement, sometimes requiring ventilatory support. Muscle pain, tenderness, and swelling, if present, tend to equate with a rapid onset.

SPECIAL FORMS
Childhood dermatomyositis
- Childhood dermatomyositis is more common than childhood and adolescent polymyositis.
- Onset is usually insidious and mistaken for a viral-type illness or dermatitis, but a fulminant onset and course may occur.
- It is commonly characterized as a vasculitis and has greater potential for calcinosis than adult disease.

DIFFERENTIAL DIAGNOSIS
Muscle weakness
- Muscular dystrophy.
- Myotonic dystrophy.
- Steroid myopathy.
- Neuropathy.

Heliotrope rash and photosensitive poikilodermatous eruption
- Systemic lupus erythematosus: a heliotrope rash is rarely seen.
- Scleroderma: a heliotrope rash is rarely seen.

Gottron's papules
- Systemic lupus erythematosus.
- Psoriasis: distinct histopathology.
- Lichen planus: distinct histopathology.

Scalp erythematous to violaceous psoriasiform dermatitis
- Psoriasis.
- Seborrheic dermatitis.

Facial erythema
- Systemic lupus erythematosus.
- Rosacea.
- Seborrheic dermatitis.
- Atopic dermatitis.

INVESTIGATIONS
Diagnosis
ESR is usually elevated

Serum muscle enzymes
CK, aldolase, lactate dehydrogenase, alanine aminotransferase levels:
- CK is the most specific and widely used.
- It is helpful in the diagnosis and monitoring the response to therapy.
- Levels may be raised up to 20 times normal, particularly in acute cases, whereas levels may be normal or only moderately raised (up to five times normal) in polymyositis, and are often normal in inclusion body myositis.

Serologic tests
- Antinuclear antibody: commonly positive.
- Antibodies to Mi-2, and antinuclear antibody, are specific but not sensitive, being found in only about 25% of patients.
- Antibodies to Jo-1 are predictive of pulmonary involvement but are rare.
- Antibodies to Ro (SS-A) are found in rare cases.

EMG
- EMG is useful for confirming active or inactive myopathy and for excluding neurogenic disorders.
- Shows a myopathic pattern of increased spontaneous activity with fibrillations, positive sharp waves, and complex repetitive discharges; and myopathic potentials characterized by short-duration, low-amplitude polyphasic motor units on voluntary activation. These findings are non-specific and occur in a variety of acute, toxic and active myopathic processes.
- Mixed myopathic and neurogenic potentials (polyphasic units of short and long duration) may also be present as a consequence of the regeneration of muscle fibers and chronicity of the disease.

Muscle biopsy
- Biopsies are obtained under local anesthetic from a moderately involved muscle, typically quadriceps or deltoid (see Pathology, above).
- Light microscopy shows microvascular injury with perifascicular fiber atrophy, a perimysial inflammatory infiltrate dominated by B and T4 lymphocytes; deposits of membrane attack complex confirm the role of complement.

Skin biopsy

PROGNOSTIC TESTS
Tests and examinations are determined by the patient's age and gender, and commonly include rectal, vaginal and breast examination for assessment of malignant disease. Tests include mammography, sigmoidoscopy, EKG, chest x-ray and pulmonary function tests, barium swallow and esophageal motility studies, abdominal scanning (ultrasound or CT), testing for fecal occult blood and basic hematologic and biochemical studies. Repeat each year for the first 3 years after diagnosis or whenever new symptoms arise.

DIAGNOSIS
Based on clinical features, supported by laboratory investigations, of which the most important is muscle biopsy.

TREATMENT
General
- Bedrest combined with a range-of-motion exercise programme if patients have progressive weakness.
- Raise the head of the bed and avoid meals before bedtime in patients with dysphagia.

Muscle disease
Treatment for muscle disease is controversial because of the absence of controlled clinical trials.

First line therapy
Oral prednisolone 0.5–1 mg/kg bodyweight/day for at least 1 month after myositis has become clinically and enzymatically inactive. The dose is then gradually reduced, generally over a period lasting 1.5 to two times as long as the period of active intense treatment, but depending on clinical progress and, to some extent, serum CK levels. Convert to an alternate day regime after a few months.

N.B. It is easier to manage patients who have presented acutely or subacutely, in whom the response to treatment is usually more obvious and a high CK levels falls, than those with a slowly progressive disorder: if a response occurs at all, it is slow, and the CK level may have been normal or little elevated at presentation.

Adjunct or second line therapy
Immunosuppressive agents: about 25% of patients will not respond to systemic corticosteroids and 25–50% will develop substantial steroid-related adverse effects. Therefore, early intervention with steroid-sparing agents, such as methotrexate, azathioprine (2.5 mg/kg bodyweight), cyclophosphamide, mycophenolate mofetil, chlorambucil, or cyclosporine may be effective in inducing or maintaining a remission.

About 50–75% of patients respond to an immunosuppressive agent with an increase in strength, a decrease in enzyme concentrations, or a decrease in corticosteroid dosage.

Other therapy
- High-dose intravenous immunoglobulin has been shown to be effective for recalcitrant dermatomyositis in a double-blind, placebo-controlled trial (*N. Engl. J. Med.*, 1993; **329**: 1993–2000). The indications are usually resistance to steroids and second line agents, adverse reactions to immunosuppressants and severe relapses. The regimen may be 0.4 g/kg/day for 5 days followed by monthly three day courses for up to 6 months (unless no response within 3 months).
- Largely anecdotal reports have described success with pulsed methylprednisolone, combination immunosuppressive therapy and whole body irradiation.
- Plasmapheresis was ineffective in a placebo-controlled trial (*N. Engl. J. Med.*, 1992; **326**: 1380–1384).

Skin disease
- Patients should avoid sunlight or use a broad-spectrum sunscreen with a high sun protective factor, if they are photosensitive.
- Hydroxychloroquine hydrochloric acid 200–400 mg/day is effective in about 80% of patients when used as a steroid-sparing agent.
- Chloroquine phosphate 250–500 mg/day can be used if patients are not responsive to hydroxychloroquine.
- Periodic ophthalmologic examinations and blood counts are required for patients on continuous antimalarial therapy.
- Methotrexate 15–35 mg/week can also be used.

PROGNOSIS
Adverse prognostic factors
- Increasing age.
- Severe myositis (frequently correlates with the degree of weakness and the serum CK concentrations).
- Dysphagia or dysphonia.
- Cardiopulmonary involvement.
- Malignant disease.
- Poor response to corticosteroid therapy.

Prognosis
- If treated early, most patients will respond well, with many showing full recovery of muscle function. In most cases the disease will burn itself out, although this may take many years during which time treatment has to be continued.
- Interstitial lung disease and other pulmonary disorders are an important but under-recognized cause of late morbidity. Similarly, cardiac involvement is common with conduction defects, rarely leading to complete heart block, arrhythmias and congestive heart failure.

Malignancy
The myositis may follow the course of malignant disease (a paraneoplastic course) or may follow its own course independent of treatment of the malignant disease.

INCLUSION BODY MYOSITIS (IBM)

DEFINITION
Inclusion body myositis is an idiopathic inflammatory myopathy.

EPIDEMIOLOGY
- Prevalence: uncommon but the most common cause of acquired myositis in patients over 50 years of age.
- Age at onset: after 50 years of age.
- Gender: M>F (3:1).
- Race: more common in whites than blacks.

PATHOLOGY
- Inflammatory infiltrates (predominantly T cells) surrounding or invading individual non-necrotic muscle fibers (endomysial inflammation) (like that seen in polymyositis) are often present but rarely extensive.
- Basophilic granular inclusions are distributed around the edge of slit-like vacuoles (rimmed vacuoles) (**836**).
- Eosinophilic cytoplasmic inclusions.
- Angulated fibers, often in small groups.
- Intranuclear or intracytoplasmic 15–18 nm tubulofilaments in muscle fibers on electron microscopy.

ETIOLOGY AND PATHOPHYSIOLOGY
Sporadic
- Uncertain; autoimmune, viral and degenerative theories prevail.
- Partly mediated by cytotoxic T cells, with a secondary inflammatory response to degenerating muscle (which is why the amount of inflammation is variable and the response to immunosuppression is poor).
- Multiple mitochondrial DNA deletions are present in 75% of patients.
- Amyloidogenic protein deposition has been reported in affected muscle and increased cellular prion protein has also been described.

Hereditary
Autosomal recessive rimmed vacuolar myopathies
Gene locus 9p1-q1.

Autosomal dominant rimmed vacuolar myopathies
- Gene locus 14q.
- Oculopharyngeal muscular dystrophy.

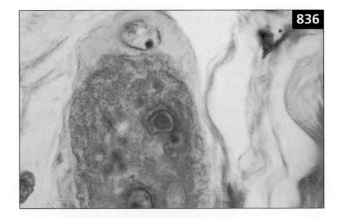
836

836 Eosinophilic (pink) cytoplasmic inclusions and basophilic (blue) granular inclusions located at the periphery of narrow vacuoles (rimmed vacuoles) in a muscle fiber of a patient with inclusion body myositis.

CLINICAL FEATURES
- Gradual onset.
- Painless weakness of distal and proximal muscles (particularly long finger flexors [flexor digitorum profundus], wrist flexors and quadriceps femoris) which may be asymmetric.
- Dysphagia in up to 30% of cases.
- Muscle wasting can be marked.
- Early loss of deep tendon reflexes.
- Numbness and sensory symptoms may suggest an associated peripheral sensory neuropathy.

DIFFERENTIAL DIAGNOSIS
- Polymyositis.
- Neuropathy: e.g. diabetic amyotrophy.

INVESTIGATIONS
Blood
- Serum CK level: often normal or mildly raised.
- ESR: normal in 80% of cases.

EMG
- A mixed neuromyopathic pattern may be seen.
- 30% of patients have EMG signs of axonal neuropathy.

Muscle biopsy
Biopsy may show inflammation, predominantly an endo-mysially-located mononuclear infiltrate with cytotoxic T cells invading non-necrotic muscle fibers; rimmed vacuoles and filamentous inclusions in muscle are characteristic. The inclusions contain ubiquitin and tau protein, and are pathologically similar to Alzheimer neurofibrillary tangles.

DIAGNOSIS
Highly likely if a clinical phenotype of asymmetric muscle weakness with prominent wrist flexor, finger flexor and knee extensory muscle involvement is present. A definitive diagnosis requires electron microscopy of muscle biopsy specimens showing muscle fibers with rimmed vacuoles containing 15–18 nm tubulofilaments and small amyloid deposits, in addition to light microscopy evidence of endomysial T cell infiltration of non-necrotic muscle fibers.

An accurate diagnosis is important because inappropriate treatment can cause adverse effects.

TREATMENT
- Numerous forms of immunosuppressive treatment have been tried without benefit: most patients are resistant to immunosuppressive treatment. High-dose steroids are rarely beneficial clinically despite often reducing a raised CK.
- In some who are not old and frail, the condition may stabilize with a 3–6 month trial of prednisolone combined with methotrexate (or azathioprine).
- Anabolic steroids (e.g. clenbuterol 20 µg/day–20 µg bd) are being trialled.
- A physiotherapy/strength training program is also important.

PROGNOSIS
Gradual deterioration is usual, with increasing weakness of the neck, trunk, and distal arm muscles, and extensive weakness and wasting in the legs. The disease can progress to severe generalized weakness and disability.

METABOLIC AND ENDOCRINE MYOPATHIES

DEFINITION
Metabolic and endocrine myopathies are a large, heterogeneous group of inherited and acquired disorders of muscle due to a disturbance of metabolism.

EPIDEMIOLOGY
- Uncommon.
- Age: usually infants and children, but may present in adulthood (particularly endocrine myopathies).
- Gender: usually M=F.

ETIOLOGY AND PATHOPHYSIOLOGY
Disorders of glycogen metabolism
Acid maltase deficiency
- An autosomal-recessive glycogen storage disorder.
- Caused by a deficiency of lysosomal alpha-glucosidase which results in impaired lysosomal conversion of glycogen to glucose so that glycogen accumulates in the liver, heart, CNS and muscle.
- The genetic abnormality maps to chromosome 17.

McArdle's disease
- Autosomal recessive.
- Caused by a myophosphorylase (a-1,4-glucan ortho-phosphate glycosyltransferase) deficiency, which results in impaired conversion of glycogen to glucose-1-phosphate in muscle.
- The gene for myophosphorylase maps to chromosome 11q13. At least 16 different mutations have been identified, the most frequent of which is a nonsense mutation in exon 1 (R49X), which causes the substitution of an arginine (CGA) with a stop codon (TGA), and a missense mutation (W797R) in exon 20.
- Glycogen breakdown is impossible during a sudden burst of muscle activity; ATP generation is compromised; muscle cell pH is shifted to alkaline.

Phosphofructokinase deficiency
- Autosomal recessive.
- Caused by impaired conversion of fructose-6-phosphate to fructose-1,6-diphosphate in muscle.

Debranching enzyme system deficiency
- Autosomal recessive.
- Caused by impaired hydrolysis of glycogen to glucose-1-phosphate.

Disorders of lipid metabolism
- Long chain fatty acids are a major source of muscle energy and are consumed during muscular activity.
- Carnitine is involved in the transport of free fatty acids into mitochondria.

Muscle carnitine deficiency
Lipids accumulate in muscle which is deficient in carnitine.

Carnitine-O-palmitoyltransferase deficiency
- Autosomal recessive.
- Caused by impaired transport of free fatty acids into mitochondria.

- The abnormal gene maps to chromosome 1.

Mitochondrial myopathies (see p.162)
Reduced ATP generation by oxidative phosphorylation.

Endocrine disorders
Thyrotoxic myopathy
Muscle stiffness and weakness.

Thyrotoxic periodic paralysis (see p.694)

Dysthyroid eye disease (exophthalmic ophthalmoplegia) (**837**)

Hypothyroid myopathy

Muscle weakness
Thyroid hormone has a regulatory role on the transcription of numerous muscle genes encoding both myofibrillar and calcium-regulatory proteins.

Steroid myopathy (**838**)
- About 70% of patients with Cushing's syndrome have muscle weakness.

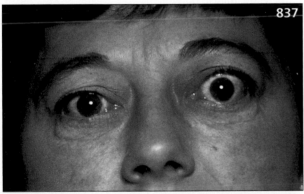

837 Dysthyroid eye disease (exophthalmic ophthalmoplegia) showing left eyelid retraction, and exophthalmos. Dysconjugate vertical eye movements were present.

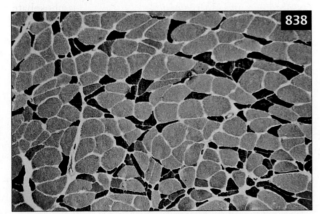

838 Muscle biopsy of a patient with a steroid myopathy showing Type II muscle fiber atrophy, which may be seen in disuse, cachexia, myasthenia gravis as well as a steroid effect. Myosin ATPase stain, pH 9.4. Type I fibers are pale and Type 2 fibers are darkly stained. Fibers showing an intermediate reaction are usually Type I.

- Fluorinated corticosteroids, such as dexamethasone and triamcinolone, have more myopathic potential. The dose required to cause myopathy varies among individuals.

Addison's disease and other forms of hypoadrenalism
May occur as one component of adrenoleukodystrophy (see p.166).

Acromegaly

Electrolyte disorders
Calcium
- Hyperparathyroidism:
- Primary hyperparathyroidism: adenoma.
- Secondary hyperparathyroidism: typically secondary to renal disease.
- Osteomalacia.

Potassium
- Iatrogenic usually.
- Secondary periodic paralyses (see p.693).
- Primary hyperaldosteronism.

Malignant hyperthermia
- An autosomal dominant susceptibility to a number of drugs, particularly anesthetics such as halothane and succinylcholine. Other drugs include tricyclic antidepressants, monoamine oxidase inhibitors, methoxyflurane, ketamine, enflurane, diethyl ether, and cyclopropane.
- Due to a malfunction of the calcium channel of the sarcoplasmic reticulum (the ryanodine receptor). The abnormal ryanodine receptor may accentuate calcium release.
- The gene for the ryanodine receptor maps to chromosome 19 (13-1).
- Fast, uncontrolled increase in skeletal muscle metabolism associated with rhabdomyolysis occurs and may occur in association with dystrophinopathies and central core congenital myopathy.

CLINICAL FEATURES
Disorders of glycogen metabolism
Acid maltase deficiency
- Infantile form: Pompe's disease: a generalized glycogenosis with severe cardiomyopathy, hypotonia, macroglossia, cardiomegaly and hepatomegaly. Death occurs in infancy.
- Adult form: a slowly progressive myopathy affecting predominantly the diaphragm (hence respiratory failure), biceps, shoulder, and thigh adductor muscles. There is little or no heart disease.

McArdle's disease
- Males are affected more than females (4:1).
- Onset in childhood or adolescence usually.
- Attacks of exercise intolerance with muscle pain (myalgia) and stiffness, often precipitated by brief, strong exercises.
- Fatigue.
- Cramps and dark urine (myoglobinuria) usually develop during adulthood.
- Seizures.
- Renal failure may occur secondary to myoglobinuria.
- Not progressive usually.

Phosphofructokinase deficiency:
- Clinically similar to McArdle's disease.
- A mild hemolytic tendency is sometimes present.

Debranching enzyme system deficiency
- Infancy: growth retardation, hepatomegaly, mild myopathy, and seizures which tend to improve after puberty.
- Adults: mild weakness of hands and legs. Cardiomyopathy is a late complication.

Disorders of lipid metabolism
Muscle carnitine deficiency
Myopathy develops in infants or children.

Carnitine-O-palmitoyltransferase deficiency
- Most patients are male and present in adolescence.
- Intermittent attacks occur without warning; precipitated by prolonged exertion, fasting or a high fat diet. Muscle cramps, muscle pain, and dark urine (myoglobinuria) are present, with normal muscle strength during attacks.
- Exposure to cold, viral infections, and general anesthesia can also precipitate rhabdomyolysis.
- Renal failure (due to myoglobinuria) and respiratory failure may ensue.
- Patients have a normal capacity to perform short, demanding exercise.

Endocrine disorders
Typically mild to moderate proximal muscle weakness.

Thyrotoxic myopathy
- Common.
- Proximal muscle weakness and some wasting occurs; occasionally the bulbar and respiratory muscles only are affected (cf. myasthenia, p.657).
- Fatigue.
- Heat intolerance.
- Normal or augmented reflexes.
- Fasciculations sometimes (cf. motor neuron disease, p.534).
- Associated with hypokalemic periodic paralysis and myasthenia gravis.

Thyrotoxic periodic paralysis (see p.694)
- Very rare.
- Orientals particularly are affected.

Dysthyroid eye disease (exophthalmic ophthalmoplegia) (**837**)
- Can be quite asymmetric.
- Difficulty of upgaze initially (inferior rectus infiltrated early).
- Diplopia.
- Lid retraction.
- Exophthalmos.
- Conjunctival and lid edema.
- Exposure keratopathy.
- Ptosis often.
- Little pain (grittiness or fullness).
- Eventually raised intraocular pressure and blindness may occur.
- The patient is usually but not necessarily thyrotoxic.

Hypothyroid myopathy
- More common in women.
- Aching and painful muscles.
- Cramps.
- Enlarged muscles.
- Muscle weakness (rare).
- Myedema (ridging of muscle on percussion).
- Respiratory muscle weakness may be present.
- Slow-recovery reflexes.

Steroid myopathy
- Proximal muscle weakness, earlier and worse in the lower limbs than upper limbs, and sometimes painful. Wasting is late.
- Difficulty climbing stairs.

Addison's disease and other forms of hypoadrenalism:
- Myalgia and muscle cramps.
- Proximal muscle weakness.
- Painful flexion contractures in the legs sometimes.
- Fatigue and lassitude.
- Postural hypotension.
- Confusional state, stupor and coma.

Acromegaly
- Increased muscle bulk.
- Improved strength initially but later muscle wasting and weakness occur.
- Non-specific headache.
- Associated entrapment neuropathy (e.g. carpal tunnel syndrome).
- Sensorimotor peripheral neuropathy (sometimes with enlarged nerves).
- Visual field defects.
- Hypopituitarism.
- Obstructive sleep apnea.
- Complications of diabetes and hypertension.

Electrolyte disorders
Hyperparathyroidism and osteomalacia
Proximal and often painful muscle weakness, mainly affecting the legs and associated with mild wasting.

Hypokalemia and hyperkalemia
Cause of generalized weakness.

Malignant hyperthermia
- During general anesthesia or after exposure to a causal drug.
- Rapid elevation of temperature which may rise to 43°C (109°F).
- Tachycardia.
- Muscle rigidity (e.g. begins with trismus).
- Areflexia.
- Coma.

DIFFERENTIAL DIAGNOSIS
Muscle cramps or pain on exercise
- Disorders of glycogenolysis or glycolysis (e.g. McArdle's disease).
- Carnitine-O-palmitoyltransferase deficiency.
- Mitochondrial myopathies, including zidovudine toxicity.
- Toxic myopathy caused by clofibrate and related drugs.
- Hypothyroid myopathy.

Myoglobinuria

Myoglobin is found in muscle and if there is severe and acute muscle injury it is released into the blood and appears in the urine (myoglobinuria). The urine is colored brown in severe cases and reacts to benzidine; if there is neither hematuria nor hemoglobinemia a positive test strongly suggests myoglobinuria. The muscle enzymes are always raised and the muscles are tender, weak and sometimes swollen. In severe cases acute renal failure occurs.

- Disorders of glycogenolysis or glycolysis (e.g. McArdle's disease).
- Carnitine-O-palmitoyltransferase deficiency.
- Duchenne muscular dystrophy after anesthetic exposure.
- Acute alcoholic myopathy.
- Acute viral myositis and other acute fulminating inflammatory myopathies.
- Malignant hyperthermia crisis.
- Neuroleptic malignant syndrome (see p.133).
- Status epilepticus.
- Excessive exercise.
- Heat stroke.
- Crush injury of muscle.
- Snake bite.

Myotonia clinically
- Myotonic dystrophy (adults).
- Myotonia congenita (dominant and recessive forms).
- Paramyotonia congenita ± hyperkalemic periodic paralysis.
- Hypothyroid myopathy.

Respiratory insufficiency (possible and prominent)
- Acid maltase deficiency (adult-onset).
- Acute myopathy after administration of high-dose corticosteroids and muscle paralysing agent (e.g. status asthmaticus).
- Myotonic dystrophy.
- Nemaline myopathy.
- Centronuclear myopathy.
- Myopathy with cytoplasmic bodies.

Thyrotoxic myopathy
- Hypokalemic periodic paralysis.
- Myasthenia gravis.
- Motor neuron disease.

Malignant hyperthermia
Neuroleptic malignant syndrome (see p.133): also present with high fever, rigidity, tachycardia, and rhabdomyolysis, but it is of slower onset over days to weeks, not familial, and usually triggered by drugs that block central dopaminergic pathways, such as phenothiazines, lithium and haloperidol, or can occur after discontinuation of L-dopa (levodopa) for Parkinson's disease.

INVESTIGATIONS
Disorders of glycogen metabolism
Acid maltase deficiency
- Serum CK: slightly elevated.
- EMG: non-specifically myopathic but myotonic discharges may occur (although patients do not have myotonia).
- Blood leukocyte or urine: acid maltase deficiency.

- Muscle biopsy: vacuolar myopathy with high glycogen content, and acid maltase deficiency.
- Chorionic villi biopsy: for prenatal diagnosis.

McArdle's disease
- Serum CK: elevated after exercise.
- Urine: myoglobinuria occasionally.
- EMG: myopathic.
- Forearm ischemic exercise produces no increase in venous lactate levels.
- Muscle biopsy: subsarcolemmal deposits of glycogen at the periphery, undetectable histochemical reaction of phosphorylase.

Phosphofructokinase deficiency
Forearm ischemic exercise produces no increase in venous lactate levels.

Debranching enzyme system deficiency
- Infancy: fasting hypoglycemia and ketonuria.
- Adults: serum CK: elevated.
- Forearm ischemic exercise produces no increase in venous lactate levels.
- Muscle biopsy: excess glycogen.

Disorders of lipid metabolism
Muscle carnitine deficiency
- Normal blood level of carnitine.
- Muscle biopsy: accumulation of lipid which is deficient in carnitine.

Carnitine-O-palmitoyltransferase deficiency
- Urine: myoglobinuria.
- Serum CK: normal but often raised following the attacks.
- Muscle biopsy at the time of an attack: may show lipid accumulation and little CPT activity.

Endocrine disorders
Typically a myopathic EMG and the non-specific finding of Type II fiber atrophy on muscle biopsy.

Thyrotoxic myopathy
- Serum CK: normal.
- EMG: myopathic.

Thyrotoxic periodic paralysis (see p.694)
Plasma potassium is usually low but can be normal.

Dysthyroid eye disease (exophthalmic ophthalmoplegia)
- Thyroid function tests: the patient is usually but not necessarily thyrotoxic.
- Thyroid antibodies: often positive.
- Response to thyrotrophin releasing hormone: abnormal.
- CT scan of the orbits: enlarged extraocular muscles.

Hypothyroid myopathy
- Serum CK: may be grossly elevated.
- Thyroid function tests: low thyroxine. TSH may be elevated if primary hypothyroidism.
- Urine myoglobin: rhabdomyolysis may be present.

Steroid myopathy
- Serum CK: normal.
- EMG: normal insertional activity and no spontaneous activity.
- Muscle biopsy (**838**).

Addison's disease and other forms of hypoadrenalism
Serum electrolytes: hyponatremia and hyperkalemia.

Acromegaly
Serum CK: sometimes elevated.

Hyperparathyroidism and osteomalacia
Serum CK: usually normal.

Malignant hyperthermia
- Arterial blood gases: metabolic acidosis.
- Serum CK: precipitous rise, sometimes to 10 000 times the normal values.
- Blood coagulation profile: disseminated intravascular coagulation.
- Urine: myoglobinuria.

DIAGNOSIS
The diagnosis usually depends on histochemistry or biochemical assay of muscle biopsy material.

PREVENTION
Malignant hyperthermia
- Screen the relatives of affected patients by muscle biopsy; abnormal muscle contracture *in vitro* is induced by caffeine or halothane.
- Barbiturate, nitrous oxide, and opiate non-depolarizing relaxant anesthesias should not induce malignant hyperthermia.

TREATMENT
Correct the metabolic defect if possible.

Disorders of glycogen metabolism
Acid maltase deficiency
- No specific therapy at present but promising results of myophosphorylase gene transfer in myoblasts *in vitro* have been reported in McArdle's disease.
- Inspiratory exercises are useful.

McArdle's disease
Oral creatine supplementation may improve skeletal muscle function.

Disorders of lipid metabolism
Carnitine-O-palmitoyltransferase deficiency
No specific therapy.

Endocrine disorders
Thyrotoxic myopathy
- Correct the hyperthyroidism
- Symptomatic therapy with beta-blockers.
- Glucocorticoids can be used in thyroid storm to block the peripheral conversion of T4 to T3.

Thyrotoxic periodic paralysis (see p.694)
Correct the thyrotoxicosis and plasma potassium if low.

Dysthyroid eye disease (exophthalmic ophthalmoplegia)
- Restore the euthyroid state.
- Tarsorrhaphy to protect the cornea.
- Surgical correction of diplopia if necessary.
- Severe cases: high doses of corticosteroids, cyclosporine, and even orbital decompression have been used to save sight.

Hypothyroid myopathy
Restore the euthyroid state.

Steroid myopathy
- Change to a non-fluorinated steroid.
- Reduce steroid dose to the lowest possible therapeutic level.
- Administer the steroid on an alternate daily basis if needed.
- Adequate diet and exercise should assist recovery.

Hyperparathyroidism
- Primary hyperparathyroidism: remove the adenoma.
- Secondary hyperparathyroidism (typically to renal disease):
- Partial parathyroidectomy.
- 1,25 dihydroxycholecalciferol.
- 1-alpha tocopheral.
- Osteomalacia: vitamin D therapy.

Malignant hyperthermia
Treatment depends on the severity, which is often related to the dosage and duration of anesthesia.

Mild cases
Discontinue the anesthetic.

More severe cases
- Dantrolene 2 mg/kg i.v. every 5 min, up to 10 mg/kg: inhibits calcium release from the sarcoplasmic reticulum.
- Correct associated hyperkalemia (*not* with calcium).
- Increase ventilation.
- Correct the acid–base disturbance: give i.v. sodium bicarbonate 2–4 mg/kg.
- Cool the patient: cooling blankets and cold i.v. fluids until temperature reaches 38°C (100°F).
- Volume load with diuretics if myoglobinuria is present.
- Give steroids for the acute stress reaction.

PROGNOSIS
In most cases, the weakness reverses when the metabolic defect is corrected but improvement may take weeks to months.

The prognosis for malignant hyperthermia is more guarded but mortality can be greatly diminished by recognizing the syndrome and treating it appropriately.

HYPOKALEMIC PARALYSIS

DEFINITION
A rare but treatable clinical syndrome, representing a heterogeneous group of disorders, characterized by acute systemic weakness and low serum potassium.

EPIDEMIOLOGY
- Rare.
- Age: youth and young adults predominantly.
- Gender: M>F.

ETIOLOGY AND PATHOPHYSIOLOGY
- Symptomatology results from the increased ratio between intra- and extracellular potassium concentrations, which modifies membrane polarization and thereby alters the function of excitable tissues such as nerve and muscle.
- Most cases are due to alteration in the transcellular distribution of potassium and the others to actual potassium depletion from renal or extrarenal losses.

Causes of hypokalemia
Transcellular shift of K (no depletion)
- Familial or primary hypokalemic periodic paralysis (most cases).
- Thyrotoxic periodic paralysis (**839, 840**).
- Barium poisoning.
- Insulin excess.
- Alkalosis.

Actual K depletion
Renal losses:
- Excessive mineralocorticoids (primary and secondary aldosteronism, liquorice ingestion, glucocorticoid excess).
- Renal tubular diseases (renal tubular acidoses, leukemia, Liddle's syndrome, antibiotics, carbonic anhydrase inhibitors).
- Diuretics.
- Magnesium depletion.

Extra-renal losses:
- Dietary deficiency.
- Diarrhea.
- Rectal villous adenoma.
- Fistulas.

- Uterosigmoidostomy.
- Laxative abuse.

CLINICAL FEATURES
- Muscular weakness, particularly of the lower extremities is present, which can be severe and generalized with marked potassium depletion (e.g. virtually total paralysis including respiratory, bulbar and cranial musculature).
- Deep tendon reflexes may be decreased or absent.
- Consciousness and sensation are preserved.
- Underlying etiology may be determined from the age of onset, race, family history, medications and underlying disease states.

SPECIAL FORMS
Familial (primary) periodic paralysis (FPP)
Epidemiology
- Age of onset: early in life (e.g. puberty), rarely after 25 years of age.
- Gender: M>F.
- Race: Caucasians typically.

Etiology and pathophysiology
- Autosomal dominant inheritance (2/3 of all cases of periodic paralysis).
- Mutations in the gene (on chromosome 1q32) encoding the skeletal muscle voltage-gated calcium channel α-1 subunit (CACNL1A3) account for most cases.
- Mutations in the gene coding for the skeletal muscle voltage-gated sodium channel α subunit (SCN4A) account for a minority of cases.
- Weakness occurs in association with hypokalemia (but can also occur with normokalemia, or hyperkalemia). However, alterations in potassium regulation are well documented. Total body potassium stores remain adequate, but serum potassium decreases due to potassium migration into muscle cells which causes the muscles to become electrically inexcitable.
- The exact method of potassium translocation is not known but is secondary to an abnormality in muscle membrane. (? An increase in muscle membrane sodium or calcium permeability associated with an inherited defect within skeletal muscle voltage-gated sodium or calcium channels.)

Continued overleaf

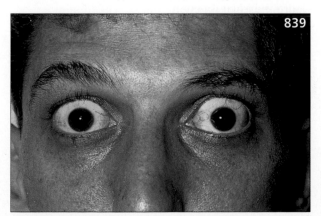
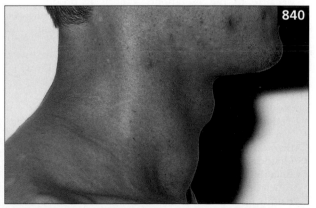

839, 840 Thyrotoxic patient presenting with periodic paralysis. Exophthalmos due to thyrotoxicosis (**839**). Lateral view of the neck showing thyroid goiter (**840**).

Etiology and pathophysiology (continued)
- Also associated with paramyotonia congenita, myotonia congenita, and generalized myotonia (i.e. both hyperkalemia and hypokalemia can cause paralysis).

Clinical features
- Episodic attacks of muscle weakness with no stiffness.
- Precipitants: decrease in blood potassium levels, rest, sleep, carbohydrate intake or insulin administration (attacks almost never occur during vigorous physical activity).
- Frequency: varies from daily to yearly.
- Duration: from 3–4 hours to a day or more.

Differential diagnosis
Hyperkalemic familial periodic paralysis:
- Usually starts in infancy or childhood.
- Attacks can be precipitated or induced by fasting, cold, pregnancy and potassium loading.
- Muscles can be stiff and in some patients there is myotonia of the eyelids, tongue, thumb and forearm muscles.
- During attacks the serum potassium is often raised (above 5.0 mmol/l [0.5 mEq/l]), as is the urine excretion of potassium and the CK level.
- Associated with a genetic abnormality at chromosome 17q.

Diagnosis
Low serum potassium during a paralytic attack, and exclusion of secondary causes of hypokalemia.

Treatment
- Oral potassium 0.2–0.4 mmol/kg (0.2–0.4 mEq/l), repeated at 15–30 minute intervals depending on the response of the patient (muscle strength), EKG, and serum potassium level.
- If the patient is unable to swallow, or is vomiting, intravenous potassium chloride 20 mmol per 100 ml normal saline hourly, while monitoring clinical status and serum potassium, may be necessary.
- Glucose in the diluent should be avoided as it can cause a further intracellular shift of potassium and reduction in serum potassium levels.

Prophylaxis against recurrent periodic attacks
- Acetazolamide 250–750 mg/day (agent of choice), or spironolactone 100–200 mg/day or triamterine.
- Acetazolamide abolishes attacks in most patients, perhaps because of the metabolic acidosis it produces. As acetazolamide lowers serum potassium, it may be necessary in some patients to supplement potassium and to avoid high carbohydrate meals.
- Chronic acetazolamide therapy may be associated with renal calculus (for which patients should be monitored).

Thyrotoxic periodic paralysis (TPP)
Epidemiology
- The most common acquired form of periodic paralysis.
- Age of onset: second to fourth decades (similar to thyrotoxicosis).
- Gender: M>F (20:1).
- Race: Orientals (90% of cases), Caucasians, native American Indians, Blacks, and Aborigines.
- Family history of TPP: rare.

Etiology
Any cause of thyrotoxicosis but usually Graves disease. Attacks only occur during hyperthyroidism.

Pathogenesis
Uncertain; perhaps a decrease in activity of the calcium pump.

Clinical features
Similar to FPP, but also signs of hyperthyroidism, which are frequently, but not always subtle (**839, 840**). Paralytic attacks can be induced by the thyrotoxic state, and carbohydrate and insulin administration but only if the patient is hyperthyroid, and not euthyroid.

Treatment
- Acute attack: potassium administration. Concurrently, begin to correct the hyperthyroid state and avoid precipitating factors (e.g. extreme exertion, heavy carbohydrate intake, and alcohol ingestion).
- Prophylaxis: beta-adrenergic blocking agents reduce the frequency and severity of attacks while measures to control thyrotoxicosis are being instituted. As serum potassium levels are normal between paralytic attacks, prophylactic potassium administration is unlikely to be helpful. Furthermore, acetazolamide is not helpful (unlike in FFP), and may even exacerbate attacks of paralysis in TPP.

Barium poisoning
- A rare cause of hypokalemic paralysis.
- Most cases are due to suicidal or accidental ingestion of barium.
- The mechanism of hypokalemia is transcellular shift of K^+.
- The paralysis is treated with potassium replacement.

DIFFERENTIAL DIAGNOSIS
CNS
- Cataplexy.
- Sleep paralysis associated with narcolepsy.
- Multiple sclerosis.
- Transient ischemic attack of the brain.
- Hyperventilation syndrome.
- Poliomyelitis.

Peripheral nerve
Guillian–Barré syndrome (see p.588).

Neuro-muscular junction
- Myasthenia gravis (see p.657).
- Lambert–Eaton myasthenic syndrome (see p.664).
- Botulism.
- Diphtheria.

Muscle
- Polymyositis.
- Dermatomyositis.
- Acute inflammatory myopathy (viral/parasitic).

Metabolic/toxic
- Electrolyte abnormalities.
- Porphyria.
- Medications (e.g. opiates).
- Alcoholism.
- Hypoglycemic disorders.
- Endocrine disorders.

INVESTIGATIONS
- Serum potassium.
- EKG.
- Thyroid function tests.

DIAGNOSIS
- Consider the diagnosis of hypokalemic paralysis in any patient presenting with a sudden onset, areflexic, pure motor weakness involving one or more limbs, without alteration in level of consciousness or sphincter function.
- Serum potassium is <3.5 mmol/l (3.5 mEq/l) during an attack (usually much lower).
- EKG shows U waves, ST segment sagging, and flattening and inversion of T waves, but these changes do not correlate well with the severity of the hypokalemia.
- Response of muscle power to provocative testing with glucose, insulin, potassium, and cold: for patients whose attacks are infrequent, but potentially hazardous and patients must be carefully monitored during their performance.

TREATMENT
- Identify and treat the cause (e.g. correction of the hyperthyroid state).
- Replace potassium: oral potassium 0.2–0.4 mmol/kg (0.2–0.4 mEq/l), repeated at 15–30 minute intervals depending on the response of the patient (muscle strength), EKG, and serum potassium level.
- Avoid precipitating factors (e.g. extreme exertion, heavy carbohydrate intake and alcohol ingestion).

PROGNOSIS
- Generally favorable, if appropriately diagnosed and managed.
- Deaths from respiratory failure and arrhythmia have been reported.

FURTHER READING

X-LINKED DYSTROPHINOPATHIES
Dubowitz V (2000) What is muscular dystrophy? *J. R. Coll. Physicians Lond.*, **34**: 464–468.
Emery AEH (1998) The muscular dystrophies. *BMJ*, **317**: 991–995.
Emery AEH (2000) Emery-Dreifuss muscular dystrophy – a 40 year retrospective. *Neuromuscular Disorders*, **10**: 228–232.
Fenichel GM, Griggs RC, Kissel J, et al. (2001) A randomized efficacy and safety trial of oxandrolone in the treatment of Duchenne dystrophy. *Neurology*, **56**: 1075–1079.
Flanigan KM (1999) The muscular dystrophies: update on genetics and appropriate testing. *Neurologist*, **5**: 113–121.
Griggs RC (2000) Techniques for ventilatory support. Clinical equipoise. *Neurology*, **55**: 615.
Jay V, Vajsar J (2001) The dystrophy of Duchenne. *Lancet*, **357**: 550–552.
Mendell JR, Buzin CH, Feng J, et al. (2001) Diagnosis of Duchenne dystrophy by enhanced detection of small mutations. *Neurology*, **57**: 645–650.
Nomori H, Ishihara T (2000) Pressure-controlled ventilation via a mini-tracheostomy tube for patients with neuromuscular disease. *Neurology*, **55**: 698–702.

FACIO-SCAPULO-HUMERAL MUSCULAR DYSTROPHY
Ricci E, Galluzzi G, Deidda G, et al. (1999) Progress in the molecular diagnosis of facioscapulohumeral muscular dystrophy and correlation between the number of *Kpn*I repeats at the 4q35 locus and clinical phenotype. *Ann. Neurol.*, **45**: 751–757.
Tawil R, Figlewicz DA, Griggs RC, Weiffenbach B, and the FSH Consortium (1998) Facioscapulohumeral dystrophy: a distinct regional myopathy with a novel molecular pathogenesis. *Ann. Neurol.*, **43**: 279–282.

LIMB-GIRDLE MUSCULAR DYSTROPHIES
Bushby KMD (1999) Making sense of the limb-girdle muscular dystrophies. *Brain*, **122**: 1403–1420.
Chou F-L, Angelini C, Daentl D, et al. (1999) Calpain III mutation analysis of a heterogeneous limb-girdle muscular dystrophy population. *Neurology*, **52**: 1015–1020.

Gamez J, Navarro C, Andreu AL, et al. (2001) Autosomal dominant limb-girdle muscular dystrophy. A large kindred with evidence of anticipation. *Neurology* **56**. 450–454.
Pollitt C, Anderson LVB, Pogue R, et al. (2001) The phenotype of calpainopathy: diagnosis based on a multidisciplinary approach. *Neuromuscular Disorders*, **11**: 287–296.
66th/67th ENMC Sponsored International Workshop (1999) The limb-girdle muscular dystrophies. 26–28 March 1999, Naarden, The Netherlands. *Neuromuscular Disorders*, **9**: 436–445.

MYOTONIC DYSTROPHY
Moxley RT III, Udd B, Ricker K (1998) Proximal myotonic myopathy (PROMM) and other proximal myotonic syndromes. *Neuromuscular Disorders*, **8**: 519–520.
Thornton CA, Ashizawa T (1999) Getting a grip on the myotonic dystrophies. *Neurology*, **52**: 12–13.

POLYMYOSITIS
Amato A, Barohn RJ (2000) Evaluation and treatment of the idiopathic inflammatory myopathies. *The Neurologist*, **6**: 267–287.
Callen JP (2000) Dermatomyositis. *Lancet*, **355**: 53–57.
Dalakas MC (1991) Polymyositis, dermatomyositis, and inclusion-body myositis. *N. Engl. J. Med.*, **325**: 1487–1498.
Dalakas MC, Illa I, Dambrosia JM. (1993) A controlled trial of high dose intravenous immune globulin as treament for dermatomyositis. *N. Engl. J. Med.*, **329**: 1993–2000.
Dalakis MC (2001) Progress in inflammatory myopathies: good but not good enough. *J. Neurol. Neurosurg. Psychiatry*, **70**: 569–573.
Miller FW, Leitman SF, Cronin ME (1992) Controlled trial of plasma exchange and leukapheresis in polymyositis and dermatomyositis. *N. Engl. J. Med.*, **326**: 1380–1384.

INCLUSION BODY MYOSITIS
Askanas V, Engel WK (2001) Inclusion-body myositis: newest concepts of pathogenesis and relation to aging and Alzheimer disease. *J. Neuropathol. Exp. Neurol.*, **60**: 1–14.
Dalakis MC, Koffman B, Fujii M, et al. (2001) A controlled study of intravenous immunoglobulin combined with prednisone in the treatment of IBM. *Neurology*, **56**: 323–327.
Nakano S, Shinde A, Kawashima S, et al. (2001) Inclusion body myositis. Expression of extracellular signal-regulated kinase and its substrate. *Neurology* **56**: 87–93.

Webster G, Beynon H (1999) Weak at the knees. *Lancet*, **354**: 1696.

METABOLIC AND ENDOCRINE MYOPATHIES
Duyff RF, Van den Bosck J, Laman DM, et al. (2000) Neuromuscular findings in thyroid dysfunction: a prospective clinical and electrodiagnostic study. *J. Neurol. Neurosurg. Psychiatry*, **68**: 750–755.
Fernández R, Navarro C, Andreu AL, et al. (2000) A novel missense mutation (W797R) in the myophosphorylase gene in Spanish patients with McArdle disease. *Arch. Neurol.*, **57**: 217–219.
Haller RG (2000) Treatment of McArdle disease. *Arch. Neurol.*, **57**: 923–924.
Klein I, Ojamaa K (2000) Thyroid (neuro)myopathy. *Lancet*, **356**: 614.
Pari G, Crerar MM, Nalbantoglu J, et al. (1999) Myophosphorylase gene transfer in McArdle's disease myoblasts *in vitro*. *Neurology*, **53**: 1352–1354.
Preedy VR, Adachi J, Veno Y, et al. (2001) Alcoholic skeletal muscle myopathy: definitions, features, contribution of neuropathy impact and diagnosis. *Eur. J. Neurol.*, **8**: 677–687.
Selim MH (2001) Neurologic aspects of thyroid disease. *The Neurologist*, **7**: 135–146.
Vorgerd M, Kubisch C, Burwinkel B, et al. (1998) Mutation analysis in myophosphorylase deficiency (McArdle's disease). *Ann. Neurol.*, **43**: 326–331.
Vorgerd M, Grehl T, Jäger M, et al. (2000) Creatine therapy in myophosphorylase deficiency (McArdle disease). A placebo-controlled crossover trial. *Arch. Neurol.*, **57**: 956–963.

HYPOKALEMIC PARALYSIS
Ahlawat SK, Sachdev A (1999) Hypokalaemic paralysis. *Postgrad. Med. J.*, **75**: 193–197.
Benatar (2000) Neurologic potassium channelopathy. *Q. J. Med.*, **93**: 787–797.
Griggs RC, Ptácek LJ (1999) Mutations of sodium channels in periodic paralysis. Can they explain the disease and predict treatment? *Neurology*, **52**: 1309–1310.
Lin S-H, Lin Y, Halperin ML (2001) Hypokalaemia and paralysis. *Q. J. Med.*, **94**: 133–139.
Ptácek LJ (1998) The familial periodic paralyses and nondystrophic myotonias. *Am. J. Med.*, **104**: 58–70.
Sternberg D, Maisonobe T, Jurkat-Rott ET (2001) Hypokalaemic periodic paralysis type X caused by mutations at codon 672 in the muscle sodium channel gene SCN4A. *Brain*, **124**: 1091–1099.

Index